2004
YEAR BOOK OF
OBSTETRICS, GYNECOLOGY,
AND WOMEN'S HEALTH®

The 2004 Year Book Series

Year Book of Allergy, Asthma, and Clinical Immunology™: Drs Rosenwasser, Boguniewicz, Milgrom, Routes, and Spahn

Year Book of Anesthesiology and Pain Management™: Drs Chestnut, Abram, Black, Lang, Roizen, Trankina, and Wood

Year Book of Cardiology®: Drs Gersh, Cheitlin, Graham, Kaplan, Sundt, and Waldo

Year Book of Critical Care Medicine®: Drs Dellinger, Parrillo, Balk, Bekes, Dries, and Roberts

Year Book of Dentistry®: Drs Zakariasen, Boghosian, Burgess, Hatcher, Horswell, McIntyre, and Zakariasen

Year Book of Dermatology and Dermatologic Surgery™: Drs Thiers and Lang

Year Book of Diagnostic Radiology®: Drs Osborn, Birdwell, Dalinka, Gardiner, Groskin, Levy, Maynard, and Oestreich

Year Book of Emergency Medicine®: Drs Burdick, Cone, Cydulka, Hamilton, Handly, and Quintana

Year Book of Endocrinology®: Drs Mazzaferri, Becker, Kannan, Kennedy, Kreisberg, Meikle, Molitch, Osei, Poehlman, and Rogol

Year Book of Family Practice®: Drs Bowman, Apgar, Dexter, Miser, Neill, and Scherger

Year Book of Gastroenterology™: Drs Lichtenstein, Dempsey, Ginsberg, Katzka, Kochman, Morris, Nunes, Reddy, Rosato, and Stein

Year Book of Hand Surgery®: Drs Berger and Ladd

Year Book of Medicine®: Drs Barkin, Frishman, Klahr, Loehrer, Mazzaferri, Phillips, Pillinger, and Snydman

Year Book of Neonatal and Perinatal Medicine®: Drs Fanaroff, Maisels, and Stevenson

Year Book of Neurology and Neurosurgery®: Drs Gibbs and Verma

Year Book of Nuclear Medicine®: Drs Coleman, Blaufox, Royal, Strauss, and Zubal

Year Book of Obstetrics, Gynecology, and Women's Health®: Drs Mishell, Kirschbaum, and Miller

Year Book of Oncology®: Drs Loehrer, Arceci, Glatstein, Gordon, Morrow, Schiller, and Thigpen

Year Book of Ophthalmology®: Drs Rapuano, Cohen, Eagle, Grossman, Myers, Nelson, Penne, Regillo, Sergott, Shields, and Tipperman

Year Book of Orthopedics®: Drs Morrey, Beauchamp, Peterson, Swiontkowski, Trigg, and Yaszemski

Year Book of Otolaryngology-Head and Neck Surgery®: Drs Paparella, Keefe, and Otto

Year Book of Pathology and Laboratory Medicine®: Drs Raab, Grzybicki, Bejarano, Bissell, and Stanley

Year Book of Pediatrics®: Dr Stockman

Year Book of Plastic and Aesthetic Surgery™: Drs Miller, Bartlett, Garner, McKinney, Ruberg, Salisbury, and Smith

Year Book of Psychiatry and Applied Mental Health®: Drs Talbott, Ballenger, Frances, Jensen, Markowitz, Meltzer, and Simpson

Year Book of Pulmonary Disease®: Drs Phillips, Barker, Blanchard, Dunlap, Lewis, and Maurer

Year Book of Rheumatology, Arthritis, and Musculoskeletal Disease™: Drs Panush, Hadler, Hellmann, Hochberg, Lahita, and Seibold

Year Book of Sports Medicine®: Drs Shephard, Alexander, Cantu, Nieman, Sanborn and Shrier

Year Book of Surgery®: Drs Copeland, Bland, Cerfolio, Daly, Eberlein, Howard, Luce, Mozingo, and Seeger

Year Book of Urology®: Drs Andriole and Coplen

Year Book of Vascular Surgery®: Dr Moneta

2004

Year Book of OBSTETRICS, GYNECOLOGY, AND WOMEN'S HEALTH

Editors

Daniel R. Mishell, Jr, MD
The Lyle G. McNeile Professor and Chairman, Department of Obstetrics and Gynecology, Keck School of Medicine, University of Southern California; Chief of Women's Services, Women's and Children's Hospital, Los Angeles County and University of Southern California Medical Center, Los Angeles, California

Thomas H. Kirschbaum, MD
Professor of Obstetrics and Gynecology, University of Alabama at Birmingham, Alabama

David Scott Miller, MD
Director and Dallas Foundation Chair in Gynecologic Oncology, Professor of Obstetrics and Gynecology, University of Texas Southwestern Medical Center at Dallas; Medical Director of Gynecologic Oncology, Parkland Health and Hospital System, Dallas, Texas

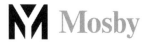

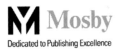

Dedicated to Publishing Excellence

Vice President, Continuity Publishing: Timothy M. Griswold
Publisher: Barton Dudlick
Managing Editor: David Orzechowski
Administrative Coordinator: Nell McShane Wulfhart
Senior Manager, Continuity Production: Idelle L.Winer
Issue Manager: Donna M. Skelton
Composition Specialist: Betty Dockins
Illustrations and Permissions Coordinator: Chidi C. Ukabam

Printed in the United States of America
Composition by Thomas Technology Solutions, Inc.
Printing/binding by Sheridan Books, Inc.

Editorial Office:
Elsevier
300 East
170 South Independence Mall West
Philadelphia, PA 19106-3399

International Standard Serial Number: 1090-798X
International Standard Book Number: 0-323-02086-0

Contributing Editors

Raquel D. Arias, MD

Associate Dean of Women, Associate Professor of Obstetrics and Gynecology, Keck School of Medicine, University of Southern California; Women's and Children's Hospital, Los Angeles County and University of Southern California Medical Center, Los Angeles, California

William H. Hindle, MD

Professor Emeritus, Department of Obstetrics and Gynecology, Keck School of Medicine, University of Southern California; Founder, Breast Diagnostic Center, Women's and Children's Hospital, Los Angeles County and University of Southern California Medical Center, Los Angeles, California

Morton A. Stenchever, MD

Professor and Chair Emeritus, Department of Obstetrics and Gynecology, University of Washington, Seattle, Washington

Table of Contents

Journals Represented

Mosby and its editors survey approximately 500 journals for its abstract and commentary publications. From these journals, the editors select the articles to be abstracted. Journals represented in this YEAR BOOK are listed below.

Acta Obstetricia et Gynecologica Scandinavica
American Journal of Epidemiology
American Journal of Medicine
American Journal of Obstetrics and Gynecology
American Journal of Ophthalmology
American Journal of Surgery
Anesthesia and Analgesia
Annals of Periodontology
Annals of Rheumatic Diseases
Archives of Pediatrics and Adolescent Medicine
Australian and New Zealand Journal of Obstetrics and Gynaecology
British Journal of Obstetrics and Gynaecology
British Journal of Urology International
Cancer
Cancer (Cancer Cytopathology)
Circulation
Clinical Chemistry
Clinical Endocrinology (Oxford)
Clinical Infectious Diseases
Contraception
Diabetes
Digestive Diseases and Sciences
European Heart Journal
European Journal of Cancer
European Journal of Obstetrics, Gynecology and Reproductive Biology
European Urology
Fertility and Sterility
Gynecologic Oncology
Heart
Human Reproduction
Infectious Diseases in Obstetrics and Gynecology
International Journal of Cancer
International Journal of Gynaecology and Obstetrics
International Journal of Gynecological Cancer
International Journal of Obesity
Journal of Bone and Joint Surgery (British Volume)
Journal of Clinical Endocrinology and Metabolism
Journal of Clinical Investigation
Journal of Clinical Microbiology
Journal of Clinical Oncology
Journal of Infectious Diseases
Journal of Maternal-Fetal and Neonatal Medicine
Journal of Pediatric Gastroenterology and Nutrition
Journal of Pediatric Surgery
Journal of Pediatrics
Journal of Periodontology
Journal of Reproductive Medicine

Journal of Ultrasound in Medicine
Journal of Urology
Journal of the American Board of Family Practice
Journal of the American College of Surgeons
Journal of the American Medical Association
Journal of the National Cancer Institute
Lancet
Maturitas
Medicine
Menopause: The Journal of The American Menopause Society
Nature Medicine
New England Journal of Medicine
Obstetrics and Gynecology
Pediatric Research
Perspectives on Sexual and Reproductive Health
Placenta
Prenatal Diagnosis
Radiology
Scandinavian Journal of Plastic and Reconstructive Surgery and Hand Surgery
Science
Stroke
Transfusion
Ultrasound in Obstetrics and Gynecology
Urology

STANDARD ABBREVIATIONS

The following terms are abbreviated in this edition: acquired immunodeficiency syndrome (AIDS), cardiopulmonary resuscitation (CPR), central nervous system (CNS), cerebrospinal fluid (CSF), computed tomography (CT), deoxyribonucleic acid (DNA), electrocardiography (ECG), health maintenance organization (HMO), human immunodeficiency virus (HIV), intensive care unit (ICU), intramuscular (IM), intravenous (IV), magnetic resonance (MR) imaging (MRI), and ribonucleic acid (RNA) and ultrasound (US).

NOTE

The YEAR BOOK OF OBSTETRICS, GYNECOLOGY, AND WOMEN'S HEALTH is a literature survey service providing abstracts of articles published in the professional literature. Every effort is made to assure the accuracy of the information presented in these pages. Neither the editors nor the publisher of the YEAR BOOK OF OBSTETRICS, GYNECOLOGY, AND WOMEN'S HEALTH can be responsible for errors in the original materials. The editors' comments are their own opinions. Mention of specific products within this publication does not constitute endorsement.

To facilitate the use of the YEAR BOOK OF OBSTETRICS, GYNECOLOGY, AND WOMEN'S HEALTH as a reference tool, all illustrations and tables included in this publication are now identified as they appear in the original article. This change is meant to help the reader recognize that any illustration or table appearing in the YEAR BOOK OF OBSTETRICS, GYNECOLOGY, AND WOMEN'S HEALTH may be only one of many in the original article. For this reason, figure and table numbers will often appear to be out of sequence within the YEAR BOOK OF OBSTETRICS, GYNECOLOGY, AND WOMEN'S HEALTH.

Introduction

The YEAR BOOK OF OBSTETRICS, GYNECOLOGY, AND WOMEN'S HEALTH contains abstracts of the most clinically relevant scientific articles published during the preceding year in the area of women's health, followed by editorial comments discussing the relevance of each article for the reader. Topics covered include care of the pregnant, parturient, and postpartum woman and diagnosis and treatment of disorders of the female reproductive organs. Articles reviewed include those involving endocrinologic disorders and infertility as well as benign and malignant neoplasias. Other areas covered include breast disease, disorders of the urinary tract, contraception, and surveillance and treatment of the post-menopausal woman.

Throughout the year, the editors of the YEAR BOOK OF OBSTETRICS, GYNECOLOGY, AND WOMEN'S HEALTH periodically review articles published in medical journals focusing upon obstetrics, gynecology, and other areas of women's health, as well as relevant articles appearing in other medical journals. The editors select those articles that provide the most pertinent clinical information for clinicians, and write comments discussing the relevance of the findings for the reader. Once abstracts are written, they are sent for final review to the editor who selected the article for placement in the YEAR BOOK.

By reading the YEAR BOOK, clinicians with limited time will gain knowledge of the most important articles on women's health published in the previous year.

As in past years, Dr Thomas H. Kirschbaum, a specialist in maternal and fetal medicine, reviewed the articles concerning obstetrics for this volume. Dr David Scott Miller, an oncologist, reviewed and selected articles on gynecologic oncology and pelvic surgery, and I have reviewed and selected articles in the areas of reproductive endocrinology, infertility, menopause, contraception, and gynecologic infection. Drs William H. Hindle and Morton A. Stenchever are experts in the field of breast disease and gynecologic urology, respectively, and have selected the most relevant articles published in these areas.

During the past year, after receiving numerous scientific journals, the authors selected 327 articles from 72 journals for publication in this volume of the YEAR BOOK.

The editors believe that reading this volume will enhance each clinician's knowledge of advances in women's health. We welcome suggestions to improve our efforts in providing clinically relevant information to our readers.

Daniel R. Mishell, Jr, MD

OBSTETRICS

1 Maternal and Fetal Physiology

Derivation of Oocytes From Mouse Embryonic Stem Cells

Hübner K, Fuhrmann G, Christenson LK, et al (Univ of Pennsylvania, Kennett Square, Pa; FRE 2373 CNRS, Strasbourg, France; Univ of Pennsylvania, Philadelphia)

Science 300:1251-1256, 2003   1-1

Background.—The germ line and soma are indistinguishable from each other in the early mammalian embryo. Germ cell competence in the mouse is induced at embryonic day 6.5. Even during the specification period, precursor cells spur the development of primordial germ cells and certain somatic cells. The potential of embryonic stem (ES) cells to generate all lineages of the embryo in vivo has been widely reported. However, there is a significant lack of data concerning the derivation of germ cells from ES cells in vitro. This study was conducted on the hypothesis that the inability to demonstrate the derivation of germ cells from ES cells in culture is a result of the lack of an adequate reporter system for the noninvasive visualization of germ cell formation. Such a reporter system was descrubed.

Methods.—The *Oct 4* gene is present in the mouse, bovine, and human and contains a specific germ cell enhancer segment (CR4) and 2 enhancers for ectodermal stimulation (CR2 and CR3). In this experiment, the CR2 and CR3 regions were removed and a green fluorescent pigment was added to a fragment of the *Oct 4* gene. This procedure produced a molecule capable of complimentary bonding to DNA in cells destined to become oocytes. This coupling had the ability to distinguish such cells in culture by their fluorescence.

Results.—ES cell cultures were then transfected with this marker and implanted into oviducts of pseudopregnant animals. Cells containing the transfected marker were then cultured, and 25% to 40% showed the green fluorescent pigment germ cell marker after 7 to 8 days. Markers of postmigratory and meiotic cells were then used to identify clones consisting of postmeiotic cells on the verge of entering prophase. With culture to day 12, these cells showed formation of primordial follicles and enveloping stromal cells. Estrogen production was evident by day 12. Blastocytes were confirmed in culture by day 43, and the addition of follicle-stimulating hormone and human chorionic gonadotropin to the median caused extrusion of oocytes and the formation of polar bodies.

Conclusion.—These findings show that mouse embryonic stem cells have the capacity to differentiate into oocytes and form structures very similar, if not identical, to blastocytes. This capacity demonstrates that mouse ES cells are in fact totipotent, even in vitro. Future studies will indicate whether these cells have underdone a gender-specific resetting of the epigenetic marks and whether they can be used as starting material from which ES cell lines can be derived after nuclear transfer.

▶ This remarkable achievement has important implications for study of the cell biology of embryogenesis and for future developments in assisted reproductive technology and fetal gene therapy. ES cells have been viewed to be pluripotent, not totipotent, by virtue of their apparent inability to produce germ cells in vitro. Surely they do in vivo, since among embryonic undifferentiated cells at some point—day 6.5 of the embryonic life in the mouse and days 26 to 28 in humans—primordial germ cells become discernable. Prior recognition of germ cells has failed for lack of an adequate reporter system for embryonic germ cells in culture. These authors provide that system.

The *Oct 4* gene, present in the mouse, bovine, and human, contains a specific germ cell enhancer segment (CR4) and 2 enhancers for ectodermal stimulation (CR2 & CR3). The authors removed regions CR 2 and CR 3 and added a green fluorescent pigment to a fragment of the *Oct 4* gene, producing a molecule capable of complimentary bonding to DNA in cells destined to become oocytes. This coupling carried with it the ability to discern such cells in culture by their fluorescence.

ES cell cultures were transfected with this marker by injection into the pronuclei of fertilized ova, then implanted into oviducts of pseudopregnant animals after it was proved that the marker localizes in germ cells but not in blastocysts or ectodermal cells in transgenic animals. Cells containing the transfected marker were grown in culture and, after 7 to 8 days, somewhere between 25% and 40% showed the fluorescent germ cell marker. Selected markers of postmigratory and meiotic cells were then used to select clones consisting of postmeiotic cells just entering their prophase. At this point, they lose cell-cell adhesion molecules, allowing atraumatic separation from neighboring cells.

The functional verification of the oocytes was extensive. With culture to day 12, these cells showed the formation of primordial follicles with the development of enveloping stromal cells. Estrogen production by day 12 proved the capacity to convert androgens to estrogen by the supporting granulocytic cells. Free-floating oocytes with zona-pellucidae were seen at embryonic day 26, and production of protein mediators of meiosis was found by reverse transcription polymerase chain reaction at day 16. By day 43, blastocystes were proven to be present in culture by morphology and molecular markers. Addition of follicle-stimulating hormone and human chorionic gonadotropin to the media resulted in the extrusion of oocytes and the formation of polar bodies.

Chapter 1–Maternal and Fetal Physiology / **5**

This is very convincing evidence for the capacity of ES cells to produce oocytes. Further studies will explore their capacity for fertilization. What application of this approach to human material may show is a compelling question.

T. H. Kirschbaum, MD

Cytokine Concentrations in the Amniotic Fluid During Parturition at Term: Correlation to Lower Uterine Segment Values and to Labor
Kemp B, Winkler M, Maas A, et al (Univ of Aachen, Germany; Univ of Tübingen, Germany; Technical Univ of Aachen, Germany)
Acta Obstet Gynecol Scand 81:938-942, 2002   1–2

Background.—As the cervix dilates with the approaching birth, the concentrations of interleukin-6 (IL-6) and IL-8 in the lower uterine segment increase significantly, and IL-8 increases are of particular importance because it functions in the neutrophil influx into the cervical stroma and in the subsequent release of collagenases and proteases. Amniotic fluid concentrations of IL-8, tumor necrosis factor-alpha (TNF-α), IL-1β, and IL-6 rise significantly after labor begins, and cervical tissue is possibly the source of IL-8 in the amniotic fluid. Whether a relationship exists between the concentrations of IL-6 and IL-8 in the lower uterine segment and the concentrations in the amniotic fluid was evaluated, along with any possible connection to the duration of labor.

Methods.—Twenty-nine patients undergoing cesarean section at term were the source for specimens of amniotic fluid and the lower uterine segment from which IL-6 and IL-8 concentrations were determined with the use of enzyme immunoassay. Based on cervical dilatation and labor duration, patients were divided into groups as follows: less than 2 cm, 2 to 3.9 cm, 4 to 6 cm, and more than 6 cm; and 0 hours, 0 to 12 hours, and more than 12 hours.

Results.—The median amniotic fluid concentration of IL-6 was 654 pg/mg total protein (TP) at less than 2 cm dilatation and increased to 13,029 pg/mg TP when dilatation exceeded 6 cm. The amniotic IL-6 concentrations correlated with the duration of labor. For the median lower uterine segment, the values rose from 13 pg/mg TP at less than 2 cm to 1226 pg/mg TP at 4 to 6 cm. The median concentrations of IL-8 in amniotic fluid increased from 316 pg/mg TP at less than 2 cm to 16,799 pg/mg TP when dilatation exceeded 6 cm. For the lower uterine segment values, an increase was noted from 17 pg/mg TP at less than 2 cm to 2081 pg/mg TP at 4 to 6 cm; then a fall to 1627 pg/mg TP occurred when dilatation exceeded 6 cm. The IL-8 concentrations showed a significant increase in both the amniotic fluid and the lower uterine segment at 4 to 6 cm dilatation, but no correlation was found between these compartments. Similarly, no correlation was found between the amniotic concentration of IL-8 and the duration of labor.

Conclusions.—IL-6 concentrations rose earlier in amniotic fluid than in the lower uterine segment and correlated with the duration of labor as determined by measures of cervical dilatation. The greatest increase in IL-8 concentrations in amniotic fluid occurred after those in the lower uterine segment and did not correlate with the duration of labor. Thus, IL-6 seems to play a critical role both in promoting labor and in the biochemical degradation processes that takes place in the lower uterine segment, but IL-8 seems to play only a minor role in initiating parturition by its amniotic fluid concentration.

▶ Clearly, infections like chorioamnionitis, pyelonephritis, and bacterial pneumonia may result in preterm birth, but they represent a small fraction of the 11% national prevalence of preterm birth in this country. Nearly three fourths of preterm births occur without evident cause, and 1.5% to 1.7% occur after preterm premature rupture of membranes. Approximately 28% are iatrogenic, designed to salvage fetuses presumed to be at jeopardy in utero. A great deal of interest in the prevention of preterm delivery through antimicrobial therapy of possible latent subclinical infections in women at risk of preterm birth has failed to yield positive results (see 1995 YEAR BOOK OF OBSTETRICS, GYNECOLOGY, AND WOMEN'S HEALTH, pp 46-47, pp 60-62; 1997 YEAR BOOK OF OBSTETRICS, GYNECOLOGY, AND WOMEN'S HEALTH, pp 31-33; 1999 YEAR BOOK OF OBSTETRICS, GYNECOLOGY, AND WOMEN'S HEALTH, pp 38-40; 2001 YEAR BOOK OF OBSTETRICS, GYNECOLOGY, AND WOMEN'S HEALTH, pp 29-36; and 2002 YEAR BOOK OF OBSTETRICS, GYNECOLOGY, AND WOMEN'S HEALTH, pp 35-38). Because it is difficult to prove that antibiotic therapy isn't effective, attention has turned to identification of products of innate or native immunity as indicators of activation of the inflammatory reaction before the presence of infection as a better means of identifying women who might benefit from antimicrobial therapy (see 2000 YEAR BOOK OF OBSTETRICS, GYNECOLOGY, AND WOMEN'S HEALTH, pp 69-71).

The indicators of innate immunity include phagocytes (eg, neutrophils and macrophages), cells that function to release mediators of special functions (eg, eosinophils, basophils, and mast cells) and natural killer cells (large granular lymphocytes) with the capacity to destroy infected cells without the specific antigen recognition characteristic of acquired immunity. Cell products responsible, in part, for native immunity are complement, which reacts with antibody to perforate cell membranes and lyse infectious agents, acute phase proteins, and cytokines. These endogenous cell mediators are part of the response to external invasion by infectious agents, and the interleukin family of cytokines has been intensively studied in this connection (see 2000 YEAR BOOK OF OBSTETRICS, GYNECOLOGY, AND WOMEN'S HEALTH, pp 69-71, pp 164-165; and 2002 YEAR BOOK OF OBSTETRICS, GYNECOLOGY, AND WOMEN'S HEALTH, pp 43-45, pp 38-43, pp 200-202).

IL-1β is a master cytokine serving to initiate the production of an array of other cytokines active in infectious and immune challenges. It is absent in amniotic fluid normally but is seen in amniotic fluid in one third of cases of preterm labor and in equal numbers of normal term births, which makes it clinically uninteresting. IL-6 is produced especially in the cervix but also in the uterus in normal labor and serves to stimulate prostaglandin production by the placenta and membrane. IL-8 stimulates neutrophil production and a series of proteases and collagenases that alter the connective tissue matrix. TNFα is produced by cervical fibroblasts in response to IL-8 and produces matrix metallo-proteinases (MMP-8 and MMP-9), which function to increase connective tissue matrix permeability to cell migration.

In this study, the concentration of IL-6 and IL-8 are studied in sections of lower uterine segments and in amniotic fluid in 19 women delivering after the onset of preterm labor and in 10 delivering surgically without labor, to investigate the probable origin and time of onset of cytokine production in labor. As Figure 1 shows, IL-6 appears in amniotic fluid before its increase in uterine tissue, in proportion to cervical dilation, whereas IL-8 appears in high concentration in amniotic fluid before its modest concentration increase in uterine tissue itself. Neither cytokine concentration changes correlated with the duration of labor, which suggests that IL-8 is formed as an inflammatory component of advanced cervical dilation and not as a factor in the initiation of labor. The earlier appearance of IL-6 in the uterus and then in the amniotic fluid may denote a role in the promotion of labor and, then later, in the matrix remodeling of the lower uterine segment and cervix. The same sort of study needs, as the authors point out, to be applied to changes in the placenta and membranes during labor. The aim of this sort of work is to be able to differentiate the inflammatory consequences of labor from early infection, which is a goal long sought by many investigators.

T. H. Kirschbaum, MD

Gestation-Related and Betamethasone-Induced Changes in 11β-Hydroxysteroid Dehydrogenase Types 1 and 2 in the Baboon Placenta
Ma XH, Wu WX, Nathanielsz PW (Cornell Univ, Ithaca, NY)
Am J Obstet Gynecol 188:13-21, 2003   1–3

Background.—Glucocorticoids have an important role in the growth and differentiation of fetal organs and tissues in late gestation, and inappropriately high concentrations of fetal glucocorticoids can slow fetal growth and cause abnormalities. The interconversion of biologically active cortisol and inactive cortisone is a fundamental mechanism that regulates the amount of biologically active glucocorticoids available to placental and fetal target tissues. The interconversion is catalyzed by the enzyme 11β-hydroxysteroid (HSD). There are 2 functionally distinct isoforms of 11β-HSD. The developmental and labor-related changes in 11β-HSD 1 and 2 expression in baboon placentas were determined during the final third of gestation and labor. Whether maternal administration of glucocorticoid alters placental 11β-HSD 2 expression was examined.

Methods.—Maternal and fetal plasma cortisol concentrations were measured in 5 baboons. In addition, types 1 and 2 11β-HSD messenger RNA (mRNA) and protein in placentas obtained at 121 to 185 days' gestation (term approximately 185 days' gestation) (16 animals), during labor between 141 and 193 days' gestation (8 animals), and after maternal administration of 4 doses of 87.5 μg/kg of betamethasone (5 animals) at 12-hour intervals at 121 to 135 days' gestation were analyzed by Northern and Western blot.

Results.—Cortisol levels were 4-fold higher in maternal plasma than in fetal plasma. Placental 11β-HSD 2 mRNA and protein declined after 0.9 gestation, whereas 11β-HSD 1 mRNA levels were unchanged (Fig 2). Labor had no effect on placental 11β-HSD 1 or 2 mRNA protein levels. Maternal betamethasone administration dramatically increased 11β-HSD 2 mRNA and protein without affecting 11β-HSD 1 mRNA and protein expression (Fig 4).

Conclusions.—The late-gestation baboon maternal plasma cortisol concentration is 4-fold greater than the fetal plasma concentration. Decreased placental 11β-HSD 2 may enhance passage of maternal cortisol to the fetus

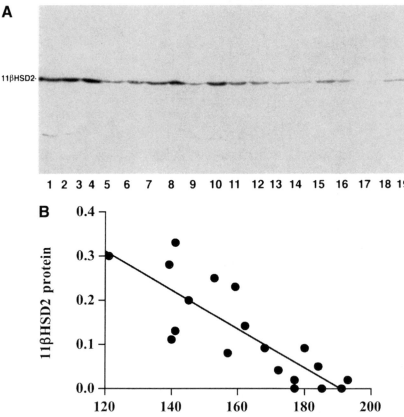

FIGURE 2.—Gestation-associated change of placental 11β-HSD 2 protein. **A,** Western blot analysis of 11β-HSD 2 in the baboon placenta throughout the period 121-193 days' gestation (dGA) (*lane 1,* 121, *2-*139, *3-*140, *4-*141, *5-*141, *6-*145, *7-*153, *8-*157, *9-*159, *10-*162, *11-*168, *12-*172, *13-*177, *14-*177, *15-*180, *16-*184, *17-*185, *18-*191, *19-*193 dGA). **B,** Densitometric analysis of 11β-HSD 2 protein in the placenta. Placental 11β-HSD 2 protein decreased significantly throughout the final third of gestation ($P < .001$, $r^2 = 0.72$). (Courtesy of Ma XH, Wu WX, Nathanielsz PW: Gestation-related and betamethasone-induced changes in 11β-hydroxysteroid dehydrogenase types 1 and 2 in the baboon placenta. *Am J Obstet Gynecol* 188:13-21. Copyright 2003 by Elsevier.)

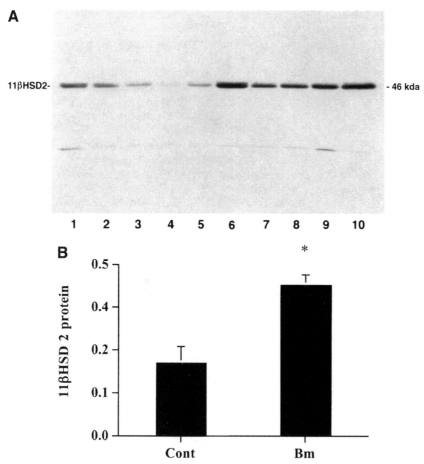

FIGURE 4.—The effect of maternal administration of betamethasone (*Bm*) on placental 11β-HSD 2 protein expression. **A,** Western analysis of placental 11β-HSD 2 protein in five betamethasone-treated baboons (*lanes 6-10*) compared with five gestational age-controlled baboons (*Cont, lanes 1-5*). **B,** Densitometric analysis of 11β-HSD 2 protein. Placental 11β-HSD 2 protein increased significantly after maternal administration of betamethasone. *Asterisk, P* < .05. (Courtesy of Ma XH, Wu WX, Nathanielsz PW: Gestation-related and betamethasone-induced changes in 11β-hydroxysteroid dehydrogenase types 1 and 2 in the baboon placenta. *Am J Obstet Gynecol* 188:13-21. Copyright 2003 by Elsevier.)

at the end of gestation, which contributes to cortisol-mediated changes within the placenta and cortisol in fetal plasma at this stage of fetal development. The positive effect of betamethasone on placental 11β-HSD 2 induction suggests that the placenta may have the ability to regulate glucocorticoid transfer in the presence of elevated maternal glucocorticoid.

▶ Maternal glucocorticoids are essential in early pregnancy for placental development and growth as they provide vascular endothelial growth stimulation and the capacity for decidual remodeling. In later pregnancy, the capacity of glucocorticoids to inhibit fetal growth and metabolism and its proteolytic properties, together with the need for fetal pituitary adrenal autonomy, mean that the fetus must in part be protected from the increasing maternal blood concentrations of corticoids as pregnancy continues. Some have attributed the imperfect placentation of preeclampsia to a defect in this protection.[1] This fine experimental group, using a chronic pregnant baboon preparation for which it is nationally known, offers help in understanding the interrelationships between maternal and fetal glucocorticoid regulation in pregnancy, a growing concern as maternal cortisol is so widely used in preterm labor to enhance fetal lung maturity.

11β-HSD 2, which unidirectionally converts cortisol to cortisone, renders it relatively inactive and is a key enzyme. In 5 chronic pregnant preparations, the authors simultaneously measured maternal and fetal blood cortisol concentrations after administration of maternal corticoid in doses comparable to those used in humans, and at the same time measured mRNA by using complementary DNAs (cDNAs) for isoform-1 and isoform-2 of 11β-HSD, employing ^{32}P-labeling hybridization and radioautography. They also measured protein concentrations of both isoforms with the use of monoclonal antibodies on a gel electrophoresis and chemiluminescence system. Blood and placental tissues from 8 animals laboring spontaneously at 141 to 193 days of gestational age and 16 pregnancies delivered abdominally without labor between 121 and 185 days were studied. Term is approximately 185 days in this species. Blood and placental specimens were subject to measurement of mRNA and protein for the 2 enzyme isoforms, and comparisons with respect to labor and maternal cortisol effects were made.

Maternal 11β-HSD 2 was the dominant isoform and progressively decreased in blood concentration, placental mRNA, and protein through the course of pregnancy, reaching very low levels close to term; maternal 11β-HSD 1 showed no changes with gestation. Maternal cortisol normally exists in blood concentrations that are roughly 4 times those of the fetus, and are unaffected by labor. Maternal cortisol administration sharply increased both placental 11β-HSD 2 mRNA and protein but left 11β-HSD 1 unchanged. The role of maternal 11β-HSD 2 appears to be to protect the fetus from increasing concentrations of maternal cortisol and also to free the fetal pituitary from adrenal suppression by that means during pregnancy, at least through 165 days of gestation. This allows fetal development to proceed relatively free of the growth-inhibiting properties of high maternal glucocorticoid concentrations through the bulk of pregnancy. On the other hand, the virtual absence of 11β-HSD 2 in the last 2 weeks of pregnancy in maternal blood allows fetal pituitary triggering of fetal cortisol production, serving to synchronize maternal and fetal circadian cortisol cycles. Reduced maternal 11β-HSD 2 allows increased maternal to fetal transfer of cortisol in late pregnancy and enables fetal pituitary suppression in the last few weeks. The authors posit increased endogenous fetal adrenal stimulation related to the onset of prelabor and labor as an important factor in maintaining the balance of fetal cocorticoids before parturition. This interplay conceivably could play a role in the onset of labor. It's an interesting potentially very important set of observations and a very useful hypothesis for future work.

T. H. Kirschbaum, MD

Reference

1. 2002 Year Book of Obstetrics, Gynecology, and Women's Health, pp 58-59.

Oxygen Regulation of Placental 11β-Hydroxysteroid Dehydrogenase 2: Physiological and Pathological Implications

Alfaidy N, Gupta S, DeMarco C, et al (Univ of Toronto)
J Clin Endocrinol Metab 87:4797-4805, 2002   1–4

Background.—Preeclampsia (PE) causes significant maternal and fetal morbidity and mortality. Histologic examination has revealed limited trophoblast migration and invasion of maternal spiral arteries and uterine artery remodeling failure in PE. This leads to impaired placental perfusion and hypoxia. In early pregnancy, the placenta develops under low oxygen conditions, approximately 20 mm Hg, which increase at 10 to 12 weeks' gestation to approximately 55 mm Hg. At this time, trophoblast cells change from a proliferative to an invasive phenotype, penetrate endometrial vessels, and access maternal blood. Glucocorticoid (GC) metabolism is also altered in PE placentas through reduction of 11β-hydroxysteroid dehydrogenase type 2 (11β-HSD2) activity. With the use of human villous explant culture, the relationship between oxygen tension, 11β-HSD2 expression and activity, and GC metabolism was explored in PE.

Methods.—Preeclamptic and age-matched control placentas were obtained from elective terminations. Term placentas were obtained from elective cesarean deliveries. Five- to 8-week gestation placentas were processed for villous explant cultures and maintained at either standard tissue culture conditions or 3% oxygen. Placental trophoblast cells were obtained from term placentas and cultured under either standard conditions or 3% oxygen. Placental tissues were also processed for immunohistochemical staining with a polyclonal antibody to 11β-HSD2 and for assays of 11β-HSD2 activity.

Results.—Both expression and activity of 11β-HSD2 were significantly reduced in PE placenta tissue compared with control placenta tissue. 11β-HSD2 was detected in 5-week placental tissue in the syncytiotrophoblast. Expression increased at 10 to 12 weeks and was also detected in the cytotrophoblast and extravillous trophoblast. Villous explants and term trophoblasts cultured under 20% oxygen had greater 11β-HSD2 activity and expression than explants cultured under 3% oxygen conditions.

Conclusions.—Placental 11β-HSD2 expression and activity are reduced in preeclampsia. Expression and activity of 11β-HSD2 are oxygen-dependent throughout gestation. This suggests that hypoxia induced by the vascular changes of PE causes reduced 11β-HSD2 expression and activity during pregnancy that result in increased glucocorticoid activity in the placenta and fetus, which contributes to altered placental development and increased fetal morbidity and mortality.

▶ Normal early placentation consists of trophoblastic proliferation into a decidua in a low p02 environment of approximately 20 mm of mercury through the first 9 weeks of gestation. Thereafter, as the trophoblast changes from proliferative to invasive characteristics associated with the expression of cell adhesion molecules characteristic of stromal tissues,[1,2] the trophoblast contacts spiral arterioles, remodels, and dilates maternal arterial inflow vessels incorporating maternal blood into trophoblastic clefts, the primordial intervillous space. At this point interstitial p02 increases into the range of 40 to 50 mm of mercury.[3] At the same time, decidual remodeling and trophoblastic behavior are protected from the proteinase and epithelial growth-stimulating properties after increased tissue cortisol concentration purveyed by increased maternal blood flow by the dominant oxidative effects of 11β-HSD2, which converts cortisol to more endocrinologically inactive cortisone in situ.[4] These authors have demonstrated that the expression of the dehydrogenase enzyme is oxygen sensitive and is diminished by the effects of hypoxia.

This extensive experience in human villous explant culture explores the possible role of hypoxemia in 11β-HSD2 suppression on the tendency for superficial trophoblastic invasion and incomplete decidual and maternal vascular remodeling seen in preeclampsia to occur.

Human placental material was obtained from 5- to 17-week and 25- to 36-week samples of placental tissue. The latter tissue was obtained from preeclamptics and age-matched normotensive controls. Explants were cultured on millipore filters, trophoblasts were collected and trypsinized and filtered, and cytotrophoblast and syncytium were identified by differential centrifugation. Additional tissue was embedded and sectioned for histochemical analysis using an 11β-HSD2 antibody and an avitin-biotin chromogram complex. Western blotting was used to estimate the quantity of the protein enzyme, and tritium-labeled cortisol conversion was used to measure changes in dehydrogenase enzyme activity.

Preeclamptic explants showed approximately 50% reduction in the steroid dehydrogenase activity and protein production compared with controls. Through 17 weeks of gestational age, 11β-HSD2 was increased in activity shown by histochemistry and Western blot; it was shown to decrease in 3% oxygen and to be restored by exposure to 20% oxygen in vitro. The authors' hypothesis is that maternal uterine arteriole development is decreased in preeclampsia as result of the failure of increase of p02 at approximately 18 to 20 weeks of gestational age[5] as high cortisol concentration, lacking the protective oxidative properties of 11β-HSD2, impairs the attainment of invasive trophoblastic properties. This prevents the vascular connection to the maternal circulation and failure of maternal vascular dilation and remodeling that follows normal trophoblast contact with spiral arterials at maternal vascular inflow sites and with intervillous space. This is excellent work and provides strong support for this broad hypothesis of the mechanisms of origin of the abnormal placentation associated with preeclampsia.

T. H. Kirschbaum, MD

References

1. 1994 YEAR BOOK OF OBSTETRICS, GYNECOLOGY, AND WOMEN'S HEALTH, pp 59-60.
2. 1998 YEAR BOOK OF OBSTETRICS, GYNECOLOGY, AND WOMEN'S HEALTH, p 51.
3. Jauniaux E, Watson AL, Hempstock J, et al: Onset of maternal arterial blood flow and placental oxidative stress. *Am J Pathol* 157:2111, 2000.
4. Hardy DB, Yang K: Trophoblastic 11β-HSD2 has been shown to be decreased in vitro by hypoxia, simultaneous with the reduction in hCG production. *J Clin Endocrinol Metab* 87:3696-3701, 2002.
5. 1999 YEAR BOOK OF OBSTETRICS, GYNECOLOGY, AND WOMEN'S HEALTH, pp 8-9.

Relaxin Causes Proliferation of Human Amniotic Epithelium by Stimulation of Insulin-Like Growth Factor-II
Millar LK, Reiny R, Yamamoto SY, et al (Univ of Hawaii, Honolulu)
Am J Obstet Gynecol 188:234-241, 2003   1–5

Introduction.—Insulin-like growth factors I and II (IGF-I and IGF-II) play key roles in fetal and placental growth. Both IGF-II and human relaxin mRNA have been found in human fetal and placental tissues. A series of experiments were performed to assess the proliferative effects of relaxin and IGF-II in human amniotic epithelial (WISH) cells.

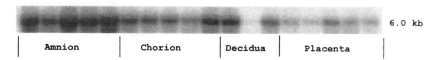

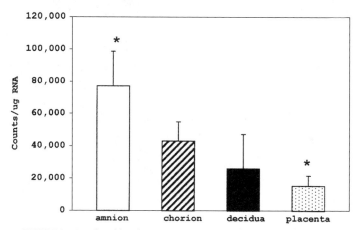

FIGURE 2.—Northern blot of IGF-II mRNA expression in amnion (n = 5), chorion (n = 5), decidua (n = 3), and placenta (n = 5) obtained after cesarean delivery at term. Quantitation is based on counts per microgram RNA (*asterisk*; *P* < .01) because there is no housekeeping gene appropriate for fetal membrane and placenta. (Courtesy of Millar LK, Reiny R, Yamamoto SY, et al: Relaxin causes proliferation of human amniotic epithelium by stimulation of insulin-like growth factor-II. *Am J Obstet Gynecol* 188:234-241. Copyright 2003 by Elsevier.)

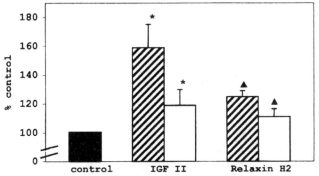

FIGURE 4.—Effect of a blocking antibody to insulin-like growth factor II (*IGF-II*) on proliferation of human amniotic epithelial cells treated with proliferative dose of IGF-II (30 ng/mL) (*asterisk*; $P < .0001$; n = 12) or relaxin (100 ng/mL) (*triangle*; $P = .006$; n = 13)(expressed as percentage of control). (Courtesy of Millar LK, Reiny R, Yamamoto SY, et al: Relaxin causes proliferation of human amniotic epithelium by stimulation of insulin-like growth factor-II. *Am J Obstet Gynecol* 188:234-241. Copyright 2003 by Elsevier.)

Methods and Findings.—In WISH cells as in amniotic epithelial and cytotrophoblast cells, significant expression of IGF-II was demonstrated (Fig 2). When WISH cells were treated with either IGF-II or relaxin, cell proliferation increased significantly and in dose-related fashion over the next several days. When treatment with an IGF-II–blocking antibody was given, the proliferative response to IGF-II was significantly lessened (Fig 4). In response to treatment with relaxin, there was a significant increase in IGF-II transcription over 24 hours. Fetal membrane expression of the relaxin gene was significantly correlated with the fetal membrane surface area. Relaxin gene levels

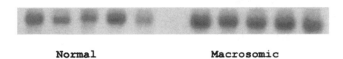

Normal   Macrosomic

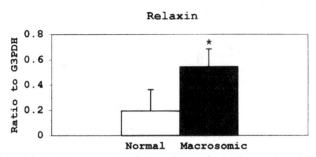

FIGURE 6.—Relaxin mRNA expression in fetal membranes of normally grown (n = 5) and macrosomic (n = 5) infants ($P = .008$) (expressed as ratio to G3PDH). (Courtesy of Millar LK, Reiny R, Yamamoto SY, et al: Relaxin causes proliferation of human amniotic epithelium by stimulation of insulin-like growth factor-II. *Am J Obstet Gynecol* 188:234-241. Copyright 2003 by Elsevier.)

were significantly higher in membranes from macrosomic versus normal-weight infants (Fig 6).

Conclusion.—These in vitro studies demonstrate proliferation of WISH cells in response to IGF-II or relaxin. The proliferative effects are reduced by treatment with an IGF-II–blocking antibody. Relaxin appears to affect IGF-II transcription, and its expression in the fetal membranes is associated with membrane surface area and birth weight. The findings point to a role of relaxin as a fetal membrane growth factor.

▶ This group has recently reported the results of subjecting human amnion, chorion, and decidua from pregnancies with premature preterm rupture of membranes without infection to complimentary DNA macroarrays, designed to demonstrate changes in expression of genes responsible for growth stimulation and regulation, mitogen control, and matrix remodeling, with and without labor (see Abstract 6–8). They demonstrated consistent significant upregulation of expression of genes for relaxin and IGF- binding proteins in IGFBP1, IGFBP2, and IGFBP3. This is an attempt to understand the biological significance of those changes.

IGF-2 is a somatomedin and a mitogen which regulates fetal and placental growth through stimulatory effects on carbohydrate and protein metabolism and production, with a strong correlation to neonatal birthweight.[1] Six binding proteins serve to stimulate IGF-2 effects upon binding.[2] Here the authors report on a series of in vitro cell culture studies using human amniotic epithelial-like cells and an in vivo study in human fetal membranes designed to explore the relationship between relaxin and IGF-2. They and others have demonstrated the growth-stimulant properties of relaxin in a variety of human and other experimental animal tissues.[3-7]

Immunostaining proved localization of IGF-2 in all cell types of human fetal membranes and in amniotic stromal matrix. Northern blots identified the general presence of mRNA for IGF in placenta with maximum distribution in the amnion (see Fig 2) and IGF-2 and relaxin growth stimulation in vitro, as well as its inhibition by blocking antibody to IGF-2 also demonstrated (see Fig 4). Relaxin proved to stimulate IGF-2 production by upregulating its gene expression in vitro, and, finally, relaxin gene expression in human and fetal membranes from human fetal macrosomic pregnancies was significantly greater than that seen with newborns of normal weight (see Fig 6).

Altogether, this work nicely demonstrates the capacity for relaxin to serve as growth stimulant by increasing the gene expression of IGF-2. What role upregulation of this growth stimulating somatomedia plays in premature preterm rupture of membranes remains to be determined.

T. H. Kirschbaum, MD

References

1. 1998 Year Book of Obstetrics, Gynecology, and Women's Health, pp 6-8; pp 218-220.
2. 2000 Year Book of Obstetrics, Gynecology, and Women's Health, pp 79-83.

3. McMurtry JP, Floersheim GI, Bryant-Greenwood GD: Characterization of the binding of ^{125}I-labelled succinylated porcine relaxin to human and mouse fibroblasts. *J Reprod Fertil* 58:43-49, 1980.
4. Hall JA, Cantley TC, Day BN, et al: Uterotropic actions of relaxin in prepubertal gilts. *Biol Reprod* 42:769-774, 1990.
5. Klonisch I, Hombach-Klonisch S: Review: Relaxin expressed at the feto-maternal interface. *Reprod Dom Anim* 35:149-152, 2000.
6. Garibay-Tupas JL, Maaskant RA, Greenwood FC, et al: Characteristics of the binding of ^{32}P-labelled human relaxins to the human fetal membranes. *J Endocrinol* 145:441-448, 1995.
7. Ohleth KM, Zhang Q, Lenhard JA, et al: Trophic effects of relaxin on reproductive tissue: Role of the IGF system. *Steroids* 64:634-639, 1999.

Cerebral Blood Flow and Metabolism in Relation to Electrocortical Activity With Severe Umbilical Cord Occlusion in the Near-Term Ovine Fetus

Kaneko M, White S, Homan J, et al (Miyazaki Med College, Japan; Univ of Western Ontario, London, Canada)
Am J Obstet Gynecol 188:961-972, 2003   1–6

Background.—Variable fetal heart rate (FHR) decelerations suggestive of umbilical cord occlusion are reported to be observed in 2% to 10% of antepartum FHR recordings and are the most common nonreassuring FHR pattern observed intra partum. These short-term hypoxic events are gener-

TABLE 1.—Cerebral Blood Flow Before, During, and After Severe Umbilical Cord Occlusion

Blood Flow (mL/100 g/Min)	3 Min Before Umbilical Cord Occlusion	During Umbilical Cord Occlusion		3 Min After Umbilical Cord Occlusion
		2 Min	3.5 Min	
Cerebral cortex	202 ± 30	472 ± 75*	549 ± 89*	311 ± 69
Gray matter	208 ± 32	486 ± 76*	567 ± 91*	319 ± 72
White matter	185 ± 24	427 ± 66*	477 ± 75*	280 ± 47
Subcortex	261 ± 37	1008 ± 198*	953 ± 171*	508 ± 115†
Corpus striatum	176 ± 30	608 ± 133*	606 ± 127*	344 ± 74†
Thalamus	286 ± 48	1032 ± 208*	984 ± 178*	550 ± 138
Hippocampus	169 ± 20	632 ± 111*	656 ± 123*	317 ± 69†
Colliculi	343 ± 45	1349 ± 269*	1224 ± 214*	634 ± 123†
Midbrain RF	307 ± 48	1457 ± 298*	1229 ± 213*	656 ± 142†
Sub.nigra/LGB	238 ± 36	1094 ± 231*	1043 ± 204*	500 ± 116†
Brainstem	321 ± 45	1492 ± 324*	1317 ± 261*	676 ± 164†
Pons	288 ± 40	1397 ± 296*	1240 ± 239*	629 ± 155†
Medulla	347 ± 49	1575 ± 351*	1386 ± 279*	710 ± 170†
Cerebellum	266 ± 32	702 ± 134*	708 ± 101*	425 ± 67†
Hemisphere	235 ± 26	671 ± 128*	657 ± 89*	391 ± 57†
Vermis	289 ± 34	723 ± 137*	744 ± 107*	453 ± 77†

Note: Data are presented as mean ± SEM; blood flow data from first cord occlusion includes 8 patients, except for 3 minutes after umbilical cord occlusion, where there were 7 patients.
*$P < .01$ versus the value 3 minutes before umbilical cord occlusion.
†$P < .05$ versus the value 3 minutes before umbilical cord occlusion.
Abbreviations: RF, Reticular formation; *LGB*, lateral geniculate body.
(Courtesy of Kaneko M, White S, Homan J, et al: Cerebral blood flow and metabolism in relation to electrocortical activity with severe umbilical cord occlusion in the near-term ovine fetus. *Am J Obstet Gynecol* 188:961-972. Copyright 2003 by Elsevier.)

ally well tolerated, but when they become more severe or more frequent, they may be associated with an increased incidence of neonatal acidosis, low Apgar scores, and nuchal cord involvement at delivery. These severe hypoxic events may also be associated with long-term adverse sequelae that involve the brain. The purpose of this study was to determine the change in cerebral blood flow and substrate metabolism in relation to electrocortical activity in the near-term ovine fetus after repeated severe occlusion of the umbilical cord.

Methods.—Eight near-term fetal sheep were studied for a 2-hour control period, a 6-hour experimental period with repeated cord occlusion of 4 minutes every 90 minutes, and a 16-hour recovery period. Regional cerebral blood flow was measured by the microsphere technique before, during, and after the first cord occlusion. Blood flow in the superior sagittal sinus, the cerebral perfusion pressure, and the electrocortical activity were monitored continuously. Brachiocephalic arterial and sagittal venous blood were sampled at various time points for blood gas and pH, oxygen content, and glucose and lactate levels.

Results.—Severe umbilical cord occlusion resulted in profound hypoxemia, with modest hypercapnia and acidemia to a similar degree with each insult (Table 1). There was a return to preocclusion values after release of the occluder. Glucose values dropped by approximately 30% with each cord occlusion but showed an overall increase through the experimental period. Lactate values increased from 1.21 to 6.10 mmol/L (Table 2). There was significant disruption of fetal electrocortical activity, with a sudden flattening of the electrocortical amplitude by an average of 1.5 minutes of each cord occlusion and an overall increase in indeterminate state activity during the experimental and through the recovery periods.

TABLE 2.—Cerebral Substrate Delivery and Fractional Extraction Before, During, and After Severe Umbilical Cord Occlusion

Substrate Delivery (μ mol/100 g/Min)	3 Min Before Umbilical Cord Occlusion	During Umbilical Cord Occlusion			3 Min After Umbilical Cord Occlusion
		0.5 Min	2 Min	3.5 Min	
Oxygen delivery (n = 8/7)	634 ± 63		408 ± 96*		1248 ± 269†
Glucose delivery (n = 8/7)	168 ± 31		273 ± 49*		390 ± 103†
Oxygen fractional extraction (n = 7)	0.28 ± 0.02	0.27 ± 0.05	0.00 ± 0.09†	−0.02 ± 0.20	0.15 ± 0.01*
Glucose fractional extraction (n = 7)	0.14 ± 0.02	0.09 ± 0.03	0.28 ± 0.04†	0.31 ± 0.07†	0.07 ± 0.02*
Lactate fractional extraction (n = 7)	0.02 ± 0.02	0.01 ± 0.02	−0.04 ± 0.03†	−0.03 ± 0.02†	0.00 ± 0.01

Note: Data are presented as mean ± SEM; substrate delivery data are from first cord occlusion, whereas substrate fractional extraction data are from second and fourth occlusions.
*$P < .01$ versus the value 3 minutes before umbilical cord occlusion.
†$P < .05$ versus the value 3 minutes before umbilical cord occlusion.
(Courtesy of Kaneko M, White S, Homan J, et al: Cerebral blood flow and metabolism in relation to electrocortical activity with severe umbilical cord occlusion in the near-term ovine fetus. *Am J Obstet Gynecol* 188:961-972. Copyright 2003 by Elsevier.)

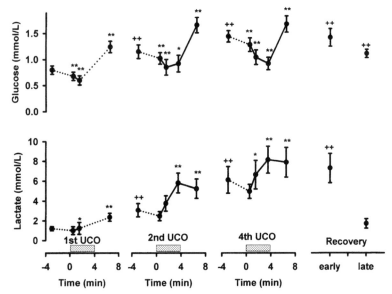

FIGURE 3.—Fetal arterial glucose and lactate measurements. Values are means ± SEM. Note that no blood sample was obtained at 3.5 minutes of first occlusion. *Asterisk* indicates P < .05, compared with respective preocclusion values; *double asterisk*, P < .01, compared with respective preocclusion values; *double dagger*, P < .01, compared with first preocclusion value. *Abbreviation: UCO*, Umbilical cord occlusion. (Courtesy of Kaneko M, White S, Homan J, et al: Cerebral blood flow and metabolism in relation to electrocortical activity with severe umbilical cord occlusion in the near-term ovine fetus. *Am J Obstet Gynecol* 188:961-972. Copyright 2003 by Elsevier.)

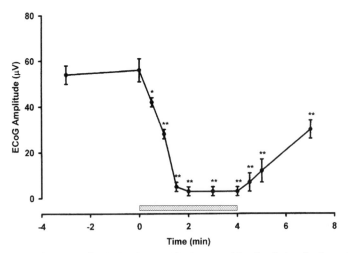

FIGURE 4.—Electrocortical (*ECoG*) voltage amplitude averaged for all occlusions for time points indicated before, during, and after umbilical cord occlusion (*hatched bar*). Values are mean ± SEM. *Asterisk* indicates P < .05, compared with preocclusion value at time 0; *double asterisk*, P < .01, compared with preocclusion value at time 0. (Courtesy of Kaneko M, White S, Homan J, et al: Cerebral blood flow and metabolism in relation to electrocortical activity with severe umbilical cord occlusion in the near-term ovine fetus. *Am J Obstet Gynecol* 188:961-972. Copyright 2003 by Elsevier.)

Cerebral blood flow increased by approximately 2.5- and 2.8-fold at 2 and 3.5 minutes, respectively, during the first cord occlusion and with the regional flow increase greater in the subcortex and brain stem (Fig 3). Cerebral extraction of oxygen was nearly zero at 2 minutes during the second and fourth occlusions, with oxygen uptake no longer measurable. Glucose extraction was increased approximately 2-fold at this time, which indicates that the anaerobic metabolism of glucose must be the predominant energy source at this time (Fig 4).

Conclusion.—Severe occlusion of the umbilical cord in the near-term sheep fetus resulted in a rapid decline in the availability of oxygen to the brain. The low partial pressure of oxygen gradient from blood to tissue limits oxygen consumption by 2 minutes after insult in spite of the significant increase in blood flow and indicates a shift to anaerobic metabolism, the suppression of electrocortical activity, and the likely shutdown of other energy-using processes.

▶ This study of the detailed impact of periodic cord occlusion on the fetal brain, of necessity done in experimental animals, is done with unusual depth of detail. The issue gains importance from the variable decelerations, which appear in 5% to 40% of labor, depending on how closely one looks. Variable decelerations in the late first and second stages of labor are the most commonly noted nonreassuring fetal heart rate patterns. Coupled with a realization that roughly 70% of cases of neonatal encephalopathy occur prior to labor onset adds urgency to understanding their impact.[1]

New information comes from isotope-labeled microsphere technology using 4 different istopes, which allows measurement of changes in regional cerebral blood flow to be made coupled with changes in whole fetal respiration and nutrition in the general circulation, together with fetal electrocorticograms expressing cortical neuronal activity. Recordings during 4 intervals of 4 minutes of cord occlusion at 90-minute intervals following a 2-hour control period, then followed by an overnight recovery period provide the fetal perturbations and data for analysis.

During cord occlusion, though cerebral blood flow, superior sagittal sinus blood flow, and oxygen delivery to the brain increased, a decrease in arterial oxygen content led to a 35% overall decrease in cerebral oxygen consumption. Cerebral cortical voltage decreased to near zero levels during occlusion and returned somewhat short of control values during recovery (see Fig 4). Blood glucose and lactate concentrations increased and rates of fetal nutrient delivery increased correspondingly. The increase indicates the glycogenolytic effect of catecholamines and the resulting glucose increased compensatory anaerobic glycolysis.

Changes in regional blood flows occurred within the brain, with smaller compensatory increases in the corpus striatum and hippocampus, both known to be sensitive to neuronal loss in hypoxemia.[2] Increased cerebral (2.5-fold) and sagittal sinus (1.5-fold) blood flow rates were driven by increased perfusion pressure and vasodilatation, the latter driven by the progressive increase in partial pressure of carbon dioxide throughout the cord obstruction intervals (see Fig 3). After cord occlusion, electrocorticogram values, and therefore cerebral cortical cell activity, returned to normal, though blood glucose, fetal oxygen delivery rates, cerebral blood perfusion pressure, and superior sagittal blood flow rates remained elevated. Fetuses showed the capacity to tolerate 4 minutes of full cord occlusion every 90 minutes over a 6-hour period with only temporary interruption of cortical electrical activity and without apparent neuronal destruction.

This level of fetal compromise does not exceed the effect of compensatory mechanisms activated. Longer periods of cord compromise and/or less effective compensatory capacity would likely result in permanent brain injury. Finding those thresholds for brain injury are important future goals for these talented investigators.

T. H. Kirschbaum, MD

References

1. Neonatal Encephalopathy in Cerebral Palsy. Report of the ACOG task force. ACOG, Washington, DC, January 2003.)
2. 1996 YEAR BOOK OF OBSTETRICS, GYNECOLOGY, AND WOMEN'S HEALTH, pp 134-137.

Magnesium Sulfate Inhibits the Oxytocin-Induced Production of Inositol 1,4,5-Trisphosphate in Cultured Human Myometrial Cells
Hurd WW, Natarajan V, Fischer JR, et al (Wright State Univ, Dayton, Ohio; Johns Hopkins School of Medicine, Baltimore, Md; Indiana Univ, Indianapolis)
Am J Obstet Gynecol 187:419-424, 2002   1–7

Background.—Magnesium sulfate is commonly used to stop premature labor. However, the mechanisms by which it inhibits contractility are not well understood. The effects of magnesium sulfate on inositol trisphosphate production were investigated.

Methods.—Myometrium was obtained from women undergoing cesarean delivery before labor at term. After stimulation with oxytocin, sodium fluoride, or Bay K 8644 with or without preincubation with magnesium sulfate or nifedipine, inositol trisphosphate was assessed in primary myometrial cell cultures. Experiments were conducted in calcium-containing or calcium-free medium containing egtazic acid and also after preincubation with the intracellular calcium chelator BAPTA-acetoxymethylester. Changes in intracellular calcium concentrations were assessed in separate experiments, using Fura-2 and spectrophotofluorometry.

Findings.—The production of inositol trisphosphate exposed to oxytocin, sodium fluoride, and Bay K 8644 was increased 2- to 4-fold. Preincubation with magnesium sulfate for 5 minutes or longer reduced oxytocin-, sodium fluoride-, and Bay K 8644-induced inositol trisphosphate production in media with or without calcium. In addition, preincubation with BAPTA-acetoxymethylester reduced oxytocin-stimulated inositol trisphosphate production by 78% in media containing calcium and completely prevented oxytocin response in media without calcium. Magnesium sulfate reduced inositol trisphosphate production in media containing calcium but produced no additional effects in calcium-free media. Oxytocin and Bay K 8644 increased intracellular calcium concentrations in media with or without calcium. Magnesium sulfate reduced the concentrations in both settings.

Conclusions.—Magnesium sulfate appears to inhibit phosphatidylinositol-4, 5-bisphosphate-specific phospholipase C activity, and subsequent calcium release in cultured myometrial cells. The mechanism underlying this effect appears to be a direct effect on phospholipase C.

▶ The thrust of this study is to remind investigators concerned with tocolytic development and evaluation of the value of exploring possibilities in both of the 2 existing sets of mechanisms for regulation of intracellular free calcium. The calcium ion serves as a key to myometrial irritability and contractility and requires an increase in calcium ion concentration from 10^{-7} to 10^{-6} mol/L for normal contractile activity. To maintain quiescence during pregnancy, cellular energy stores must be called upon to sequester calcium in the endopolasmic reticulum where it is inactive in determining cell irritability.[1] Adenosine trisphosphate (ATP) is ubiquitously distributed and serves to store, transport, and liberate activated protons derived from aerobic glycolysis in the form of high-energy phosphate bonds covalently bound to adenosine. Plasma membrane-based ATPase converts ATP to ADP and liberates the stored energy needed to transport calcium into endoplasmic sites where it cannot phosphorylate actin and myosin filaments and influence contractility. Oxytocin, coupled to its receptor, decreases ATP activity and allows calcium to enter the intracellular fluid volume. Beta-adrenergic agents, such as epinephrine and ritodrine, combined with their beta$_2$ receptor rendered stimulatory by its guanine nucleotide dependent regulatory protein (Gs) generates adenylate cyclase, which increases ATP activity and results in increased calcium storage. Regrettably, manifestation of this ATP-regulated mechanism has proven to be of very limited value in tocolysis in the human.

An alternative pathway involves phosphatidyl inositol, a plasma membrane component that, when bound to its receptor, generates a hydrolytic enzyme, phospholipase C. This enzyme degrades phosphoinositide to diacyl glycerol and inositol triphosphate. IP$_3$ is active in intracellular release of calcium stored in the endoplasmic reticulum. Diacyl glycerol, in turn, generates protein kinase C that modulates the action of IP$_3$ in its release of stored calcium. Magnesium sulfate inhibits the production of IP$_3$ from oxytocin which normally stimulates it, perhaps part of its transient tocolytic effect. Perhaps more important, several other antagonists of phospholipase C are known and are candidates for clinical testing as tocolytics. There is some optimism here since so many investigators feel that advancing pregnancy is associated with increasing dominance of the IP$_3$ pathway over the ATP-driven pathway in regulating myometrium irritability. It may well be agents that alter IP$_3$ production may lead to the development of a more clinically fruitful inhibitor of uterine contractions and premature labor than is currently available.

T. H. Kirschbaum, MD

Reference

1. 1990 YEAR BOOK OF OBSTETRICS AND GYNECOLOGY, pp 13-14.

Pregnancy-Associated Plasma Protein A Proteolytic Activity Is Associated With the Human Placental Trophoblast Cell Membrane
Sun IYC, Overgaard MT, Oxvig C, et al (Stanford Univ, Calif; Univ of Aarhus, Denmark)
J Clin Endocrinol Metab 87:5235-5240, 2002   1–8

Background.—Pregnancy-associated plasma protein A (PAPP-A) is expressed by human placental trophoblasts. PAPP-A is well known as a secreted placental product with an unknown function that is useful as a first-trimester marker for Down syndrome. A function for PAPP-A as a protease for insulin-like growth factor (IGF)-binding protein (IGFBP)-4 has recently been identified. The functions of PAPP-4 at the maternal-fetal interface are thought to be to proteolyze IGFBP-4 and thus to increase IGF bioavailability locally in the placenta, to promote IGF-II–mediated trophoblast invasion into the maternal decidua, and to modulate IGF regulation of steroidogenesis and glucose and amino acid transport in the villous. The possibility that IGFBP-4 proteolysis may occur on the trophoblast cell membrane, presumably to increase local bioavailable IGF for interactions with cognate IGF membrane receptors, was investigated.

Methods.—Sixteen human placentas were collected at 10 to 18 weeks at elective termination of genetically normal pregnancies. Trophoblasts were cultured, and trophoblast plasma membranes were isolated and solubilized. IGFBP-4 protease activity and PAPP-A immunoreactivity in the solubilized plasma membrane fraction were investigated.

Results.—IGFBP-4 protease activity was detected in solubilized human trophoblast membranes. This activity resulted in the cleavage of recombinant human IGFBP-4 into 18- and 14-kd fragments that were detected by Western blot analysis. This protease activity depended on the presence of IGF-II, and its metal ion dependence was demonstrated by inhibition of the protease by the metal chelators ethylenediaminetetraacetic acid (EDTA) and ethyleneglycoltetraacetic acid (EGTA). PAPP-A was demonstrated in solubilized human trophoblast membranes by Western immunoblotting (Fig 4). Immunocytochemical analysis showed PAPP-A on the cell membrane and in the cytoplasm of human trophoblasts in culture.

Conclusions.—These findings demonstrate the presence of an IGF-II–dependent and metal-dependent IGFBP-4 protease activity in human trophoblast plasma membranes, identified as PAPP-A. The location of PAPP-A at the maternal-placental interface allows it to proteolyze IGFBP-4 and to facilitate IGF action at the villous surface, at the invading extravillous cytotrophoblast, or at both locations.

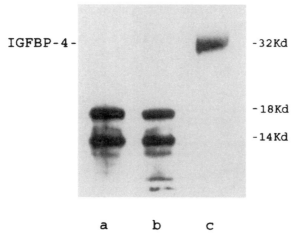

FIGURE 4.—Identification of the trophoblast membrane IGFBP-4 protease as PAPP-A. Shown is a representative Western immunoblot of IGFBP-4 in the IGFBP-4 protease assay using solubilized trophoblast membranes (*lane a*), trophoblast membrane fraction immunodepleted of PAPP-A with PAPP-A polyclonal antibodies (*lane c*), and treated with nonimmune IgG (*lane b*). Molecular weight markers are shown on the **right.** *Abbreviations: IGFBP-4*, Insulin-like growth factor (IGF)-binding protein; *PAPP-A*, pregnancy-associated plasma protein A. (Courtesy of Sun IYC, Overgaard MT, Oxvig C, et al: Pregnancy-associated plasma protein A proteolytic activity is associated with the human placental trophoblast cell membrane. *J Clin Endocrinol Metab* 87[11]:5235-5240, 2002. Copyright The Endocrine Society.)

▶ PAPP-A has been recognized as a placental secretory product of unknown function since the early 1980s. Known to increase in concentration in maternal pregnancy plasma in normals and in decreased concentration in the presence of a fetus with Down syndrome, PAPP-A has occasionally been used as a biochemical marker for that trisomy over the past 10 years. This group of investigators includes members of each of the 2 independent sets of scientists who first identified PAPP-A as a protease that acts to inactivate IGFBP-4 in the presence of IGF-2. In this study, they provide further information about its biological significance in pregnancy.

IGF-2 is a polypeptide mitogen secreted by trophoblastic epithlium and has the capacity to stimulate cellular proliferation, growth, and differentiation. Its concentration in fetal blood is strongly correlated with fetal birth weight and with placental growth. It also plays a role in steroidogenesis and developmental placentation. The IGFBPs, present in 6 isoforms, are produced by the decidua and are variously distributed among other organs sites, many but not all serving to inhibit activity of the IGF isoforms IGF-1 and IGF-2. IGFBP-4 is produced by the decidua and is capable of inhibiting the mitogenic effect of IGF-2 in serum. Since the binding protein is inhibitory, the effect of its protease PAPP-A is to free bound IFG-2 and to increase its role in growth and development. The role of IGF-1 and IGF-2 and their 6 binding proteins has been discussed here repeatedly.[1-6] The work presented here proves the specificity of PAPP-A's specific inactivating activity on IGFBP-4 by inhibition with competitive monoclonal antibody to PAPP-A. By using trophoblastic cell membrane preparations, the authors prove the comigration of native PAPP-A and trophoblast with solubilized membrane preparations, and using immunocytochemistry, they localize PAPP-A in trophoblastic cells and cell membranes in 10- to 18-week placental sections. Their findings strongly suggest that the normal role of PAPP-A in pregnancy is to increase IGF-2 in active form.

T. H. Kirschbaum, MD

References

1. 1996 YEAR BOOK OF OBSTETRICS, GYNECOLOGY, AND WOMEN'S HEALTH, pp 17-21.
2. 1998 YEAR BOOK OF OBSTETRICS, GYNECOLOGY, AND WOMEN'S HEALTH, pp 3-8, 218-220.
3. 1999 YEAR BOOK OF OBSTETRICS, GYNECOLOGY, AND WOMEN'S HEALTH, pp 163-166.
4. 2000 YEAR BOOK OF OBSTETRICS, GYNECOLOGY, AND WOMEN'S HEALTH, pp 79-83.
5. 2001 YEAR BOOK OF OBSTETRICS, GYNECOLOGY, AND WOMEN'S HEALTH, pp 231-232.
6. 2002 YEAR BOOK OF OBSTETRICS, GYNECOLOGY, AND WOMEN'S HEALTH, pp 19-20, 236-238.

Nitric Oxide: Does It Have an Etiological Role in Pre-Eclampsia?: A Study of Decidual Biopsies and Fetal Membranes

Rajagopal M, Moodley J, Chetty R (Univ of Natal, Durban, South Africa)
Acta Obstet Gynecol Scand 82:216-219, 2003   1–9

Background.—The etiology of preeclampsia/eclampsia remains elusive, but most studies indicate that the pathogenesis of preeclampsia likely involves the placental bed. In humans, normal pregnancy is characterized by the transformation of the spiral arteries into wide-bore tortuous vessels of low resistance. The mechanism for this transformation is not understood, but it has been suggested that the presence of interstitial cytotrophoblast produces vasoactive mediators, which cause vascular dilation before invasion of the spiral arteries, by endovascular trophoblast. Nitric oxide (NO) is a small molecular weight mediator. Among the diverse functions of NO are vasodilation, inhibition of platelet aggregation, and vascular remodeling. This study sought evidence of NO in decidual biopsy specimens and fetal membranes of women with preeclampsia.

Methods.—A total of 42 women with 28 weeks' gestation or more were included in the study. Of these women, 20 were normotensive and 22 had preeclampsia. Women with chronic hypertension, diabetes, or multiple pregnancies were excluded. Maternal blood samples were obtained prior to cesarean section, and decidual biopsy specimens were obtained during cesarean section. Fetal membrane specimens were also obtained. Tissue specimens were fixed immediately in formalin, washed, and embedded in paraffin. Immunohistochemical staining for NO synthases I, II, and III was performed and reviewed.

Results.—No statistically significant difference was observed between the normotensive and hypertensive patients in the level of immunostaining of NO synthases.

Conclusion.—This study of the role of NO in preeclampsia found that the severity of blood pressure in pregnant women does not affect the expression of NO synthases.

▶ With recognition of the important signaling and vasodilatory role of endo- thelial NO, many investigators sought in vain for deficient NO production to explain the increased peripheral vascular resistance in preeclampsia. On fur- ther evaluation, NO synthesis and its metabolic products were found to be in- creased in the blood and several other tissues of preeclamptics,[1,2] though it was not clear whether increased NO production was derived from the pla- centa and its decidual implantation site or from the general vasculature.

Vascular shear stress is an important stimulant of endothelial NO produc- tion.[3,4] Shear forces are generated by 2 separate oppositely directed but paral- lel forces acting at a phase interface as, for instance, generated by blood flow through endothelial lined blood vessels. Shear stress and, therefore, NO synthase–directed conversion of arginine to NO and citrulline might be expect- ed to be enhanced by the vasoconstriction responsible for the increased pe- ripheral vascular resistance in preeclampsia.

This study of 42 women, half of them preeclamptics, all scheduled for re- peat cesarean section confirms the primacy of increased NO production as a result of peripheral vasoconstriction associated with hypertensive disease. At the time of cesarean section, decidual biopsy specimens, including myo- metrium at the placental attachment site as well as sections of placenta membranes, were obtained and compared with respect to the density of nuclear staining by immmunohistochemistry using monoclonal antibody to 3 isoforms of NO synthetases. There were no significant differences between the hypertensives and normal controls except for mean blood pressure and newborn birth weights. No significant differences were noted either for de- cidual, myometrial, or endothelial biopsy specimens or for fetal membrane biopsy specimens for any of the 3 NO synthetase isoforms nor the density of nuclear staining. It has become quite clear that increased placental produc- tion is not a result of pregnancy hypertension but a result of changes of pe- ripheral vascular resistance as the result of something, as yet unspecified, that produces preeclampsia.

T. H. Kirschbaum, MD

References

1. 1997 Year Book of Obstetrics, Gynecology, and Women's Health, pp 24-25.
2. 1998 Year Book of Obstetrics, Gynecology, and Women's Health, pp 23-25.
3. 2002 Year Book of Obstetrics, Gynecology, and Women's Health, pp 128-131.
4. 2003 Year Book of Obstetrics, Gynecology, and Women's Health, pp 10-12.

Human Placental Vascular Development: Vasculogenic and Angiogenic (Branching and Nonbranching) Transformation Is Regulated by Vascular Endothelial Growth Factor-A, Angiopoietin-1, and Angiopoietin-2
Geva E, Ginzinger DG, Zaloudek CJ, et al (Univ of California, San Francisco)
J Clin Endocrinol Metab 87:4213-4224, 2002   1–10

Background.—Vessel formation occurs during placental development. Human placental vascular development includes 3 stages: an initial stage of

TABLE 2.—Vascular Endothelial Growth Factor A, Angiopoietin 1, and Angiopoietin 2 (Messenger RNA and Protein) Localization in the Human Placenta (Chorionic Villi) During Pregnancy

mRNA	Protein
VEGF-A	
Cytotrophoblast	Cytotrophoblast
Syncytiotrophoblast	Syncytiotrophoblast
Perivascular cells	Endothelial cells
Stromal macrophages	Stromal macrophages
Ang1	
Syncytiotrophoblast	
Perivascular cells	
Stromal macrophages	
Ang2	
Syncytiotrophoblast	Syncytiotrophoblast
Perivascular cells	Endothelial cells
Stromal macrophages	Stromal macrophages

(Courtesy of Geva E, Ginzinger DG, Zaloudek CJ, et al: Human placental vascular development: Vasculogenic and angiogenic (branching and nonbranching) transformation is regulated by vascular endothelial growth factor-A, angiopoietin-1, and angiopoietin-2. *J Clin Endocrinol Metab* 87(9):4213-4224, 2002. Copyright The Endocrine Society.)

vasculogenesis and branching, and nonbranching angiogenesis. Vascular endothelial growth factor A (VEGF-A) has been shown to initiate vasculogenesis and angiogenesis, with angiopoietin (Ang)1 and Ang2 acting in concert with VEGF-A in the later stages of angiogenesis. The transcript profiles of VEGF-A and Ang2 and how these molecules regulate placental vascular development at the transcriptional level were investigated.

Methods.—Human placental tissue from 24 normotensive pregnancies and 5 pregnancies with severe preeclampsia were used for RNA and protein analyses. No difference in relative VEGF-A and Ang transcription was found among the placentas.

FIGURE 1.—A, The development of villi is initiated during the first 28 days postconception (p.c.), during which the primary villi, composed of trophoblast cells, develop. Approximately 15 to 22 days p.c., invasion of the primary villi by extra-embryonic mesodermal cells (*EEMs*) occurs, leading to the formation of the secondary villi. During the next 7 days, mesenchymal cells, derived from the extra-embryonic mesoderm, differentiate into hemangioblasts (*HBLs*), which further differentiate into angioblastic and endothelial cells (*ECs*) and hematopoietic stem cells (*HSs*) (day 28 p.c.), which delaminate from the primitive vessel wall into the early lumen. The fetoplacental vascular lumina form by dilation of the intracellular clefts, creating a primitive capillary network (*PCN*), the hallmark of the tertiary villus. Before the formation of the primitive vessels, mesenchyme-derived macrophages (Hofbauer cells), which express angiogenic growth factors, appear in the mesenchyme of the secondary villi, suggesting a paracrine role in initiation of vasculogenesis. In contrast, expression of angiogenic growth factors in decidual cells (*DCs*) and maternal macrophages suggest a paracrine mechanism mediating trophoblast invasion of the maternal circulation. From this stage of development until the end of the first trimester of pregnancy, the new fetal vessels are generated via branching angiogenesis, resulting in the formation of a capillary network within the stem and immature intermediate villi (*IMV*). Once the primary vascular plexus is formed, new capillaries form by sprouting and nonsprouting angiogenesis. During sprouting angiogenesis, endothelial cells degrade the basement membrane, migrate, proliferate, and reassemble into tubes. In nonsprouting angiogenesis, new vessels are formed by intussusceptive growth. The formed vasculature is further differentiated by recruitment of pericytes and smooth muscle cells and remodeled into a tree-like hierarchy containing vessels of different sizes. From the beginning of the third trimester until term, villous vascular architecture undergoes change from branching to nonbranching angiogenesis in which the existing vessels increase in size through intercalated growth, due to the formation of mature intermediate (*MMV*) and terminal villi (*TV*). The decrease in trophoblast proliferation and increase in endothelial cell proliferation along the entire length of the capillary leads to a final coil and bulge

(*Continued*)

FIGURE 1 (cont.)

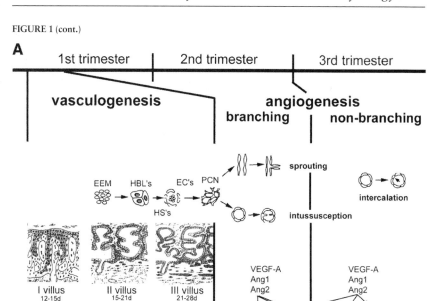

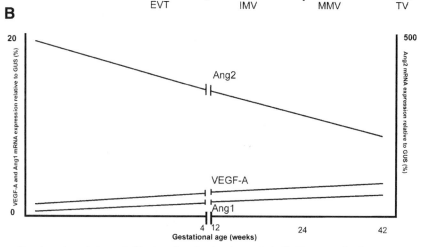

capillary loop through the trophoblastic surface, forming the terminal villi. There specialized structures are the main site of diffusional gas exchange between the fetal and maternal circulations. As gestation proceeds, these terminal capillaries focally dilate to form large sinusoids which, with increasing fetal blood pressure, counterbalance the effects of the long, poorly branched capillaries on total fetal-placental vascular imped-ance (10-12, 25 in the original journal article). B, Vascular endothelial growth factor A (*VEGF-A*), angiopoi-etin 1 (*Ang1*), and angiopoietin 2 (*Ang2*) mRNA expression (real-time quantitative polymerase chain reac-tion analysis). Illustrated congruent with panel A. See also Fig 2 in the original journal article. (Courtesy of Geva E, Ginzinger DG, Zaloudek CJ, et al: Human placental vascular development: Vasculogenic and angio-genic (branching and nonbranching) transformation is regulated by vascular endothelial growth factor-A, angiopoietin-1, and angiopoietin-2. *J Clin Endocrinol Metab* 87(9):4213-4224, 2002. Copyright The En-docrine Society.)

Results.—VEGF-A, Ang1, and Ang2 messenger RNA (mRNA) were measured with real-time quantitative polymerase chain reaction analysis. The analysis showed that VEGF-A and Ang1 mRNA increased by 2.5% and 2.8% per week, respectively, whereas Ang2 decreased by 3.5% per week. The localization of VEGF-A, Ang1, and Ang2 mRNA in the human placenta was in the villous cytotrophoblast and syncytiotrophoblast, perivascular cells, and stromal macrophages (VEGF-A mRNA), and villous syncytiotrophoblast, perivascular cells, and stromal macrophages (Ang1 and Ang2 mRNA) (Table 2). The decrease in Ang2 mRNA expression throughout the pregnancy may allow villous vessels a more plastic form for transformation from branching to nonbranching angiogenesis and prevent the vessels from undergoing destabilization, whereas VEGF-A and Ang1 stabilize the blood vessels (Fig 1).

Conclusion.—VEGF-A, Ang1, and Ang2 gene expression in the human placenta during pregnancy have been suggested as having autocrine/paracrine effects on vasculogenic-angiogenic transformation. The correlation between mRNA and protein concentrations of these vascular endothelial-specific growth factors suggest that regulation of placental vascular development occurs at the genetic level for both normotensive and preeclampsic pregnancies.

▶ Knowing the cell biology of placental development is important to understanding normal fetal nutrition, growth retardation, and possibly preeclampsia. The early development of trophoblastic invasion and organization by changes in trophoblastic epithelial cell adhesion molecular phenotypes has been well researched.[1,2] That fine work describes the control and development of umbilical vasculization, which is essential to normal villus formation. The bulk of differential development takes place in the first 28 days of pregnancy. Vasculogenesis or the de novo development of new vessels must be differentiated from angiogenesis in which established vascular channels are further extended by endothelial proliferation and sprouting into straight and branched capillary structures inside trophoblastic buds. Tissue culture techniques have identified 2 classes of mitogens involved in this process.

VEGF-A is a protein that results in new endothelial proliferation, migration, sprouting, and formation of tubular primordial structures. Ang1 acts in conjunction with VEGF-A to produce maturation and stabilization of endothelial growth stimulation produced by VEGF-A. Ang2 antagonizes the effects of ANG1 and delays or disrupts angiogenesis to allow further endothelial sprouting and increased plasticity and remodeling of endothelial structures previously produced by VEGF-A. VEGF-A and Ang2 are both upregulated in hypoxia.

Here a series of 29 placentas was obtained from women in each of the 3 trimesters of pregnancy, including 5 placentas from preeclamptics with growth retarded fetuses at the lower 5% of expected weight at gestational age. RNA and protein were extracted from each placenta and reverse transcription done to yield cDNA and DNA quantitation done by the TaqMAN polymerase system using primers specific to VEGF-A, Ang1, and Ang2 cDNA.[3] These cRNA were conjugated to monoclonal antibodies for use in fluorescent in situ hybridization localization of mRNA for all 3 of the angiogenic factors, and the corresponding proteins were localized immmunohistochemically using analagous techniques.

In normals, VEGF-A and Ang1 mrnas both increased linearly through pregnancy at rates of 2.5% to 2.8% per week while Ang2 progressively declined at a rate of 3.5% per week. Rnas for Ang1 and Ang2 and their proteins were localized primarily to syncytiotrophoblast, perivascular cells, and stromal macrophages and, in the case of Ang2, in endothelial cells. VEGF-A RNA and protein were found in both trophoblastic layers and in perivascular and Hoffbauer cells. Preeclamptic preparations showed a 3.1-fold increase in VEGF-A and a 1.5-fold increase in Ang2, presumably a result of relatively low PO2 in situ in the placenta. No change in Ang2 compared to normals was seen.

In normals, the decline of the Ang2 with gestation allows for initial vasculogenic plasticity of placental vasculature during the first 2 trimesters and in increasing stabilization thereafter to term. Chronic low intensity vascular development is supported by progressive lower-level increases in VEGF-A and Ang1. Analysis of preeclamptic specimens supports the failure of increases in tissue level PO2 associated with that disease.[4] Increased VEGF-A and Ang1, as well as increased expression of several other angiogentic factors, is associated with increases in the numbers of nonbranching angiogentic structures, apparently in attempt to increase PO2 and oxygen therapy in response to hypoxia. This work is a major step in understanding placental vascular development and the compensatory capacity that it possesses.

T. H. Kirschbaum, MD

References

1. 1994 Year Book of Obstetrics, Gynecology, and Women's Health, pp 59-60.
2. 1998 Year Book of Obstetrics, Gynecology, and Women's Health, pp 18-21, 50-51.
3. 1999 Year Book of Obstetrics, Gynecology, and Women's Health, pp 193-196.
4. 1999 Year Book of Obstetrics, Gynecology, and Women's Health, pp 8-9.

The Thrombomodulin–Protein C System Is Essential for the Maintenance of Pregnancy

Isermann B, Sood R, Pawlinski R, et al (Blood Research Inst, Milwaukee, Wis; Scripps Research Inst, La Jolla, Calif; Children's Hosp Research Found, Cincinnati, Ohio; et al)
Nature Med 9:331-337, 2003   1–11

Background.—The thrombomodulin–protein C pathway is an inhibitory feedback loop that suppresses excessive activation of coagulation. Thrombomodulin-deficient ($Thbd^{-/-}$) mice die at 8.5 days post coitum (dpc) due to a placental defect. This report demonstrates that $Thbd^{-/-}$ lethality is caused by a tissue factor–initiated activation of the coagulation cascade at the maternal-fetal interface.

Methods and Results.—$Thbd^{-/-}$ embryos were examined in situ at 8.5 dpc for evidence of cell death and altered proliferation. The diploid trophoblast cells of the ectoplacental cone had significantly reduced 5-bromo-2-deoxy-uridine, a marker of growth and replication, compared with controls. This is consistent with a growth defect in the mutant cells and selective cell death of giant trophoblast cells. Pregnant mice were treated with anticoagulation therapy to determine whether this would rescue $Thbd^{-/-}$ embryos. Anticoagulation successfully prevented embryo resorption, but the embryonic growth defect persisted.

To determine whether a complete anticoagulation block would rescue these embryos, Thbd-Tf mice were produced. These coagulation-negative mice embryos survived until the point of $Tf-$ lethality, indicating that complete coagulant loss rescued Thbd embryos. Heterozygous $Thbd^{-/-}$ mice were bred to fibrinogen mutant ($Fg^{-/-}$) mice to evaluate whether the conversion of fibrinogen to fibrin is involved in $Thbd$ lethality.

Trophoblast cell death and $Thbd^{-/-}$ lethality were dependent on the generation of fibrin degradation products, but the growth defect persisted in the absence of fibrin degradation products. Therefore, the embryo growth defect must occur through a different mechanism. Reverse transcriptase–polymerase chain reaction analysis of cultured $Thbd^{-/-}$ trophoblast cells demonstrated that protease activated receptor (PAR)-1, -2, -3, and -4 transcripts were produced in these placentas, suggesting that PAR-1 expression is either ineffective or overcome by the growth inhibiting response to PAR-2 and PAR-4 in the $Thbd$ embryos.

Conclusion.—These experiments demonstrate that $Thbd^{-/-}$ embryonic lethality is caused by the tissue factor–initiated activation of the blood coagulation cascade at the fetal-maternal interface. Activated coagulation factors induce both cell death and growth inhibition of placental trophoblast cells, but by 2 distinct mechanisms. Giant trophoblast cell death is caused by the formation of fibrin degradation products. The growth arrest of trophoblasts appears to be due to the activation of PAR-2 and PAR-4 by coagulation factors. These results reveal a new function for the thrombomodulin–protein C system in the maintenance of pregnancy in this mouse model. Whether similar mechanisms may contribute to unexplained first trimester fetal loss in humans remains to be investigated.

▶ In a series of gene knockout experimental animals[1] using in vitro cell cultures, TUNEL assays of apoptosis[2] (Abstract 7–6) histopathology and pharmacologic therapeutics, these investigators establish important new roles for thrombomodulin and protein C in the balance of blood coagulation and fluidity as well as the regulation of placental and fetal development. Thrombomodulin is a cell surface thrombin receptor with 2 separate roles in the cell biology of pregnancy. In addition to an anti-inflammatory property, it acts to complex with thrombin, serving thereby to inhibit the role of that enzyme in initiating the coagulation cascade and fibrin formation. Secondly, it forms a complex with protein C, activating it and influencing thrombus substrate regulation, initiating its anticoagulant activity.

Gene knockout animals in which the gene for thrombomodulin is homozygously deleted experienced fetal deaths at 8.5 dpc (gestational duration, 20 to 24 days), resorption, and placental degeneration without evidence of placental fibrin deposition or coagula. Histomorphology of the placenta shows decreased proliferation of extraplacental trophoblast and apoptosis of giant trophoblast cells which make up the fetal part of the hemochorial mouse placenta. Anti-coagulant treatment prevents embryo resorption, but growth retardation of the embryo and placenta persists in the absence of thrombomodulin.

Through use of gene knockout preparations for tissue factor (tissue thromboplastinogen to some), and for fibrinogen, it is reasonably clear that thrombin unable to interact with thrombomodulin with the thrombomodulin–protein C complex in gene knockout animals reacts with placental PARs and initiates fibrin formation, which rapidly yields inactive fibrin split products, which in turn produce placental pathology. Tissue factor is a necessary part of that process. Genetically manipulated tissue factor absence allows survival of the embryo until it succumbs later to inadequate yoke sac development, a product of its tissue factor deficiency. Though thrombin inhibits trophoblastic proliferation, its complex to PAR results in trophoblastic proliferation.

In this admittedly complex fashion, thrombomodulin plays an important role in modulating the thrombophylic properties of pregnancy hematology, preventing excessive fibrin formation and deposition and assuring normal embryogenesis while simultaneously avoiding placental damage from fibrin split products. These relationships need to be confirmed in human pregnancy where it seems likely they also exist.

T. H. Kirschbaum, MD

References

1. 2002 YEAR BOOK OF OBSTETRICS, GYNECOLOGY, AND WOMEN'S HEALTH, pp 3-5.
2. Almog O, Fainaru O, Gamzu, R, et al: Placental apoptosis in discordant twins. *Placenta* 23:331-336, 2002.

Soluble Adhesion Molecule Profile in Normal Pregnancy and Pre-Eclampsia

Chaiworapongsa T, Romero R, Yoshimatsu J, et al (Natl Inst of Child Health and Human Development, Bethesda, Md; Wayne State Univ, Detroit; Sotero del Rio Hosp, Puente Alto, Chile)
J Matern Fetal Neonatal Med 12:19-27, 2002   1–12

Background.—Endothelial cell dysfunction is thought to be a key factor in the pathophysiology of preeclampsia. However, the mechanism responsible for the development of endothelial dysfunction in preeclampsia has not been determined. An exaggerated inflammatory response has been implicated. Adhesion molecules play a central role in the adherence of leukocytes to endothelial cells and the subsequent migration of white blood cells into perivascular tissue. Cellular forms of adhesion molecules mediate specific steps of leukocyte–endothelial cell interaction and have been implicated in the pathophysiology of preeclampsia. The soluble forms of these molecules

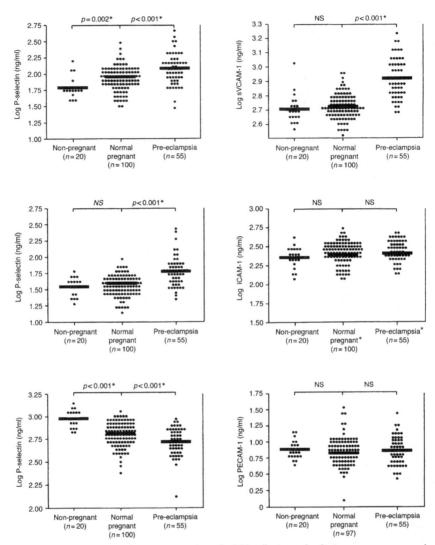

FIGURE 1.—The mean plasma concentrations of soluble adhesion molecules in nonpregnant, normal pregnant, and preeclamptic women. *Asterisk* indicates that 2 samples in the normal pregnant group and 1 sample in the preeclampsia group had nondetectable concentrations. *Abbreviations:* PECAM-1, Platelet endothelial cell adhesion molecule 1; ICAM-1, intercellular adhesion molecule 1; VCAM-1, vascular cell adhesion molecule 1. (Courtesy of Chaiworapongsa T, Romero R, Yoshimatsu J, et al: Soluble adhesion molecule profile in normal pregnancy and pre-eclampsia. *J Matern Fetal Neonatal Med* 12:19-27, 2002.)

are detectable in plasma, and their concentrations are thought to reflect the degree of activation of a particular cell type.

Elevations in soluble P-selectin (sP-selectin) indicate platelet activation, and changes in soluble L-selectin (sL-selectin) suggest leukocyte activation. An increase in the soluble forms of E-selectin (sE-selectin), vascular cell adhesion molecule 1 (sVCAM-1), intercellular adhesion molecule 1 (sICAM-

1), and platelet endothelial cell adhesion molecule (sPECAM-1) indicate endothelial cell activation/dysfunction. This study sought to determine whether normal pregnancy and preeclampsia were associated with changes in this concentrations of soluble selectins and members of the immunoglobulin superfamily of adhesion molecules.

Methods.—This cross-sectional investigation determined the plasma concentrations of sL-selectin, sE-selectin, sP-selectin, sVCAM-1, sICAM-1, and sPECAM-1 in peripheral blood. The study group comprised 20 nonpregnant women, 100 normal pregnant women, and 55 women with preeclampsia. Concentrations of soluble adhesion molecules were determined with enzyme-linked immunoassays. Parametric statistics were used for data analysis.

Results.—Normal pregnancy was associated with a significant increase in the maternal plasma concentration of sP-selectin and a decrease in sL-selectin (Fig 1). There were no changes in maternal plasma concentrations of sE-selectin, sVCAM-1, sICAM-1, or sPECAM-1. In contrast, preeclampsia was associated with a significant increase in sP-selectin, sE-selectin, and sVCAM-1; a decrease in sL-selectin; and no change in sICAM-1 or sPECAM-1 concentrations.

Conclusion.—This study demonstrated an increased concentration of sP-selectin and decreased sL-selectin, as well as no change in endothelial cell-associated soluble adhesion molecules. These findings suggest that pregnancy is associated with platelet and leukocyte activation but not endothelial cell activation. Preeclampsia, however, appears to be characterized by activation of platelets, leukocytes, and endothelial cells.

▶ The innumerable observations of abnormality in the complex relationships between thromboplastic epithelium and decidual cells and their connective tissue matrixes in preeclampsia has generated a great deal of interest in exploring the expression of connective tissue adhesion molecules amenable to enzyme-linked immunosorbent assay in normal and preeclamptic pregnancy.[1,2] The 3 classes of molecules serve to provide a structural matrix within cells (ICAMs), between cells (cadherins), and between cells and their connective tissue matrixes (integrins).

Cell adhesion molecules which function to connect endothelial cells and blood-formed elements (selectins) are of special interest. Work previously reviewed here[3] demonstrated no significant difference in the distribution and density of PECAMs, ICAM-1s, and VCAM-1s in the placental bed sections of normotensive women and those with preeclampsia. On the other hand, human umbilical vein endothelial cells grown in vitro from preeclamptics showed decreased vascular endothelial cadherin, and occludin, both endothelial junction proteins, in preeclampsia compared to normal pregnancy. These changes have been interpreted to suggest endothelial injury in preeclampsia.

This work provides longitudinal assays of 3 selectins, (leukocyte, platelet, and endothelial-derived) and VCAM-1, ICAM-1, and PECAM-1 in 20 nonpregnant women, 100 normotensive gravidas, and 55 preeclamptics. Compared with nonpregnant women, normals show increased concentrations of plasma platelet selectin, no changes endothelial selectin, and decreased leukocyte selectin activity. No other cell adhesion molecules studied were altered by pregnancy per se. Compared to normal gravidas, preeclamptics showed increased endothelial and platelet selectins as well as VCAM-1 activity.

Adhesion molecules are active in situ in tissues of origin, and their increased presence in plasma may mean increased production or increased release and, in fact, decreased presence in their in situ positions in tissue. Further, the relationship between native adhesion molecules in tissue and their soluble forms in plasma is uncertain and may not represent a simple, stable equilibrium. A further problem is that studies of preeclamptics are often not confined to primigravidas, despite strong evidence of the need to do so in studying hypertensive disease.[4]

To date it appears the changes in plasma soluble adhesion molecules in hypertensive pregnancy more likely represent changes in vascular endothelium function and endothelial receptors for platelet epitopes than they do alterations in the relationship of troploblasts to decidua and decidual vessels at their site of implantation. They appear more likely an effect than a cause.

T. H. Kirschbaum, MD

References

1. 1994 YEAR BOOK OF OBSTETRICS, GYNECOLOGY, AND WOMEN'S HEALTH, pp 59-60.
2. 1998 YEAR BOOK OF OBSTETRICS, GYNECOLOGY, AND WOMEN'S HEALTH, pp 18-21, 50-51.
3. 2003 YEAR BOOK OF OBSTETRICS, GYNECOLOGY, AND WOMEN'S HEALTH, pp 19-21.
4. Chesley LC: Recognition of the long term sequellae of pre-eclampsia. *Am J Obstet Gynecol* 182:289, 2000.

Physical Properties of the Chorioamnion Throughout Gestation
Pressman EK, Cavanaugh JL, Woods JR (Univ of Rochester, NY)
Am J Obstet Gynecol 187:672-675, 2002   1–13

Introduction.—The chorioamnion membrane is a highly specialized but underappreciated organ that has a rich portfolio of roles. It is surprising that so little is understood about how the chorioamnion, as a supporting matrix, changes through gestation. The tensile strength of the human chorioamnion was assessed between 17 to 41 weeks' gestation. These results were compared with those obtained from commercially available products used as industrial wrappings because of their uniform strength.

Methods.—Ten × 10 cm segments of chorioamnion were obtained from 35 placentas (27 singletons and 4 sets of twins) at the time of delivery. Gestational age at delivery, the presence or absence of clinical chorioamnionitis, premature rupture of membranes, onset of labor, and the indications and mode of delivery were recorded. Tensile strength (grams to burst and deflection at rupture) were measured on 2 to 16 specimens per patient. The tensile strength of several commercial products (Reynolds wax paper, Reynolds plastic wrap, Glad Cling Wrap, and Saran Cling Plus) was used for comparison.

A

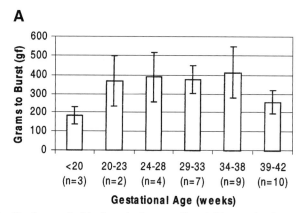

FIGURE 1.—Tensile strength of chorioamnion in grams of force (gf) by gestational age. $P = .005$ between groups by analysis of variance; $P = .04$ between <20 weeks and 24-28 weeks; $P = .008$ between 34-38 weeks and 39-42 weeks by student t test. (Courtesy of Pressman EK, Cavanaugh JL, Woods JR: Physical properties of the chorioamnion throughout gestation. *Am J Obstet Gynecol* 187:672-675. Copyright 2002 by Elsevier.)

Results.—Tensile strength increased up to 20 weeks' gestation, then plateaued until 39 weeks' gestation, at which time it dropped dramatically (Fig 1). Clinical chorioamnionitis alone did not influence tensile strength. Gross membrane inflammation caused reduced tensile strength.

Conclusion.—The tensile strength of the chorioamnion differs with gestational age. These baseline data should be useful in evaluating the effects of various conditions and therapies on membrane strength and may offer insight into spontaneous rupture of the membranes.

▶ This study uses industrial materials testing to compare chorioamnion segments with some commercial wrapping products and produces some interesting findings. Normal chorioamnion is slightly superior to commercial household wraps with respect to the grams of force delivered through a 3-mm diameter probe required to rupture membranes and far superior in terms of membrane distension prior to rupture to all but domestic plastic wrap. Physical integrity of fetal membranes increases to a maximum at 20 to 23 weeks' gestational age, presumably a result of fusion of the stromal portions of chorion and amnion, obliterating the extraembryonic coelome. Further, fusion of the decidua capsularis with the decidua parietalis, possibly connecting the decidua capsularis, the outermost layer of the fused chorioamnion to the rich vascular network underlying the decidua parietalis, occurs at that time. Though the number of cases in support of this observation is not large, it appears there is a decline in tensile strength of chorioamnion during the interval from 39 to 42 weeks' gestation. Even more interesting is the failure to alter membrane physical properties in the presence of either clinical or histologic chorioamnionitis: only in 2 cases of gross inflammation was bursting pressure of the membranes diminished. These observations oppose some long-standing dogma and raise interesting questions regarding the decrease in membrane tensile properties that occurs at term.

T. H. Kirschbaum, MD

2 Maternal Complications of Pregnancy

Prophylactic Administration of Progesterone by Vaginal Suppository to Reduce the Incidence of Spontaneous Preterm Birth in Women at Increased Risk: A Randomized Placebo-controlled Double-blind Study
da Fonseca EB, Bittar RE, Carvalho MHB, et al (Univ of São Paulo, Brazil)
Am J Obstet Gynecol 188:419-424, 2003   2–1

Introduction.—Primary prevention of preterm delivery is desirable, yet not always possible. One of the best ways to prevent preterm birth is through the early identification of pregnant females at high risk for preterm delivery. Progesterone is useful in permitting pregnancy to reach its physiologic term because at sufficient levels in the myometrium, it blocks the oxytocin effect of prostaglandin $F_2\alpha$ and α-adrenergic stimulation and therefore increases the α-adrenergic tocolytic response. The effect of prophylactic vaginal progesterone in reducing the preterm birth rate was examined in a high-risk population of 142 asymptomatic women with singleton pregnancies in a randomized, double-blind, placebo-controlled investigation.

Methods.—Patients were randomized to either progesterone (100 mg) or placebo administered daily by vaginal suppository. All patients underwent uterine contraction monitoring with an external tocodynamometer once weekly for 60 minutes between 24 and 34 weeks' gestation. Groups were compared with respect to their epidemiologic characteristics (Table 2), uterine contraction frequency, and incidence of preterm birth.

Results.—The overall preterm birth rate was 21.1% (30/142). There were differences in the progesterone and placebo groups in uterine activity (23.6% vs 54.3%; $P < .05$) and in preterm birth rates (13.8% vs 28.5%; $P < .05$). More women had delivered before 34 weeks' gestation in the placebo group than in the progesterone group (18.5% vs 2.7%; $P < .05$) (Fig 3).

Conclusion.—Prophylactic vaginal progesterone decreased the frequency of uterine contractions and the incidence of preterm delivery in females at high risk for prematurity.

TABLE 2.—Characteristics of Women at Randomization

	Placebo (n = 70)	Progesterone (n = 72)
Age (y)*	26.8	27.6
Ethnicity*		
White	71.4%	68.0%
Nonwhite	28.6%	32.0%
Parity (>1 delivery)*	97.1%	90.2%
Risk factor*		
Previous preterm delivery	97.2%	90.3%
Uterine malformation	1.4%	5.6%
Incompetent cervix	1.4%	4.1%
Gestational age at intake (wk)*	25.2	26.5

*Not significant.
(Courtesy of da Fonseca EB, Bittar RE, Carvalho MHB, et al: Prophylactic administration of progesterone by vaginal suppository to reduce the incidence of spontaneous preterm birth in women at increased risk: A randomized placebo-controlled double-blind study. *Am J Obstet Gynecol* 188:419-424. Copyright 2003 by Elsevier.)

▶ In a recent review of the management of preterm labor, R. L. Goldenberg[1] has pointed to a series of failed efforts to prevent preterm deliveries, pointing out a meta-analysis of 6 randomized, controlled trials of 17 α-hydroxy progesterone caproate that reported a reduction in the incidence of preterm birth without change in prenatal morbidity and mortality.[2] Several earlier studies failed to indicate reduction of preterm labor using progesterone or its derived compounds.[3,4] This is 1 of 2 recent articles purporting to demonstrate success in using progesterone to this purpose.

Certainly, there is strong phylogenetic support for the role of reduction of progesterone concentration in the onset of normal mammalian labor and for its role in maintaining pregnancy, particularly in ungulates and rodents.[5] In those

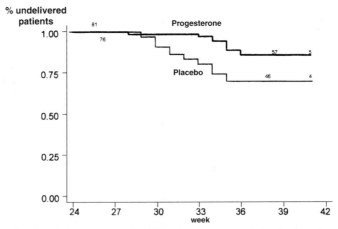

FIGURE 3.—Cumulative percentage of undelivered patients per week, by placebo and progesterone group. Log-rank $\chi^2 = 5.33$, $P = .029$. (Courtesy of da Fonseca EB, Bittar RE, Carvalho MHB, et al: Prophylactic administration of progesterone by vaginal suppository to reduce the incidence of spontaneous preterm birth in women at increased risk: A randomized placebo-controlled double-blind study. *Am J Obstet Gynecol* 188:419-424. Copyright 2003 by Elsevier.)

species, fetal cortisol production alters the enzymatic regulation in the system of metabolic processes that coverts the cyclopentanophenanthrene nucleus derived from cholesterol into adrenal steroids, progesterone, estrogen, and androgens in such a way as to increase estrogen and reduce progesterone placental production sharply, with consequences for decidual and myometrial changes and labor onset.[6] Though changes in sex hormone concentration take place in similar directions preceding the onset of human labor, the changes are smaller, subtler, and occur over weeks of time, not closely temporally related to labor onset as in other species. There's evidence that the biologic effects of estrogen and progesterone are altered by changes in receptor density or receptor-binding proteins with agonist or antagonist properties without much change in blood concentrations of the hormones.[7]

This study explores the use of vaginal progesterone 100 mg per day from 24 to 34 weeks of pregnancy in a randomly allocated, controlled, blinded experiment until labor began in 142 women. Apparently because of socioeconomic differences, the preterm birth rate at this São Paulo clinic averages 22.5%. Patient entry was restricted to women with a prior preterm birth, cervical cerclage, or presence of a uterine malformation. Cervicovaginal infections were identified by culture and treated, and uterine contraction monitoring was conducted weekly between 24 and 34 weeks. Labor was diagnosed by the presence of at least 2 uterine contractions per 10 minutes, with a cervix greater than 2 cm dilated or with progressive dilation and effacement of the cervix. Tocolysis with β-adrenergic analogs was used in the presence of preterm labor.

The primary outcome measure, preterm delivery prior to 37 weeks, was less common in progesterone-treated patients (13.8% vs 28.5%), and the overall preterm birth rate in all 142 patients was 21.1%, not markedly less than the 22.5% rate for the general population. The progesterone recipients showed no significant difference in admissions for suspected preterm birth but appeared to respond more often to β-mimetic tocolysis in terms of the number of uterine contractions and the presence of more than 72 hours of delay until the onset of labor. Progesterone recipients had fewer repeated episodes of possible labor, fewer births before 34 weeks of pregnancy, and a lower frequency of uterine contractions on weekly uterine contraction tests.

It's important that no data pertaining to perinatal morbidity or mortality were included, possibly because of the infrequency of perinatal deaths. Those data are critical since, without reducing perinatal morbidity and mortality, a significant reduction in the incidence of preterm labor and delivery may be a statistically significant observation, but it lacks clinical significance.

T. H. Kirschbaum, MD

References

1. Goldenberg RL: The management of preterm labor. *Obstet Gynecol* 100:1020-1037, 2002.
2. Keirse MJ: Progestogen administration in pregnancy may prevent preterm delivery. *Br J Obstet Gynaecol* 97:149-154, 1990.
3. Fuchs AR, Stakeman G: Treatment of threatened premature labor with large doses of progesterone. *Am J Obstet Gynecol* 79:172-176, 1960.

4. Ovlisen B, Iverson J: Treatment of threatened premature labor with 6-methyl-17 α-hydroxy progesterone. *Am J Obstet Gynecol* 86:291, 1963.
5. Casey MR, Mcdonald PC: Biomolecular processes in the initiation of parturition. In: JD Iams, ed. *Clinical Obstetrics and Gynecology*. Vol 31. Philadelphia, J. B. Lippincott, 1988.
6. McDonald PC: Placental steroidogenesis. In: RM Wynn, ed. *Fetal Homeostasis*. Vol I. New York, New York Academy of Sciences, 1965. p. 265.
7. 2003 YEAR BOOK OF OBSTETRICS, GYNECOLOGY, AND WOMEN'S HEALTH, pp 24-26.

Periodontal Disease Increases the Risk of Preterm Delivery Among Preeclamptic Women

Riché EL, Boggess KA, Lieff S, et al (Univ of North Carolina, Chapel Hill; Duke Univ, Durham, NC)

Ann Periodontol 7:95-101, 2002   2–2

Background.—Preterm births are an important public health problem, accounting for a major proportion of neonatal morbidity and mortality. About 30% of preterm births are the result of maternal or fetal medical conditions, with preeclampsia playing a major role. It was previously reported that the risk for preterm delivery and preeclampsia is increased in pregnant women with periodontal disease. Whether maternal periodontal disease in-

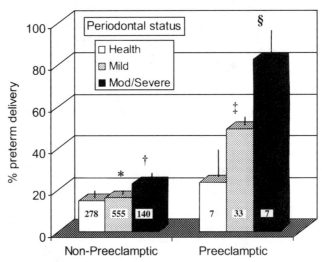

FIGURE 1.—General linear model of the effect of periodontal disease status at enrollment on the adjusted rates of preterm delivery in preeclamptic and nonpreeclamptic mothers, based upon 3 levels of periodontal disease. Estimates of prevalence rates are adjusted for maternal race; age; marital status; women, infants, and children or food stamp usage; insurance; previous preterm delivery; and chorioamnionitis for all 6 groups. The *number of subjects in each group* is indicated at the base in each column. Data are shown as mean point estimates ± standard error. *P* values are shown comparing the distribution of periodontal disease to healthy periodontal status for nonpreeclamptic and preeclamptic women. *Asterisk* indicates *P* = .60, †*P* = .046 compared to nonpreeclamptic periodontally healthy women, ‡*P* = .09, §*P* = .002 compared to preeclamptic periodontally healthy women. (Courtesy of Riché EL, Boggess KA, Lieff S, et al: Periodontal disease increases the risk of preterm delivery among preeclamptic women. *Ann Periodontal* 7:95-101, 2002.)

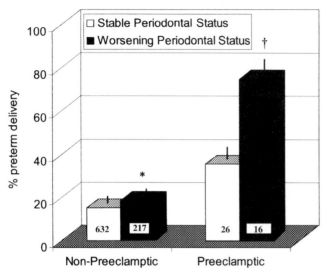

FIGURE 2.—General linear model of the effect of changes in periodontal status during pregnancy on the adjusted rates of preterm delivery in preeclamptic and nonpreeclamptic mothers. Estimates of prevalence rates are adjusted for maternal race; age; marital status; women, infants, and children programs or food stamp usage; insurance; previous preterm delivery; and chorioamnionitis for all 4 groups. The number of subjects in each group is indicated in each *column*. Data are shown as mean point estimates ± standard error. *P* values are shown comparing the levels of worsening periodontal status to stable periodontal status for each of the 2 groups. *Asterisk* indicates *P* = .26 compared to nonpreeclamptic women with stable periodontal status. †*P* = .0006 compared to preeclamptic women with stable periodontal status. (Courtesy of Riché EL, Boggess KA, Lieff S, et al: Periodontal disease increases the risk of preterm delivery among preeclamptic women. *Ann Periodontal* 7:95-101, 2002.)

creases the risk for preterm delivery among preeclamptic women was investigated.

Methods.—The Oral Conditions and Pregnancy study was a prospective cohort study that enrolled women before their 26th week of gestation. Oral health examinations were performed on the first or second prenatal visit and within 48 hours post partum, and periodontal status was defined as healthy, mild, or moderate-to-severe.

Results.—The study enrolled a total of 1020 women, of whom 47 had preeclampsia. There was a strong association between periodontal disease status at enrollment and the rate of premature delivery among preeclamptic women (Fig 1). Preterm deliveries occurred in 99.3% of preeclamptic women with mild periodontal disease and in 82.6% of preeclamptic women with moderate-to-severe disease (Fig 2). Periodontal disease worsened during pregnancy in the preeclamptic women and was associated with an increased risk of preterm birth.

Conclusion.—These findings suggest that pregnant women with preeclampsia may be at greater risk for preterm delivery if they have periodontal disease early in pregnancy or if there is progression of existing periodontal disease during pregnancy.

▶ This is a large, prospective noninterventional study conducted by the University of North Carolina School of Dentistry to explore the impact of periodontal disease on occurrence of preeclampsia and preterm birth. The reader may wish to compare with a controlled interventional study reviewed here recently (see Abstract 2–3).

One thousand twenty women were enrolled prior to 26 weeks' gestational age and subject to dental exams at entry, later compared with examinations done 24 hours post partum. Comparisons were made between the presence and severity of periodontal disease and both preterm birth and preeclampsia. Gingival probe depth (normal less than 4 mm), gingival attachment level, and bleeding on probing were used to rate women as periodontally healthy (27.9%) and mildly (57.7%) and severely (14%) afflicted with periodontitis. Two thirds of the enrollees were African-American; the preterm birth rate was 18.2% and preeclampsia incidence was 4.6% of this population. Deepening probe depth post partum was used to denote worsening periodontal status through the course of pregnancy.

Evidence for a relationship of periodontitis to preterm birth was not striking. Normotensive women with mild to severe periodontal disease showed a significantly increased risk of preterm birth prior to 37 weeks of gestation compared to those with mild or absent disease, and worsening findings after pregnancy had no relationship to an increased risk of preterm birth. Comparative analysis of 47 preeclamptics is subject to concern for small case numbers and the use of univariate statistics. The 7 women with severe periodontal disease and the 16 with worsening findings had higher preterm birth rates than normotensive periodontally healthy women or than preeclamptic women with stable disease. Worsening adverse periodontal findings had no apparent relationship to preterm birth rates in nonhypertensive women.

In brief, though periodontal disease may not be related to the likelihood of developing preeclampsia, its severity may. Though that conclusion rests solely with 7 cases (see Fig 1), preeclampsia is strongly and independently related to preterm birth since labor induction is such a frequent therapeutic. In the relationship between periodontal disease and preterm birth, precclampsia is a confounding variable with probably little impact, as multivariate statistical techniques might have shown here.

T. H. Kirschbaum, MD

Periodontal Therapy May Reduce the Risk of Preterm Low Birth Weight in Women With Periodontal Disease: A Randomized Controlled Trial
López NJ, Smith PC, Gutierrez J (Univ of Chile, Santiago; Hosp San José)
J Periodontol 73:911-924, 2002   2–3

Background.—Maternal infection has been linked to the birth of preterm low birth weight (PLBW) infants. While genitourinary infections have been the principal focus of investigation, 2 case-control studies and a cohort study have identified periodontal disease as a potential independent risk factor for both preterm birth (PTB) and low birth weight (LBW). The possible connection between periodontal disease and PLBW was explored, along with the possible benefit to be derived from periodontal therapy in pregnant women with respect to reducing the risk of PLBW.

Methods.—The 400 participants had a singleton gestation and were undergoing prenatal care in Santiago, Chile. All had periodontal disease; they ranged in age from 18 to 35 years. Two hundred were assigned to receive periodontal treatment before 28 weeks of gestation and 200 to receive periodontal treatment after delivery. Delivery at less than 37 weeks of gestation or birth of an infant weighing under 2500 g were the primary outcomes evaluated.

Results.—Thirty-seven in the treatment group and 12 in the control group were excluded. In addition to the mechanical treatment, antibiotics were prescribed for 29 women receiving periodontal treatment because of the severity of their disease. Of the 351 live births, 22 were PTB or LBW infants (Table 4). Women who had periodontal disease had an incidence of PLBW and PTB more than 5 times higher than women without periodontal disease. LBW was also more prevalent among the women with periodontal disease, but the difference was not statistically significant. Infants with PLBW whose mothers had received periodontal care during pregnancy had a greater gestational age and a higher mean birth weight than were noted in the control group, but the difference did not reach a significant level. Women whose infants were PLBW showed significantly more severe and extensive gingival inflammation and poorer periodontal status than was found among women whose infants were not PLBW. A significant association was found between periodontal disease and PLBW, with women who had periodontal disease having a risk of PLBW over 4 times greater than women who had no periodontal disease. Women who had periodontal disease, a previous PLBW infant, low weight gain, and fewer than 6 prenatal visits had an increased probability of having a second PLBW of 70.4% (Table 8).

TABLE 4.—Incidence of Preterm Births (PTB), Low Birth Weight (LBW), and Preterm/Low Birth Weight (PLBW)

	Treatment Group (N = 163)		Control Group (N = 188)		
	N	%	N	%	*P* Value
Intention-to-treat analysis					
PTB	2	1.10	12	6.38	0.017
LBW	1	0.55	7	3.72	0.083
PLBW	3	1.63	19	10.11	0.001
Protocol analysis					
PTB	2	1.22	12	6.38	0.001
LBW	1	0.61	7	3.72	0.11
PLBW	3	1.84	19	10.11	0.003

(Courtesy of López NJ, Smith PC, Gutierrez J: Periodontal therapy may reduce the risk of preterm low birth weight in women with peridontal disease: a randomized controlled trial. *J Periodontal* 73:911-924, 2002.)

TABLE 8.—Multivariate Logistic Regression Model for Preterm/Low Birth
Weight (PLBW)

Risk Factor	Parameter Estimate	Standard Error	Adjusted Odds Ratio	95% CI	P Value
Periodontal disease	1.5483	0.6595	4.70	1.29-17.13	0.018
Previous PLBW	1.3830	0.6486	3.98	1.11-14.21	0.033
Less than 6 prenatal visits	1.3097	0.4741	3.70	1.46-9.38	0.005
Low maternal weight gain	1.2310	0.5484	3.42	1.16-10.03	0.024

(Courtesy of López NJ, Smith PC, Gutierrez J: Periodontal therapy may reduce the risk of preterm low birth weight in women with periodontal disease: a randomized controlled trial. *J Periodontal* 73:911-924, 2002.)

Conclusions.—Women who gave birth to PLBW infants tended to have more severe periodontal disease than did women who had normal births. Evaluation of the relationship between potential risk factors and PLBW revealed 4 significant associations: periodontal disease, previous PLBW infant, making fewer than 6 prenatal visits, and low maternal weight gain. The strongest association was found for periodontal disease, suggesting that it is an independent risk factor for PLBW; the risk of PLBW was over 4 times greater for women with periodontal disease. Therapy for periodontal disease was able to significantly reduce the rate of PLBW in women with periodontal disease.

▶ Periodontal disease has been identified by factor analysis in 3 studies[1-3] as a possible independent risk factors for preterm birth and low birth weight. Hypothetically, foci of chronic infection might result in immune activation and pro-inflammatory protein production, as well as periodic general seeding of infectious pathogens, which might in turn play a role in preterm premature rupture of membranes and preterm labor. Those who have lived in the mid 20th century recognize this as a partial return to the concept of chronic focal infection as a cause of a variety of otherwise unexplainable diseases. This is a randomized, prospective controlled but unblinded study of 351 gravidas with singlet pregnancies. The women ranged in age from 18 to 35 years, and were attending a free public health service clinic for low socioeconomic Chilean gravidas in Santiago. Women selected for study first had a dental entry examination, including probing periodontal depths, measuring the degree of tooth mortality, and the extent of dental plaque. Those randomized to control and treatment groups showed no significant difference in the nature and severity of periodontal disease, but the treatment group contained significantly more single women than did the control. The periodontal therapy group received plaque control therapy, scaling, root planing when needed, as well as antibiotics for severe periodontitis. Therapy was completed at 28 weeks of gestational age and return visits given every 2 to 3 weeks to term. Results of therapy showed significant evidence of improved dental status; the control group women received the same dental care postpartum. As table 4 demonstrates, univariate analyses either defined by intent to treat or adherence to protocol showed a significant decrease in the incidence of preterm birth and low birth weight in the treated group compared with control patients. The presence of only 1 low weight birth infant not delivered preterm interferes with the analysis of growth retardation in this study. Multivariate analyses against preterm low birth weight outcomes yield statically significant risk ratios for periodontal disease, previous preterm low birth infant and infrequent prenatal visits as well as low maternal weight gain as covariants.

This appears to be a thoughtful, well-conducted study which deserves to be taken seriously, despite the lack of evaluator blinding in an important preventable obstetrical concern where we have so little else to offer.

T. H. Kirschbaum, MD

References

1. Offenbacher S, Katz V, Fertik G, et al: Periodontal infection as a possible risk factor for preterm low birth weight. *J Periodontal* 67:1103-1113, 1996.
2. Dasanayake AP: Poor periodontal health of the pregnant woman as a risk factor for low birth weight. *Ann Periodontal* 3:206-212, 1996.
3. López NJ, Smith PC, Gutierrez J: Higher risk of preterm birth weight in women with periodontal disease. *J Dent Res* 81:58-63, 2002.

Randomized Clinical Trial of Metronidazole Plus Erythromycin to Prevent Spontaneous Preterm Delivery in Fetal Fibronectin–Positive Women

Andrews WW, for the National Institute of Child Health & Human Development Maternal–Fetal Medicine Units Network (Univ of Alabama at Birmingham; et al)

Obstet Gynecol 101:847-855, 2003   2–4

Background.—Preterm birth is a complication in 11% of all pregnancies and the primary cause of perinatal mortality and long-term neurologic morbidity. Reports in the literature have strongly linked clinically silent upper genital tract bacterial infection or inflammation with preterm birth and adverse pregnancy outcomes. Whether antibiotic treatment of asymptomatic women with a positive cervical or vaginal fetal fibronectin test in the second trimester would reduce the risk of spontaneous preterm delivery was investigated.

Methods.—Women undergoing routine prenatal care at 13 participating centers were screened between 21 weeks 0 days and 25 weeks 6 days of gestation for cervical and vaginal fetal fibronectin. Women with a positive test were randomly assigned to receive metronidazole (250 mg orally 3 times per day) and erythromycin (250 mg orally 4 times per day) or identical placebo for 10 days. The primary outcome was spontaneous delivery before 37 weeks' gestation after preterm labor or premature membrane rupture.

Results.—From a total of 16,317 women screened, 6.6% had a positive test for fetal fibronectin. Of these women, 715 consented to randomization, and outcome data were available for 703 women (347 in the antibiotic group and 356 in the placebo group). There were no significant differences between the antibiotic and placebo groups in maternal age, ethnicity, marital status, education, or presence of bacterial vaginosis.

TABLE 2.—Pregnancy Outcomes According to Treatment Group

Outcome	Active Drug Group (%) (n = 347)	Placebo Group (%) (n = 356)	Relative Risk (95% CI)
Spontaneous* preterm delivery			
Before 37 wk	14.4	12.4	1.17 (0.80, 1.70)
Before 35 wk	6.9	7.5	0.92 (0.54, 1.56)
Before 32 wk	4.3	2.2	1.94 (0.83, 4.52)
Preterm delivery			
Before 37 wk	16.4	16.6	0.99 (0.71, 1.38)
Before 35 wk	8.1	9.5	0.85 (0.53, 1.37)
Before 32 wk	4.9	3.1	1.60 (0.76, 3.36)
Birth weight			
Less than 2500 g	12.7	14.3	0.88 (0.60, 1.29)
Less than 1500 g	3.5	3.2	1.12 (0.50, 2.50)

*Due to spontaneous onset of preterm labor or spontaneous preterm premature rupture of membranes.
Abbreviation: CI, Confidence interval. (Reprinted with permission from The American College of Obstetricians and Gynecologists from Andrews WW, for the National Institute of Child Health & Human Development Maternal-Fetal Medicine Units Network: Randomized clinical trial of metronidazole plus erythromycin to prevent spontaneous preterm delivery in fetal fibronectin–positive women. Obstet Gynecol 101:847-855, 2003.)

There were no differences observed between the 2 groups in spontaneous preterm birth before 37 weeks', less than 35 weeks', or less than 32 weeks' gestation. Among women with a prior spontaneous preterm delivery, the rate of repeat spontaneous preterm delivery at less than 37 weeks' gestation was significantly higher in the antibiotic group than in the placebo group (46.7% vs 23.9%) (Table 2).

Conclusion.—There was no evidence that the use of metronidazole plus erythromycin for asymptomatic women with positive cervical or vaginal fetal fibronectin in the late second trimester will decrease the incidence of spontaneous preterm delivery.

▶ This effort, sponsored by the National Institute of Child Health & Human Development Maternal–Fetal Medicine Units Network , attempts—despite prior failed efforts at using antimicrobial therapy to prevent preterm labor—to explore the possible benefit in studying a new subset of asymptomatic women using broader antimicrobial therapy (see Abstract 7–3). Women were screened for entry at 21 to 26 weeks' gestational age. Fetal fibronection determination done on vaginal swabs and those with symptoms and other pregnancy abnormalities were removed by exclusion factors, with the ultimate selection of 5.4% (715 women) from the available population. Random allocation divided them between placebo and metronidazole 0.25 g 3 times a day plus erythromycin 0.25 g 4 times a day for 10 days.

The hope was that metronidazole, an agent effective in overt pelvic infection, coupled with an often used antibiotic might provide broad coverage against the presumed covert infection/colonization which has long been an enticing correlate of preterm delivery. The choice of onco-fetal fibronectin as a predictor of preterm labor is probably unfortunate because it is linked to a false-positive rate ranging from 50% to 80% and has proven to be an ineffective predicter of preterm labor in numerous trial.[1-5] Outcome results showed no significant benefit from the drug therapy compared to placebo. Interesting but unexplained is the 46.7% incidence of preterm delivery in 30 women receiving drug with a prior history of preterm delivery, compared to 23.9% of 48 women in the placebo group with the same past history. This has to be listed as another failure in the pursuit of antimicrobial prophylaxsis of preterm delivery with or without ruptured membranes.

T. H. Kirschbaum, MD

References

1. 1996 YEAR BOOK OF OBSTETRICS, GYNECOLOGY, AND WOMEN'S HEALTH, pp 129-130.
2. 1997 YEAR BOOK OF OBSTETRICS, GYNECOLOGY, AND WOMEN'S HEALTH, 146-148.
3. 1998 YEAR BOOK OF OBSTETRICS, GYNECOLOGY, AND WOMEN'S HEALTH, pp 53-54.
4. 2000 YEAR BOOK OF OBSTETRICS, GYNECOLOGY, AND WOMEN'S HEALTH, pp 47-48.
5. 2002 YEAR BOOK OF OBSTETRICS, GYNECOLOGY, AND WOMEN'S HEALTH, pp 45-48.

Early Pregnancy Threshold Vaginal pH and Gram Stain Scores Predictive of Subsequent Preterm Birth in Asymptomatic Women
Hauth JC, for the National Institute of Child Health and Human Development Network of Maternal-Fetal Medicine Units (Univ of Alabama at Birmingham; et al)
Am J Obstet Gynecol 188:831-835, 2003   2–5

Background.—Bacterial vaginosis (BV) is a syndrome characterized by alterations in vaginal flora and an increase in vaginal pH. The association between vaginosis and preterm birth was examined.

Study Design.—The study group consisted of pregnant women who were screened for vaginosis as part of the National Institute of Child Health and Human Development Network of Maternal-Fetal Medicine Units Network BV/*Trichomonas vaginalis* treatment trials. Vaginal swabs were obtained and used for analysis of vaginal pH. Those women with pH greater than 4.4 had a Gram's stain applied to a slide from their swab. BV was defined as vaginal pH of at least 4.5 and a vaginal Gram's stain score of at least 7. There were 12,010 women with BV in this study group. A documented pregnancy

TABLE 2A.—Total Preterm Births in Relation to Early Pregnancy Vaginal Gram's Stain Score (Nugent Criteria) in 6838 Women

| Birth (wk GA) | Gram Score | | | |
	0-6 (n = 3158)	7-8 (n = 2015)	9-10 (n = 1665)	*P* Value*
<37 (No. [%])	423 (13.4)	269 (13.4)	290 (17.4)	.0006
<35 (No. [%])	230 (7.3)	153 (7.6)	167 (10.0)	.0090
<32 (No. [%])	140 (4.4)	114 (5.7)	111 (6.7)	.2035

*For the comparison of 7-8 versus 9-10.
Abbreviation: GA, Gestational age.
(Reprinted by permission of the publisher, courtesy of Hauth JC, for the National Institute of Child Health and Human Development Network of Maternal-Fetal Medicine Units: Early pregnancy threshold vaginal pH and Gram's stain scores predictive of subsequent preterm birth in asymptomatic women *Am J Obstet Gynecol* 188: 831-835. Copyright 2003 by Elsevier.)

TABLE 2B.—Spontaneous Preterm Birth in Relation to Early Pregnancy Vaginal Gram's Stain Score (Nugent Criteria) in 6831 Women

Birth (wk GA)	Gram Score 0-6 (n = 3155)	7-8 (n = 2012)	9-10 (n = 1664)	P Value*
<37 (No. [%])	317 (10.1)	209 (10.4)	209 (12.6)	.0388
<35 (No. [%])	168 (5.3)	117 (5.8)	121 (7.3)	.0741
<32 (No. [%])	100 (3.2)	90 (4.5)	79 (4.8)	.6925

*For the comparison of 7-8 versus 9-10.
Abbreviation: GA, Gestational age.
(Reprinted by permission of the publisher, courtesy of Hauth JC, for the National Institute of Child Health and Human Development Network of Maternal-Fetal Medicine Units: Early pregnancy threshold vaginal pH and Gram's stain scores predictive of subsequent preterm birth in asymptomatic women *Am J Obstet Gynecol* 188: 831-835. Copyright 2003 by Elsevier.)

outcome was available for 6838 of these women. The relationship between vaginosis and preterm birth was investigated.

Findings.—Preterm delivery and low birth weight were significantly increased in women with BV (Table 2). Women with a vaginal pH of at least 5.0 had a significantly greater prevalence of vaginal fetal fibronectin, but this was not related to Gram's stain.

Conclusion.—Pregnant women with BV, defined as elevated pH and a Gram's stain score of 9 to 10, had significantly increased preterm births and low birth weight babies. Trials of antimicrobial intervention may be warranted in this high-risk population to reduce preterm birth.

▶ There's no question of the presence of an associative relationship between BV and preterm delivery, but it seems to be neither a direct nor strongly predictive one. These data obtained in the study of metronidazole therapy to prevent preterm delivery in asymptomatic women with BV[1] confirms those prior conclusions. Here, BV was diagnosed by relative vaginal alkalosis (pH = 4.5) and a Gram's stain evaluation of vaginal secretions after Nugent,[2] with maximum association with Nugent score 9 to 10.

Pregnancy outcomes were based on the records of 6838 women with BV. Preterm delivery was significantly more common among women with pH = 4.5 and Nugent scores 7 to 10 than in those with lower pH and Nugent scores, but predictive indexes for preterm delivery were poor. Among 2305 women with vaginal pH ≥4.5, false positive rates of prediction were 90.5%; among the 1605 women with Nugent score 9 to 10, the false-positive rate was 82.6%. As the authors indicate, using the diagnosis of BV to predict preterm delivery has a sensitivity of only 30%.[3]

The several prospective, randomized trials that have failed to support the value of antimicrobial therapy for pregnant asymptomatic women with BV in order to prevent preterm delivery, including the ones for which these data were obtained,[4] are consonant with this poor predictive capacity.[5-10] The sole exception[7] contains questions of interpretation which complicate its evaluation. Its seems unlikely there is a direct relationship between BV and preterm delivery and likely that future trials of antimicrobial therapy based on patient subsets with various elements of the diagnosis, which these authors suggest, will be similarly unproductive.

T. H. Kirschbaum, MD

References

1. 2001 YEAR BOOK OF OBSTETRICS, GYNECOLOGY, AND WOMEN'S HEALTH, pp 29-31.
2. Nugent RP, Krohn MA, Hillier SL: Reliability of diagnosing bacterial vaginosis by a standard method of Gram stain interpretation. *J Clin Microbiol* 29:297, 1991.
3. 1997 YEAR BOOK OF OBSTETRICS, GYNECOLOGY, AND WOMEN'S HEALTH, pp 146-148.
4. 2001 YEAR BOOK OF OBSTETRICS, GYNECOLOGY, AND WOMEN'S HEALTH, pp 29-31.
5. 1992 YEAR BOOK OF OBSTETRICS, GYNECOLOGY, AND WOMEN'S HEALTH, pp 78-79.
6. 1995 YEAR BOOK OF OBSTETRICS, GYNECOLOGY, AND WOMEN'S HEALTH, pp 41-42.
7. 1997 YEAR BOOK OF OBSTETRICS, GYNECOLOGY, AND WOMEN'S HEALTH, pp 31-33.
8. 1999 YEAR BOOK OF OBSTETRICS, GYNECOLOGY, AND WOMEN'S HEALTH, pp 38-40.
9. 2001 YEAR BOOK OF OBSTETRICS, GYNECOLOGY, AND WOMEN'S HEALTH, pp 29-31.
10. 2002 YEAR BOOK OF OBSTETRICS, GYNECOLOGY, AND WOMEN'S HEALTH, pp 37-38.

Transvaginal Sonographic Examination of the Cervix in Asymptomatic Pregnant Women: Review of the Literature
Rozenberg P, Gillet A, Ville Y (Univ Paris V)
Ultrasound Obstet Gynecol 19:302-311, 2002   2–6

Background.—Various strategies have been used to predict the risk of preterm delivery in asymptomatic women. Transvaginal sonography is used to assess the length and shape of the cervix. Clinical studies involving transvaginal sonographic assessment of the cervix in asymptomatic women at high risk of preterm delivery and in the general population of pregnant women were reviewed.

Review.—Three US signs suggest cervical incompetence: dilation of the internal os; sacculation or prolapse of the membranes into the cervix, with shortening of the functional cervical length, either spontaneously or induced by transfundal pressure; and short cervix in the absence of uterine contractions. Transvaginal sonography has demonstrated that cerclage results in a measurable increase in cervical length, which may contribute to this procedure's efficacy in decreasing the risk of preterm delivery. Several published nonrandomized interventional studies involving patients with cervical incompetence have defined a new group of patients needing cerclage in the presence of progressive cervical modifications on transvaginal sonography. In other studies, cerclage performed on the basis of these findings did not prevent premature delivery. One prospective, randomized trial in asymptomatic, high-risk women demonstrated that performing cerclage after transvaginal sonographic indications would result in fewer prophylactic cerclages in high-risk women and that therapeutic cerclage before 27 weeks may decrease the incidence of premature delivery before 34 weeks.

Conclusions.—The risk of preterm delivery correlates inversely with cervical length. Routine transvaginal sonography of the cervix between 18 and

22 weeks' gestation can help identify patients at risk of perterm delivery, but the prevalence of preterm births is so low that screening would result in either a high false-positive rate or a low sensitivity. In the general obstetric population, transvaginal sonography may help clinicians identify asymptomatic women at high risk. However, the benefits of performing cerclage for sonographic indications have not been established.

▶ This is a review and interpretation of the literature of this topic that is unusual for its thoroughness and completeness. The authors reason that failure to impact very low birth weight delivery incidence either in France or America is a failure both of therapeutics and of high-risk case findings, and for the latter, transvaginal US at least results in minimal invasiveness and does not necessarily mandate subsequent invasive strategies. The approach is supported by the ability to discern cervical dilatation and shortening and membrane prolapse, spontaneously or pressure-induced, as well as the effects of cerclage. Many—but not all—the studies referenced here have been reviewed earlier in the YEAR BOOK OF OBSTETRICS, GYNECOLOGY, AND WOMEN'S HEALTH.[1-7] Here the role of transvaginal US in asymptomatic women was used to investigate the natural course of cervical change during pregnancy, and the results of randomized and nonrandomized trials of cerclage following presumed pathology on ultrasonic cervical examination in clinical trials applied to screened gravidas were compared.

There is no question that cervical shortening and some other cervical changes are associated with preterm delivery, but trials of intervention, most specifically using cerclage, result in no significant difference in preterm delivery rates from controls or general population norms. In general, such an experience results in high specificity and positive values of negative findings, which are functions of the low prevalence of preterm and very preterm delivery. Though it has been impossible to prove the value of cerclage compared with controls, there is little evidence of harm beyond a tendency for amnionitis before and during labor in such women. The authors suggest that ultrasonic screening of the cervix at 22 to 24 weeks should be supported, perhaps in the forlorn hope that someday, the findings may have proven clinical relevance.

T. H. Kirschbaum, MD

References

1. 1995 YEAR BOOK OF OBSTETRICS, GYNECOLOGY, AND WOMEN'S HEALTH, pp 52-55.
2. 1997 YEAR BOOK OF OBSTETRICS, GYNECOLOGY, AND WOMEN'S HEALTH, pp 27-28.
3. 1998 YEAR BOOK OF OBSTETRICS, GYNECOLOGY, AND WOMEN'S HEALTH, pp 54-56.
4. 1999 YEAR BOOK OF OBSTETRICS, GYNECOLOGY, AND WOMEN'S HEALTH, pp 70-71.
5. 2000 YEAR BOOK OF OBSTETRICS, GYNECOLOGY, AND WOMEN'S HEALTH, pp 41-44.
6. 2001 YEAR BOOK OF OBSTETRICS, GYNECOLOGY, AND WOMEN'S HEALTH, pp 157-158.
7. 2002 YEAR BOOK OF OBSTETRICS, GYNECOLOGY, AND WOMEN'S HEALTH, pp 50-51.

Pregnancy in the Sixth Decade of Life: Obstetric Outcomes in Women of Advanced Reproductive Age

Paulson RJ, Boonstanfar R, Saadat P, et al (Univ of Southern California, Los Angeles)
JAMA 288:2320-2323, 2002   2–7

Background.—Although oocyte donation was originally developed as a therapy for young women who had premature ovarian failure, it is now also used for women older than 40 years with high success rates. Concern arises regarding the incidence of obstetric complications in women of advanced reproductive age and the possibility that perinatal and maternal morbidity or mortality may be increased. The pregnancy outcomes of women 50 years or older who conceived after in vitro fertilization with donor oocytes were documented.

Methods.—The 77 women who participated had no chronic medical conditions and underwent 121 embryo transfer procedures, of which 89 were fresh and 32 were frozen, over a period of 11 years. Chart review and telephone interviews were used to follow up with the women and their neonates.

Results.—Fifty-five clinical pregnancies were achieved, which yielded a rate of 45.5%. Forty-two live births occurred, and 3 women had 2 consecutive pregnancies. These 3 women were all in their 50s during both pregnancies. In 58% of cases, the delivery was the mother's first. Thirty-one of the births were singletons, 12 were twins, and 2 were triplets. At 1 and 5 minutes, the mean Apgar scores were 8.2 and 9.1, respectively. For the multiple gestations, the mean gestational ages were significantly younger than for the singleton births. Cesarean delivery was used for 78% of the cases. Sixty-eight percent of the singleton births were by cesarean, 6% were by vacuum-assisted vaginal delivery, and 26% were by normal spontaneous vaginal delivery. All the multiple births were accomplished by cesarean section. Of the 40 cases in which perinatal data were available, mild preeclampsia was noted in 25% and severe preeclampsia was noted in 10%; no cases of eclampsia developed. Preeclampsia occurred in 26% of the women younger than 55 years and in 60% of those older than 55 years. The incidence of preeclampsia was the same whether the delivery was the woman's first or a subsequent delivery. In 17.5% of patients, gestational diabetes required dietary modifications; 2.5% of the patients needed insulin. Women older than 55 years were more likely to have gestational diabetes than those younger than 55 years (40% vs 13%). One patient required hospitalization for premature rupture of membranes over the 10 days preceding delivery, 1 patient had twins delivered at 30 weeks' gestation because of early onset of severe preeclampsia, 1 patient required a hysterectomy for placenta accreta, and 1 patient needed a blood transfusion after cesarean delivery for placenta previa. None of the neonates or mothers died.

Conclusions.—Healthy women in their 50s were able to conceive, maintain pregnancies, and successfully deliver healthy neonates. The pregnancy rates, rates of multiple gestation, and spontaneous abortion rates were comparable with those of younger women, but preeclampsia and gestational diabetes occurred at a higher rate among the older women. Cesarean delivery should be expected for most of these women. Thus, age alone should not be a barrier to pregnancy in women older than 50 years.

▶ In this remarkable publication, Paulson and his colleagues report on their use of ovum donation, in vitro fertilization, replacement sex hormone provision, and oocyte transfer in a group of 77 postmenopausal women with a mean age of 52.8 years and a maximum of 63 years. It's very important that the women were thoroughly studied with respect to the biological features of the uterus and cervix, endometrial response to estrogen and progesterone, and cardiovascular reserve and that they were screened for infectious diseases and psychological status. Ovum donors received the same medical and psychological appraisal. Candidates for ovum transfer with hypertension, diabetes mellitus, or chronic medical illness were rejected. The diagnosis of pregnancy was based on β-human chorionic gonadotropin assays confirmed by US visualization of the corpus luteum of pregnancy.

A total of 89 women received fresh ovum zygotes, and 32 received frozen embryos. The pregnancy rates were 54.5% with the use of fresh embryos and 6.8% with the use of frozen embryos, which yielded an overall incidence of 37.2% pregnancies. Thirty-one percent had multiple pregnancies, and the neonates had normal mean gestational ages and normal mean Apgar scores at birth; the low birth rate incidence was also normal for these multiple pregnancies. Seventy-eight percent of the women delivered by cesarean section, and the incidence of preeclampsia was 35%. Gestational diabetes mellitus requiring a special diet occurred in 17.5%, and 2.5% ultimately required insulin therapy. No neonatal or maternal mortality occurred.

This is a benchmark experience in this undertaking and is clear evidence of the adaptability of the postmenopausal uterus and the ability to sustain pregnancy in the postmenopausal uterus. Clearly, the careful preliminary screening is important. There are serious ethical considerations here, but if a couple understands the cost of increased hazards and the imponderability present in the outcome, physicians with the skill of the University of Southern California group are capable of fulfilling what the couple see as something they need, with relative safety.

T. H. Kirschbaum, MD

Smoking Before Pregnancy and Risk of Gestational Hypertension and Preeclampsia

England LJ, Levine RJ, Qian C, et al (Natl Inst of Child Health and Human Development, Bethesda, Md; Allied Technology Group, Rockville, Md; Oregon Health Sciences Univ, Portland; et al)
Am J Obstet Gynecol 186:1035-1040, 2002   2–8

Background.—Although women who smoke during pregnancy have an increased risk of several adverse outcomes, they also have a reduced risk of

TABLE 2.—Association Between Smoking History and Risk of Hypertension During Pregnancy

Smoking History	Normotensive (n = 3227) No. (%)	Gestational Hypertension (n = 736)			Preeclampsia (n = 326)			Gestational Hypertension or Preeclampsia (n = 1062)		
		No. (%)	ARR*	95% CI	No. (%)	ARR*	95% CI	No. (%)	ARR*	95% CI
Never smoked (n = 3010)	2214 (73.5)	550 (18.3)	—	—	246 (8.2)	—	—	796 (26.4)	—	—
Quit before LMP (n = 326)	242 (74.2)	60 (18.4)	1.1	0.9-1.4	24 (7.4)	1.1	0.7-1.7	84 (25.8)	1.1	0.9-1.3
Quit after LMP (n = 445)	354 (79.6)	64 (14.4)	0.9	0.7-1.1	27 (6.1)	0.9	0.6-1.3	91 (20.4)	0.9	0.7-1.1
Smoking at enrollment (n = 508)	417 (82.1)	62 (12.2)	0.7	0.6-0.9	29 (5.7)	0.7	0.5-1.1	91 (17.9)	0.8	0.6-0.9

Abbreviation: ARR, Adjusted relative risk.
Adjustment variables include maternal age, race, type of health insurance, study center, and body mass index at the time of study enrollment.
(Reprinted by permission of the publisher, courtesy of England LJ, Levine RJ, Qian C, et al: Smoking before pregnancy and risk of gestational hypertension and preeclampsia. *Am J Obstet Gynecol* 186:1035-1040. Copyright 2002 by Elsevier.)

hypertension. A large, prospectively collected dataset was used to examine the relation between smoking and hypertension during pregnancy.

Study Design.—Data were obtained from a large, randomized, multicenter clinical trial, Calcium for Preeclampsia Prevention (CPEP). This study included 4589 healthy nulliparous women who were followed from 12 to 21 weeks' gestation until the end of their pregnancy. All participants were normotensive and free of proteinuria at enrollment. Smoking history was obtained at baseline, and women were divided into 4 categories: never smoked, smoked before pregnancy, smoked but quit during pregnancy, and smoked during pregnancy. Blood pressure and proteinuria were measured at each follow-up visit. Multiple logistic regression analyses were performed to calculate adjusted odds ratios for hypertensive disorders of pregnancy for women in each smoking category.

Findings.—After adjustment for maternal age, race, body mass index, health insurance type, and clinical center, women smoking during pregnancy had a reduced risk of hypertension (Table 2). Women who quit smoking before pregnancy did not have this reduced relative risk. Results for gestational hypertension and for preeclampsia were similar.

Conclusions.—Smoking during pregnancy is associated with a reduced risk of hypertensive disorders of pregnancy, but smoking before pregnancy does not appear to be associated with reduced risk.

▶ The consistent evidence that smoking is associated with a decreased rate of development of hypertensive disease of pregnancy is an intriguing, utterly unexplained phenomenon. This study is another serendipitous use of earlier data that failed to demonstrate a preventive role for calcium supplementation in preeclampsia.[1] Records of 4289 women seen periodically from 13 to 21 weeks' gestational age to delivery were queried about smoking habits before and during pregnancy, and the incidence of hypertensive disease compared among 4 classes of smoking experiences. Interpretation of the results depends on how you feel about gestational hypertension as defined here (diastolic blood pressure greater than 90 mm Hg on 2 occasions at least 4 hours apart), seen in 12.1% of women. Preeclampsia (hypertension with albuminuria during pregnancy) was seen in 7.6%. The adjusted risk ratio among nonsmokers for preeclampsia was numerically larger, but not statistically significantly so, when compared with smokers. When those with gestational hypertension and gestational preeclampsia were combined, risk ratios were larger among nonsmokers than smokers at the time of enrollment, supporting a protective role for smoking. No amelioration of risk occurred among those who quit smoking before or shortly after pregnancy onset. This is evidence that however smoking influences hypertensive disease, there is no carryover from early pregnancy events and suggests changes taking place during and after the first trimester of pregnancy are responsible. It's at least a hint of when during pregnancy the search for protective mechanisms against pregnancy-related hypertension should be mounted.

T. H. Kirschbaum, MD

Reference

1. 1998 Year Book of Obstetrics, Gynecology, and Women's Health, pp 45-47.

The Likelihood of Placenta Previa With Greater Number of Cesarean Deliveries and Higher Parity

Gilliam M, Rosenberg D, Davis F (Univ of Illinois, Chicago)
Obstet Gynecol 99:976-980, 2002   2–9

Background.—The cause of placenta previa continues to be controversial. A relationship between placenta previa and cesarean delivery has been hypothesized but is unclear. The possibility of an association between a previous cesarean delivery and placenta previa was investigated in a hospital-based, case-control study.

Methods.—The study included 316 multiparous women with placenta previa (case group) and 2051 multiparous women with spontaneous vaginal deliveries (control group). Data on previous cesarean delivery were assessed as dichotomous variables, ordinal variables, and as a set of 3 indicator variables for 1, 2, and 3 or more cesarean deliveries.

Findings.—Compared with women with no previous cesarean delivery, women with a prior cesarean delivery were more likely to have a placenta previa (odds ratio [OR], 1.59). The likelihood of placenta previa increased with an increase in parity and number of cesarean deliveries. The adjusted OR for a primiparous woman with 1 cesarean delivery was 1.28 but increased to 1.72 for a woman with 4 or more deliveries with only a single cesarean delivery. The OR of placenta previa for a woman with parity greater than 4 with more than 4 previous cesarean deliveries was 8.76 (Table 4).

TABLE 4.—The Association Between the Number of Cesarean Deliveries and Placenta Previa Based on an Ordinal Variable for Number of Prior Cesarean Deliveries (Adjusted Odds Ratios and 95% Confidence Intervals* Stratified by Parity)

Number of Prior	Parity			
Cesarean Deliverest	1 ($n = 1171$)	2 ($n = 675$)	3 ($n = 265$)	4+ ($n = 171$)
0	1.0	1.0	1.0	1.0
1	1.28	1.40	1.60	1.72
	0.82, 1.99	1.06, 1.84	1.15, 2.22	1.12, 2.64
2		1.95	2.56	2.96
		1.13, 3.39	1.33, 4.93	1.26, 6.97
3			4.09	5.09
			1.53, 10.96	1.41, 18.39
4+				8.76
				1.58, 48.53

*Age ≥ 35 vs other, smoker vs nonsmoker, and any prior induced abortion are included in the adjusted model.
†The sample sizes for each parity level differ from those shown previously because of missing values.
(Courtesy of Gilliam M, Rosenberg D, Davis F: The likelihood of placenta previa with greater number of cesarean deliveries and higher parity. *Obstet Gynecol* 99:976-980, 2002. Reprinted with permission from The American College of Obstetricians and Gynecologists.)

Conclusions.—Previous cesarean delivery is associated with placenta previa. The combined effect of parity and prior cesarean delivery is greater than that of either variable alone.

▶ This is an exploration of the relationship between a prior cesarean section and placenta previa in a subsequent pregnancy that makes it clear that both the number of prior cesarean sections and patient parity are significant independent contributors to the risk. This case control study is based on a retrospective review of data from the University of Illinois and Cook County medical centers from 1986 to 1989 containing, in many cases, information on 450 variables. The diagnosis of previa was based on a recorded statement that the placenta partially or totally covered the cervix. Three hundred sixteen such cases were compared with data from 2081 normal singlet pregnancies delivered spontaneously and vaginally in this same time span. Statistical analysis was complex.

First, a univariate analysis was done on each independent variable viewed as dichotomous (ie, primiparas—yes or no). Then, variables, appropriately viewed as ordinal, were collected and stratified, although the range was large (maternal age in units in 5 of 10 years), looking for evidence of confounding relationships among the sea of possibilities. Finally, multivariate regression was applied to each of the variables: dichotomous, ordinal, and stratified, showing likely strong relationships to the incidence of placenta previa.

The clearest result (see Table 4) shows both parity and number of cesarean sections independently and significantly bear on the increase in the likelihood of placenta previa with a subsequent pregnancy. An exception applies to primiparas delivered by cesarean section for the first pregnancy for which the risk of previa is the same as in nulliparas, that is, approximately 0.5%. The analysis is a more accurate reflection of the probabilities, which for incidence, some authors derive from risk ratios based on populations of 2 to 5 cases.[1,2] As Table 4 shows, as risk ratios increase, their confidence intervals become so large because of the small numbers of cases in most extreme subsets that all one can say is that the greater the parity and the larger the number of prior cesarean sections, the greater is the risk of subsequent previa.

T. H. Kirschbaum, MD

References

1. 1987 YEAR BOOK OF OBSTETRICS, GYNECOLOGY, AND WOMEN'S HEALTH, pp 132-133.
2. 1994 YEAR BOOK OF OBSTETRICS, GYNECOLOGY, AND WOMEN'S HEALTH, pp 198-199.

Sexual Intercourse Association With Asymptomatic Bacterial Vaginosis and *Trichomonas vaginalis* Treatment in Relationship to Preterm Birth

Berghella V, for the National Institute for Child Health and Development Maternal Fetal Medicine Units Network (Thomas Jefferson Univ, Philadelphia; et al)
Am J Obstet Gynecol 187:1277-1282, 2002   2–10

Introduction.—Both bacterial vaginosis (BV) and *Trichomonas vaginalis* (TV) have been linked with increased risk of preterm birth. A secondary analysis of 2 multicenter, double-blind, placebo-controlled trials in which metronidazole treatment of BV or TV did not decrease preterm birth was performed to ascertain whether sexual intercourse was correlated with treatment efficacy or the incidence of preterm birth.

Methods.—In both trials, participants took 2 g of metronidazole or placebo in the presence of a nurse (first dose) and were given a second dose to take 48 hours later at 16 to 23 weeks' gestation. The third and fourth doses were repeated at 24 to 29 weeks gestation. Specimens of BV and TV were obtained at the time of the third dose. Patients in the metronidazole group were evaluated for BV and TV at 24 to 29 weeks and for preterm birth of less than 37 weeks gestation.

Results.—Sexual intercourse between the first and second doses or between the second and third doses did not influence the incidence of BV (18% vs 24%; relative risk [RR], 0.7; 95% confidence interval [CI], 0.5-1.1; and 23% vs 20%; RR, 1.2; 95% CI, 0.9-1.6, respectively) or TV (4% vs 8%; RR, 0.5; 95% CI, 0.1-3.6; and 5% vs 10%; RR, 0.5; 95% CI, 0.1-1.2, respectively) at 24 to 29 weeks' gestation versus no intercourse.

In the TV trial, sexual intercourse between the first and second doses or between the second and third doses did not influence the incidence of preterm birth (13% vs 17%; RR, 0.8; 95% CI, 0.3-2.1; and 16% vs 17%; RR, 1.0; 95% CI, 0.6-1.6, respectively) versus no intercourse. In the BV group, although sexual intercourse between the first and second doses did not impact the incidence of preterm birth (11% vs 12%; RR, 0.9; 95% CI, 0.6-1.5), sexual intercourse between the second and third doses was correlated with a decrease in the incidence of preterm birth (10% vs 16%; RR, 0.6; 95% CI, 0.4-0.9) vs no intercourse.

Conclusion.—Sexual intercourse was not correlated with the efficacy of metronidazole treatment of BV or TV or preterm birth. In the BV trial, intercourse between the second and third doses had a negative correlation with preterm birth.

▶ To the consternation of many, 2 large, prospective, randomized trials of treatment and prophylaxsis of BV[1] and TV[2] failed to alter the incidence of preterm birth. This is a secondary analysis of that data collected from 2570 women in those 2 trials, both with similar protocol construction, designed to investigate whether differences in coital frequency before and/or after treatment may have influenced those conclusions. The data were collected in each case by research nurses during the course of the studies. The implicit question is whether differing coital activities among treated and nontreated groups may have biased the apparently negative results of drug treatment. The results reveal that sexual intercourse did not alter the efficacy of either drug treatment in eliminating infection or in reducing the incidence of preterm birth. Indeed, in the bacterial vaginosis trial, provided metronidazole was administered, coital activity appeared to be associated with a decreased incidence of preterm birth.

T. H. Kirschbaum, MD

References

1. 2001 Year Book of Obstetrics, Gynecology, and Women's Health, pp 29-31.
2. 2003 Year Book of Obstetrics, Gynecology, and Women's Health, pp 29-30.

Effect of Serologic Status and Cesarean Delivery on Transmission Rates of Herpes Simplex Virus From Mother to Infant
Brown ZA, Wald A, Morrow RA, et al (Univ of Washington, Seattle; Fred Hutchinson Cancer Research Ctr, Seattle)
JAMA 289:203-209, 2003   2–11

Introduction.—Neonatal herpes usually is caused by fetal exposure to infected maternal genital secretions at the time of delivery. The risk of transmission from mother to infant as it relates to maternal herpes simplex virus (HSV) serologic status and exposure to HSV in the maternal genital tract at the time of labor has yet to be quantified. There are no data regarding whether cesarean delivery, the standard of care for women with genital herpes lesions at the time of delivery, diminishes the transmission of HSV. The effects of viral shedding, maternal HSV serologic status, and delivery route on the risk of HSV transmission from mother to infant were examined in a prospective cohort of pregnant women enrolled between January 1982 and December 1999.

Methods.—A prospective cohort of 58,362 pregnant women was enrolled between January 1982 and December 1999. Of these, 40,023 had HSV cul-

TABLE 2.—Delivery Route and Acquisition of Neonatal Herpes in Women With Herpes Simplex Virus Isolated From the Genital Tract, Stratified by Presence of Lesions

	Neonatal Infection	No Neonatal Infection	Total
Women with lesions present at delivery			
Cesarean	0	60	60
Vaginal*	0	14	14
Women with subclinical viral shedding			
Cesarean	1	24	25
Vaginal	9	94	103
Overall			
Cesarean	1	84	85
Vaginal	9	108	117
Total	10	192	202

*Lesions noted immediately postpartum or too late for cesarean delivery.
(Courtesy of Brown ZA, Wald A, Morrow RA, et al: Effect of serologic status and cesarean delivery on transmission rates of herpes simplex virus from mother to infant. *JAMA* 289:203-209, 2003. Copyright 2003, American Medical Association.)

TABLE 3.—Transmission Rates of Neonatal HSV by Maternal HSV Serologic Status Among Women Who Delivered at the University of Washington and Madigan Army Hospitals

Maternal HSV Serostatus	No./Total (%) of Infants With Neonatal HSV	Rate per 100,000 Live Births (95% Confidence Interval)
HSV seronegative	6/11 115 (0.054)	54 (19.8-118)
HSV-1 seropositive only	6/23 480 (0.026)	29 (9.3-56)
All HSV-2 seropositive	3/13 795 (0.022)	22 (4.4-64)
HSV-2 only	2/5761 (0.035)	35 (4.2-126)
HSV-1 and HSV-2	1/8034 (0.012)	12 (0.3-70)

Abbreviation: HSV, Herpes simplex virus.
(Courtesy of Brown ZA, Wald A, Morrow RA, et al: Effect of serologic status and cesarean delivery on transmission rates of herpes simplex virus from mother to infant. *JAMA* 289:203-209, 2003. Copyright 2003, American Medical Association.)

tures obtained from the cervix and external genitalia, and 31,663 had serum samples that were tested for HSV. The primary outcome measure was rates of neonatal HSV infection.

Results.—Of 202 women from whom HSV was isolated at the time of labor, 10 (5%) had neonates with HSV infection (odds ratio [OR], 346; 95% confidence interval [CI], 125-956 for neonatal herpes when HSV was isolated vs not isolated). Cesarean delivery significantly diminished the HSV transmission rate among women for whom HSV was isolated (1 [1.2%] of 85 cesarean vs 9 [7.7%] of 117 vaginal; OR, 0.14; 95% CI, 0.02-1.08; *P* = .047) (Table 2). Other risk factors for neonatal HSV were first-episode infection (OR, 33.1; 95% CI, 6.5-168), HSV isolation from the cervix (OR, 32.6; 95% CI, 4.1-260), HSV-1 vs HSV-2 isolation at the time of labor (OR, 16.5 ; 95% CI, 4.1-65), invasive monitoring (OR, 6.8; 95% CI, 1.4-32), delivery before 38 weeks (OR, 4.4; 95% CI, 1.2-16), and maternal age less than 21 years (OR, 4.1; 95% CI, 1.1-15). Neonatal HSV infection rates per 100,000 live births were 54 (95% CI, 19.8-118) in HSV-seronegative women, 26 (95% CI, 9.3-56) in women who were HSV-1 seropositive only, and 22 (95% CI, 4.4-64) among all HSV-2–seropositive women (Table 3).

Conclusion.—The incidence of neonatal HSV infection can be decreased by preventing maternal acquisition of genital HSV-1 and HSV-2 infection near term. Cesarean delivery and limiting the use of invasive monitors in women shedding HSV at the time of delivery may also reduce these rates.

▶ This retrospective study of data obtained over a period of 18 years, ending in 1999, is designed to answer some questions still pending after more than 3 decades of study regarding the 2% of gravidas who seroconvert to positive HSV-2 status during pregnancy with prior antibody to HSV-1, HSV-2, or both. The data consist of records of genital viral cultures and DNA–polymerase chain reaction for identification of HSV-1 and HSV-2 coupled with antibody determination by Western blot, both compared by evidence of neonatal infection during pregnancy. Eighteen cases of acquired neonatal HSV were identified during that time, 10 cases with HSV-2 (7 primary infections) and 8 with HSV-1 (4 primary cases). Primary infection was manifest by newly acquired maternal positive cultures with negative antibody studies; virus reactivation by neonatal infection by virus with a mother positive for the type-specific antibody for the same virus at the onset of pregnancy. From a population of more than 55,000 deliveries, 202 women (0.5%) had positive HSV cultures, 26 exhibiting primary infection and 151 (85% of the 177 with corresponding serology) showing reactivation of prepregnancy infection. None of the women with reactivation infection transmitted the disease to their infants. Cases of neonatal transmission occurred among 10 of the 202 women found to be culture positive, asymptomatically shredding virus proven by culture. Half of them had no prior history of HSV infection. Neonatal primary transmission was seen in 3 of 3 cases of HSV-1, 1 of 6 of HSV-2, and 4 of 16 with nonprimary first infections (culture positive, antibody negative) in 2 of 11 with reactivation HSV-1 infection. Of 202 women with positive HSV cultures, of those delivered vaginally, neonatal infection occurred in 9 of 117 neonates, while in women delivered by caesarean section largely for the presence of vulvovaginal lesions, only 1 of 85 neonates were infected, a statistically significant decrease compared with those delivered vaginally. Of 74 women with lesions not noted preoperatively, there were no cases of fetal transmission, and for those with external vulva lesions, the odds ratio for cesarean section was 5.7 times more likely than for those without lesions, demonstrating the clinical application of what has become common knowledge. Neonatal infection was largely confined (10 of 128 cases) to women without lesions who were culture positive, but more likely than not lacking a history of prior infection.

In general, the risk for fetal transmission was highest in women who lacked prepregnancy HSV antibody. HSV-2 antibody appears to protect against both HSV-1 and HSV-2 transmission. Cesarean section protects against fetal transmission by women shedding the virus, and HSV-1 appears to be more readily transmitted than HSV-2. As the authors point out, routine screening for HSV-2 virus will only identify large numbers of seropositive women with a risk primarily of reactivation transmission, but the risk of infant infection in that group is very small. The best prospects for preventing neonatal infection appear to rest with the detection of viral DNA in early to mid pregnancy, with careful detection of maternal vulvar lesions together with consideration of cesarean section for those without antibody or history of infection found to be shedding virus without symptoms or lesions. This is a small subset, 11 of 31,663 (0.03%) in this study.

T. H. Kirschbaum, MD

3 Medical Complications of Pregnancy

Troponin I in the Diagnosis of Acute Myocardial Infarction in Pregnancy, Labor, and Post Partum

Shade GH Jr, Ross G, Bever FN, et al (St John Detroit Riverview Hosp; St John Macomb Hosp, Warren, Mich; St John Hosp and Med Ctr, Warren, Mich)

Am J Obstet Gynecol 187:1719-1720, 2002   3–1

Background.—Cardiac-specific troponin I (cTnI) has proved useful in the diagnosis of acute, evolving, or recent myocardial infarction (MI) and is the marker of choice for diagnosing cardiac injury in pregnant women. Its advantages include never rising above the upper limit of normal in healthy pregnant women 30 minutes, 12 hours, and 24 hours after delivery; not being influenced by obstetric anesthesia; and not being affected by the uterine contractions and cell breakdown that normally take place during labor and delivery.

 Case Report.—Woman, 18, gravida 2, para 1, went into labor at 39 weeks of gestation. The placenta was spontaneously delivered after oxytocin administration. Although the patient had no history of heart disease and no complaints of chest discomfort before or during delivery, she experienced an unusual sensation in the chest area, and supraventricular tachycardia was detected immediately after delivery. The patient was given adenosine, which successfully converted the heart rhythm to sinus rhythm; blood pressure was stable, and the electrocardiogram after conversion showed completely normal findings. The patient was given heparin, β-blockers, and aspirin. Ten hours after delivery, the patient's first cTnI result was 11.6 ng/mL; the diagnostic criteria for acute MI is a result over 4.5 ng/mL. Four subsequent assessments, taken up to 32 hours after delivery, showed a classic pattern of cTnI in acute MI. Three days after delivery, the patient underwent a nuclear isotope myocardial perfusion scan with wall motion analysis and ejection fraction assessment. Her estimated ejection fraction was 61%, and the anterior wall demonstrated mild to moderately reduced activity during both phases of the evaluation. Thallium was used at rest, and tetrofosmin was used during peak exercise. The valvular structure was normal, pericardial effusion was absent, the left ventricle was only mildly dilated, systolic left ventricular functioning was normal, paradoxical septal motion at the base was detected, and atrial or ventricular septal defects were absent.

Conclusions.—The sensitivity and specificity of cTnI simplified the diagnosis of acute MI in this woman. Its pattern of a rapid rise and a gradual fall after acute MI was clearly shown. Under appropriate conditions, cTnI is the marker of choice for the diagnosis of acute MI in women during the peripartum period.

► This brief report is helpful in introducing some obstetricians to the use of measurements of cTnI, a serum marker for MI that has come to be the preferred choice among other serum markers in contemporary cardiology. Troponin I is 1 of 3 isoforms that facilitate myocardial excitation through calcium activation of the actin–myosin reactions in cardiomyocytes associated with myocardial contraction. Troponin C binds to calcium ions after undergoing steric alteration. Troponin I binds to actin, troponin T stabilizes its complex with troponin C and, in turn, binds to tropomyosin, and contractual activity ensues. All 3 isoforms are amenable to quantitation with specific monoclonal antibodies. What is clinically useful about troponin I are the dynamics of its changes in concentration as it is released into the circulation after myocardial necrosis. Troponin I is barely identifiable in normal serum but increases sharply in concentration, about 20-fold, after MI. Further, it remains elevated for a period of 7 to 10 days after the myocardial injury. Its serum activity is unchanged by normal pregnancy, labor and delivery, anesthesia, prolonged labor, or operative vaginal or abdominal birth. In those respects, it is far more specific than are changes in serum myoglobin, lactic dehydrogenase, creatinine, and phosphokinase and its M and B isoenzymes. The case report is a nice example of its usefulness in establishing the diagnosis in cases in which normal EKG and echocardiographic findings are present in puerperal women but in which the diagnosis is ultimately later proven by echocardiography. It's the most sensitive and reliable serum marker we have for MI at present.

T. H. Kirschbaum, MD

Resistin Is Expressed in the Human Placenta
Yura S, Sagawa N, Itoh H, et al (Kyoto Univ, Japan)
J Clin Endocrinol Metab 88:1394-1397, 2003   3–2

Background.—Energy metabolism is altered during pregnancy to meet the developing fetus's increasing demands for energy. Postprandial hyperglycemia is usually observed in gestation due to decreased insulin sensitivity.

It has been proposed that placenta-derived hormones are involved in this metabolic adaptation, but the mechanism for decreased insulin sensitivity in pregnant women has not been fully elucidated. Resistin is a novel peptide hormone that is specifically expressed in the human placental tissue, primarily in trophoblastic cells. Expression of the resistin gene was measured in maternal adipose tissue, placenta, and fetal membranes to determine whether resistin has a role in pregnancy in humans.

Methods.—Chorionic villous tissue and decidua tissue were obtained in the first trimester from 5 pregnant women who underwent artificial termination of pregnancy. In addition, the placenta and fetal membranes were collected from 8 women who underwent noncomplicated elective cesarean section. Subcutaneous adipose tissue around previous surgical scars was also obtained from 3 premenopausal nonpregnant and 4 pregnant women at repeated laparotomy for gynecologic or obstetric reasons. Plasma samples were obtained from 12 normal premenopausal nonpregnant women and 15 noncomplicated pregnant women in the third trimester, before the onset of labor.

Results.—Resistin gene expression in term placental tissue was more prominent than in the first trimester chorionic tissue (Fig 4). However, resistin gene expression was somewhat weak in adipose tissue and remained unchanged during pregnancy (Fig 5).

Conclusion.—Resistin, a novel placental hormone, may modulate insulin sensitivity during pregnancy.

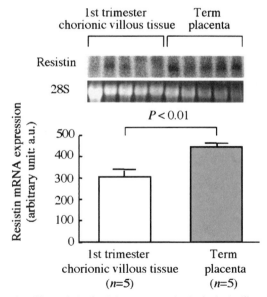

FIGURE 4.—Northern blot analysis of resistin gene expression in chorionic villous tissue in the first trimester (5 patients) and placental tissue at term (5 patients). Total RNA (30 µg/lane) was loaded. (Courtesy of Ura S, Sagawa N, Itoh H, et al: Resistin is expressed in the human placenta. *J Clin Endocrinol Metab* 88(3): 1394-1397, 2003. Copyright The Endocrine Society.)

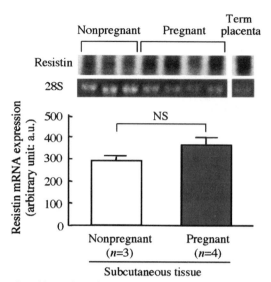

FIGURE 5.—Northern blot analysis of resistin gene expression in adipose tissue from nonpregnant women (3 patients) and pregnant women at term (4 patients). Total RNA (8 μg/lane) was loaded. Term placenta was blotted on the same sheet, the same sample loaded on Fig 1 in the original journal article. *Abbreviation: NS,* Not significant difference. (Courtesy of Ura S, Sagawa N, Itoh H, et al: Resistin is expressed in the human placenta. *J Clin Endocrinol Metab* 88(3):1394-1397, 2003. Copyright The Endocrine Society.)

▶ The World Health Organization predicts a doubling in the worldwide incidence of diabetes from an estimated 150 million cases to 300 million cases over the years 1995 to 2025, the majority of them type II diabetics.[1] Type II diabetes mellitus evolves as dietary and other environmental factors overwhelm the ability of an individual to sustain chronically high insulin blood levels appropriate to counterbalance insulin resistance. In pregnancy, insulin resistance is enhanced by the increase in placental production of human placental lactogen, prolactin, and sex steroids, and elevated leptin concentrations are rendered relatively ineffective in increasing insulin sensitivity as pregnancy progresses (see Abstract 1–6). Leptin apparently serves primarily to prevent hypoglycemia in pregnancy rather than responding to hyperglycemia. Clearly, identifying an agent(s) responsible for increased insulin resistance in pregnancy, which might then be altered pharmacologically to decrease insulin resistance, is theoretically a high desirable. The use of metformin in this connection is handicapped by uncertainty about its effects on the fetus.[2,3]

Resistin, a peptide hormone expressed in adipose tissue in mice and important in obesity in that species, is currently under investigation in that role. In humans, it appears to be suppressed by thiazolidinediones, such as pioglitazone, and rosiglitazone, both of which have the capacity to reduce blood sugar without increasing insulin concentration in humans. In a group of 13 samples of placental tissues from the first and third trimesters, fat biopsy specimens from pregnant and postmenopausal women, and plasma samples from 27 women pregnant or not, the authors explored the origin of resistin in human females. Using reverse transcription–polymerase chain reaction (a technique which allows RNA replication without cloning intermediates by using the polyadenine 3-prime DNA tail as a promoter for reverse transcription of an RNA segment attached to it as a hybrid) they found mRNA for resistin in placenta and amniotic epithelium but little in decidua.

Trophoblastic cell culture produces abundant mRNA, which is found in syncytiotrophoblast by immunocytochemistry. Gene expression of mRNA from trophoblast cultures increases with gestation (see Fig 4), and plasma leptin is present in greater mean concentration in term pregnancy (68.2 µg/mL) than in nonpregnant women (5.4µ/mL). Adipose tissue contains resistin, but there's no significant difference between its concentration in pregnancy compared with blood from postmenopausal women (see Fig 5).

Increase in insulin resistance which appears in pregnancy seems to come predominantly from the trophoblast. In earlier works, these authors have shown early placental expression of leptin and subsequent decreases with gestation as resistin activity increases, suggesting resistin may play a role in limiting insulin sensitivity imposed by other hormones.[4] All this explains the interest in resistin as a potentially important mediator of insulin resistance in gestational diabetes and type II diabetes mellitus.

T. H. Kirschbaum, MD

References

1. King H, Aubert R, Herman W: Global burden of diabetes 1995 - 2025. *Diabetes Care* 21:1414, 1998.
2. 1998 YEAR BOOK OF OBSTETRICS, GYNECOLOGY, AND WOMEN'S HEALTH, pp 99-100.
3. 2002 YEAR BOOK OF OBSTETRICS, GYNECOLOGY, AND WOMEN'S HEALTH, pp 112-113.
4. Yura S, Sagawa N, Ogawa Y, et al: Augmentation of leptin synthesis through activation of protein kinases A and C in cultured human trophoblastic cells. *J Clin Endocrinol Metab* 83:3609, 1998.

The Relative Contributions of Birth Weight, Weight Change, and Current Weight to Insulin Resistance in Contemporary 5-Year-Olds: The EarlyBird Study

Wilkin TJ, Metcalf BS, Murphy MJ, et al (Peninsula Med School, Plymouth, England; Derriford Hosp, Plymouth, England)
Diabetes 51:3468-3472, 2002   3–3

Background.—Type 2 diabetes is the outcome of the process of insulin resistance. The "Barker" hypothesis suggests that low birth weight, a surrogate for poor gestational environment, is correlated with insulin resistance later in life through fetal programming coupled with later catch-up weight gain. Low birth weight is now rare in industrialized society, but insulin resistance and type 2 diabetes are not. The relationship between insulin resistance and birth weight, catch-up weight, and current weight in British children was examined.

Study Design.—The EarlyBird study is a noninterventional, prospective cohort study monitoring 300 healthy children from Plymouth, England from school entry (4 to 5 years) to age 16. All are ethnically white. At school entry, baseline assessments were made of fasting insulin, glucose, insulin resistance, height, weight, and subcutaneous fat. Body mass index was calculated. Birth weights were obtained from the registry and catch-up weight was calculated by weight standard deviation scores. Premature infants were excluded from the study group.

Findings.—Insulin resistance at 5 years of age was not correlated with birth weight but was significantly correlated with current weight and weight catch-up. Girls were significantly more insulin resistant than boys. Weight change (catch-up weight gain) was also correlated with current weight and was not an independent predictor of insulin resistance. Insulin resistance at 5 years of age was the same in children with a high birth weight and in those lighter at birth who then experienced catch-up weight gain.

Conclusion.—There appears to be no relationship among contemporary children between birth weight and insulin resistance. Girls are significantly more insulin resistant than boys. Insulin resistance is the same in those who are born heavy and remain heavy as it is in those who become heavy later. These findings indicate that some neonates are too heavy at birth and other are gaining too much weight. Childhood over-nutrition is a problem that can be avoided or corrected to maintain insulin sensitivity in young children.

▶ This is an attempt to test the Barker hypothesis which links term low birth weight and "catch-up" weight to type 2 diabetes, dyslipidemia, hypertension, and atherosclerosis using contemporary data.[1] In brief, Barker's view is that term low birth weight infants undergo in utero programming, which renders them insulin resistant in later life, with serious propensity for metabolic implications then. In his view, this tendency is particularly strong for a subset of low birth weight infants who undergo rapid catch-up growth as neonates.

As the authors point out, Barker's relationships were formulated from data from aging males born before 1930, many of them born into impoverished environments. In the intervening 75 years, low birth weight at term become much less common. Further, since birth weight and subsequent weight are highly mutually correlated, metabolic disturbances after infancy may be just as significant in determining the incidence of diabetes and its covariants as are fetal events.

The basic data here are a collection of semi-annual observations on 279 infants born at term and followed up through 5 years of age from 1988 to 1998. At each observation, fasting insulin, insulin resistance, blood glucose, height, weight, body mass index, and skin-fold thicknesses were measured. Birth weights were obtained from a regional National Health Service child registry that also contained mean values and trends of change for the first 5 years of age, from which rates of changes and compositions could be made, reflecting relatively contemporary life in the United Kingdom. These data showed that no relationship between birth weight and insulin resistance exists. Girls were more often insulin resistance than were boys, even when the values were controlled for weight at 5 years of age and having greater body mass index, skin-fold thickness, and hip circumferences than boys. No significant differences could be demonstrated in insulin resistance related to height or weight.

Finally, insulin resistance is the same in children with high birth weights who remain at high birth weight percentiles as it is in those born with low birth weight who undergo "catch-up" growth to a subsequently higher percentile. Though birth weight has increased slowly over the past decade in the United Kingdom, body weight at age 5 has increased much more rapidly. Though the influence of low birth weight in a nutritionally less than optimal population is not precluded, these data indicate that low birth weight is no longer related to insulin resistance and its apparent consequences in modern children, as it may have been prior to World War II.

T. H. Kirschbaum, MD

Reference

1. 2002 YEAR BOOK OF OBSTETRICS, GYNECOLOGY, AND WOMEN'S HEALTH, pp 73-77; pp 254-256.

TNF-α Is a Predictor of Insulin Resistance in Human Pregnancy
Kirwan JP, Hauguel-De Mouzon S, Lepercq J, et al (Case Western Reserve Univ, Cleveland, Ohio; Institut Cochin de Génétique Moléculaire, Paris; Hôpital Cochin-Saint Vincent-de-Paul, Paris; et al)
Diabetes 51:2207-2213, 2002   3–4

Introduction.—Insulin resistance during pregnancy has been linked to increased production of placental hormones and cortisol. The longitudinal changes in concentrations of reproductive hormones (HPL, progesterone, human chorionic gonadotropin [hCG], prolactin, and estradiol), tumor necrosis factor [TNF]-α, leptin, and cortisol with the corresponding changes in maternal insulin sensitivity, as determined by the euglycemic-hyperinsulinemia clamp, were prospectively examined. The placenta was evaluated as a potential contributing source of maternal circulating TNF-α, using the dual perfusion model of human placental cotyledon.

Methods.—Insulin resistance was evaluated in 15 females (5 with gestational diabetes mellitus and 10 with normal glucose tolerance) using the euglycemic-hyperinsulinemic clamp procedure before pregnancy (pregravid) and during early (12-14 weeks) and late (34-36 weeks) gestation. Body composition, plasma TNF-α, leptin, cortisol, and reproductive hormones (hCG, estradiol, progesterone, human placental lactogen, and prolactin) were determined in conjunction with the clamps. Placental TNF-α was determined in vitro using dually perfused human placental cotyledon from 5 additional patients.

Results.—Compared with pregravid, insulin resistance was obvious during late pregnancy in all patients (12.4 vs 8.1 mg kg^{-1} fat-free mass minutes^{-1} microU^{-1} mL^{-1}) (Fig 1). In late pregnancy, TNF-α, leptin, cortisol, all reproductive hormones, and fat mass were increased ($P < .001$). In vitro, nearly all of the placental TNF-α (94%) was released into the maternal side. During late pregnancy, there was an inverse relationship between TNF-α and insulin sensitivity (r = -0.69; $P < .006$). Of all the hormonal changes observed, the

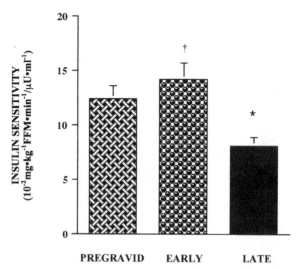

FIGURE 1.—Insulin sensitivity measured during euglycemic-hyperinsulinemic clamps performed pregravid and during early (12-14 weeks) and late (34-36 weeks) pregnancy. Data are means +/− SE; n = 15. Glucose disposal rates and insulin concentration were calculated for the final 150-180 minutes of the clamp. Units are expressed relative to fat-free mass. *Significantly increased from pregravid, P < .02. †Significantly decreased from pregravid, P < .0001. (Courtesy of Kirwan JP, Haugeul-De Mouzon S, Lepercq J, et al: TNF-α is a predictor of insulin resistance in human pregnancy. *Diabetes* 51:2207-2213, 2002. Copyright by the American Diabetes Association.)

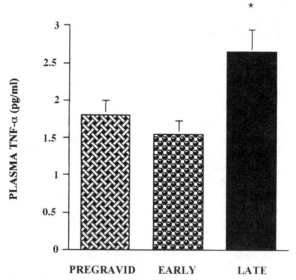

FIGURE 2.—Plasma TNF-α concentrations of all women pregravid and during early (12-14 weeks) and late (34-36 weeks) pregnancy. Data are mean +/− SE; n = 15. Fasting blood samples were collected before each corresponding clamp. *Significantly higher than pregravid, P < .004. (Courtesy of Kirwan JP, Haugeul-De Mouzon S, Lepercq J, et al: TNF-α is a predictor of insulin resistance in human pregnancy. *Diabetes* 51:2207-2213, 2002. Copyright by the American Diabetes Association.)

change in TNF-α from pregravid to late pregnancy was the only significant change in insulin sensitivity (r = −0.60; $P < .02$) (Fig 2). The placental reproductive hormones and cortisol were not correlated with insulin sensitivity in late pregnancy. Multivariate stepwise regression analysis showed that TNF-α was the most significant independent predictor of insulin sensitivity (r = −0.67; $P < .0001$), even after adjusting for fat mass by covariance (r = 0.46; $P < .01$). These findings are not in keeping with the view that the classical reproductive hormones are the primary mediators of change in insulin sensitivity during gestation and offer a basis for including TNF-α in a new paradigm to explain insulin resistance in pregnancy.

▶ This is a significant contribution from this productive group of investigators at Case Western Reserve University exploring the mechanisms of insulin resistance in pregnancy. They report a longitudinal study of 10 gravidas (5 obese) with normal early pregnancy glucose tolerance and 5 women with the propensity for gestational diabetes based on Carpenter and Coustans glucose testing criteria in early pregnancy. The study gains its significance from evidence that increases in insulin resistance play a role in the development of gestational diabetes mellitus, type II diabetes, fetal macrosomia, preeclampsia, and, possibly, endovascular diseases. Studies were done on 2 occasions, the first at 12 to 14 weeks and the second at 34 to 36 weeks of gestation. Each patient survey included a euglycemic-hyperinsulinemic clamp procedure to measure insulin resistance, fasting blood sugar, plasma determination of TNF-α, leptin, and a variety of reproductive endocrine products, including human placental lactogen, progesterone, estradiol, human chorionic gonadotropin, prolactin, and corticosterone. All of the endocrine products at one time or another have had attributed a role in increasing insulin resistance in pregnancy. TNF-α is cytokine which, like leptin, is produced by the placenta and adipose tissue. It was measured by Elisa and HCG was measured by immnoassay; the remaining endocrine assays were done by radioimmunoassay.

In vitro cotyledonary perfusion experiments were performed to determine cotyledonary TNF-α production (an average of 123.1 pg/m per placenta) and the relative secretions of product into maternal (94%) and fetal (6%) circulations. Insulin resistance did not differ between fat and lean normal subjects through pregnancy but insulin resistance increased in those who were destined to become gestational diabetics. Overall, insulin sensitivity increased by 14% in early pregnancy but decreased by a mean of 65% in late pregnancy coupled with increases in plasma insulin at that time. In parallel, TNF-α in maternal plasma decreased by 13% after the end of the first trimester but increased by 45% in third trimester subjects. When stepwise linear regression was employed, for multvariant analysis, inverse changes in TNF-α plasma concentration accounted for 45% of the variance noted in insulin sensitivity. Leptin increased concentration accounted for 9% of the variance and plasma cortisol for 7%. No significant linear correlations occurred between insulin sensitivity and any of the other endocrine products.

The observations would have benefited by more than 2 insulin insensitivity measurements per pregnancy. What the authors present are measures of covariability of insulin resistance and TNF-α with the duration of gestation which cannot be used to say anything about direct casual relationships nor mechanisms. Their data does suggest that the cytokine TNF-α and leptin production from the placenta may be more important than endocrine products to which are usually ascribed the changes in insulin sensitivity during pregnancy.

T. H. Kirschbaum, MD

Prospective Delivery of Reliably Dated Term Infants of Diabetic Mothers Without Determination of Fetal Lung Maturity: Comparison of Historical Control

Kjos SL, Berkowitz KM, Kung B (Univ of Southern California, Los Angeles; Univ of California, Irvine)
J Matern Fetal Neonatal Med 12:433-437, 2002   3–5

Background.—Management of the pregnancies of women with diabetes has included testing of fetal lung maturity (FLM) to determine whether elective delivery of term or near-term infants should be performed, for the purpose of decreasing the risk of respiratory distress syndrome (RDS) and stillbirth. Even with the advances made in diabetic management that have lowered the rates of stillbirth to those of the general obstetric population and made the occurrence of RDS in a term infant of a mother with diabetes a rarity, FLM testing has persisted. Whether routine FLM testing serves any purpose in the reliably dated term pregnancies of women with diabetes was investigated. In addition, it was determined whether the occurrence of RDS appreciably increases when such testing is omitted.

Methods.—The 1457 women enrolled had accurately dated pregnancies and had completed 37 weeks of gestation. All were followed up prospectively through delivery; no FLM testing was performed. Results of the prevalence of RDS and other outcomes were compared with those of a historical control group of 713 women who had lecithin–sphingomyelin testing performed before delivery at term. Independent predictors of RDS were identified with the use of logistic regression analysis.

Results.—Fewer of the control women had diet-controlled gestational diabetes mellitus (GDM), and more had probably undiagnosed diabetes in comparison with the study group. The control group also had significantly higher rates of poor glycemic control in the third trimester and less frequent insulin use. Women in the control group delivered at significantly earlier gestational age, less frequently had a trial of labor, and had cesarean delivery more often than those in the study group. A higher rate of large-for-gestational-age infants were born to study group women than to those in the control group. No significant difference in RDS rates was found between the 2 groups, and the rate of RDS in infants of women with diagnoses of glucose intolerance during pregnancy was the same in the 2 groups. Cesarean delivery was the only obstetric, medical, or neonatal characteristic found to be significantly linked to RDS; RDS occurred in 0.5% of infants delivered vaginally and in 1.5% of those delivered by cesarean section. Thus, cesarean delivery was the only independent predictor of RDS.

Conclusions.—Comparing a group of pregnant women who did not have FLM testing to a group that had it in the preceding 2 years did not reveal any link with RDS risk. RDS rates were not significantly different between the 2 groups. Only cesarean delivery was an independent predictor of an increased risk of RDS. Thus, eliminating FLM testing in reliably dated diabetic pregnancies should not increase the risk of RDS.

▶ The prevalence of RDS in infants of diabetic mothers has steadily decreased in recent decades, making it increasingly difficult to justify management recommendations first made decades earlier. This review of the management of patients with pregestational or GDM A1 at term with reliable pregnancy dating calls into question the need for routine FLM assays as part of that management. The authors present results from a group of 1457 such pregnancies managed without pulmonary maturity testing from 1990 to 1991 and compare results of that care with the results from 713 similar women treated in 1988-1989 with pulmonary maturation studies. Historical controls are proposed because the low prevalence of RDS makes it difficult to enroll concurrent controls.

Comparing the test and control groups makes it clear how diabetic management has changed with time in this large unit. Obstetricians now see fewer pregnancies with problems in diabetic control and fewer that require insulin to supplement dietary changes. At the same time, the University of Southern California group is moving in the direction of greater mean gestational age at delivery with more spontaneous labor and fewer labor inductions (55.8%-38.1%) achieved by an increasing occurrence of cesarean section (26.7%-51.2%).

RDS is defined by clinical findings within the first 3 hours of life that last for greater than 24 hours and that are confirmed by chest radiographs together with the exclusion of other potential causes of neonatal pulmonary compromise. The authors found no increase in RDS prevalence (0.8% compared with 1% in controls) as a result of abolishing pulmonary maturity testing. Further, and just as significant, they found no impact on the occurrence rate of RDS based on either management of women with GDM first diagnosed during the pregnancy at issue or its occurrence in prior pregnancies, thereby raising questions regarding the value of routine diabetic testing in pregnancy. Of a list of 11 existing or potential confounding variables treated with multivariate analysis, only the incidence of cesarean section proved to be statistically, significantly associated both with an increased risk of RDS (1.5% vs 0.5% in vaginal deliveries) and as an independent predictor of RDS (odds ratio, 2.21; 95% CI, 2.04-2.27) compared with the control group. Perhaps, that points to a need for an initiative to decrease the cesarean section rate that may result in an even further reduction of RDS in future patients.

T. H. Kirschbaum, MD

Combination Antiretroviral Therapy in 100 HIV-1–Infected Pregnant Women

Bucceri AM, Somigliana E, Matrone R, et al (Univ of Milan, Italy)

Hum Reprod 17:436-441, 2002   3–6

Background.—Combination antiretroviral therapy has markedly improved the prognosis of those with HIV-1 infection in recent years. However, data on the effects of these regimens during pregnancy are limited. The adverse effects, vertical transmission rates, and neonatal outcomes associated with different combination therapies for HIV-1 infection were evaluated.

Methods and Findings.—One hundred pregnant women with HIV-1 infection were included in the study (Table 3). Antiretroviral treatment was begun at a median 16 weeks' gestation, with a range of prepregnancy to 31 weeks' gestation. Twenty-three women continued their prepregnancy treatments in their first trimester. Twenty-three of the final treatment regimens included protease inhibitors. In 25 women, treatment regimens did not include zidovudine. Ninety-seven percent of the women delivered by cesarean section. None of the women breastfed. Nineteen percent of the babies were born prematurely. However, after the exclusion of women actively using illicit drugs, the premature birth rate was only 10% (Table 4). The rate of congenital malformations did not seem to differ significantly from that reported for the general population. Of the 102 live newborns, only 1 was infected with HIV-1.

Conclusions.—These data confirm the efficacy of combination antiretroviral treatment, cesarean delivery, and the avoidance of breast-feeding in reducing the rate of vertical HIV-1 transmission. These findings also suggest that combination antiretroviral therapy may not cause major neonatal toxicity.

▶ This experience from the University of Milan is the largest consecutive account of the treatment of HIV-1–positive gravidas using combined antiretroviral therapy supplemented by protease inhibitors and elective cesarean section I have seen to date. These data come from patients treated from 1998-2000. The combination of zidovudine and lamivudine (Combivir), 2 synthetic nucleoside analogs found to be synergistic in impeding HIV retroviral activity,

TABLE 3.—Maternal Immunological and Virological Data

	n	First Test	Last Test	P
CD4 cell count (mean + SD)	95	418 + 256	466 + 258	0.02
Viral load titre (median and range)	87	5982	188	0.001
		(neg −236 000)	(neg −51 000)	
Undetectable viral load (n and %)	87	15 (17)	39 (45)	0.001

"First test" refers to the first blood sample examination during pregnancy and "Last test" to the last test before delivery. CD4 cell counts and viral load titer are expressed as cells/mm³ and number of copies/mL, respectively. *neg*, Undetectable viral load. Paired analysis was performed. Total number varies because of missing information.

(Courtesy of Bucceri AM, Somigliana E, Matrone R, et al: Combination antiretroviral therapy in 100 HIV-1-infected pregnant women. *Hum Reprod* 17:436-441, 2002. Copyright European Society for Human Reproduction and Embryology, by permission of Oxford University Press.)

TABLE 4.—Newborn Outcomes: Prematurity and Low Birth Weight

Outcome	n (%)
Preterm delivery	18/96 (19)
Use of illicit drugs and/or methadone	
Active use	11/27* (41)
Non active use	7/69 (10)
Small for gestational age	10/96 (10)

*$P < .001$ compared with nonactive users.

Twin pregnancy newborns were not considered. *Preterm delivery* was defined as the birth of an infant before 37 completed gestational weeks. Small for gestational age newborns were defined as infants whose weight at birth was below the 10th percentile.

(Courtesy of Bucceri AM, Somigliana E, Matrone R, et al: Combination antiretroviral therapy in 100 HIV-1-infected pregnant women. *Hum Reprod* 17:436-441, 2002. Copyright European Society for Human Reproduction and Embryology, by permission of Oxford University Press.)

were given to 75 women; 25 were unable to tolerate its side effects. Twenty-three women also received protease inhibitors (indinavir, saquinavir, nelfinavir, etc), largely on indication of drug failure and side effects. Nine of 23 women with AIDS received protease inhibitors. Eighteen of the subject women had delivered 21 infants prior to enrollment in this program, with 2 (10%) delivering infected infants. The median onset of therapy was 21 weeks of gestational age, and the duration of therapy averaged 16 weeks. Forty-six women had no retroviral therapy prior to pregnancy and received Combivir as a drug of first choice. The pattern of drug options was complex, being driven by measures of CD4 cell counts, HIV-1 RNA viral loads, and drug tolerance. Twenty two percent of women on protease inhibitors discontinued the drug because of gastrointestinal intolerance. Abdominal delivery was conducted in 97 women—electively in 72 cases—to decrease the risk of THE transfer of virus from mother to fetus. Breast-feeding was interdicted.

The results of therapy showed a clear increase in mean CD4 cell counts and decrease in mean HIV-1 viral loads among women treated, the viral loads becoming undeterminable in 39, or 45%, of women through the course of therapy. Though the results are not conclusive, there was no apparent increase in fetal anomalies noted. Birth before 37 weeks occurred in 19% of women. The active use of illicit drugs during pregnancy in 41% of these subjects may be an important contributing factor to the relatively high preterm birth rate noted. Newborn AZT was given only for infants less than 34 weeks' gestational age or in cases of failed maternal therapy. Two women developed AIDS on therapy (chorioretinitis, pancytopenia, *Candida* esophagitis), and there were 25 coincidental infections (eg, herpes simplex, hepatitis B, and pneumonia) as well. Fetal transmission occurred in a single pregnancy for a rate of 1%.

Despite the laudable decrease of newborn transmission reported here, several management questions remain. More data are needed on the relationship between protease inhibitors and preterm birth. Whether drug therapy during the first trimester has positive risk benefits of value or may impede normal pregnancy development is uncertain and whether AZT should be given routinely to all gravidas remains to be settled. Both the excellent results in preventing maternal-to-fetal transfer and the cost and effort needed to obtain that result are noteworthy in this experience.

T. H. Kirschbaum, MD

Antiretroviral Therapy During Pregnancy and the Risk of an Adverse Outcome
Tuomala RE, Shapiro DE, Mofenson LM, et al (Brigham and Women's Hosp, Boston; Harvard School of Public Health, Boston; Natl Inst of Child Health and Human Development, Rockville, Md; et al)
N Engl J Med 346:1863-1870, 2002   3–7

Background.—Combination antiretroviral therapy in pregnant women with HIV-1 infection may increase the risk of premature birth and other adverse pregnancy outcomes. Data on pregnant women with HIV-1 infection enrolled in 7 large studies were analyzed to assess the risk of premature delivery and other adverse outcomes associated with antiretroviral drugs.

Methods.—The study included 2123 women who gave birth between 1990 and 1998. Antiretroviral monotherapy was given to 1590 women, combination treatment without protease inhibitors to 396, and combination therapy with protease inhibitors to 137.

Findings.—After adjusting for the CD4+ cell count and use of tobacoo, alcohol, and illicit drugs, the premature delivery rate was comparable for women with and without antiretroviral therapy—16% and 17%, respectively. In both groups, the rate of low birth weight was 16%. Very low birth weight occurred in 2% of infants born to mothers receiving antiretroviral therapy and in 1% of infants born to women who did not. The 2 groups were comparable in rates of low Apgar scores and stillbirths. After adjusting for multiple risk factors, no correlation was noted for the combination antiretroviral treatment and an increased risk of premature delivery and delivery of a low-birth-weight infant compared with monotherapy. Five percent of women receiving combination therapy with protease inhibitors had infants with very low birth weight, compared with 2% of those receiving combination therapy without protease inhibitors (Table 3).

Conclusions.—Compared with no antiretroviral treatment or monotherapy, combination therapy for HIV-1 infection in pregnant women is apparently not related to increased rates of premature delivery or to low birth weight, low Apgar scores, or stillbirth. Further research is needed to confirm the relationship between combination therapy with protease inhibitors and an increased risk of very low birth weight.

▶ The addition of protease inhibitors to the treatment of HIV-1 infection has, by virtue of their effectiveness in inhibiting replication of virions in intracellular loci, resulted in dramatic reduction of HIV-1-RNA copy numbers and patient symptomatology. This article marks the beginnings of what will certainly be an exhaustive investigation of risk-benefit implications for maternal to fetal transmission rates and pregnancy complications, especially preterm birth, as a result of their use. These investigators were stimulated by a Swiss HIV cohort

TABLE 3.—Risks of Adverse Pregnancy Outcomes According to the
Antiretroviral Regimen*

Outcome	Odds Ratio (95% CI)	
	Adjusted for All Risk Factors Except Prior Premature Delivery (N = 1936)†	Adjusted for All Risk Factors, Including Prior Premature Delivery (N = 1598)‡
Premature delivery (<37 wk)		
Combination vs. monotherapy	0.96 (0.66-1.40)	1.08 (0.71-1.62)
Combination without PI vs. monotherapy	0.87 (0.58-1.30)	0.95 (0.60-1.48)
Combination with PI vs. monotherapy	1.28 (0.74-2.13)	1.45 (0.81-2.50)
Combination with PI vs. without PI	1.58 (0.86-2.87)	1.80 (0.94-3.43)
Very premature delivery (<32 wk)		
Combination vs. monotherapy	0.83 (0.38-1.77)§	1.17 (0.49-2.72)§
Combination without PI vs. monotherapy	0.71 (0.29-1.62)§	0.97 (0.36-2.41)§
Combination with PI vs. monotherapy	1.78 (0.61-4.53)§	1.96 (0.64-5.28)§
Combination with PI vs. without PI	2.22 (0.70-6.58)§¶	2.70 (0.82-8.49)§¶
Low birth weight (<2500 g)		
Combination vs. monotherapy	0.76 (0.50-1.13)	1.03 (0.64-1.63)
Combination without PI vs. monotherapy	0.59 (0.37-0.93)‖	0.86 (0.51-1.42)
Combination with PI vs. monotherapy	1.52 (0.89-2.54)	1.45 (0.79-2.56)
Combination with PI vs. without PI	2.31 (1.21-4.39)#	2.00 (0.98-4.05)
Very low birth weight (<1500 g)		
Combination vs. monotherapy	1.11 (0.47-2.56)	1.64 (0.59-4.35)§
Combination without PI vs. monotherapy	0.82 (0.29-2.11)	1.23 (0.36-3.73)§
Combination with PI vs. monotherapy	2.93 (1.03-7.47)‖	3.03 (0.93-8.83)§
Combination with PI vs. without PI	3.15 (1.04-9.40)¶**	3.56 (1.04-12.19)§¶**

*CI denotes confidence interval, and PI protease inhibitors.

†These odds ratios are for the subgroup of 1936 treated women for whom data were available on all risk factors except prior premature delivery. Unless otherwise noted, these odds ratios were adjusted for the study; the CD4+ cell count (<200, 200-499, or ≥500/mm³); age (<18, 18-34, or >34 years); race or ethnic group; and use or nonuse of tobacco, alcohol, and illicit drugs. The odds ratios for combination therapy as compared with monotherapy and for combination therapy without protease inhibitors as compared with monotherapy were also adjusted for the year of delivery.

‡These odds ratios are for the subgroup of 1598 treated women for whom data were available on all risk factors, including prior premature delivery. Unless otherwise noted, the odds ratios for this subgroup were adjusted for the study; the CD4+ cell count (<200, 200-499, or ≥500/mm³); age (<18, 18-34, or >34 years); race or ethnic group, use or nonuse of tobacco, alcohol, and illicit drugs; and the presence or absence of a history of premature delivery. The odds ratios for combination therapy as compared with monotherapy and for combination therapy without protease inhibitors as compared with monotherapy were also adjusted for the year of delivery.

§The odds ratio was adjusted for age as a 2-category variable (≤34 or >34 years) instead of a 3-category variable because there were no events in some strata.

‖P = .03.

¶The odds ratio was not adjusted for the study because there were no events in some strata.

#P = .01.

**P = .04.

(Reprinted by permission of *The New England Journal of Medicine* from Tuomala RE, Shapiro DE, Mofenson LM, et al: Antiretroviral therapy during pregnancy and the risk of an adverse outcome. *N Engl J Med* 346:1863-1870, 2002. Copyright 2002, Massachusetts Medical Society. All rights reserved.)

study of 43 women, which suggested that women receiving combination antiretroviral agents and protease inhibitors had a higher incidence of preterm birth than those who did not receive protease inhibitors. The investigators here used data from the perinatal AIDS collaborative transmission study,[1] the Women's and Infants Transmission study,[2] and 3 additional single site studies. A total of 2123 gravid women receiving therapy included 1590 women receiving only AZT, 396 women who with combination therapy excluding protease inhibitors and 137 receiving combination therapy with protease inhibitors compared with 1143 HIV-1 antibody positive women receiving no antiretroviral therapy during pregnancy.

In general, there were no significant differences with respect to very low birth weight and low birth weight occurrence rates, Apgar scores, or fetal death rates among the 4 groups. No differences were noted between those treated or not with antiretrovirals and those treated with single versus multiple combinations with or without protease inhibitors. Outcome data were adjusted for mothers CD4 counts and use of tobacco, alcohol, and illicit drugs, but only unadjusted rates showed a decreased risk of preterm birth in women receiving therapy versus those not treated during pregnancy. However, the risk of very low birth weight and low birth weight birth was higher for women receiving combination therapy with protease inhibitors than for those treated with monotherapy or combination therapy without protease inhibitors. Bear in mind that relatively few cases were treated with this new agent. What this means is that further work on demonstrating whether protease inhibitors play a role in increasing the chances of preterm birth when added to a treatment regimen for HIV-1 gravidas will be required because this risk result certainly doesn't exclude the possibility.

T. H. Kirschbaum, MD

References

1. 1996 YEAR BOOK OF OBSTETRICS, GYNECOLOGY, AND WOMEN'S HEALTH, pp 85-87.
2. Sheon AR, Fox HE, Rich KC, et al: The Women's and Infants Transmission Study (WITS) of maternal-infant HIV transmission: Study design, methods, and baseline data. *J Womens Health* 5:69-78, 1996.

Time Trends in Primary HIV-1 Drug Resistance Among Recently Infected Persons

Grant RM, Hecht FM, Warmerdam M, et al (Univ of California, San Francisco; ViroLogic, South San Francisco)
JAMA 288:181-188, 2002   3–8

Introduction.—Primary HIV-1 resistance to antiretroviral therapy has been reported. The rate of multidrug resistant–HIV-1 may rise with the wider use of antiretroviral therapy. Trends in the prevalence of HIV-1 drug resistance among recently infected persons was examined in a hospital in a geographic area with a high concentration of antiviral treatment.

Methods.—A consecutive case series of 225 patients with recent HIV-1 infection referred between June 1996 and June 2001 was evaluated. Patients were assessed for genotypic resistance, defined as the presence of viral mutations associated with impaired drug susceptibility or virologic response, as specified by the International AIDS Society-USA mutations panel. Time trends in the prevalence of genotypic and phenotypic primary drug resistance were examined.

Results.—The rate of mutations associated with resistance to nonnucleoside reverse transcriptase inhibitors (NNRTIs) steadily rose from 0% in 1996 to 1997 to 13.2% (n = 12) in 2000 to 2001 ($P = .01$). One mutation was correlated with protease inhibitor resistance in 1996 to 1997 (2.5%);

there were 7 (7.7%) in 2000 to 2001 ($P = 0.25$). Genotypic resistance to nucleoside reverse transcriptase inhibitors (NRTIs) initially diminished, then returned to prior levels ($P = .007$ for test of homogeneity). Genotypic resistance to 2 or more classes of drugs rose from 1 (2.5%) to 12 (13.2%) ($P = .004$). Only 1 infection (1.2%) in the latter period was resistant to all 3 classes of agents ($P = .58$). Primary phenotypic resistance for NRTIs dropped from 21% to 6.2% ($P = .03$) and rose for NNRTIs from 0 to 8 (9.9%) ($P = .02$). Phenotypic resistance rose for protease inhibitors from 2.6% to 6.2% ($P = .32$). The median time to virologic suppression (<500 copies/mL) during treatment was 12 weeks for patients with genotypic evidence of resistance compared with 5 weeks for patients with drug-sensitive infections ($P = .02$).

Conclusion.—The frequency of primary resistance to NNRTIs in increasing, although resistance to all available classes of antiretroviral therapy continues to occur rarely. Genotypic resistance testing in recently infected persons may be used to predict time to viral suppression during therapy.

▶ It's been clear from the start that the high mutability of HIV-1 predisposes to drug resistance during its chemotherapy.[1] The problem has been complicated by the development of 3 classes of therapeutic agents, each capable of inactivation by 3 series of different mutational sites in the virus. The first class of agents, NRTIs, which block transcription of DNA from RNA and the reverse, act by incorporation of an synthetic nucleoside, a base-sugar-phosphoric acid complex, into the DNA chain to be replicated and disrupt the sequence of the incorporating DNA strand. Examples are zidovudine, lamivadine, and abacavir. NNRTIs disrupt the catalytic site for both RNA and DNA incorporation of the reverse transcriptase enzyme and inactivate several other DNA polymerases as well (eg, abacavir and nevirapine). Protease inhibitors block the enzymatic steps necessary for virion capsule formation and therefore virus replication. Examples are amprenavir, saquinavir, and indinavir.

This is a study of 141 patients with acute recent HIV-1 infection, most with 2 or more sets of symptoms, supported by laboratory evidence of HIV-1-RNA in blood, Western blots positive for HIV-1 antibody, or positive enzyme immunoassay together with positive Western blot. Individuals receiving antiretrovirals for more than 7 days prior to contact were excluded from the study. Patients were followed through three 2-year intervals from 1996 to 2001. Drug resistance was characterized by genotypic identity of any of a series of 8 mutational sites for NRTIs, 5 sites for NNRTIs, or 4 sites for protease inhibitors. Phenotypic analysis of drug resistance was accomplished through measurements of CD4 cell counts, HIV-1-RNA copy numbers per unit of blood volume, or a 50% increase in the concentration of an agent necessary to inhibit replication of the viral strain in vitro. A common pattern for drug resistance was an increase in RNA copy numbers with preservation of near normal CD4 cell counts together with clinical progression, often substantially delayed past the point of treatment. Genotypic evidence of resistance appeared in 23.1% of all individuals but varied by drug type. Over the time of the study, NRTI agent resistance decreased from 25% from 1996 to 1997 to 7.4% from 1998 to 1999 to 20.9% from 2000 to 2001, reflecting, perhaps, the decreased use of NRTI as evidence that NNRTI agents were as effective as protease inhibitors in decreasing HIV-1-RNA copy numbers and symptoms.[2] NNRTI drug resistance increased rapidly from 0% to 15% in the 6 years they were available, while resistance of protease inhibitors was relatively consistent throughout, ranging from 2.6% to 6.2% over 6 years. The drug resistance problem is destined to worsen with time and highlights the need for effective counseling to maintain the drug compliance so important in preventing drug resistance and drug adjustment to improve patient tolerance to side effects.

T. H. Kirschbaum, MD

References

1. 2003 YEAR BOOK OF OBSTETRICS, GYNECOLOGY, AND WOMEN'S HEALTH, p 64.
2. Staszewski S, Morales-Ramirez J, Tashima KT, et al: Treatment of HIV infection in adults. *N Engl J Med* 341:1865-1873, 1999.

Antiretroviral-Drug Resistance Among Patients Recently Infected With HIV

Little SJ, Holte S, Routy J-P, et al (Univ of California, San Diego; Univ of Washington, Seattle; McGill Univ, Montreal; et al)

N Engl J Med 347:385-394, 2002   3–9

Introduction.—Potent antiretroviral therapy reduces morbidity and mortality in patients with HIV-1 infection, but transmission of drug-resistant virus limits the response to treatment in an estimated 1% to 11% of patients. A cohort of treatment-naive patients with primary HIV infection was studied retrospectively for the prevalence of transmitted drug-resistant virus. The association between baseline susceptibility to anti-HIV drugs and the virologic response to therapy was also examined.

Methods.—Study subjects had been referred to programs in 10 North American cities between May 1995 and June 2000. The response to treatment could be evaluated in 202 of 377 patients identified with early HIV infection. A pretreatment plasma sample was obtained in all cases and analyzed for drug susceptibility. The choice of initial regimen was based on the protocols of clinical studies or the standard of care.

Results.—Patients were predominantly non-Hispanic white men whose risk factor for HIV infection was having had sex with men. Baseline antiretroviral-susceptibility testing was performed a median of 71 days after the estimated date of HIV infection; the potent antiretroviral regimen was started at a median of 97 days after this date. The frequency of transmitted drug resistance increased significantly over the 5-year period, from 3.4% during the years from 1995 to 1998 to 12.4% in the 1999 to 2000 period (Fig 1B). Multidrug resistance increased from 1.1% to 6.2%, and a significant increase was seen in the frequency of resistant mutations detected by sequence analysis (from 8.0% to 22.7%). Patients who were infected with drug-resistant virus had a longer time to viral suppression after antiretroviral therapy was started and a shorter time to virologic failure (Fig 2A).

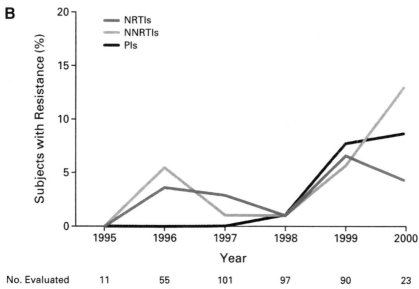

No. Evaluated   11   55   101   97   90   23

FIGURE 1B.—Changes in the prevalence of reduced drug susceptibility over time and according to drug class. The 50% inhibitory concentration (IC_{50}) ratio is the ratio of the IC_{50} for the subject's virus to the IC_{50} for a drug-sensitive reference virus. Panel **B** shows the percentages of subjects identified each year with an IC_{50} ratio of more than 10 for 1 or more nucleoside reverse-transcriptase inhibitors (*NRTIs*), nonnucleoside reverse-transcriptase inhibitors (*NNRTIs*), or protease inhibitors (*PIs*). The Mantel-Haenszel χ^{-2} test was used to evaluate the probability that observed changes were significant during the period of study. (Reprinted by permission of *The New England Journal of Medicine* from Little SJ, Holte S, Routy J-P, et al: Antiretroviral-drug resistance among patients recently infected with HIV. *N Engl J Med* 347:385-394. Copyright 2002, Massachusetts Medical Society. All rights reserved.)

Conclusion.—An increase has been seen in the proportion of new HIV infections involving drug-resistant virus in North America. Patients with a drug-resistant virus are more likely to fail to respond to initial antiretroviral therapy. These findings have important implications for prevention and treatment strategies.

▶ It's been known for about a decade that use of highly effective antiretroviral therapy is associated with viral selection and the appearance of mutations, which result in relative drug resistance. This retrospective cohort study of 377 primary acute infections gives a clear look at the size and impact of the problem and its rate of change. Patients were selected who showed positive HIV-RNA or P24 antigen in blood prior to HIV-1 antibody conversion or who showed recent seroconversion. In some cases, the duration of the infection was estimated from records of serial Western blots. Persons with prior therapy or HIV-RNA copy numbers less than 400/mL were excluded from study. Time to viral suppression was defined as the time from the onset of therapy to the reduction of HIV-RNA copy numbers to less than 500/mL of plasma. Drug susceptibility to an agent was defined by the concentration of agent required for 50% inhibition of viral growth in vitro divided by the concentration needed for 50% inhibition of a known susceptible virus. When the new viral culture showed 10

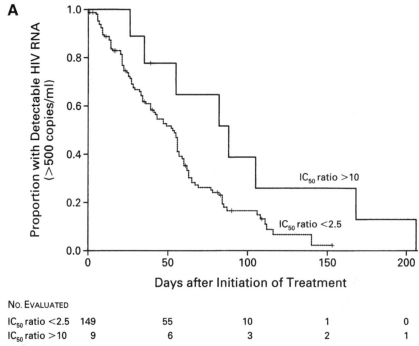

No. Evaluated

IC$_{50}$ ratio <2.5	149	55	10	1	0
IC$_{50}$ ratio >10	9	6	3	2	1

FIGURE 2A.—Kaplan-Meier estimates of the time to viral suppression and subsequent virologic failure relative to baseline drug susceptibility. The time from the initiation of antiretroviral therapy to viral suppression was shorter for subjects with drug-susceptible viral isolates at baseline (a value <2.5 of the 50% inhibitory concentration [IC$_{50}$] for the subject's virus to the IC$_{50}$ for a reference virus) than for subjects with an IC$_{50}$ ratio of more than 10 for one or more antiretroviral drugs ($P = .05$) (panel A). (Reprinted by permission of *The New England Journal of Medicine* from Little SJ, Holte S, Routy J-P, et al: Antiretroviral-drug resistance among patients recently infected with HIV. *N Engl J Med* 347:385-394. Copyright 2002, Massachusetts Medical Society. All rights reserved.).

times more drug concentration needed than for the reference virus, it was deemed to have lost susceptibility to drug. Data were segregated for patients seen from 1995 to 1998 (period 1) and those seen from 1999 to 2000 (period 2). On the basis of phenotypic studies, viral susceptibility, and time to suppression, that is, less than 500 RNA copies per milliliter, viral resistance occurred in 6.1% of the patients, 3.4% in period 1 and 12.4% in period 2. Based on identification of genotype mutations known to be associated with viral drug resistance, they were found in12% in primary cases, 8% in period 1 and 22.7% in period 2. Despite the increasing drug resistance, only 1 case (0.3%), failed viral suppression after 24 weeks of therapy as defined. Time between onset of therapy and viral suppression was shorter and time to uncontrolled viral copy numbers was longer with virus with reduced susceptibility.

This study reveals viral drug resistance to be a progressively more common complication, perhaps accelerating with time, with clinical implications at least so far manageable. There seems to be no difference between the effects of nucleoside or nonnucleoside retroviral transcriptase inhibitors or protease inhibitors.

In an editorial comment on the same issue, Dr Martin Hirsch points to the relationship between suboptimal compliance with treatment programs and increased viral resistance. He believes that drug resistance testing should now be increasingly available and employed as part of all optimal therapy for HIV infections, especially important for those with opportunistic infections, pregnancy, or prior failed therapy. Just as with bacterial infection therapeutics, our hope is that new drugs and drug combinations will enable control of this threat that looms in the future.

T. H. Kirschbaum, MD

A Multicenter Randomized Controlled Trial of Nevirapine Versus a Combination of Zidovudine and Lamivudine to Reduce Intrapartum and Early Postpartum Mother-to-Child Transmission of Human Immunodeficiency Virus Type 1

Moodley D, for the South African Intrapartum Nevirapine Trial (SAINT) Investigators (Univ of Natal, KwaZulu Natal, South Africa; et al)

J Infect Dis 187:725-735, 2003   3–10

Background.—The report in 1994 that a long, complex regimen of zidovudine would reduce mother-to-child transmission of HIV type 1 (HIV-1) prompted an ongoing search for a practical and effective short-course antiretroviral regimen for the prevention of mother-to-child transmission of HIV-1 in developing countries. Most mother-to-child transmission occurs during labor and delivery (intrapartum) and after delivery through breast-feeding (postpartum). Antiretroviral regimens administered in the last 4 weeks of pregnancy have cut the rates of mother-to-child transmission in half in non–breast-feeding populations. This study assessed the efficacy and safety of 2 inexpensive and easily deliverable antiretroviral regimens for the prevention of mother-to-child transmission of HIV-1 during labor and delivery.

Methods.—Pregnant women infected with HIV-1 were screened at 11 maternity health institutions in South Africa and enrolled in an open-label, short-course antiretroviral regimen of either nevirapine (Nvp) or multiple-dose zidovudine and lamivudine (Zdv/3TC) (Fig 2).

Results.—A total of 1331 infants were born to 1317 women enrolled in the study. The overall estimated HIV-1 infection rates by 8 weeks were 12.3% for Nvp and 9.3% for Zdv/3TC. After exclusion of infections detected within 72 hours (intrauterine infections), new HIV-1 infections were detected in 5.7% and 3.6% of infants in the Nvp and Zdv/3TC groups, respectively, in the 8 weeks after birth (Table 2). No drug-related maternal or pediatric serious adverse events occurred. The most frequent complications were obstetrical in mothers (24.3% in the Nvp group and 26.3% in the Zdv/3TC group) and respiratory in infants (16.1% in the Nvp group and 17% in the Adv/3TC group) (Table 3).

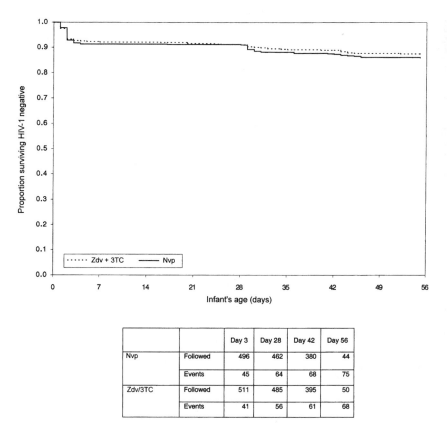

		Day 3	Day 28	Day 42	Day 56
Nvp	Followed	496	462	380	44
	Events	45	64	68	75
Zdv/3TC	Followed	511	485	395	50
	Events	41	56	61	68

FIGURE 2.—Kaplan-Meier estimates of HIV-type 1–free survival through 8 weeks. *Abbreviations: Nvp*, Nevirapine; *Zdv*, zidovudine; *3TC*, lamivudine. (Courtesy of Moodley D, for the South African Intrapartum Nevirapine Trial (SAINT) Investigators: A multicenter randomized controlled trial of nevirapine versus a combination of zidovudine and lamivudine to reduce intrapartum and early postpartum mother-to-child transmission of human immunodeficiency virus type 1. *J Infect Dis* 187:725-735. © 2003 by the Infectious Diseases Society of America. All rights reserved. Published by the University of Chicago.)

Conclusion.—These findings provide further evidence of the safety and efficacy of short-course antiretroviral regimens in reducing mother-to-child transmission of HIV-1 in developing countries.

▶ The release of the report of the Pediatric Aids Clinical Trial Protocol 076 demonstrated that azidothymidine (AZT) given to HIV-1–infected women for 12 weeks during pregnancy, intrapartum and postpartum, coupled with newborn therapy reduced fetal transmission of HIV-1 by two thirds. After that, the search for a less expensive option better suited to African and Asian epidemic sites was on.[1-3] When demonstration that maternal Nvp, 200 mg, at the onset of labor and neonatal administration within the first 72 hours of life reduced fetal infection rates to 8.2% at birth at a cost of $4 compared to an estimated cost of $48,000.00 per pregnancy using the 076 protocol as initially proposed, Nvp appeared to be a partial solution.[4] If an HIV-1–positive women nurses her

TABLE 2.—Rates of Infant HIV Type 1 Infections by 4 Weeks and From 4 to 8 Weeks in Mother-Infant Pairs Given Either Nevirapine or Zidovudine and Lamivudine

Timing of Transmission	Nvp Observed for Time Interval*	Nvp Kaplan-Meier Infection Rate/ 100 Infants	Zdv/3TC Observed for Time Interval*	Zdv/3TC Kaplan-Meier Infection Rate/ 100 Infants	Difference/ 100 Infants
Intrauterine Positive PCR result at birth	45	7.0 (5.0-9.0)	38	5.9 (4.1-7.7)	1.1 (−1.6-3.8)
Intrapartum Positive PCR result 4 weeks after birth	18	10.4 (7.9-12.8)	11	7.9 (5.8-10.1)	2.4 (−0.8-5.7)
Early postpartum Positive PCR result 4-8 weeks after birth	10	12.3 (9.7-15.0)	7	9.3 (7.0-11.6)	3.0 (−0.5-6.6)
Intrapartum, early postpartum Positive PCR result 8 weeks after birth	28	5.7 (3.7-7.8)	18	3.6 (2.0-5.3)	2.1

Note: Data are percentage (95% confidence interval), unless otherwise indicated.
*Data are no. of observed infections are new HIV-1 infections defined as positive by HIV-1 DNA/RNA polymerase chain reaction analysis at birth and/or positive DNA polymerase chain reaction result at subsequent visits.
Abbreviations: Nvp, Nevirapine; Zdv/3TC, zidovudine and lamivudine.
(Courtesy of Moodley D, for the South African Intrapartum Nevirapine Trial (SAINT) Investigators: A multicenter randomized controlled trial of nevirapine versus a combination of zidovudine and lamivudine to reduce intrapartum and early postpartum mother-to-child transmission of human immunodeficiency virus type 1. J Infect Dis 187:725-735. © 2003 by the Infectious Diseases Society of America. All rights reserved. Published by the University of Chicago.)

newborn, it increases the risk of perinatal infection by about 14% and the cultural, microbiological, and economic factors that motivate nursing in third world countries remain a serious problem.[5]

Subsequently the PETRA study using AZT and lamivudine, beginning at 36 weeks of pregnancy through 7 days post partum, demonstrated reduced fetal transmission through 3 months of life but a loss of protection by 18 months, due apparently to the impact of nursing.[6] Nvp, however, proved to have longer lasting effects in reducing infant transmission through nursing in comparison.[7]

This is an important next step in the evaluation of Nvp therapy when a multicenter, randomized but unblinded case comparison between its single dose intrapartum and postpartum use is compared with the augmented AZT protocol beginning at 36 weeks as in the PETRA study.[8] The 2 approaches were compared with respect to rates of fetal transmission, clinical complications, and markers of infection. Because of the controversial role of cesarean section in infant HIV transmission, such women were excluded from the study.

There were approximately 500 women in each arm of the study, 470 with complete data including 68-week infant follow-up. The mean HIV-1 RNA copy number per milliliter was slightly higher in those receiving the Nvp than the AZT group. Results based on indicators of infection in cord blood and intrapartum and early postpartum maternal blood evaluation showed no significant difference between the 2 groups (see Table 2). Similarly, no significant differences were noted in clinical complications (see Table 3).

TABLE 3.—Adverse Events of Clinical Importance Occurring in Trial Participants

Events	Zdv/3TC	Nvp	Total
Maternal	662	655	1317
Deaths*	4 (0.6)	5 (0.8)	9 (0.7)
Obstetrical procedures	174 (26.3)	159 (24.3)	333 (25.3)
Rash	5 (0.8)	4 (0.6)	9 (0.7)
Cesarean section	208 (31.4)	182 (27.8)	390 (29.6)
Prolonged labor	129	119	248
Fetal compromise	63	50	113
Other indications	16	13	29
Infant	666	663	1329
Respiratory disorders	113 (17.0)	107 (16.1)	220 (16.6)
Infections	60 (9.0)	51 (7.7)	111 (8.4)
Serious events†	21 (3.2)	17 (2.6)	38 (2.9)
Hepatic adverse events	22 (3.3)	18 (2.7)	40 (3.0)
Neonatal jaundice	20 (3.0)	13 (2.0)	33 (2.5)
Hepatosplenomegaly	2 (0.3)	3 (0.5)	5 (0.4)
Hepatomegaly	0 (0)	1 (0.2)	1 (0.1)
Increased SGPT	0 (0)	1 (0.2)	1 (0.1)
Rash‡	17 (2.6)	10 (1.5)	27 (2.0)
Deaths§	19 (2.9)	19 (2.9)	38 (2.9)
Neonatal death	8	4	12
Diarrhea/gastroenteritis	4	6	10
Pneumonia	1	4	5
Birth aphyxia	3	1	4
Other‖	3	4	7

Note: Data are no. or no./total no. (%) of trial participants. Adverse events occurred from labor to 28 days post partum, except for deaths, which are represented from labor through 8 to 12 weeks post partum.

*Causes of maternal death in the 2 groups were as follows: Nevirapine (*Nvp*) group, unknown causes (2), meningitis (1), sudden death (1), and dyspnea (1); zidovudine and lamivudine (*Zdv/3TC*) group, sepsis (2), pulmonary tuberculosis (1), and cerebral vascular accident (1).

†Serious adverse events of infection are a subset of all adverse events of infection.

‡Skin rashes that occurred in 2 participants in the Nvp group and 2 in the Zdv/3TC group were determined by the investigators to be treatment related.

§In addition, there were 2 stillbirths reported in this study (Zdv/3TC group). Of the 38 reported deaths, 18 occurred among infants who were positive for HIV type 1 (4 in the Zdv/3TC group and 14 in the Nvp group).

‖"Other" includes septicemia (1 in the Zdv/3TC group and 2 in the Nvp group), congenital heart disease (1 in the Nvp group), and intracranial hemorrhage (1 in the Zdv/3TC group).

Abbreviaiton: SGPT, Serum glutamic pyruvic transaminase.

(Courtesy of Moodley D, for the South African Intrapartum Nevirapine Trial (SAINT) Investigators: A multicenter randomized controlled trial of nevirapine versus a combination of zidovudine and lamivudine to reduce intrapartum and early postpartum mother-to-child transmission of human immunodeficiency virus type 1. *J Infect Dis* 187:725-735. © 2003 by the Infectious Diseases Society of America. All rights reserved. Published by the University of Chicago.)

In brief, both modes of therapy proved to be safe and efficient though the Nvp approach was the simpler. Marketing and other factors have reduced the cost differential to $3 for the Nvp and $41 for the PETRA approach. Members of the study group raise cautions regarding the role of cesarean section in reducing transmission further because of the high incidence of cesarean section for obstructed, prolonged, and infected labor in Africa and the high incidence of postpartum infection. On balance, at this point, the Nvp alternative seems at least as good as the PETRA mode of prevention of infant infection and may prove to be more valuable with time.

T. H. Kirschbaum, MD

References

1. 1995 Year Book of Obstetrics, Gynecology, and Women's Health, pp 76-77.

2. 1996 YEAR BOOK OF OBSTETRICS, GYNECOLOGY, AND WOMEN'S HEALTH, pp 84-85.
3. 1997 YEAR BOOK OF OBSTETRICS, GYNECOLOGY, AND WOMEN'S HEALTH, pp 84-86.
4. 2001 YEAR BOOK OF OBSTETRICS, GYNECOLOGY, AND WOMEN'S HEALTH, pp 87-89.
5. 2001 YEAR BOOK OF OBSTETRICS, GYNECOLOGY, AND WOMEN'S HEALTH, pp 97-98.
6. 2003 YEAR BOOK OF OBSTETRICS, GYNECOLOGY, AND WOMEN'S HEALTH, pp 65-70.
7. 2001 YEAR BOOK OF OBSTETRICS, GYNECOLOGY, AND WOMEN'S HEALTH, pp 87-90.
8. 2003 YEAR BOOK OF OBSTETRICS, GYNECOLOGY, AND WOMEN'S HEALTH, pp 65-70.

Two-Dose Intrapartum/Newborn Nevirapine and Standard Antiretroviral Therapy to Reduce Perinatal HIV Transmission: A Randomized Trial

Cunningham CK, for the International PACTG 316 Team (Univ of California, San Francisco; et al)

JAMA 288:189-198, 2002   3–11

Introduction.—A 2-dose intrapartum/newborn nevirapine regimen has been shown to decrease perinatal HIV transmission in Ugandan women not receiving antenatal anteretroviral therapy (ART). It is not known if a 2-dose, nevirapine regimen can reduce the perinatal transmission of HIV in non-breast-feeding women undergoing standard ART. This combined therapy was evaluated in 1270 women between May 1997 and June 2000 in an international, blinded, placebo-controlled, phase III trial providing care for HIV infection throughout the United States, Europe, Brazil, and the Bahamas.

Methods.—Women receiving standard ART were randomly assigned to additionally receive either nevirapine 200 mg or placebo (642 and 628 patients, respectively) after onset of labor and a 2-mg/kg dose of oral nevirapine; a dose was administered to their newborns between 48 and 72 hours after birth. Infants were monitored for 6 months to ascertain HIV status; information was available for 1248 deliveries. The primary outcome measures were identification of HIV infection in infants and grade 3/4 toxic effects in women and newborns.

Results.—The trial was stopped early by the data and safety board because the overall transmission rates were significantly lower than assumed for the study design. The antenatal ART regimen included zidovudine alone in 23% of patients, combinations without protease inhibitors in 36%, and combinations with protease inhibitors in 41%. Elective cesarean delivery was performed in 345. No significant safety concerns were observed in mothers or infants. HIV was identified in 9 (1.4%; 95% confidence interval [CI], 0.6%-2.7%) of 631 nevirapine group deliveries and 10 (1.6%; 95% CI, 0.8%-2.9%) of 617 placebo group deliveries. The 95% CI for the difference in transmission rate (−0.2) between the 2 study arms ranged from −1.5% in favor of nevirapine versus 1.2% in favor of placebo ($P = 0.82$). The transmission rate was higher in women with lower baseline CD4 cell counts and higher delivery HIV RNA levels. There were no statistically significant differences between treatment arms in any subgroup.

Conclusion.—The risk of perinatal HIV transmission was low. No additional benefit was afforded from the addition of intrapartum/newborn nevirapine when women received prenatal care, antenatal ART, and elective cesarean was available.

▶ This is the report of the Pediatric AIDS Clinical Child Group 316, an international multicenter, randomized, double-blind study including 67 sites designed to test whether maternal use of nevirapine 200 mg orally during active labor and parenteral nevirapine in dose of 2 mg/kg given to the infant within 72 hours of life[1] offers any additional benefits to woman receiving the standard zidovudine regimen. This latter regimen consists of zidovudine given antepartum and intrapartum plus 1 mg/kg given to the infant 1 hour after birth in accordance with the protocol PACTG 076.[2]

The former abbreviated dosage given alone in the HIV NET 012 trial reduced infant transmission rates from 25.1% to 13.1%, while the latter standard zidovudine regimen 076 resulted in transmission rates from 5% to 8%.

This study reports 642 women receiving nevirapine and 628 placebo controls, all 1270 women receiving zidovudine as per PACTG 076. The entry requirements were age at least 13 years with gestational age at least 20 weeks.

Nevirapine dosage was accomplished in 92% of gravidas and 98% of infants. At the time of entry, those likely to produce infected infants (CD4 cells less than 200 per mm^3, HIV-1-RNA greater than 10,000 copies per milliliter) constituted 11% to 12% in the treatment and control groups. An additional agent used in this series was protease inhibitors, used in 41% of women, and use of elective cesarean section in 34%, more often in European than American sites. The incidence of preterm birth was 19%, the same with or without protease inhibitors. The maternal-to-fetal transmission rate was 1.6% in the zidovudine group 016 recipients and 1.4% of those receiving nevirapine, as per the 076 protocol, a statistically insignificant difference. Severe drug toxicity was rare and there were 8 infant deaths, only 1 of them HIV positive. The decrease in transfer rates in the zidovudine recipients compared with earlier studies probably reflects use of protease inhibitors.

This study provides proof that protease inhibitors do not increase preterm birth rates and sets a new standard for treatment of HIV-infected gravidas and reduction of maternal-to-fetal HIV transfer rates.

T. H. Kirschbaum, MD

References

1. 2001 YEAR BOOK OF OBSTETRICS, GYNECOLOGY, AND WOMEN'S HEALTH, pp 87-89.
2. 1996 YEAR BOOK OF OBSTETRICS, GYNECOLOGY, AND WOMEN'S HEALTH, pp 84-85.

Ureteroscopy and Holmium:YAG Laser Lithotripsy: An Emerging Definitive Management Strategy for Symptomatic Ureteral Calculi in Pregnancy

Watterson JD, Girvan AR, Beiko DT, et al (Univ of Western Ontario, London, Canada; Univ of Alberta, Edmonton, Canada)
Urology 60:383-387, 2002   3–12

Background.—Urolithiasis can usually be managed conservatively during pregnancy, but in those patients for whom conservative treatment fails, either percutaneous nephrostomy (PCN) or ureteral stenting has been employed. These treatment options have associated morbidity risks and do not provide definitive stone management. Holmium laser lithotripsy is a newer treatment option that can safely fragment calculi. The use of holmium: yttrium-aluminum-garnet (YAG) laser lithotripsy in the treatment of pregnant patients with urolithiasis is described.

Study Design.—A chart review was conducted at 2 tertiary stone centers from January 1996 to August 2001 and identified 8 patients with 10 symptomatic calculi and 2 encrusted stents who were treated with ureteroscopic holmium laser lithotripsy during pregnancy. The average age of these patients was 29 years, and the mean gestational age was 22 weeks. The overall average stone size was 8.1 mm. The results of treatment of these patients with holmium:YAG laser lithotripsy were reviewed.

Findings.—Stone fragmentation or stent removal was accomplished in all patients with holmium:YAG laser lithotripsy. The overall procedure success rate was 91%, and the overall stone-free rate was 89%. There were no urologic or obstetric complications. All patients delivered at term without adverse fetal outcomes.

Conclusions.—Ureteroscopy combined with holmium:YAG laser lithotripsy is a safe and effective treatment for pregnant patients with symptomatic calculi that do not respond to conservative management. This treatment method avoids the undesirable features and risks associated with either ureteral stents or nephrostomy tubes and provides definitive management with minimal risk to either mother of fetus.

▶ Perhaps because of the dilation of the urinary collecting system during pregnancy, nephroureterolithiasis relatively rarely causes serious problems. Approximately 70% to 80% of pregnant women with urinary stones pass them spontaneously. When that's not the case, however, and urinary obstruction or recurrent infection complicates the picture. Use of nephrostomy, ureteral stenting, and rarely surgical ureterotomy may be necessary but are fraught with serious management problems. The use of the holmium:YAG laser coupled with fiberoptic ureteroscopy for lithotripsy in situ offers real advantages. The procedure, introduced in the mid-1990s, has been well reported in men and nonpregnant women.[1] This is the authors' first report of its use in 8 pregnant women.

Development of the technique rests on improvements in flexible fiberoptical systems and miniaturization, which would allow a 2-lumen tube of 6.9

to 7.5F diameter to be employed for urethral catherization, avoiding the need for urethral orifice dilation in all but 4% of the nonpregnant group cited. Holmium, a rare earth element, when incorporated in the yttrium-aluminum-garnet crystal (hence YAG) yields a laser ouput with a wavelength of approximately 2100 Ångstroms, enabling the near infrared laser light impulse to be transmitted through silica quartz fibers with relatively little energy loss. Energy dissipation at the fiberoptic tip extends no further than 0.5 mm, allowing the incision and fragmentation of calculi of any chemical composition with precision and safety in a liquid medium.

In the article by Sofer et al,[1] calculi averaging 11.3 mm in diameter were reduced to 2- to 3-mm fragments, which then passed the urinary tract spontaneously. In 598 patients, one third of them women, 97% were rendered stone free, 94% after a single procedure, with an 84% success rate for stones in the renal pelvis. Complications were noted in 4%, only 4 related solely to the lithotripsy itself. Here in 8 gravidas ranging from 10 to 35 weeks' gestational age, 91% were rendered stone free, 89% on the first attempt, without complications noted in either fetus or mother. This contribution from the University of Western Ontario may well change our approach to the management of this uncommon but potentially grave complication of pregnancy.

T. H. Kirschbaum, MD

Reference

1. Sofer M, Watterson JD, Wollin TA, et al: Holmium:YAG laser lithotripsy for upper urinary tract calculi in 598 patients. *J Urol* 167:31, 2002.

Pregnancy in Women Who Undergo Long-term Hemodialysis
Chao A-S, Huang J-Y, Lien R, et al (Chang Gung Mem Hosp, Tao-Yuan, Taiwan; Chang Gung Children's Hosp, Tao-Yuan, Taiwan)
Am J Obstet Gynecol 187:152-156, 2002   3–13

Background.—Pregnancy is risky in women requiring long-term hemodialysis. The management of pregnancy in 1 series of women undergoing long-term hemodialysis was reported.

Method.—Data on 18 pregnancies occurring in 15 patients undergoing hemodialysis between 1990 and 2000 were analyzed. The mean duration of hemodialysis before pregnancy was 5.3 years for all but 1 woman, who began hemodialysis at 16 weeks' gestation. In almost all patients, hemodialysis was delivered by a high-flux dialyzer with volume-controlled ultrafiltration. During pregnancy, the hemodialysis schedule was increased to 4 hours 4 to 6 times a week. The blood flow rate was 250 to 300 mL/min, and the dialysate flow, 500 to 600 mL/min.

Findings.—Five of the 18 pregnancies were terminated electively. The remaining 13 pregnancies resulted in 12 live births. Nine of these infants survived. One fetus died in utero, and 3 infants died in the neonatal period. There were no fetal anomalies. The mean gestational age at delivery was 32 weeks, ranging from 23 to 36 weeks. Newborn weights ranged from 512 to

1660 g. Intrauterine growth restriction occurred in 7 of the 9 survivors. Treatment for anemia with recombinant human erythropoietin or transfusion, or both, was needed in all patients. During 13 pregnancies, increased blood pressure developed in all the women, 7 of whom required antihypertensive drugs. Six of the 9 surviving infants had polyhydramnios, which was partially relieved after hemodialysis. Six of 13 deliveries were cesarean. After delivery, all women returned to prepregnancy dialysis therapy levels.

Conclusions.—Advances in dialysis, obstetrics, and neonatal care have improved the success rates of pregnancy in women requiring long-term hemodialysis. The current patient series had a success rate of 60%.

▶ Though there is abundant evidence for reproductive efficiency after allograft renal transplant[1,2] and for a low incidence of transplant deterioration during pregnancy,[3] there is little current information regarding the outcomes for the roughly 2% of women undergoing chronic renal dialysis who conceive. The largest experience reported 115 such pregnancies,[4] with a 23% pregnancy viability rate. Though based on a smaller population sample, this experience of 18 pregnancies in 15 women on chronic dialysis points out a somewhat more favorable picture. Five pregnancies were terminated by therapeutic abortion, perhaps a reflection of the reported low success rates published 20 years earlier. In the remaining 13 women, there was 1 fetal death and all but 1 conceived after beginning dialysis on average 5.3 years after the onset of recognition of uremia-bearing mean serum urea concentrations of 65 mg/dL and hemoglobin levels of 7.2 g/dL. Of the 12 live births (67%), there were 9 surviving infants, or 50%. The usual complications were seen among the mothers: that is, pregnancy hypertension, polyhydramnios, preterm rupture of membranes, growth retardation, and preterm labor. It appears that the availability of recombinant erythropoietin in uremic gravidas and advances in prenatal care over the past 25 years have brightened the prospects for reproduction in such women.

T. H. Kirschbaum, MD

References

1. 1994 Year Book of Obstetrics, Gynecology, and Women's Health, pp 113-115.
2. 2000 Year Book of Obstetrics, Gynecology, and Women's Health, pp 151-152.
3. 1995 Year Book of Obstetrics, Gynecology, and Women's Health, pp 97-98.
4. Successful pregnancies in women treated by dialysis and kidney transplantation. Report from the Registration Committee of the European Dialysis and Transplant Association. *Br J Obstet Gynaecol* 87:839-845, 1980.

Pregnancy Outcome of Female Survivors of Childhood Cancer: A Report From the Childhood Cancer Survivor Study

Green DM, Whitton JA, Stovall M, et al (State Univ of New York, Buffalo; Fred Hutchinson Cancer Research Ctr, Seattle; Children's Hosp and Regional Med Ctr, Houston; et al)

Am J Obstet Gynecol 187:1070-1080, 2002   3–14

Background.—Children and adolescents who are successfully treated for cancer may have subsequent adverse reproductive sequelae. The effect of prior treatment for childhood cancer on a woman's pregnancy outcome was investigated.

Methods.—The study group included 1915 women, less than 21 years old at cancer diagnosis, who participated in the Childhood Cancer Survivor Study (CCSS) and reported being pregnant. They answered a questionnaire about their pregnancy. Information on their previous cancer treatment was available from medical records. The proximity of the ovaries to the radiation field was also noted. Questionnaires were also sent to siblings of study participants to serve as control answers.

Findings.—Among the 1915 women, 4029 pregnancies were reported: live births, 63%; stillbirths, 1%; miscarriages, 15%; abortions, 17%; and unknown, 3%; or in gestation. No significant differences were noted in pregnancy outcome by treatment. The neonates of those treated with pelvic irradiation were more likely to have low birth weight (Figs 1 and 2).

Conclusions.—Childhood chemotherapy does not appear to effect subsequent pregnancy of adult survivors. A small, but significant, adverse affect of prior pelvic irradiation was noted on birth weight.

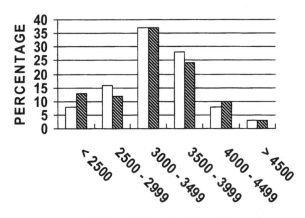

BIRTHWEIGHT (GRAMS)

FIGURE 1.—Distribution of birth weight by treatment with (*hatched*) or without (*solid*) pelvic radiation therapy. (Reprinted by permission of the publisher courtesy of Green DM, Whitton JA, Stovall M, et al: Pregnancy outcome of female survivors of childhood cancer: A report from the Childhood Cancer Survivor Study *Am J Obstet Gynecol* 187:1070-1080. Copyright 2002 by Elsevier.)

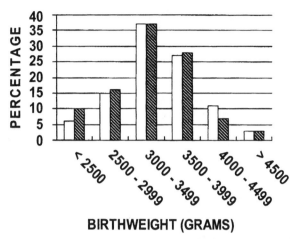

BIRTHWEIGHT (GRAMS)

FIGURE 2.—Distribution of birth weight by treatment with (*hatched*) or without (*solid*) nonalkylating agent chemotherapy. (Reprinted by permission of the publisher courtesy of Green DM, Whitton JA, Stovall M, et al: Pregnancy outcome of female survivors of childhood cancer: A report from the Childhood Cancer Survivor Study *Am J Obstet Gynecol* 187:1070-1080. Copyright 2002 by Elsevier.)

▶ Treatment of pregnant women with chemotherapy for malignant disease has few if any acute adverse affects on pregnancy outcome and fetal development, provided it is begun after the first trimester is completed. X-ray therapy may or may not influence the outcome of subsequent pregnancy, depending on dosage and pelvic field exposure. This study, the collaboration of 6 cancer therapy centers, has for 17 years identified 1915 women treated with chemotherapy or x-ray therapy for malignant disease, resulting in 4029 subsequent pregnancies, 95% at or prior to maternal age 35. This large number of cases allows evaluations to be made regarding combinations of therapy, types of chemotherapeutic agents, and degrees of pelvic field x-ray exposure on long-term pregnancy outcomes in their subsequent pregnancies. Outcome variables studied were the incidence of fetal death, preterm birth, live birth, and induced abortion compared with the outcomes of pregnant women, age specific, not treated for cancer. Results were expressed in risk ratios using both uni- and multi-variate analysis.

There was a significant surplus of therapeutic abortion experience among women treated for cancer during their ages of 21 to 25 years. On univariate analysis of all patients treated for malignant disease aggregated, the risk ratio for normal pregnancy outcomes were lower than controls. Multivariate analysis was used to control for variable birth number, maternal age, education, smoking, and drinking. Those treated with chemotherapy showed no decrease in the incidence of live births, no increase in fetal deaths or abortion as a consequence (see Fig 2). With radiation directed to the pelvis or through fields less than 5 cm distant from the pelvis, there is an increased risk of birth weight less than 2.5 kg (see Fig 1), which is relatively minor and did not appear otherwise to influence pregnancy outcome. Data comparing 11 chemotherapeutic agents are included with this article and may be of interest to some readers. Generally, the results support the contention that chemotherapy does not adversely affect subsequent pregnancy outcome, provided it is given after the first trimester and that x-ray therapy insufficient to destroy ovarian function leads only to growth retardation as a possible long-term consequence.

T. H. Kirschbaum, MD

A Comparison of Magnesium Sulfate and Nimodipine for the Prevention of Eclampsia

Belfort MA, for the Nimodipine Study Group (Univ of Utah, Salt Lake City; et al)

N Engl J Med 348:304-311, 2003   3–15

Objective.—Magnesium sulfate has been shown to be effective in preventing eclampsia in women with preeclampsia, perhaps by decreasing cerebral vasospasm and ischemia. As a specific cerebral vasodilator, the calcium channel–blocking agent, nimodipine, might be effective as well. Magnesium sulfate and nimodipine were compared for prevention of eclampsia.

Methods.—The randomized, nonblinded trial included 1650 women at 14 centers with severe preeclampsia. One group received oral nimodipine, 60 mg every 4 hours, while the other received IV magnesium sulfate given according to the protocol of the participating institution. Treatment continued until 24 hours post partum, with IV hydralazine given to control high blood pressure if necessary. The study definition of eclampsia was a witnessed tonic-clonic seizure.

Results.—The mean patient age was 25 years; about 40% of patients were black. Seizures occurred in 2.6% of women receiving nimodipine compared with 0.8% of those receiving magnesium sulfate. Thus, nimodipine was associated with approximately a 3-fold increase in the risk of eclampsia. The nimodipine group also had a higher rate of antepartum seizures (1.1% vs 0%); however, this difference was nonsignificant. Neonatal outcomes were not significantly different between groups. Women receiving nimodipine were more likely to require hydralazine (54.3% vs 45.7%).

Conclusion.—For women with severe preeclampsia, magnesium sulfate is more effective than nimodipine in preventing eclampsia. As established by recent clinical trials, magnesium sulfate is the standard prophylactic treatment in this situation. The inefficacy of nimodipine is consistent with the theory that eclampsia results not from reduced cerebral blood flow, but from cerebral overperfusion.

▶ In several comparative studies, magnesium sulfate has been found to be superior to most other agents in seizure prevention and termination in hypertension disease of pregnancy.[1] There's strong evidence that magnesium sulfate acts by partially inactivating the n-methyl d-aspartate receptor which, in turn, decreases calcium flux through voltage-regulated calcium channels.[2] It's therefore possible that direct use of calcium channel blockers might be similarly effective and, despite concerns for possible fetal effects,[3-5] might be a useful replacement for seizure prophylaxis in view of its potent antihypertension effect and ease of oral administration.

This is an unblinded, randomly controlled study of women with severe preeclampsia planned for delivery in about half of the cases by cesarean section. A total of 819 women received nimodipine, 60 mg per mouth every 4 hours, and 831 received magnesium sulfate either at a dose of 6-g IV loading dose followed by 2 g per hour IV or a 4-g loading dose followed by 1 g per hour IV. The impact of the difference in magnesium sulfate dosage was not studied.

Predelivery characteristics of the 2 groups were nearly identical. The incidence of seizures during or up to 24 hours post partum was 2.6% for nimodipine and 0.8% for magnesium sulfate. The risk ratio for nimodipine versus magnesium sulfate for seizure occurrence—after adjustment for covariants such as blood pressure, age, history of prior antihypertensive agents, and systolic blood pressure greater than 180—was 3.15 times. Women receiving magnesium sulfate exhibited the usual vasomotor flushing, more often requiring hydralazine for blood pressure control and, somewhat unexpectedly, had a higher risk of postpartum hemorrhage than those with nimodipine.

Serum magnesium concentrations were not measured and that's regrettable since, in the experience of most of us, the incidence of seizures with magnesium ion concentration in the effective range is far less common than 0.8% reported here. It was a worthwhile trial but, once again, magnesium sulfate proves to be the superior eclamptic prophylatic.

T. H. Kirschbaum, MD

References

1. 1997 Year Book of Obstetrics, Gynecology, and Women's Health, pp 67-68.
2. 1998 Year Book of Obstetrics, Gynecology, and Women's Health, pp 12-13.
3. 1992 Year Book of Obstetrics, Gynecology, and Women's Health, pp 47-48.
4. 1997 Year Book of Obstetrics, Gynecology, and Women's Health, pp 41-43.
5. 1998 Year Book of Obstetrics, Gynecology, and Women's Health, pp 8-12.

Platelet Activation in the Hypertensive Disorders of Pregnancy
Harlow FH, Brown MA, Brighton TA, et al (Univ of New South Wales, Sydney, Australia)
Am J Obstet Gynecol 187:688-695, 2002   3–16

Introduction.—Platelets have an early pathogenetic role in preeclampsia. Only 2 small trials have used flow cytometry to identify the extent of platelet activation in patients with established preeclampsia. Both trials (total of 18 patients) concluded that platelet activation was significantly increased in women with proteinuric preeclampsia compared with normal pregnant women. One hundred forty women were evaluated to determine if platelet activation is enhanced by the third trimester of normal pregnancy or was exclusive to preeclampsia or occurred in other hypertensive disorders of pregnancy.

Methods.—Of the 140 patients evaluated, 30 had preeclampsia, 30 had gestational hypertension, 20 had essential hypertension in the third trimester of pregnancy, 30 were normotensive, and 30 were not pregnant. Venous blood was obtained for measures of platelet activation, as determined by flow cytometry.

Results.—Platelet activation was similar for all groups, with the exception of the preeclampsia group. Compared with normal pregnant women, those with preeclampsia had significantly greater CD62 expression (1.35% vs 0.61%; *P* = .002), CD63 expression (1.73% vs 0.95%; *P* < .0001), and annexin V binding (1.03% vs 0.66%; *P* = .03), and significantly fewer circulating platelet microparticles (33 vs 49 × 10^9/L; *P* = .001) (Fig). This was

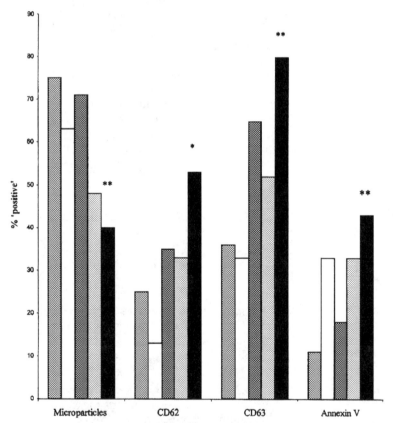

FIGURE.—Proportion of each group that had positive test results for each of the platelet activation markers. The 9 gestational women with hypertension in whom preeclampsia later developed have been excluded from these study groups. *Positive* denotes that >40 × 10^9/L microparticles or >1% surface expression of activation marker was present. Threshold values were derived from distribution of data in normal subjects. *Diamond-filled columns* denote control subjects (normal pregnant women); *dark grey columns* denote pregnant women with essential hypertension; *black columns* denote women with preeclampsia; *white columns* denote control individuals (nonpregnant women); and light grey columns denote women with gestational hypertension. *One asterisk* denotes *P* < .05; *2 asterisks* denote *P* < .01 vs nonpregnant control group. (Courtesy of Harlow FH, Brown MA, Brighton TA, et al: Platelet activation in the hypertensive disorders of pregnancy. *Am J Obstet Gynecol* 187:688-695. Copyright 2002 by Elsevier.)

not associated with other parameters, including platelet counts. Women with gestational hypertension in whom preeclampsia developed did not have platelet activation profiles.

Conclusion.—Platelet activation is increased during preeclampsia and not during other hypertensive disorders or during normal pregnancy. It may have a role in the pathophysiologic factors of preeclampsia complications. Platelet activation is not predictable by the platelet count and is not apparent in all women with preeclampsia.

▶ This study of platelet activation in pregnancy and pregnancy-induced hypertension is unusual for the large number of patients employed and its methodology. Platelet activation is important because it serves as an initial phase of interaction between platelets, endothelium, immune cells, and other leukocytes, which may, in some cases, result in altered vessel reactivity and morphology. Activation is marked by platelet budding and release of platelet microparticles, degranulation and cell surface expression of CD62 and CD63 cell selectins or adhesion molecules present in platelet secretory granules, which serve to bind platelets to leukocytes. Here, flow cytometry with fluorescein isothiocyanate beads conjugated to monoclonal antibody recognize the 2 selectin isoforms: annexin V, which is a marker for platelet expression of phosphotidyl serine, and platelet microparticles. Preeclampsia is defined here after the Australian Society for the Study of Hypertension in Pregnancy, which includes evidence of multisystem organ involvement but does not require primigravidity. The 30 women with preeclampsia showed significant increase in all 4 markers for platelet activation, whereas 9 women with gestational hypertension and 17 with essential hypertension did not. No increase in platelet activation was seen in 28 normal control gravidas compared with 30 nonpregnant controls. Not all those with preeclampsia showed platelet activation—anywhere from 40% to 80% did, but the changes were far more common in preeclampsia than in other forms of hypertension. It's important that these changes were not reflected in thrombopenia or in gross changes in platelet morphology or the quantity of activation expression. Further, they are clearly not due to hypertension per se. The reasons for platelet activation and the mechanisms involved remain obscure.

T. H. Kirschbaum, MD

Cell-Free Hemoglobin Limits Nitric Oxide Bioavailability in Sickle-Cell Disease
Reiter CD, Wang X, Tanus-Santos JE, et al (NIH, Bethesda, Md; Med College of Wisconsin, Milwaukee)
Nature Med 8:1383-1389, 2002   3–17

Background.—The deleterious vasoconstrictive effects of cell-free, hemoglobin-based blood substitutes are well described; however, the systemic effects of chronic hemolysis on nitric oxide (NO) bioavailability have not been considered or quantified. At the center of such an investigation is the understanding that NO reacts at least 1000 times more rapidly with free hemoglo-

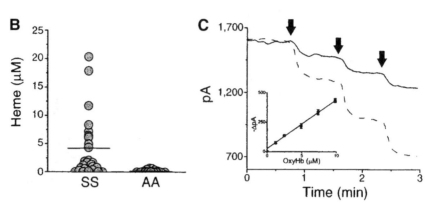

FIGURE 1.—Plasma of patients with sickle-cell disease contains elevated hemoglobin and heme and consumes micromolar concentrations of nitric oxide (NO). B, Arterial plasma collected from patients with sickle-cell disease contains on average 4.2 ±1.1 µM heme compared with 0.2 ±0.1 µM heme in plasma collected from normal volunteers (P = .004). C, Arterial plasma collected from a patient with sickle-cell disease (*dashed trace*) consumes more NO than plasma collected from a normal volunteer (*solid trace*). NO was generated in situ, which was measured using amperometrics (current in picoamperes [pA]). Plasma was added at times indicated by the *arrows*. (Courtesy of Reiter CD, Wang X, Tanus-Santos JE, et al: Cell-free hemoglobin limits nitric oxide bioavailability in sickle-cell disease. *Nature Med* 8:1383-1389, 2002.)

bin solutions than with erythrocytes. This study investigated the hypothesis that sickle-cell disease, which is characterized by high concentrations of decompartmentalized hemoglobin caused by acute and chronic hemolysis, would limit NO bioavailability as a direct result of cell-free hemoglobin-mediated NO dioxygenation and nitrosylation.

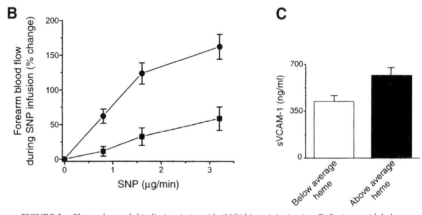

FIGURE 3.—Plasma hemoglobin limits nitric oxide (NO) bioactivity in vivo. B, Patients with below average heme levels (*circles*) had robust blood flow responses to all doses of nitroprusside (P < .005 by 2-way analysis of variance), whereas patients with above average heme levels (*squares*) had limited responses. In the original journal article, points are filled with red, green or blue corresponding to 0.8, 1.6 or 3.2 µg/min-infusions of nitroprusside, respectively. *Editor's note:* The 0.8, 1.6, and 3.2 µg/min-infusions of nitroprusside are pictured from left to right. C, The plasma of patients with below average heme (*white bar*) contained less soluble vascular cell adhesion molecule (sVCAM)-1 than patients with above average heme (*black bar*; P = .02). Concentrations of the soluble adhesion molecule, sVCAM-1, in the plasma of patients with sickle-cell disease correlated with plasma concentrations of heme (r = 0.46; P = .02; n = 25). *Error bars* indicate SEM. (Courtesy of Reiter CD, Wang X, Tanus-Santos JE, et al: Cell-free hemoglobin limits nitric oxide bioavailability in sickle-cell disease. *Nature Med* 8:1383-1389, 2002.)

Methods.—Blood was obtained from the brachial artery of 27 patients with sickle-cell disease and 16 control subjects. Large-bore angiocatheters were used to prevent artifactual hemolysis. Whole blood was centrifuged at 750*g* for 5 minutes, and plasma samples were tested for NO consumption. *Results.*—The plasma of patients with sickle-cell disease consumed 6.7 ±1.2 µM NO, while arterial plasma from the normal control subjects consumed 2.2 ±0.1 µM NO (Fig 1). This study also found that NO transcriptionally downregulates the soluble vascular cell adhesion molecule. Elevated levels of this adhesion molecule have been suggested as contributing to the pathophysiology of sickle-cell disease.

Conclusion.—This study demonstrated that plasma from patients with sickle-cell disease contains cell-free ferrous hemoglobin, which stoichiometrically consumes micromolar quantities of NO and abrogates forearm blood flow responses to NO donor infusions (Fig 3). NO bioavailability is restored by therapies that inactivate plasma hemoglobin by oxidation or NO ligation. Decompartmentalization of hemoglobin and the resulting dioxygenation of NO may account for the vascular complications shared by acute and chronic hemolytic disorders.

▶ In a set of 3 experiments, these investigators, many from the intramural program of the National Institute of Diabetes, Digestive Disorder, and Kidney Diseases, help clarify the pathophysiology of NO in sickle-cell disease. Endothelial cells convert arginine to citrulline, water, and NO by means of NO synthetase. NO then activates guanylyl cyclase, in turn increasing cGMP synthetase from guanylyl triphosphate in smooth muscle cells.

This source of energy induces vasodilation. NO also functions in inhibiting platelet agglutination and serves as a messenger for immune modulation. Cell-free oxyhemoglobin has a strong affinity for NO, converting it into nitrate and itself to physiologically inactive methemoglobin, thereby scavenging and destroying NO by forming a heme-nitrosyl hemoglobin complex. Normally, hemoglobin is enclosed in the red cell envelope and has only 0.2% of the capacity to inactive NO as does cell-free hemoglobin. NO is normally efficiently partitioned from hemoglobin and protected from inactivation by the diffusion resistance of the red cell envelope and the 1 to 2 µm zone free of red cells at the endothelial surface of arterial structures greater than 20 in diameter, conferred by virtue of its rheology.

Normally, hemoglobin serves to bind and stabilize NO by combining with it in a ferrous state and releasing NO on oxidation to its ferric state or by reduction to deoxyhemoglobin at sites of oxygen release or methemoglobin production. The effect can be demonstrated in vitro using ferricyanide added to blood samples.

Inactive sickle-cell disease disrupts this balance of NO metabolism through the hemolysis that follows hemoglobin polymerization during sickling, which results in destruction of about 10% of a sickle-cell patient's red cell mass per day and raises plasma free hemoglobin concentration from the range of 1 to 2 µmol to 20 µ, as these authors showed in a group of 27 sickle-cell patients. They also demonstrated the increased NO scavenging capacity of blood containing increased free heme from sickle-cell patients in comparison to normals, following treatment in vitro with ferricyanide, which released 3 times more NO than in controls as ferrous ion was oxidized. Increased NO scavenging prevents NO from maintaining its role in vasodilation and platelet fluidity.

Finally, the authors measured forearm blood flow by venous occlusion plethysmography and showed vasodilation with infusion of nitroprusside, an NO donor, in normals. In presence of plasma heme concentrations of at least 6 μmol, however, up to an 80% decrease in blood flow marked the deactivation of endothelial NO by the increased heme concentration associated with sickle-cell hemolysis. Further, those patients showed down regulation of expression of sVCAM-1, increasing the capacity for white cell and platelet and agglutination and endovascular coagulation. In animal studies referenced here, infusion of cell-free hemoglobin resulted in pulmonary and systemic hypertension, decreased organ perfusion, and death.

This evidence supports the hypothesis that hemoglobin polymerization in vivo results in hemolysis and high cell-free plasma hemoglobin concentrations which, as a result of hemoglobin concentration reduction, increases nitrosylation and increases NO scavenging; reduces the normal role of NO in vasoregulation; and results in vasoconstriction, reduced perfusion, thrombotic occlusion, ischemia, and pain. Further, the authors' data help explain the large phenotypic heterogeneity among those with sickle-cell disease who share at least a simple thymine for adenine homozygous substitution in the gene for betaglobin. This phenotypic variability may well be due to mutational differences in the 3 NO synthetase isotypes, heme catabolizing enzymes such as bilirubin reductase, and hemoglobin scavenging proteins such as haptoglobins among those with sickle-cell disease. This is the clearest view we have of the vascular pathology of this disease.

T. H. Kirschbaum, MD

Maternal Immunity and Prevention of Congenital Cytomegalovirus Infection
Fowler KB, Stagno S, Pass RF (Univ of Alabama, Birmingham)
JAMA 289:1008-1011, 2003   3–18

Introduction.—Congenital cytomegalovirus (CMV) infection can be transmitted to the fetus during primary maternal infection during pregnancy and can also be transmitted when maternal infection has occurred years before conception. It is not known whether maternal immunity reduces the incidence of the transplacental transmission of CMV. The uncertainty over the ability of naturally acquired immunity to prevent future infection is an important impediment to the development of vaccines for the prevention of congenital CMV infection. The rates of congenital infection were compared in terms of maternal CMV serology status ascertained years before delivery in a cohort investigation.

Methods.—A total of 3461 multiparous women from a population with a high rate of congenital CMV infection who delivered newborns were screened for congenital CMV infection between 1993 and 1998; all had cord serum specimens from a previous delivery that could be retrieved and tested for antibody to CMV. The primary outcome measures were congenital CMV infection according to maternal immune status, age, race, parity, and socioeconomic status.

Results.—Of 604 newborns born to initially seronegative mothers, congenital CMV infections were identified in 18 (3.0%). By comparison, 28 (1.0%) of 2857 newborns born to immune mothers had congenital CMV infection. Only 2 factors were highly protective against congenital CMV infection: preconception maternal immunity (adjusted risk ratio, 0.31; 95% confidence interval, 0.17-0.58) and maternal age of 25 years or older (adjusted risk ratio, 0.19; 95% confidence interval, 0.07-0.49).

Conclusion.—Naturally acquired immunity resulted in a 69% decrease in the risk of congenital CMV infection in future pregnancies. A vaccine that could achieve protection similar to that of immunity from naturally acquired infection could decrease the rate of congenital CMV infection by at least 70%.

▶ CMV is the most common cause of fetal infection, occurring in 1% to 2% of American births, and resulting, especially where primary infection strikes young gravidas without protective antibody, in impaired hearing, vision, and brain injury in some fetuses.[1] Maternal CMV IgG antibody is increasingly prevalent with age, occurring earlier among women from lower socioeconomic strata than others. Though the maternal antibody does not prevent fetal infection, it appears to decrease the likelihood of severe fetal consequences somewhat.[2,3] Currently, attempts at drug prophylaxis to prevent or abort fetal infection[4] and vaccine development to produce maternal antibody in those without immunity are under consideration. This study making use of the archival collection of maternal and neonatal sera maintained over nearly 30 years by this group of investigators is aimed at estimating the effectiveness of a potential CMV vaccine.

Data were obtained from multiparous women delivering from 1993 to 1998 whose newborns were screened for congenital CMV and had 1 or more prior siblings born in Birmingham for whom an archival cord sample was available for testing for CMV IgG. Of the 3461 such women, the most current pregnancy resulted in 46 cases of newborn infection. Eighteen were born to the 604 women who were initially seronegative for CMV IgG (3%) during this pregnancy, and 28 were born to the 2857 women with prior immunity (1%). Of the 604 seronegative gravidas, 23.5% seroconverted to positive and all the infected fetuses from seronegative women occurred in this subset of new primary infection. Conferring immunity by vaccination of women seronegative for CMV, whether pregnant or contemplating pregnancy, might well decrease the risk of congenital CMV infection by as much as 69%. Potentially, this would reduce the number of infected newborns at a rate of 30 per thousand live births to women who were seronegative at the onset of pregnancy and might further reduce their 23.5% risk of seroconversion. These data need to be confirmed by studies in primigravid women. The possibility of seropositive women producing congenital CMV in their offspring by infection with a new viral strain different to that causing the primary infection persists as an occasional complicating problem.[5]

T. H. Kirschbaum, MD

References

1. 1993 YEAR BOOK OF OBSTETRICS AND GYNECOLOGY, pp 232-233.
2. 1993 YEAR BOOK OF OBSTETRICS AND GYNECOLOGY, pp 119-120.
3. 1995 YEAR BOOK OF OBSTETRICS AND GYNECOLOGY, pp 147-149.
4. 2000 YEAR BOOK OF OBSTETRICS, GYNECOLOGY, AND WOMEN'S HEALTH, pp 75-78.
5. 2002 YEAR BOOK OF OBSTETRICS, GYNECOLOGY, AND WOMEN'S HEALTH, pp 100-101.

High Risk Pregnancies in Hypopituitary Women
Overton CE, Davis CJ, West C, et al (Univ College London; Middlesex Hosp, London)
Hum Reprod 17:1464-1467, 2002   3–19

Introduction.—Only scant information is available concerning pregnancy outcomes of women with established hypopituitarism. Some reports have indicated that pregnancies in these women are at high risk. A prospectively gathered database that recorded fertility treatment cycles in 9 women (18 pregnancies) with panhypopituitarism who had successfully conceived after undergoing ovulation induction was examined. Median patient age was 35.5 years (range, 29-42 years). Complete data were available for 8 patients. All patients had received complete pituitary replacement with thyroxine, corticosteroids, and estrogen replacement; full pituitary testing with standard insulin intolerance, gonadotropin-releasing hormone, and thyroid-releasing hormone was documented in 8 patients. One patient subsequently underwent repeat pituitary testing, and cortisol replacement was successfully withdrawn. Four patients were also taking vasopressin for diabetes insipidus. Two patients had uneventful earlier pregnancies; 1 had a normal delivery and 1 underwent cesarean section. All 9 women were amenorrheic and needed ovulation induction to be able to conceive. Two women had a response to the gonadotropin-releasing hormone pump and both conceived; 1 ended in miscarriage and 1 resulted in a live birth. The remaining patients received treatment with gonadotropins and human chorionic gonadotropin.

Results.—Of 18 pregnancies, 14 (78%) were singletons and 4 were twin births. Eleven (61%) pregnancies resulted in a live birth, 5 (28%) were first trimester miscarriages, and 2 (11%) were second trimester intrauterine deaths. There were no survivors among the 4 sets of twins. All deliveries were by cesarean section; half of the live births were at or below the tenth percentile for weight. One woman was able to breast-feed successfully.

Conclusion.—Women with hypopituitarism have high-risk pregnancies, possibly because of a uterine defect caused by endocrine deficiency. It is recommended that fertility treatments strive for singleton pregnancies and use strict criteria to prevent twin pregnancies. Early elective cesarean section is probably needed in these patients.

▶ Achieving pregnancy in women with panhypopituitarism is a endocrinologic triumph that reflects skill in ovulation induction and early pregnancy endocrine support. Accounts of subsequent pregnancy results are rare and this group of 9 such pregnancies, all amenorrheic before therapy, seen at London's University College Hospital from 1980 to 2000 equals the entire number reported previously from 1965 to 1980. The majority of cases stem from surgery for pituitary tumors or hyperplasia; there were 2 cases of Sheehan's syndrome and 1 case resulting from tuberculosis meningitis. The women received thyroxine, estrogen, and corticosterone replacement therapy, and vasopressin was needed in 4 cases to regulate water balance. Among the women with median age 35.5 years and body mass index of 23 kg/m², there were 11 live births (61%), 2 of them preterm. Though the incidence of spontaneous abortion was not exceptional, there were 2 second trimester fetal deaths. Half of the infants were born small for gestational age and the 4 sets of twins all succumbed either from abortion or intrauterine fetal death. Only 1 spontaneous vaginal delivery occurred; cesarean section was done on the remaining 8 cases, 2 for failed induction or inadequate labor. It is regrettably impossible to judge the labor performance among these women. Lactation was successful in 3 cases and most women required prolactin supplementation. The adequacy of endogenous growth hormone production was not regularly tested and supplementation might have improved pregnancy outcomes. Clearly, twin pregnancies were not well tolerated in the uteri of the 4 women who bore them and there may, to some, be indication here for pregnancy reduction where twins are seen in early prenatal care. The results recorded by this group were quite similar to those previous pregnancies reported over the previous 4 decades, suggesting little progress in management of these pregnancies has occurred in the last 2 decades.

T. H. Kirschbaum, MD

Prospective Screening for Pediatric Mitochondrial Trifunctional Protein Defects in Pregnancies Complicated by Liver Disease
Yang Z, Yamada J, Zhao Y, et al (Wake Forest Univ, Winston-Salem, NC; Vanderbilt Univ, Nashville, Tenn)
JAMA 288:2163-2166, 2002   3–20

Background.—Syndromes occurring in the third trimester of pregnancy include acute fatty liver of pregnancy (AFLP) and hemolysis, elevated liver enzymes, and low platelets (HELLP), which is a complication of severe preeclampsia. HELLP carries a better prognosis than AFLP, but both of these maternal disorders have been linked to an inherited fetal disorder of fatty acid oxidation, specifically, deficiency of long-chain 3-hydroxyacyl coenzyme A dehydrogenase (LCHAD), an enzyme that resides in the α subunit of the trifunctional protein. This enzyme functions as a catalyst in the third step of long-chain fatty acid β-oxidation. The frequency with which this fetal condition occurs in pregnancies complicated by AFLP or HELLP syndrome was evaluated.

Methods.—One hundred eight consecutive samples of blood from women who had either the AFLP (27 women) or HELLP syndromes (81 women), from their offspring, or from their partners were subjected to molecular screening. DNA screening was carried out seeking mutations in the α subunit of the trifunctional protein.

Results.—Three stillbirths were documented: 2 in women with AFLP and 1 in a women with HELLP syndrome. The DNA of the parents in these cases was evaluated. Five of the 27 families with AFLP had the mutation linked to LCHAD deficiency. Two newborns with LCHAD deficiency were clinically asymptomatic when evaluated 2 and 3 months after birth but were homozygous for the E474Q mutation. One other child is on a low-fat, high-carbohydrate diet and is doing well; the diagnosis in this case was compound heterozygosity for mutations in exons 4 and 15. A fourth child was homozygous for the E474Q mutation and died because of severe prematurity. In the fifth case, the mother was heterozygous for the common exon 15 mutation and the father was heterozygous for an exon 12 donor-site splice mutation; intrauterine fetal demise occurred at the thirty-sixth week of gestation. Only 1 woman with HELLP syndrome was heterozygous for the E474Q mutation. She recovered from the HELLP syndrome after induced vaginal delivery, and her newborn had no mitochondrial trifunctional protein mutations.

Conclusions.—A significant association was found between AFLP in the mother and the E474Q mutation in the fetus. Thus, pregnancies complicated by AFLP may benefit from screening for this mutation, which would allow early diagnosis and treatment of the newborn, as well as genetic counseling and prenatal diagnosis in subsequent pregnancies.

▶ This is a nice example of the price that is sometimes paid by those who study obstetric problems without obstetric consultation. AFLP is a mitochondrial disorder in which mutational changes in mitochondrial DNA interfere with β-oxidation of free fatty acids.[1-4] The result is high concentrations of plasma free fatty acids often complexed with carnitine, resulting in metabolic acidosis, hepatic fatty acid infiltration and dysfunction, compensatory glycogenolysis, and carbohydrate use to the point of hypoglycemia. The resultant effects on other organs produce a variety of additional pathologic changes. With homozygous mutations of mitochondrial DNA, the effects are devastating; heterozygotes may express the disease in the presence of infection, drug exposure, and pregnancy. HELLP syndrome is simply one of a large number of clusters of findings in severe preeclampsia in which hepatic dysfunction arises from obliterative vascular changes in multiple areas of hepatic focal necrosis. In some cases, focal interstitial hemorrhaging appears in the liver with perfusion of the necrotic foci site.

Here, the authors found restriction fragment length polymorphisms, in an exon known to interfere with free fatty acid β-oxidation in 5 of 27 (18%) of women, or their offspring, who exhibited fatty liver of pregnancy. Only 1 of 81 women with HELLP syndrome in pregnancy bore a heterozygous mutational defect not shown by the infant. Screening for this mitochondrial DNA defect is pointless in preeclampsia: most obstetricians would have pointed that out.

T. H. Kirschbaum, MD

References

1. 1992 YEAR BOOK OF OBSTETRICS, GYNECOLOGY, AND WOMEN'S HEALTH, pp 69-70.
2. 1994 YEAR BOOK OF OBSTETRICS, GYNECOLOGY, AND WOMEN'S HEALTH, pp 109-110.
3. 1994 YEAR BOOK OF OBSTETRICS, GYNECOLOGY, AND WOMEN'S HEALTH, pp 211-213.
4. 1995 YEAR BOOK OF OBSTETRICS, GYNECOLOGY, AND WOMEN'S HEALTH, pp 116-117.

4 Fetal Complications of Pregnancy

Association Between the Use of Antenatal Magnesium Sulfate in Preterm Labor and Adverse Health Outcomes in Infants
Mittendorf R, Dambrosia J, Pryde PG, et al (Loyola Univ, Maywood, Ill; NIH, Bethesda, Md; Univ of Wisconsin, Madison; et al)
Am J Obstet Gynecol 186:1111-1118, 2002   4–1

Background.—In 1995, fetal exposure to magnesium sulfate (MgSO$_4$) was reported to be associated with a decreased risk for cerebral palsy among premature infants. At that time, a randomized study was begun to determine whether, in the setting of preterm labor, antenatal exposure to MgSO$_4$ would decrease neonatal markers of brain injury, the prevalence of subsequent cerebral palsy, and overall perinatal mortality. Unexpectedly, exposure to MgSO$_4$ appeared to be associated with an increase in pediatric mortality. The current study sought to determine whether antenatal MgSO$_4$ exposure

---

TABLE 3.—Possible Risk Factors for Total Adverse Outcomes: Obstetric Variables

Variable	Adverse Outcome (No.)		P Value
	Yes	No	
Preterm premature rupture of membrane	24/34 (71%)	77/108 (71%)	>.99
Betamethasone	34/36 (94%)	86/99 (87%)	.35
Chorioamnionitis (clinical suspicion before delivery)*	13/19 (68%)	51/107 (48%)	.04
Bleeding ≤1 wk of delivery	8/37 (22%)	9/109 (8%)	.04
Meconium	1/37 (3%)	3/110 (3%)	>.99
Apgar score			
1 minute, <7	14/37 (38%)	24/110 (22%)	.08
5 minute, <7	3/37 (8%)	5/110 (5%)	.42
Gestational age <28 wk	14/37 (38%)	29/110 (26%)	.21
Birth weight <1500 g	19/36 (53%)	36/110 (33%)	.05
Individual twins	5/37 (14%)	25/110 (23%)	.35
Cesarean delivery	13/37 (35%)	30/110 (27%)	.41
Sex, male	23/37 (62%)	63/110 (57%)	.70
Funisitis	8/36 (22%)	16/110 (15%)	.30
Interleukin-6 ≥10 pg/mL	9/20 (45%)	32/74 (43%)	>.99
Ionized magnesium >0.60 mmol/L	15/40 (38%)	6/42 (14%)	.02

*Two of 3 conditions: maternal fever ≥38°C, uterine tenderness, elevated white blood cell count.
(Reprinted by permission of the publisher courtesy of Mittendorf R, Dambrosia J, Pryde PG, et al: Association between the use of antenatal magnesium sulfate in preterm labor and adverse health outcomes in infants. *Am J Obstet Gynecol* 186:1111-1118. Copyright 2002 by Elsevier.)

TABLE 5.—Multivariable Logistic Regression of Cord Ionized Magnesium Level, Steroid Usage in the Neonatal ICU, and Interaction of Cord Ionized Magnesium and Steroid Usage in the Neonatal ICU

Variable	Adjusted Odds Ratio	95% CI	P Value
Cord ionized magnesium	3.4	1.04-11.1	.04
Steroid usage in NICU	6.8	0.4-126.9	.20
Cord ionized magnesium by steroids in NICU	0.15	0.005-4.7	.28

(Reprinted by permission of the publisher courtesy of Mittendorf R, Dambrosia J, Pryde PG, et al: Association between the use of antenatal magnesium sulfate in preterm labor and adverse health outcomes in infants. *Am J Obstet Gynecol* 186:1111-1118. Copyright 2002 by Elsevier.)

prevents adverse outcomes, including neonatal intraventricular hemorrhage, periventricular leukomalacia, cerebral palsy, and death.

Methods.—One hundred forty-nine women in preterm labor before 34 weeks' gestation were enrolled in the controlled trial. The women were assigned randomly to MgSO$_4$, another tocolytic, or placebo. At delivery, umbilical cord blood was obtained for the analysis of serum ionized magnesium concentrations. In addition, neonatal cranial US scans were periodically obtained and assessed for intraventricular bleeding and periventricular leukomalacia. Cerebral palsy diagnoses were made among survivors at 18 months.

Findings.—Umbilical cord magnesium levels at delivery were greater in children with adverse outcomes. In regression analyses that adjusted for confounders, including very low birth weight, magnesium continued to be a significant risk factor, with an adjusted odds ratio of 3.7 (Tables 3 and 5).

Conclusions.—Exposure to antenatal MgSO$_4$ is associated with worse, not better, perinatal outcomes. The relationship between MgSO$_4$ and poor outcomes appears to be dose-dependent.

▶ This is the long-awaited report of the MagNET study in cell biology sponsored by the National Institute for Neurological Disorders and Stroke spurred by the suggestion by K. B. Nelson and J. K. Grether that magnesium exposure to the fetus reduces the risk of cerebral palsy in very low birth weight neonates.[1] Randomization with respect to race, age, gestational age, and singlet pregnancy status was performed on 149 gravidas delivering 165 neonates, each presenting at 24 to 34 weeks' gestational age with reassuring antenatal testing and no clinical suggestions of preeclampsia or infection. Two tandem trials with individual controls were formed. In the aggressive tocolysis trial, women in suspect preterm labor were randomized between typical intravenous MgSO$_4$ tocolysis (46 women, 9 with twins) and tocolysis by either β-adrenergic agonists or indomethacin (46 women with 5 twins). The neuroprotective trial included women with a cervix greater than 4 cm dilated who were randomized between MgSO$_4$ tocolytic doses (29 women with 1 set of twins) and saline controls (27 gravidas with 1 set of twins). Several demographic, obstetrical, and neonatal variables were measured, as well as umbilical vein and maternal veinous serum magnesium concentration and interleukin 6. Membranes were cultured for bacterial evidence of infection. US and MRI were used to supplement the clinical diagnoses of periventricular leukomalacia and cerebral palsy based on pediatric observations through the age of 18 months. Dependent variables for the study were intraventricular hemorrhage, periventricular leukomalacia, perinatal mortality, and cerebral palsy. A composite incidence of adverse effects was 42 out of 165 (25%) and for cerebral palsy, 6 of 165, or 3.6%.

In the tocolytic and neuroprotective arms, no significant differences were noted in adverse effect incidence between magnesium tocolysis and other tocolytics or between $MgSO_4$ and saline administration, based on intent to treat. In each case the incidence rate of adverse effects was greater in magnesium recipients. In the tocolytic arm, magnesium seum concentrations exhibited a higher mean value among those with adverse outcomes than in those without, and magnesium concentration was handled in a nonparametric fashion by dichotomizing patients around a value of 1.2 mEq/L. In both cases, statistical significance was claimed on the basis of nonparametric analysis (see Table 3). Note that the analysis required aggregates of frequency and several disparate variables—only 4 of which showed individual significant differences, with respect to increased adverse effects: the presence of chorioamnionitis, antepartum bleeding, birth weight of less than 1.5 kg, and maternal serum magnesium concentration greater than 1.2 mEq/L. Among the maternal variables, only elevated cord blood magnesium was significantly associated with adverse neonatal newborn outcomes. The data yielded an inconclusive suggestion of a dose-response relationship between cord blood magnesium concentration and adverse newborn outcome. Though chorioamnionitis showed a univariate association with adverse neonatal outcome, multivariate analysis abolished the significance of that finding. There was a statistically significant relationship demonstrated to the deleterious effect of magnesium when a bivariate model demonstrated its covariate relationship with elevated cord blood magnesium. Since 60% of adverse pediatric outcomes took the form of intraventricular hemorrhage and 26% were attributable to neonatal death, the authors feel that magnesium should not be used for tocolysis in very low birth weight labor routinely, but only when a clearly established benefit exists. Certainly this important study effectively refutes the purported beneficial effects of magnesium on central nervous system pathology earlier reported and should cause some concern about the possible deleterious effect of tocolysis with this agent in pregnancies in the very low birth weight range, especially in view of the absence of evidence of benefit from its use. The 6 cases of cerebral palsy reported here are too few for individual meaningful analysis.

T. H. Kirschbaum, MD

Reference

1. 1996 Year Book of Obstetrics, Gynecology, and Women's Health, pp 126-128.

Absence of Nasal Bone in Fetuses With Trisomy 21 at 11-14 Weeks of Gestation: An Observational Study

Cicero S, Curcio P, Papageorghiou A, et al (King's College Hosp, London; Ohio State Univ, Columbus)
Lancet 358:1665-1667, 2001   4-2

Background.—Prenatal diagnosis of trisomy 21 is performed on women considered at high risk after screening. The sensitivity is 85% for a combination screening consisting of maternal age, first trimester nuchal translucency scanning, and maternal serum biochemical analysis at 11 to 14 weeks. A 5% false-negative rate exists. In this observational study, nasal hypoplasia was used to improve the prenatal screening for trisomy 21.

Study Design.—This study was performed at 1 center between January and October 2001 on 701 fetuses at 11 to 14 weeks of gestation. All fetuses were considered to be at risk after screening with a combination of antenatal age and fetal nuchal translucency thickness. Parents had decided to have invasive testing. During the routine US performed before chorionic villus sampling, the presence of nasal bone was noted. For detection of the fetal nose bone, a midsagittal view, with the beam of the US transducer parallel to the nasal bone, was used. The correlation between absent nasal bone and trisomy 21 was calculated. Data from a multicenter study, including 326 fetuses with trisomy 21 and 95,476 chromosomally normal fetuses, were used to calculate the effect of screening for the nasal bone. Sensitivity and false-positive rates were also calculated.

Findings.—The fetal profile could be successfully examined by US in all cases. The nasal bone could not be detected by US in 73% of fetuses with trisomy 21 and in 0.5% of chromosomally normal fetuses. Inclusion of US examination for the nasal bone at 11 to 14 weeks' gestation, along with maternal age, maternal serum biochemical analysis, and fetal nuchal translucency scanning, could increase the sensitivity of screening for fetuses at risk for trisomy 21 to 85% and could decrease the false-positive rate to 1%.

Conclusions.—Examination for the fetal nasal bone by US at 11 to 14 weeks' gestation could be beneficial for the detection of fetuses at risk for trisomy 21. It would increase sensitivity and reduce the false-negative rate of screening while also reducing the number of fetuses exposed to invasive testing and decreasing costs.

▶ Following the suggestion by Down[1] that patients now recognized to have trisomy 21 had small noses and flat faces, these investigators looked in the first trimester of pregnancy for ultrasonic evidence of a nasal bone in 685 singlet pregnancies suspect for Down syndrome based on maternal age and nuchal ultrasonic translucency.[2] The technique requires midsagittal facial scans while taking care with transducer placement to prevent acquiring images of a nasal skin fold. Of 59 infants ultimately proven by karyotype to have trisomy 21, the nasal bone was absent in 43 or 72.9%. In this patient group, sensitivity was 93.4%, specificity 97.8%, and the prospective value of a positive finding was 72.9%. The false positive rate for absent nasal images was therefore 27%. In this group, there was no proof of the relationship of absent nasal image to maternal age, nuchal translucency, or crown rump length. The authors then returned to the earlier 1998 study and estimated the hypothetical effect of adding this variable to those data for maternal age and nuchal translucency, assuming it was independent of those 2 variables and submitted improved measures of predictability from this hypothetical combination. This is an inappropriate step since, to evaluate the usefulness of 3 pieces of data, they need to be obtained simultaneously from the same population and to do otherwise is to assume that in the earlier 95,802 patients previously reported, the nasal finding is unrelated in any way to nuchal translucency or maternal age without proof. The authors in their penultimate paragraph decry that speculation which they in turn made earlier. In a comment in the same journal issue, Dr Howard Cuckle of Leeds, England, an important contributor to prenatal diagnosis of trisomy 21, exercises excessive enthusiasm by saying that, in his view, it's time for routine first trimester Down screening. That position is not supportable by this study, I believe.

T. H. Kirschbaum, MD

References

1. Down JLH: Observations on an ethnic classification of idiots: 1866. *Ment Retard* 33:54-56, 1995.
2. Snijders RJ, Noble P, Sebire B, et al: A UK multicenter projection on assessment of risks of trisomy 21 by maternal age and fetal nuchal translucency thickness at 10 to 14 weeks' gestational age. *Lancet* 352:343-346, 1998.

Intrauterine Exposure to Infection and Risk of Cerebral Palsy in Very Preterm Infants
Grether JK, Nelson KB, Walsh E, et al (California Dept of Health Services, Oakland; NIH, Bethesda, Md; Johns Hopkins Univ, Baltimore, Md; et al)
Arch Pediatr Adolesc Med 157:26-32, 2003   4–3

Background.—Preterm infants have a much greater risk of having cerebral palsy (CP) than more mature infants, and the younger the gestational age, the greater the risk. Intrauterine exposure to infection has been postulated to produce CP, that is, children of mothers who have preterm labor or premature rupture of membranes, both of which may increase the risk of infection, may have a greater risk of CP. In addition, the gestational age group that is at highest risk of intrauterine infection is also at highest risk of CP. Very preterm infants at high risk of CP were evaluated for indicators of intrauterine infection to determine whether those exposed to infection were at higher risk of having CP.

Methods.—The children's gestational ages were less than 32 weeks, and their weights at birth were less than 1999 g. All survived until at least age 2 years. One hundred seventy children had congenital spastic CP, and 270 were control subjects randomly sampled within 250-g birth weight intervals.

Results.—The children with CP had no more clinical signs or symptoms of infection before birth than those without CP. Half of the mothers of children with CP and 41% of those whose children did not have CP had fevers exceeding 37.7°C during admission for delivery or up to 24 hours post partum. Antibiotic use before delivery and purulent amniotic fluid showed no link to CP. Acute placental inflammation was detected histologically in more than 70% of children with CP and in control children; it did not correlate with CP risk. A doubling of the risk of CP was linked to the identification of bacteria and viruses that commonly cause neonatal sepsis and death (group 1 organisms) in placental cultures. Infection indicators did not differ among women of various races/ethnicities, but white control individuals had a lower frequency of all the infection indicators in comparison with other groups. As a result, indicators of infection were significantly associated with an increased risk of CP in white children but not in other racial/ethnic groups.

Conclusions.—The very premature infants evaluated did not show any relationship between exposure to intrauterine infection and CP.

▶ This is a carefully designed and conducted study that uses data from the Northern California Cerebral Palsy Inquiry conducted from 1988-1994.[1] It deals with the relationship between intrauterine infection and CP in 170 infants with CP compared with 270 healthy control infants. The incidence of CP is inversely related to both gestational age at birth and the prevalence of fetoplacental infection,[2] and with such a strong confounding relationship, it is not surprising that an apparent correlation between CP and intrauterine infection in very premature infants has been identified by others,[3] although not uniformly so by all investigators.

Cases of CP were identified in this retrospective case–control study from 2 California registries, and details were obtained from records available in the 22 regional hospitals offering care. Controls were matched for birth weight and gestational age in a 2 to 1 ratio. The diagnosis of infection was based on placental morphological features in 76% of cases and on placental cultures in 33%, together with multiple clinical findings of fever, leukocytosis, uterine tenderness, vaginal discharge, and others. In an important step, because preeclampsia/pregnancy-induced hypertension is associated with a well-known diminution in the likelihood of CP,[4] patients were divided into a tocolytic-eligible group (ie, no pregnancy hypertension) and a tocolytic-ineligible group (ie, pregnancy hypertension) to control for that covariance. Data analysis was by multiple logistic regression yielding odds ratios of events comparing pregnancies resulting in CP with controls.

Neither infant gender nor maternal age proved to be related to an increased risk of CP. In an unanticipated finding, CP more often occurred in children of white than nonwhite mothers (see Table 1 in the original article). In the tocolytic-eligible group without pregnancy hypertension, a detailed analysis of indications of maternal infection, both clinical and histologic, showed no significant difference between infants with CP and controls (see Table 2 in the original article), nor was there an increased risk of CP in infants when all 269 pregnancies resulting in CP were compared, grouping both hypertensive and nonhypertensive pregnancies, in comparison to controls. Evidence of infection did seem to be statistically, significantly increased when white pregnancies resulting in CP were compared with nonwhite pregnancies resulting in CP. Compared with nonwhite parentage, white parentage among infants with CP had an odds ratio that was 2 to 4 times greater. It may well be that the uncontrolled impact of this racially biased differential may account for the uncertain but, in some cases, strong impact of uterine infection on the occurrence of CP previously cited. This study casts some doubt on the conclusion of a recent meta-analysis that found that chorioamnionitis is a risk factor for CP.[5] In that aggregate of 22 studies dealing with chorioamnionitis and CP, in 14, or 64%, of the studies, the diagnosis of chorioamnionitis was based solely on clinical findings without confirmatory pathologic or culture findings. Certainly, this study by Grether et al offers the most rigorous refutation of the oft-cited role of chorioamnionitis as a significant risk factor for CP.

T. H. Kirschbaum, MD

References

1. 1995 Year Book of Obstetrics, Gynecology, and Women's Health, pp 135-138.
2. 1990 Year Book of Obstetrics and Gynecology, pp 34-36.
3. 1999 Year Book of Obstetrics, Gynecology, and Women's Health, pp 126-128.
4. 1996 Year Book of Obstetrics, Gynecology, and Women's Health, pp 126-128.
5. Wu YW, Colford JM Jr: Chorioamnionitis as a risk factor for cerebral palsy. *JAMA* 284:1417-1424, 2002.

Impairment of Fetal Growth Potential and Neonatal Encephalopathy

Bukowski R, Burgett AD, Gei A, et al (Univ of Texas, Galveston)
Am J Obstet Gynecol 188:1011-1015, 2003   4–4

Background.—It is clear from the current evidence that most cases of neonatal encephalopathy and cerebral palsy result from antepartum events. While a number of these adverse events have been identified, many more are unknown, which makes it difficult to determine the total effect of adverse antenatal events on fetal neurologic development and fetal growth. The term

TABLE 2.—Proportions of Cases and Controls in Different Percentile Groups of Their Individual Growth Potential

Percentile Growth Potential	CTR (No. [%])	IP (No. [%])	OR (95% CI)	NIP (No. [%])	OR (95% CI)
<10th	1 (2.4)	7 (33.3)	20.5 (2.2-114.0)	6 (30.0)	17.6 (1.8-102.5)
<50th	18 (42.9)	11 (52.4)	1.5 (0.5-4.8)	11 (55.0)	1.6 (0.5-5.5)
<90th	37 (88.1)	16 (76.2)	0.4 (0.1-2.1)	14 (70.0)	0.3 (0.1-1.4)

Note: Data presented as number (percentage) and odds ratio (*OR*) (95% confidence interval (*CI*).
Abbreviations: CTR, Control; *IP*, intrapartum hypoxic event; *NIP*, no intrapartum hypoxic event.
(Reprinted by permission of the publisher courtesy of Bukowski R, Burgett AD, Gei A, et al: Impairment of fetal growth potential and neonatal encephalopathy. *Am J Obstet Gynecol* 188:1011-1015. Copyright 2003 by Elsevier.)

TABLE 3.—Proportions of Cases and Controls in Different Percentile Groups Using Standard Norms

Percentile Birth Weight	CTR (No. [%])	IP (No. [%])	OR (95% CI)	NIP (No. [%])	OR (95% CI)
<10th	1 (2.4)	4 (19.0)	9.6 (0.9-67.2)	4 (20.0)	10.3 (0.9-70.7)
<50th	22 (52.4)	11 (52.4)	1.0 (0.3-3.2)	14 (70.0)	2.1 (0.6-7.7)
<90th	39 (92.9)	18 (85.7)	0.5 (0.1-3.3)	18 (90.0)	0.7 (0.1-4.5)

Note: Data are presented as number (percentage) and odds ratio (OR) (95% confidence interval (CI).
(Reprinted by permission of the publisher courtesy of Bukowski R, Burgett AD, Gei A, et al: Impairment of fetal growth potential and neonatal encephalopathy. *Am J Obstet Gynecol* 188:1011-1015. Copyright 2003 by Elsevier.)

"growth potential" refers to a measure of the optimal weight a fetus should achieve in the absence of pathological conditions. It is calculated individually for each fetus and reflects its achieved proportion of individual optimal weight rather than a relationship of the fetal weight to population norms. This study tested the hypothesis that impairment of growth potential below the 10th percentile, which indicates severe antepartum fetal injury, occurs in fetuses with neonatal encephalopathy attributed to an adverse antenatal event.

Methods.—In this case-control study, 21 neonates with neonatal encephalopathy who met the criteria for an acute intrapartum hypoxic event (IHE) and 20 neonates with neonatal encephalopathy who did not meet these criteria were compared with 42 control neonates who had no complications. The control neonates were matched 2:1 for gestational age with IHE neonates. The percentile of growth potential was calculated for each fetus.

Results.—More neonates with neonatal encephalopathy with and without IHE were below the 10th percentile of growth potential compared with control neonates (33% and 30%, respectively, vs 2.4%) (Table 2). These associations remained significant after controlling for gestational age and birth weight (Table 3).

Conclusion.—A significant number of neonates with neonatal encephalopathy show signs of antepartum injury manifested in growth impairment. This association was similar in the presence and absence of an acute intrapartum hypoxic event, which indicates that antepartum injury is a causative rather than a predisposing factor in many cases of intrapartum hypoxic event.

▶ This study introduces 2 sets of concepts, both of which require some explanation. The senior author, Dr Gary Hankins, has chaired the American College of Obstetricians and Gynecologists (ACOG) Task Force on Neonatal Encephalopathy and Cerebral Palsy, and the report of the task force now available through ACOG should be part of any obstetrician's library since it provides several useful definitions and sharpens research goals in this area.[1]

Neonatal encephalopathy is defined by neurologic signs and symptoms—abnormal consciousness, muscle tone and reflexes, respiration, seizures, and feeding abnormalities—and may or may not lead to permanent injury. When associated with hypoxemia and reduced cardiac output and cerebral blood flow, that subset is correctly called hypoxic-ischemic encephalopathy. An estimated 70% of episodes of neonatal encephalopathy occur before the onset of labor.[1] Perinatal asphyxia must be marked by hypoxic-ischemic metabolic acidosis (umbilical pH 7 or less base excess greater than -12 meq/h); its clinical definition (abnormal fetal heart rate patterns, meconium, reduced Apgar scores) is such a poor prognostic basis as to be useless.

Acute intrapartum asphyxia requires the presence of all of several criteria: a sentinel event during or before labor, fetal bradycardia combined with late decelerations, Apgar score 0 to 3, multisystem abnormalities within 72 hours of birth, and abnormalities in brain scan prior to discharge. All cases of cerebral palsy pass through a phase of neonatal encephalopathy but the converse is not true. Here the question is whether neonatal encephalopathy per se during pregnancy impairs fetal growth during subsequent development.

The authors recognize that birth weight is a function both of the fetus' inherent genetically determined growth potential, and a host of maternal environmental- and pregnancy-related variables together with their pathologic variants. For this reason, they use a computer program which originated at the University of Nottingham,[2] derived from an extensive database from Queens University Medical Center.

The product of multiple regression and programming skills, it requires input of means and variances of birth weight for the population under study for scaling and specific entries important to the regression (maternal weight at first visit, height, parity, ethnicity, infant gender, and gestational age) from which it can derive weight versus gestational age plots, including data entries from each of the fetuses being studied from which the extent to which they conform to optimal fetal growth may be judged. It is an attempt to isolate fetal growth potential from all the impacts of pregnancy's maternal cofounding variables.

Twenty-one fetuses meeting criteria for an acute IHE and 20 who did not were compared with a control group in terms of the percentile of growth potential for each fetus compared to its predicted norm. This percentile figure was used as a measure of weight expected without pathology at birth, in contrast to weight expected from norms from the population used to define the nomogram. The proportion of infants below the 10th percentile of growth potential were larger in the IHE and non-IHE cases of neonatal encephalopathy than controls, and about one third of neonates with neonatal encephalopathy were below the 10th percentile of their own growth potential measured in this way.

Presence of a strong relationship between neonatal encephalopathy and impaired growth potential support the observations of others that cerebral palsy and newborn encephalopathy are predominately the results of antepartum events. The results rest on the accuracy and validity of the Nottingham statisticians' work, but, conceptually, the authors' approaches are sound.

T. H. Kirschbaum, MD

References

1. Neonatal Encephalopathy and Cerebral Palsy. ACOG Task Force on Neonatal Encephalopathy and Cerebral Palsy. Washington, DC 2003.

2. Gardosi J, Chang A, Kalyan B, et al: Customized antenatal growth charts. *Lancet* 339:283, 1992.

Decreased Vascularization and Cell Proliferation in Placentas of Intra-uterine Growth—Restricted Fetuses With Abnormal Umbilical Artery Flow Velocity Waveforms
Chen C-P, Bajoria R, Aplin JD (Mackay Mem Hosp, Taipei, Taiwan; Univ of Man-chester, England)
Am J Obstet Gynecol 187:764-769, 2002   4–5

Background.—Intrauterine fetal growth restriction (IUGR) is an impor-tant cause of perinatal death and morbidity. There are differences concern-ing the precise definition of IUGR, and it is likely that this condition is het-erogeneous. However, it has been shown in several studies that reduced umbilical artery blood flow velocity is associated with IUGR. The morpho-logical features of placentas in severe IUGR were compared with abnormal umbilical artery blood flow velocity waveforms and normal gestation.

Methods.—The study population comprised 9 pregnancies in which the diagnosis of IUGR was made on the basis of fetal birth weight below the 10th percentile with abnormal umbilical artery Doppler waveforms and re-duced amniotic fluid volume (amniotic fluid index, ≥ 5). Control deliveries were from spontaneous preterm labor and term pregnancy with no signs or symptoms of chorioamnionitis and with grossly normal placentas matched for the closest gestational age. Immunohistochemical studies evaluated cell proliferation, vascular density, and α-smooth muscle actin expression by stromal cells in both groups.

Results.—There were fewer MIB1-positive nuclei observed in both tro-phoblast and stromal cell populations from pregnancies with IUGR, indicat-ing fewer cells in cycle. In addition, a greatly reduced vascular density was observed, along with higher levels of α-smooth muscle actin expression in stromal cells.

Conclusion.—Intrauterine growth–restricted placentas show reduced cell proliferation in both trophoblast and stromal cell compartments. The find-ings suggest that increased fetoplacental vascular impedance is developed at least in part at the capillary level. However, these findings differ with those of similar studies, suggesting that intrauterine growth restriction is likely to have a heterogeneous etiology.

▶ This is a careful, apparently well-done morphological analysis of placental structure in 9 cases of IUGR associated with absent end-diastolic flow velocity (AEDFV) of the umbilical artery at a mean of 32 weeks' gestational age com-pared with a control group of normals at comparable gestation. Sections of pla-centa were subjected to immunohistochemistry using antibody to MIB1, a nuclear proliferative associated antigen expressed after G0 and G1 in the ac-tive phases of the cell growth cycle. Additional antibodies to CD34 used to stain intravillous endothelium and α-actin to detect stromal myofibroblasts were employed.

Classic morphometry was done to estimate the number of peripheral, that is, terminal and intermediate, villi. The capillary cross-sectional area as a fraction of total placental stroma and the number of capillaries per unit surface area were also calculated. In all cases, both the density of placental villi and capillary areas were decreased in placentas from growth retardation fetuses with AEDFV. Cell proliferation indexes derived from MIB1 staining showed no difference from control and α-actin proved to be significantly increased in villous stroma, indicating an increase in myofibroblast proliferation in growth retardation.

Professer Ivo Brosens, who first pointed out the abnormal placental vasculature in hypertension and growth retarded pregnancies,[1] has recently, with his colleagues, reviewed the current literature on the topic[2] in placentas associated with pregnancy hypertension or growth retardation. They feel there is little evidence of decreased placental and trophoblastic growth and invasiveness in these disturbances, and that there is reason to question whether changes in expression of trophoblastic integrins and platelet endothelial cell adhesion molecules occur in fact in either preeclampsia or growth retardation. Their opinion is that decidualization is impaired in such placentas as a result of a complex interaction of many endocrine and paracrine factors determined by ovarian steroids, corticotrophin-releasing factor, and prostaglandin E_2.

Among the paracrine factors are natural killer cells of native immunity, T lymphocytes, macrophages, monocytes, and neutrophiles. Interferon-γ expression—which in turn activates macrophage and increases expression of such agents as class 2 major histocompatibility complex proteins, nitric oxide synthetase, and endothelin—is also involved in the alteration of placental function in such cases. The latter view, supported in part by this study, makes it easier to understand the changes in umbilical artery circulation in fetuses with absent or negative end diastolic flow velocity in response to maternal steroid (see Abstract 6–6).

T. H. Kirschbaum, MD

References

1. Brosens I, Robertson WB, Dixon HG: The physiological response of the vessels of the placental bed to normal pregnancy. *J Pathol Bacteriol* 93:569, 1967.
2. Brosens JJ, Pijnenborg R, Brosens I: The myometrial junctional zone spiral arteriole in normal and abnormal pregnancies. *Am J Obstet Gynecol* 187:1416, 2002.

The Risk of Mortality or Cerebral Palsy in Twins: A Collaborative Population-Based Study

Scher AI, Petterson B, Blair E, et al (NIH, Bethesda, Md; Child Health Research, Subiaco, Western Australia; Inst for Child Health Research, Western Australia; et al)

Pediatr Res 52:671-681, 2002   4–6

Background.—There has been an increase in the prevalence of multiple births in recent years. As a result, it has become increasingly important to identify factors that influence outcomes in these infants. Infants from multiple births are at a higher risk of cerebral palsy than singleton infants. The risk of cerebral palsy is strongly associated with low birth weight or immaturity, and twin infants are on average smaller and are born earlier than singleton infants. Thus, it is necessary to separate the effects of birth weight from other factors that may be independent predictors of unfavorable outcome. Demographic and clinical factors associated with fetal or neonatal death or cerebral palsy in twins were described.

Methods.—Vital statistics gathered during the 1980s from 5 populations in the United States and Australia were combined for analysis of mortality and neurologic morbidity in multiple births. Included in these data was information on cerebral palsy diagnosed after 1 year of age. However, information on zygosity was not available. Crude rates of mortality and cerebral palsy were calculated overall and by demographic and twin factors. Mortality rates included stillbirth and death within 28 days of birth and were calculated as a percentage of all births. Rates of cerebral palsy were calculated as a percentage of all infants alive at 1 year.

Results.—In 1,141,351 births there were 25,772 twins. Significant secular trends from 1980 to 1989 included increasing prevalence of twins, increasing proportion of unlike-sex twins, and increasing maternal age. Twins were at an overall approximately 5-fold increased risk of fetal death and a 4-fold increased risk of cerebral palsy compared with singletons (Table 3). However, among infants with a birth weight of less than 2500 g, twins generally did better than singletons in both mortality and cerebral palsy rates (Fig 2, A). Second-born twins and twins from same-sex pairs were at an increased risk of early death but not of cerebral palsy (Fig 3, A). Twins from growth-discordant pairs as well as twins whose co-twin died were at an increased risk for both mortality and cerebral palsy (Fig 4, A). The highest rates of cerebral palsy were found in surviving twins whose co-twin was stillborn (4.7%), died shortly after birth (6.3%), or had cerebral palsy (11.8%) (Fig 5, A).

Conclusions.—In this large data set during a period of 10 years, the overall rates of death or cerebral palsy were higher in twins than in singletons, although small twins fared better generally than small singletons. Co-twin death was found to be a strong predictor of cerebral palsy in surviving twins. This risk was the same for same- and different-sex pairs and was found among preterm as well as term infants.

TABLE 3.—Crude Early Mortality (Still-birth and Neonatal), and Crude Cerebral Palsy (CP) Rates by Twin Factors

		BW (Mean, g)	GA* (Mean, wk)	n All Births	MORT (%)	n (1 Year)	CP (%)
Birth order	1st	2408	35.9	13235	6.38]†	12327	0.56
	2nd	2362	35.9	13274	7.40]	12197	0.61
Twin type	Same-sex	2363	35.9	18799	7.11]†	17344	0.59
	Different-sex	2453	36.1	7620	4.92]†	7203	0.56
Pair type†	M:M	2400	35.8	9536	7.91]†	8710	0.65
	M:F	2510	36.1	3810	4.93]	3604	0.64
	F:M	2395	36.1	3810	4.91]	3599	0.47
	F:F	2324	36.0	9263	6.29]	8634	0.52
Growth	No	2471	36.3	21210	2.81]†]††	20494	0.49]†
Discordance	Yes‡	2269	35.9	4000	5.03]	3769	0.77]‡
	Smaller§	1904	35.9	2000	6.00]	1854	0.76
	Larger**	2634	35.9	2000	4.05]	1915	0.78
Co-twin	Co-twin alive 28 days	2476	36.5	24741	2.15]†	24065	0.48]†
Outcome	Co-twin died	1084	27.8	1833	70.92]†	516	5.43]†
Total		2384 g	35.9 wk	26644	6.95	24632	0.58

Note: All births, including those with unknown birth weight or unknown/out of range gestational age.
*For this column only, based on infants with valid (20–46) gestational age.
†M:M, Male twins from same-sex pairs; M:F, male twins from mixed pairs; F:F, female twins from same-sex pairs; F:M, female twins from mixed pairs.
‡Twins from pairs in which the difference in birth weight exceeds 20% of the larger twin's birth weight. This comparison limited to twin pairs in which both twins were live-born.
§Comparing the smaller twin in a discordant pair with twins from nondiscordant pairs.
**Comparing the larger twin in a discordant pair with twins from nondiscordant pairs.
††$P < .005$, χ^2 (P values calculated taking into account nonindependence of twin data).
‡‡$P < .05$, χ^2 (P values calculated taking into account nonindependence of twin data).
Abbreviations: BW, Birth weight; GA, gestational age; MORT, mortality.
(Courtesy of Scher AI, Petterson B, Blair E, et al: The risk of mortality or cerebral palsy in twins: A collaborative population-based study. Pediatr Res 52(5):671-681, 2002.)

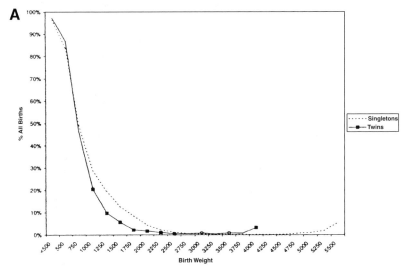

FIGURE 2.—**A**, Mortality (still-birth and neonatal) by birth weight for singletons and twins. *Solid square* indicates *P* < .002, difference between singletons and twins. *Open circle* indicates *P* < .05, difference between singletons and twins. Note: *Birth Weight* is combined above 4000 g for twins and above 5500 g for singletons. (Courtesy of Scher AI, Petterson B, Blair E, et al: The risk of mortality or cerebral palsy in twins: A collaborative population-based study. *Pediatr Res* 52(5):671-681, 2002.)

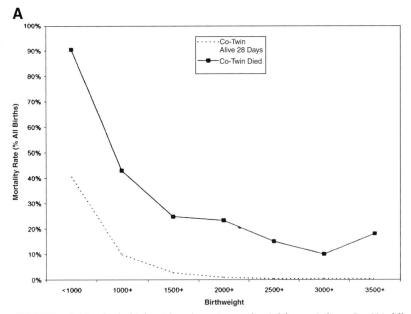

FIGURE 3.—**A**, Mortality by birth weight and co-twin mortality. *Solid square* indicates *P* < .004, difference between twins whose co-twin was a neonatal survivor and twins whose co-twin was not a neonatal survivor. (Courtesy of Scher AI, Petterson B, Blair E, et al: The risk of mortality or cerebral palsy in twins: A collaborative population-based study. *Pediatr Res* 52(5):671-681, 2002.)

A

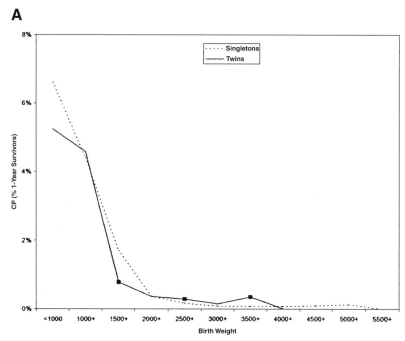

FIGURE 4.—A, Cerebral palsy (*CP*) by birth weight for singletons and twins. *Solid square* indicates *P* < .004, difference between singletons and twins. (Courtesy of Scher AI, Petterson B, Blair E, et al: The risk of mortality or cerebral palsy in twins: A collaborative population-based study. *Pediatr Res* 52(5):671-681, 2002.)

▶ It's clear that, independent of the reduced birth weight and gestational age of twins, they carry an additional incremental risk both for prenatal mortality and cerebral palsy.[1,2] As the National Center for Health Statistics Natality Data has disclosed, with an increase in incidence of multiple pregnancies over the period from 1980 to 1999 from 1.9% to 2.9% simultaneously compounded by a 6.2% increase in total births, the impact of twin morbidity on national public health services has significantly increased.[3] This collaborative review of vital and natality statistics from 3 regions in Australia and 2 from the United States, consisting of more than a million births, 25,772 of them twin pregnancies, provides a clear view of the risk factors for mortality and cerebral palsy in this looming problem.

A few findings stand out in this massive data collection, which deserves careful review by obstetricians. Twin pregnancies categorized by the number of births, not pregnancies, are associated with an increased risk of early perinatal death (5.83% vs 1.13%) and of cerebral palsy (0.59% vs 0.14%) compared with singlet births. For births during early pregnancy, from 29 to 35 weeks, with birth weights of 1 to 2.5 kg, twin newborns have lower mortality rates than singlets with no significant difference in the rates of occurrences of cerebral palsy. Early mortality rates and cerebral palsy incidence rates are lower in nonwhites when data are adjusted for differences in birth weight at gestational age. Delivery of a twin whose sibling died in utero or in the early

A

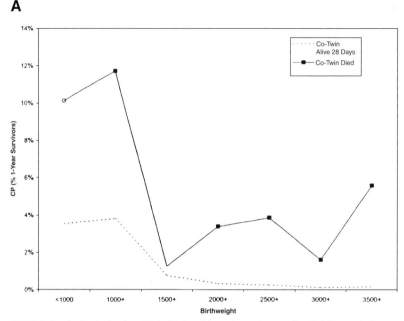

FIGURE 5.—A, Cerebral palsy (CP) by birth weight and co-twin mortality. *Solid square* indicates *P* < .002, difference between infants whose co-twin was a neonatal survivor and infants whose co-twin was not a neonatal survivor. *Open circle* indicates *P* < .05, difference between infants whose co-twin was a neonatal survivor and infants whose co-twin was not a neonatal survivor. (Courtesy of Scher AI, Petterson B, Blair E, et al: The risk of mortality or cerebral palsy in twins: A collaborative population-based study. *Pediatr Res* 52(5):671-681, 2002.)

neonatal period increases his risk of mortality from 2.15% to 70.92%, and of cerebral palsy from 0.48% to 5.43% compared with a co-twin who survived to 28 days of life. Similarly, birth weight–discordant twins differing by at least 20% in birth weight were associated with mortality rates from 2.81% to 5.03% and rates of occurrence of cerebral palsy from 0.49% to 0.77% compared with nondiscordant twins. This is by far our largest, most authoritative, and clearest comparative study of the perinatal mortality of twin pregnancies.

T. H. Kirschbaum, MD

References

1. 1995 YEAR BOOK OF OBSTETRICS, GYNECOLOGY, AND WOMEN'S HEALTH, pp 137-138.
2. 2000 YEAR BOOK OF OBSTETRICS, GYNECOLOGY, AND WOMEN'S HEALTH, pp 59-60.
3. Russell RB, Petrini JR, Damus K, et al: The changing epidemiology of multiple births in the United States. *Am J Obstet Gynecol* 101:129, 2003.

Fetal and Neonatal Mortality Among Twin Gestations in the United States: The Role of Intrapair Birth Weight Discordance

Demissie K, Ananth CV, Martin J, et al (Univ of Medicine and Dentistry of New Jersey, Piscataway; Ctrs for Disease Control and Prevention, Hyattsville, Md)
Obstet Gynecol 100:474-480, 2002   4–7

Background.—Differing twin sizes have been a cause for concern in the management of twin pregnancies. The relationship between intrapair birth weight discordance and fetal and neonatal mortality rates was investigated. *Methods and Findings.*—Data were obtained on 297,155 twins registered with the US Matched Multiple Birth File between 1995 and 1997. The weight discordance between a twin born live and its stillborn sibling was less than 5% in 29.9%, 5% to 9% in 24.2%, 10% to 19% in 29.6%, 20% to 29% in 11.1%, 30% to 39% in 3.4%, and 40% or greater in 1.8%. The rate of stillborn fetuses increased progressively with increasing birth weight discordance for same-sex smaller and larger twins (Table 2). Compared with the category of birth weight discordance of less than 5%, the odds ratios (ORs) for birth weight discordances of 5% to 9%, 10% to 19%, 20% to 29%, 30% to 39%, and 40% or greater were 0.81, 1.41, 1.74, 3.06, and 4.29, respectively, for the smaller twins. For the larger twins, the corresponding ORs were 0.78, 1.26, 1.77, 3.38, and 2.91, respectively. Comparable correlations were evident among smaller but not larger twins of the opposite sex. Among larger (but not smaller) twins of the same sex, increasing birth weight discordance correlated with overall neonatal death. This rela-

TABLE 2.—Risk of Mortality by the Percentage of Intrapair Birth Weight Discordance for Smaller and Larger Twins of Same Sex

Birth Weight Discordance (Birth Weight Centiles)	Fetal Death		Neonatal Mortality	
	n (%)	OR* (95% CI)	n (%)	OR† (95% CI)
Smaller twin				
<5%	371 (1.2)	1.00 (reference)	526 (1.7)	1.00 (reference)
5-9%	264 (1.1)	0.81 (0.58, 1.11)	411 (1.7)	1.07 (0.90, 1.28)
10-19%	472 (1.7)	1.41 (1.07, 1.84)	492 (1.8)	1.02 (0.86, 1.20)
20-29%	351 (3.4)	1.74 (1.28, 2.35)	279 (2.8)	1.21 (0.99, 1.48)
30-39%	275 (8.1)	3.06 (2.21, 4.24)	156 (5.0)	1.27 (0.99, 1.64)
≥40%	510 (26.6)	4.29 (3.05, 6.04)	179 (12.7)	1.29 (0.99, 1.68)
Larger twin				
<5%	409 (1.3)	1.00 (reference)	498 (1.6)	1.00 (reference)
5-9%	236 (1.0)	0.78 (0.57, 1.08)	364 (1.5)	1.04 (0.86, 1.26)
10-19%	356 (1.3)	1.26 (0.96, 1.66)	431 (1.5)	1.26 (1.05, 1.51)
20-29%	249 (2.4)	1.77 (1.27, 2.46)	180 (1.8)	1.41 (1.11, 1.78)
30-39%	166 (4.9)	3.38 (2.33, 4.92)	107 (3.3)	2.71 (2.08, 3.64)
≥40%	116 (6.0)	2.91 (1.89, 4.47)	109 (6.0)	3.43 (2.53, 4.65)

*Adjusted for the infant's gestational age, birth weight, gender, birth order and maternal age, race, education, parity, marital status, prenatal care utilization, placental abruption, placenta previa, anemia, chronic hypertension, and diabetes.
†Adjusted for the above factors plus the effects of cesarean and instrumental deliveries.
Abbreviations: OR, Odds ratio; CI, confidence interval.
(Courtesy of Demissie K, Ananth CV, Martin J, et al: Fetal and neonatal mortality among twin gestations in the United States: The role of intrapair birth weight discordance. *Obstet Gynecol* 100:474-480, 2002. Reprinted with permission from The American College of Obstetricians and Gynecologists.)

TABLE 3.—Risk of Mortality by the Percentage of Intrapair Birth Weight Discordance for Smaller and Larger Twins of Opposite Sex

Birth Weight Discordance (Birth Weight Centiles)	Fetal Death		Neonatal Mortality	
	n (%)	OR* (95% CI)	n (%)	OR† (95% CI)
Smaller twin				
<5%	67 (0.5)	1.00 (reference)	197 (1.5)	1.00 (reference)
5-9%	75 (0.7)	1.11 (0.55, 2.27)	152 (1.3)	1.00 (0.75, 1.34)
10-19%	113 (0.7)	1.30 (0.69, 2.47)	209 (1.3)	0.86 (0.65, 1.13)
20-29%	60 (1.0)	2.69 (1.38, 5.27)	108 (1.8)	1.42 (1.03, 1.97)
30-39%	56 (3.3)	6.16 (3.07, 12.37)	42 (2.6)	1.29 (0.83, 2.01)
≥40%	167 (22.6)	12.75 (6.26, 25.98)	54 (9.5)	1.40 (0.89, 2.21)
Larger twin				
<5%	72 (0.5)	1.00 (reference)	187 (1.4)	1.00 (reference)
5-9%	60 (0.5)	0.95 (0.48, 1.89)	157 (1.4)	1.07 (0.79, 1.47)
10-19%	105 (0.7)	1.36 (0.74, 2.48)	223 (1.4)	1.38 (1.03, 1.84)
20-29%	33 (0.5)	1.28 (0.56, 2.94)	68 (1.1)	1.44 (0.97, 2.12)
30-39%	21 (1.2)	2.79 (1.03, 7.57)	19 (1.1)	1.42 (0.77, 2.62)
≥40%	18 (2.4)	1.60 (0.40, 6.34)	20 (2.8)	2.06 (1.07, 3.97)

Abbreviations as in Table 2.
*Adjusted for the infant's gestational age, birth weight, gender, birth order and maternal age, race, education, parity, marital status, prenatal care utilization, placental abruption, placenta previa, anemia, chronic hypertension, and diabetes.
†Adjusted for the above factors plus for the effects of cesarean and instrumental deliveries.
Abbreviations: OR, Odds ratio; *CI,* confidence interval.
(Courtesy of Demissie K, Ananth CV, Martin J, et al: Fetal and neonatal mortality among twin gestations in the United States: The role of intrapair birth weight discordance. *Obstet Gynecol* 100:474-480, 2002. Reprinted with permission from The American College of Obstetricians and Gynecologists.)

tionship was not observed among smaller and larger twins of the opposite sex (Table 3). However, increasing birth weight discordance correlated with neonatal deaths associated with congenital malformations among smaller and larger twins.

Conclusions.—Increased discordance between the birth weights of twins appears to be related to an increased risk of intrauterine death. It also appears to be associated with neonatal deaths related to congenital malformations.

▶ There is no question that increasing discordance in twin birth weights is associated with increased risk of fetal and neonatal mortality, but this massive collection of data from almost 300,000 twin births, held by the CDC and its Preventive Matched Multiple Birth File affords an opportunity to set some limits for definition of what degree of discordance warrants special prenatal management. Postnatal deaths of infants weighing less than 300 g and of fetuses weighing less than 100 g were excluded from the data set. Extensive associated sociodemographic and medical data make it possible to explore covariables extensively. Because fetal and neonatal death rates are higher for same sex twins than for opposite sex twins (1.89% vs 0.87%), and for neonatal deaths (2.59% vs 1.47%), it's important to consider those subsets separately. Since half of all like sex twins come from monochorionic placentas while no unlike sex twins do, the difference in mortality rate likely stems from the vascular interrelationships in monochorionic twin pregnancies that find them shared between siblings. Among like sex twins, risk ratios for fetal deaths and neonatal deaths become statistically significantly increased in the 20% to 29% discordance range for smaller twins and in the 30% to 39% discordance range for the larger of the twins. For like sex twins, thresholds of significantly increased risk ratios begin at 10% to 19% discordance for smaller twins and 20% to 29% for larger twins. Neonatal death rates are independent of the degree of discordance for smaller like sex twins but become significantly increased for larger twins at the level of 10% to 19% discordance. The increased mortality rates related to discordance were explained almost solely by the incidence of congenital anomalies, especially in the CNS and lungs. Discordance was unrelated to neonatal death rates from respiratory distress syndrome, birth asphyxia and septicemia after adjusting for birth weight and gestational age.

It is important that a 20% to 29% disparity in twin birth weight occurs in 11.1% of twin pregnancies and that a 30% to 39% disparity occurs in only 3.4%. The increase in risk ratios increases strikingly in all categories except for neonatal mortality in the smaller of like sex twins. Those are the reasons that I choose an estimated fetal weight disparity of at least 30% to concentrate antepartum efforts for an investigation of anomalous twin development, especially in like sex twins. Others may differ. These data allow obstetricians to make their own informed decision.

T. H. Kirschbaum, MD

Placental Vascular Anastomoses Visualized During Fetoscopic Laser Surgery in Severe Mid-Trimester Twin-Twin Transfusion Syndrome
Diehl W, Hecher K, Zikulnig L, et al (AK Barmbek, Hamburg, Germany)
Placenta 22:876-881, 2001   4–8

Background.—Mid-trimester twin-twin transfusion syndrome (TTTS) develops in 10% to 20% of monochorionic twin pregnancies in which placental vascular anastomoses are present. This is a severe and life-threatening situation for both fetuses, with an 80% to 90% mortality rate. Because of an imbalance in net blood flow from one twin to the other, the recipient twin could have progressive polyhydramnios and congestive heart failure develop, whereas the donor twin becomes the "stuck twin" and experiences growth restriction. The type and number of placental vascular anastomoses identified in severe mid-trimester TTTS during fetoscopic laser coagulation were described and compared with other postnatal injection study findings.

Methods.—The study group comprised of 126 patients with severe TTTS who underwent fetoscopic laser coagulation between 16 and 25 weeks' gestation. Placental vascular anastomoses were identified as arterio-venous (AV), arterio-arterial (AA), and veno-venous (VV), with the AV anastomoses being further categorized into 4 different groups (groups 1-4). Nine of the 126 placentas had anastomoses that could not be clearly identified, leaving 117 cases for analysis.

Results.—AV anastomoses in groups 2 to 4 shunted in both directions, whereas group 1 anastomoses were shunting in only 1 direction (donor to recipient) without anastomoses in the opposite direction. Group 3 had an equal number of anastomoses shunting in both directions, whereas group 4 had more anastomoses shunting from recipient to donor than in the opposite direction. All 117 cases had AV anastomoses from donor to recipient, 36 (31%) also had AA anastomoses, and 14 (12%) had VV anastomoses. A majority of AV anastomoses (74%) showed shunting from donor to recipient compared with AV anastomoses shunting in the opposite direction. There were no cases that showed AV anastomoses shunting only from the recipient to the donor. Of the 36 cases with AA anastomoses, 27 had only a single AA, 8 had 2 AAs, and only 1 had 3 AAs.

Conclusion.—The complexity of the umbilico-placental vascular system in monochorionic placentas is reflected by the high number and different types of anastomoses found in the study. Obtaining a functionally dichorionic placenta and interrupting the circle of TTTS was the goal of fetoscopic laser coagulation of placental anastomoses. The survival rate with this minimally invasive procedure shows an effectiveness of 81% for at least 1 twin and 54% of pregnancies with 2 survivors.

▶ The observations of Bajoria et al, done on fixed placental tissues, are fundamental to understanding the vascular features present in TTTS in monochorionic diamniotic twins.[1,2] In brief, they showed that most cases were associated with a major AV shunt from donor to recipient twin at depth in the body of the placenta and relatively few recipient to donor shunts lying on the chorionic plate for compensation in the form of reverse flow. In general, AA and VV shunts appear relatively unimportant because of the small pressure gradients across the shunt structures.

These investigators provide confirmation based on visualization of the fetal surfaces of the placenta during YAG laser cauterization of shunts seen at the base of the diamniotic membrane separating monochorionic twins. The nature of the shunts was established by recognizing that umbilical arteries cross over umbilical veins on the chorionic plate and that contents viewed through these arterial vessels are darker due to the increased concentration of deoxyhemoglobin.

In 126 cases of severe TTTS failure of visualization occurred in only 7%. In all cases of TTTS, donor to recipient AV shunts were seen, and in 74% of all cases, donor to recipient AV shunts predominated over all others. No cases of simple recipient to donor shunting were seen. Its good confirmation in vivo of the role of subamniotic shunts and compensation for the deeper more important channels that lay within the body of the placenta as Bajoria first demonstrated.

T. H. Kirschbaum, MD

References

1. 1996 YEAR BOOK OF OBSTETRICS, GYNECOLOGY, AND WOMEN'S HEALTH, pp 118-119.
2. 2000 YEAR BOOK OF OBSTETRICS, GYNECOLOGY, AND WOMEN'S HEALTH, pp 65-66.

Myocardial Hypertrophy of the Recipient Twins in Twin-to-Twin Transfusion Syndrome and Cerebral Palsy
Hyodo HM, Unno N, Masuda H, et al (Univ of Tokyo; Nagano Children's Hosp, Japan; Tokyo Metropolitan Bokutoh Gen Hosp)
Int J Gynaecol Obstet 80:29-34, 2003   4–9

Introduction.—It is well known that monochorionic twins are at increased risk of neurodevelopmental disorders, including cerebral palsy (CP). This is especially true in monochorionic twins with twin-to-twin transfusion syndrome (TTTS). The etiologic factors for CP in monochorionic twin pregnancies have yet to be determined. The clinical course and neurologic prognosis of monochorionic twins with TTTS and without TTTS was examined, with particular emphasis on their cardiac functions.

Methods.—The incidence of cardiovascular and neurologic complications were examined in 33 pathologically verified monochorionic twin pregnancies that completed before 37 weeks' gestation. Data obtained from maternal and neonatal records were compared between the TTTS and non-TTTS groups. Relationships between clinical complications were also examined.

Results.—Seventeen of 33 monochorionic twins had TTTS. Seven recipient twins with TTTS had myocardial hypertrophy; none was seen in donor twins with TTTS or in those without TTTS. Six of 29 infants with TTTS and 1 of 32 without TTTS developed CP. In those with TTTS, all instances of CP occurred in the recipient twins. The development of CP was significantly linked with cardiovascular complications, including myocardial hypertrophy and hydropic changes.

Conclusion.—Myocardial hypertrophy in recipient twins with TTTS may be linked to the later development of CP. These observations may have implications for understanding the pathogenesis of CP.

▶ The reported incidence of CP in twins is usually 3 to 3½ times greater than the 0.2% of live births seen regularly among singlet pregnancies. This rate is larger than can be accounted for by the tendency for preterm delivery to occur in twin pregnancies. For preterm infants to have increased rates of CP can be seen from the 6-fold greater incidence of CP or severe mental retardation among monochorionic compared with dichorionic twins.[1] The risk of CP is even higher in the survivor when fetal death occurs, especially with monochorionic twin pregnancies. This is a second recent report of infant effects of TTTS in monochorionic pregnancies, which should focus our concern for the neonatal life of the surviving recipient twin with that syndrome.

In this collection of 33 monochorionic twin pregnancies delivered at less than 37 weeks' gestational age, TTTS was diagnosable in 17, or 51%, of cases. Nearly all were transported into the University of Tokyo center, so little predelivery therapy could be done. Among those 17 newborns delivering at a mean of 31.6 weeks' gestational age, 7 recipient twins and 2 donors showed congestive heart failure with ventricular dilation and tricuspid insufficiency. Seven recipient twins and no donors showed left ventricular hypertrophy, and

3 recipients and 1 donor twin without congenital heart disease exhibited hydropic changes. Among the 16 in whom the diagnosis of CP was made, myocardial hypertrophy was strongly predictive of that outcome (sensitivity, 71%; specificity, 89%), and logistic regression confirmed a statistically significant relationship between myocardial hypertrophy and CP. Here, as in Abstract 4–8, the TTTS- surviving recipient should be carefully followed for evidence of periventricular leukomalacia and CP, as well as congestive heart failure, for which he is at high risk.

T. H. Kirschbaum, MD

Reference

1. Minakami H, Honma Y, Matsubara S, et al: Effects of placental chorionicity on outcome in twin pregnancies: A cohort study. *J Reprod Med* 44:595-600, 1999.

Fetal Duodenal Obstructions: Increased Risk of Prenatal Sudden Death
Brantberg A, Blaas H-GK, Salvesen KÅ, et al (Univ Hosp of Trondheim, Norway)
Ultrasound Obstet Gynecol 20:439-446, 2002   4–10

Background.—Duodenal obstruction (stenosis and atresia) occurs in approximately 1 in 10,000 live births, which makes it the most common intestinal obstruction in neonates. Annular pancreas may be associated in obstructions close to the orifice of the bile duct. In addition, congenital anomalies accompany obstruction in approximately 50% of cases: 30% of infants have trisomy 21. The outcomes for these neonates have improved, but severe associated anomalies continue to cause perinatal death, and prematurity and postnatal enteral nutrition add to the management problems. Even though prenatal diagnosis of the problem allows earlier surgical intervention, which can prevent some of the complications, the ultimate outcome may not be improved.

Methods.—The participants included all fetuses given diagnoses of duodenal obstruction prenatally from January 1985 until December 2000. A prospective evaluation was carried out for each case.

Results.—Duodenal obstructions were suspected prenatally in 31 fetuses, but only 29 were eventually shown to have the problem. At the time of diagnosis, the mean gestational age was 29 + 2 weeks. All cases exhibited the "double-bubble" sign; referrals were generally based on an increased symphyseal–fundal measurement (18 of 29 cases). Twenty-four fetuses had polyhydramnios, and 12 patients had amniodrainage to relieve extensive polyhydramnios and a subjective sense of pressure; in 8 of these cases, the fetus was given the diagnosis of duodenal obstruction after 32 weeks of gestation. Six fetuses had trisomy 21 accompanying the duodenal obstruction, and, overall, 62% of fetuses had associated anomalies of some type. One pregnancy was terminated, and the fetus had trisomy 21, an atrioventricular septal defect, and signs of fetal duodenal obstruction found at 21 weeks of gestation. Intrauterine fetal death occurred in 4 pregnancies at 31 to 35 weeks of gestation; all these had diagnoses of duodenal obstruction at 31 to

34 weeks of gestation, and all had polyhydramnios; however, a normal karyotype was found. All 4 of these deaths occurred suddenly and unexpectedly, and all the infants had duodenal atresia. At delivery, the mean gestational age was 35 + 5 weeks, and 64% of the infants were delivered prematurely, including 9 before 34 weeks and 2 before 32 weeks. The mean birth weight was 2562 g (range, 1400-5050 g). Twenty-nine percent of the fetuses exhibited fetal distress during labor, leading to operative or instrumental delivery; overall, 54% of the infants were delivered operatively or with instrumentation. Three infants died postnatally, all of whom had associated anomalies. Two infants with isolated duodenal obstruction had severe neurologic dysfunction, and 2 others had impaired psychomotor development. At follow-up, 21 infants were alive, but only 6 had normal karyotypes, lacked anomalies, and had developed uneventfully after birth.

Conclusions.—Duodenal obstruction diagnosed prenatally was shown to be a serious condition presenting significant risks for the neonate. Even when the karyotype was normal and no associated anomalies were present, some infants developed bradycardia or asphyxia or died.

▶ These investigators take advantage of Norway's excellent system of tertiary obstetric referral to report on the antenatal courses of 29 pregnancies complicated by fetal duodenal atresia among patients seen at the National Center for Fetal Medicine in Trondheim over 14 years. The diagnosis was made by fetal abdominal US and the double-bubble sign and was complicated by polyhydramnios in 83%. Some form of associated developmental anomaly was seen in 62% of patients, among them trisomy 21 in 21%. Study of the anomaly, focusing on the diagnosis and care after birth, in this longitudinal study discloses an important tendency for bradycardia and transient asystole in fetal life of such fetuses. Four cases of intrauterine fetal death occurred among infants lacking other anomalies, all of whom had normal fetal heart rate tracings at 31 to 35 weeks' gestational age. One fetus showed a transient episode of asystole incidental to a US examination. Two infants who developed cerebral palsy were delivered by emergency cesarean section for fetal bradycardia, and 2 others showed impaired psychomotor development without evidence of trisomy 21, other anomalies, or adverse postnatal events. The total prenatal death rate was 38%. The authors conclude that there may be sufficient parasympathetic stimulation from the distended gastrointestinal tracts in these fetuses, which results in vagal bradycardia and periodic asystole, to explain their findings. Delivery took place at a mean gestational age of 35 weeks. This is a suggestion that is worth pursuing in the prenatal care of fetuses known to have congenital duodenal atresia.

T. H. Kirschbaum, MD

The Cervical Rib: A Predisposing Factor for Obstetric Brachial Plexus Lesions

Becker MH-J, Lassner F, Bahm J, et al (Univ of Witten-Herdecke, Wuppertal, Germany; Clinic for Plastic Surgery, Hand and Burn Surgery, RWTH Aachen, Germany; Franziskus-Hosp Aachen, Germany)

J Bone Joint Surg Br 84-B:740-743, 2002   4–11

Introduction.—Obstetrical brachial plexus lesions are often accompanied by clavicular fractures, hematoma of the sternocleidomastoid muscle, or fracture of the humerus. Traction injury is a major factor in obstetrical brachial plexus lesions, yet this explanation is not adequate for all patients. Some patients have no history of major traction during delivery, and some are delivered by cesarean section. Forty-two patients who underwent surgery for obstetric brachial plexus lesions were evaluated to determine predisposing factors for this injury.

Methods.—The study included 28 patients who had an Erb's palsy, with the paralysis being restricted to the shoulder and biceps muscles. Fourteen infants had partial or total lesions, including triceps palsy or additional lesions of the forearm and hand. Intraoperatively, the infants with Erb's palsy

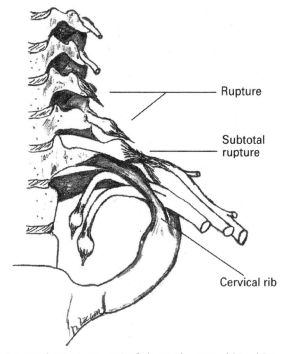

Rupture

Subtotal
rupture

Cervical rib

FIGURE 4.—Diagram showing intraoperative findings with rupture of C5 and C6, subtotal rupture of C7, and root avulsion of C8 and T1 with a complete cervical rib. (Courtesy of Becker MH-J, Lassner F, Bahm J, et al: The cervical rib: A predisposing factor for obstetric brachial plexus lesions. *J Bone Joint Surg Br* 84-B:740-743, 2002.)

had typical damage to the C5 or C6 nerve roots and the superior trunk. If damage to the lower roots was seen, it was only marginal. The remaining infants with extensive clinical findings had marked damage at the root and trunk levels. No isolated Klumpke's lesions were observed.

Results.—Complete cervical ribs were observed in 5 infants. Histologic evaluation revealed ossification and a high bone-marrow content. Four patients had a high birth weight (3890 to 4250 g), cephalic presentation, and shoulder dystocia. Apparently, the lesion was exacerbated by the cervical rib. One child was born prematurely by breech delivery with a birth weight of 1870 g, bilateral upper lesions, no regeneration on the right side, and reinnervated biceps and shoulder muscles on the left after 3 months. Intraoperatively, on the right side, an intraforaminal rupture of the C5 and C6 roots was speculated, while the caudal parts of the plexus seemed normal; the cervical rib was complete. In another patient, C8 and T1 root avulsions were noted (Fig 4). In 3 patients, fibrosis of grade B to C was seen. Thus, 4 of 5 infants with a complete cervical rib had lesions of the nerves in the narrow space between the first thoracic and eighth cervical ribs.

Conclusion.—Anatomical variations, including cervical ribs or fibrous bands, can produce narrowing of the supracostoclavicular space. This can make the adjacent nerves more susceptible to external trauma.

▶ Neonatal brachial plexus injury continues to be reported with an incidence of about 0.5 to 1 per thousand live births and has remained largely unchanged in the occurrence even with the increased incidence of abdominal birth and efforts to predict its occurrence prenatally.[1,2] This report of findings in 42 instances of attempts at surgical correction, and therefore, failures of spontaneous resolution of the neurologic injury, is a reminder of an objectively verifiable predisposing factor present in more than 10% of such infants studies here.

A cervical rib is an anomalous tranverse process of a cervical vertebral body, here, the 8th cervical, connecting with the first thoracic rib. It predisposes to brachial plexus injury with neck flexion and traction and/or compression of the infants shoulder girdle against the cervical spine. The lesion is easily seen on radiograph, which should be part of the evaluation of any newborn with brachial plexus palsy, especially, if neuromuscular surgery becomes appropriate.

T. H. Kirschbaum, MD

References

1. 1994 Year Book of Obstetrics, Gynecology, and Women's Health, pp 157-158.
2. 1997 Year Book of Obstetrics, Gynecology, and Women's Health, p 188.

Obstetric Outcome After Fetal Reduction to Singleton Pregnancies
De Catte L, Foulon W (Univ Hosp Vrije Universiteit Brussel, Brussels, Belgium)
Prenat Diagn 22:206-210, 2002   4–12

Background.—Reduction to a single fetus is considered appropriate in multiple pregnancies with structural or genetic abnormalities, uterine malformations, medical disease, cervical incompetence, or a history of repetitive preterm delivery. Fetal reduction for social/psychological indications remains controversial. This prospective study examined the obstetric outcome after multifetal pregnancy reduction (MPR) or selective feticide (SF) to singleton pregnancies.

Study Design.—The study group included 80 patients for which MFR or SF to singleton pregnancy was performed. Of the pregnancies in this group, 8 were quadruplet, 27 were triplet, and 45 were twin pregnancies. The pregnancies were divided into group 1, pregnancies complicated by congenital malformation; group 2, pregnancies with high-risk obstetric conditions; and group 3, multiple pregnancies reduced for psychological/social considerations. Prenatal diagnosis was performed by chorionic villus sampling. Perinatal outcome was recorded for all pregnancies.

Findings.—The overall pregnancy loss rate was 10%. Pregnancy failure was significantly higher when SF was performed for preterm prelabor rupture of membranes compared with other indications. MFR to singleton pregnancy for psychological reasons had a pregnancy loss rate of 5.3%. Procedures performed by 14 weeks' gestation had a significantly lower fetal loss rate, higher mean gestational age at delivery, and a decreased rate of prematurity than those performed later in gestation. Pregnancy outcome was not affected by number of fetuses reduced, chorionic villus sampling, or maternal age.

Conclusions.—Fetal reduction to singleton pregnancy has a favorable outcome, especially when performed before the fourteenth week of gestation.

▶ Experience with fetal reduction in multiple pregnancy is now extensive enough to provide some valid generalizations.[1-4] The single most authoritative source is large international experience.[5] This contribution from Brussels, however, is a clear, careful study of 80 gravidas with pregnancy reduction to singlets at a mean gestational age of 13 weeks. About half were twin pregnancies and the remainder of higher multiple order. Results were categorized into 3 classes, including 21% with a congenital anomaly in 1 twin, 31% with high-risk obstetric problems, and 48% with psychosocial indications for reductions. Fetal deaths were recorded only from pregnancies terminated past 22 weeks of gestational age with fetuses greater than 0.5 kg birth weight.

Overall, fetal loss of the singletons remaining after reduction was 10%, and in only 1 of the 3 subsets, which was composed of women with obstetric complications, was the fetal loss rate significantly higher than the overall fetal loss figure. Among those in class II with premature preterm rupture of membranes, the remaining singlets experienced a fetal death rate of 50% stemming from the presence of general chorioamnionitis and reflecting the prolonged interval between rupture of membranes and delivery of the fetuses. Fetal death rates after reduction in monochorionic twin pregnancies were more than 6 times higher than for dichorionic twins, and monochorionic preterm death rates were more than 6 times larger. This means that for triplets, reduction is best aimed at a monochorionic pair if possible. Among all the determinants of fetal death, gestational age is most important. Here for reduction to singlets at or prior to the fifteenth week of gestational age, fetal death rate of the remaining fetus was 3.3% while for those with later procedures, fetal loss was 31.6%. For pregnancies with psychosocial indications, fetal death of the remaining infant occurred in 5.3%. The advantage of early termination was also discernable for multiple pregnancies of higher order. This experience gives us a fairly clear view of some of the important guidelines in fetal reduction to procedures.

T. H. Kirschbaum, MD

References

1. 1995 Year Book of Obstetrics, Gynecology, and Women's Health, pp 119-120.
2. 2000 Year Book of Obstetrics, Gynecology, and Women's Health, pp 67-70.
3. 2001 Year Book of Obstetrics, Gynecology, and Women's Health, pp 40-42.
4. 2002 Year Book of Obstetrics, Gynecology, and Women's Health, pp 95-100.
5. Evans MI, Goldberg JD, Hornstein J, et al: Selective termination for structural, chromosomal, and Mendelian anomalies. *Am J Obstet Gynecol* 181:893-897, 1999.

Perinatal Predictors of Neurodevelopmental Outcome in Small-for-Gestational-Age Children at 18 Months of Age
McCowan LME, Pryor J, Harding JE (Univ of Auckland, New Zealand; Victoria Univ, Wellington, New Zealand)
Am J Obstet Gynecol 186:1069-1075, 2002   4–13

Background.—Small for gestational age (SGA) status is associated with adverse neurodevelopmental outcomes. The influence of perinatal variables on neurodevelopment at 18 months was prospectively examined in a group of SGA children.

Study Design.—The study group included 220 SGA children born between 1993 and 1997. Perinatal data were collected by research midwives. The Bayley Scales of Infant Development II (BSID) was used to evaluate these children at 18 months of corrected age.

Findings.—The average BSID scores were: Mental Development Index (MDI), 95.6; Psychomotor Developmental Index (PDI), 97.9; and Behavioral Rating Scale (BRS), 110.6. SGA children of mothers with pregnancy-induced hypertension were less likely to have low mental development scores than those of normotensive mothers. Low psychomotor development scores were associated with lack of breast-feeding at 3 months and long neonatal nursery stay. Low behavioral rating was associated with small head circumference (Table 2).

TABLE 2.—Pregnancy Details and BSID Scores at 18 Months

No.	MDI (n = 219)		PDI (n = 218)		BRS (n = 219)	
	Abnormal 43	Normal 176	Abnormal 31	Normal 187	Abnormal 27	Normal 192
Gestation SGA diagnosed (wk)	32.9 (3.7)	33 (3.7)	32.3 (3.9)	33.1 (3.7)	32.7 (3.7)	32.9 (3.7)
Diagnosis to delivery interval (wk)	4.3 (3.1)	3.4 (2.9)	3.7 (2.6)	3.6 (3.0)	4.3 (3.5)	3.5 (2.9)
Recruited to antenatal study	14 (33%)	75 (43%)	12 (39%)	76 (41%)	12 (44%)	77 (40%)
Antenatal corticosteroids	7 (16%)	47 (27%)	8 (26%)	46 (25%)	6 (22%)	48 (25%)
Abnormal findings on umbilical Doppler sonography	18 (42%)	70 (40%)	14 (45%)	73 (39%)	7 (26%)	81 (42%)
Pregnancy-induced hypertension	10 (23%)	78 (44%)*	9 (29%)	77 (41%)	8 (30%)	80 (42%)
Elective cesarean delivery	14 (33%)	65 (37%)	10 (32%)	69 (37%)	9 (33%)	70 (36%)

Data are expressed as mean (SD) and number (%) as appropriate.
* P = .01.

(Reprinted by permission of the publisher courtesy of McCowan LME, Pryor J, Harding JE: Perinatal predictors of neurodevelopmental outcome in small-for-gestational-age children at 18 months of age. Am J Obstet Gynecol 186:1069-1075. Copyright 2002 by Elsevier.)

Conclusions.—Few perinatal variables are predictive of outcome at 18 months in a group of SGA children.

▶ It was from one of my mentors, Dr James Low of Kingston, Ontario, that I learned that obstetric practice should be evaluated by means of developmental appraisal of resultant infants during the first 1 to 2 years of life. Thereafter, the impact of obstetric events tends to be swamped by those genetic, familial, and environmental variables, which in the absence of gross early neonatal birth injury, are ultimately more important. Here, 220 infants, originally studied in connection with 2 experiences in which umbilical artery and uterine artery Doppler evaluation of fetuses proved to be ineffective approaches to predicting and preventing preeclampsia and growth retardation in later pregnancy.[1,2] In this work, developmental appraisal of 220 infants 18 months old was compared with demographic data, records of pregnancy, and birth and socioeconomic evaluation of the earlier pregnancies. Developmental appraisal consisted of the BSID and its related MDI, PDI, and BRS. Small for gestational age infants showed a significantly lower MDI than normal controls, but women with pregnancy hypertension and growth-retarded infants had better MDI and PDI scores. Pregnancy hypertension may have protected neural development, perhaps the reason for the low cerebral palsy incidence among infants of hypertensive women. None of the variables thought to predict delayed development (abnormal umbilical Doppler signals, early growth retardation, preterm births, neonatal acidosis, and asphyxia) were useful predictors of abnormal development at 18 months. The PDI score was lower among infants not breast fed at 3 months of life, and infants with small head size at birth had lower BSID scores than normals. In general, very few perinatal observations proved to be reliable predictors of neural developmental status at 18 months of age in this group of growth-retarded infants born between 1993 and 1997.

T. H. Kirschbaum, MD

References

1. 2001 YEAR BOOK OF OBSTETRICS, GYNECOLOGY, AND WOMEN'S HEALTH, pp 161-163.
2. 2001 YEAR BOOK OF OBSTETRICS, GYNECOLOGY, AND WOMEN'S HEALTH, pp 163-164.

Absence of Association of Thrombophilia Polymorphisms With Intrauterine Growth Restriction
Infante-Rivard C, Rivard G-E, Yotov WV, et al (McGill Univ, Montreal; Université de Montreal; IMSERM Unité 535, Paris; et al)
N Engl J Med 347:19-25, 2002 4–14

Background.—Thrombophilia polymorphisms in pregnant women have been associated with an increased risk of intrauterine growth restriction (IUGR) in their babies. However, this finding is not certain. A hospital-based case-control study and a family-based study were performed to further investigate the relation.

Methods.—Four hundred ninety-three newborns with IUGR, defined as birth weight below the tenth percentile for gestational age and sex, were compared with 472 control infants, with birth weights at or above the tenth percentile. The newborns and their parents were evaluated for the polymorphisms methylenetetrahydrofolate reductase (MTHFR) C677T and A1298C, factor V Leiden G1691A, and prothrombin G20210A. In addition, the mothers were interviewed about other possible risk factors for IUGR.

Findings.—Mothers carrying a polymorphism associated with thrombophilia did not have an increased risk of IUGR newborns. The case-control study demonstrated that the odds ratios associated with 2 copies of the variant, after adjustment for newborn genotype and other risk factors, were 1.55 for MTHFR C677T and 0.49 for MTHFR A1298C. The odds ratio in heterozygotes for factor V Leiden was 1.18 and 0.92 in heterozygotes for prothrombin G20210A (Table 3). In the newborn, these polymorphisms were not related to an increased risk. Newborns homozygous for the MTHFR C677T variant had a reduced risk of IUGR, with an odds ratio was 0.52. The findings in the family-based analysis supported the results of the case-control study.

Conclusions.—These data do not suggest an association between maternal or newborn polymorphisms associated with thrombophilia and an in-

TABLE 3.—Odds Ratios for Intrauterine Growth Restriction for Maternal Polymorphisms Associated With Thrombophilia

Genotype	Basic Model†	Odds Ratio (95% CI)* Adjusted for Genotype of Newborn†	Fully Adjusted‡
MTHFR C677T			
−/+	0.84 (0.63-1.12)	0.91 (0.66-1.24)	0.98 (0.69-1.40)
+/+	1.17 (0.72-1.92)	1.48 (0.84-2.58)	1.55 (0.83-2.90)
MTHFR C677T as a single-integer variable	0.98 (0.79-1.21)	1.07 (0.84-1.38)	1.13 (0.86-1.49)
MTHFR A1298C			
−/+	0.92 (0.70-1.21)	0.81 (0.60-1.10)	0.90 (0.63-1.27)
+/+	0.72 (0.43-1.19)	0.52 (0.29-0.93)	0.49 (0.25-0.93)
MTHFR A1298C as a single-integer variable	0.88 (0.71-1.08)	0.76 (0.59-0.97)	0.78 (0.59-1.02)
Factor V Leiden			
−/+	1.24 (0.65-2.36)	1.00 (0.49-2.05)	1.18 (0.54-2.55)
Prothrombin G20210A			
−/+	1.10 (0.48-2.53)	1.02 (0.43-2.41)	0.92 (0.36-2.35)

*The comparison groups are the −/− genotypes. *CI* denotes confidence interval.

†The model includes gestational age, sex, and race or ethnic group.

‡The model includes gestational age, sex, and race or ethnic group as well as the genotype of the newborn, weight gain during pregnancy, the prepregnancy body-mass index, smoking during the third trimester, primiparity or multiparity, presence or absence of preeclampsia in the current pregnancy, and presence or absence of previous intrauterine growth restriction.

(Reprinted by permission courtesy of Infante-Rivard C, Rivard G-E, Yotov WV, et al: Absence of association of thrombophilia polymorphisms with intrauterine growth restriction. *N Engl J Med* 347:19-25. Copyright 2002, Massachusetts Medical Society. All rights reserved.)

creased risk of IUGR. A reduced risk of IUGR was observed in mothers homozygous for the MTHFR A1298C variant and in infants homozygous for the MTHFR C677T variant. Further research is needed.

▶ This is a very large study based on 472 women with growth retarded newborns compared with 493 normal controls, with thoughtful excellent statistical analysis. It is a convincing part of what seems to be a second generational evaluation of the role of genetically determined thrombophilia in pregnancy abnormality. Although a search for the mutations may be appropriate in intrauterine fetal death of uncertain origin,[1] several investigators have failed to find evidence of their role in the development of pregnancy hypertension.[2] In this study, DNA was collected from blood and, in fathers, buccal smears and PCR on epithelial cells DNA done with appropriate primers for the C6775 and A1298C sites of the methylene tetrahydrofolate reductase gene mutation (MTHFR), the Factor V Leiden mutation, and the mutation for prothrombin at the G20210A site. Controls were matched for gestational age, sex, race, ethnicity in either mother and newborn, and covariates describing weight gain, pre-pregnancy weight, parity, history of prior preeclampsia or growth retardation, and smoking. Results are expressed as odds ratios and in 95% confidence ranges, comparing women homozygous and heterozygous for gene mutations with controls. Laudably, the authors found no difference when the definition of growth retardation was set at either the 5th percentile or 10th percentile of weight at stated gestational age. Gravidas were caucasian in 70% and 24% black, largely Haitian in nationality.

In brief, none of the gene polymorphisms were associated with an increased risk of growth retardation. However, women homozygous for the A1298C mutation for MTHFR had a reduced risk of bearing a growth retarded infant. Among 201 women homozygous for the C677T MTHFR gene not taking multivitamins in the third trimester, there was an increased likelihood of newborn growth retardation (RR 12.3), presumably a result of fetal folate deficiency. Analyses based on 246 sets of data from mother, father, and newborn, and 463 controls generated the same conclusions. These results seemed largely to lay to rest concerns for growth retardation resulting from these maternal genetic thrombophilias.

T. H. Kirschbaum, MD

References

1. 2003 Year Book of Obstetrics, Gynecology, and Women's Health, pp 41-42.
2. 2002 Year Book of Obstetrics, Gynecology, and Women's Health, pp 133-134, 142-144, and 227-229.

5 Antepartum Fetal Surveillance

Venous Doppler Velocimetry in the Surveillance of Severely Compromised Fetuses
Hofstaetter C, Gudmundsson S, Hansmann M (Univ of Bonn, Germany; Univ Hosp MAS, Malmö, Sweden)
Ultrasound Obstet Gynecol 20:233-239, 2002   5–1

Background.—When the venous fetal circulation is evaluated, the normal pulsation noted in blood velocity waveforms of the central veins was found to follow a characteristic pattern during fetal heart failure, which implies that fetal venous blood velocity may help in monitoring the fetal condition during high-risk pregnancies. Normally, 20% to 30% of well-oxygenated placental blood is shunted through the fetal ductus venosus (DV) to the heart's left side, while 70% to 80% flows through the liver, mainly into the right side of the heart and through the ductus arteriosus and the descending aorta back to the placenta. When fetal compromise occurs, as much as 70% of venous blood is shunted through the DV to oxygenate essential organs, which, in turn, reduces liver perfusion to 30% and extends fetal survival. The changes in the venous velocimetry of the right hepatic vein (HV), DV, and umbilical vein (UV) were assessed in severely compromised fetuses with growth restriction. In addition, changes normally occurring before fetal demise were noted.

Methods.—Of the 154 growth-restricted fetuses evaluated prospectively, 37 had reversed flow in the umbilical artery (blood flow class [BFC] III). The right HV and DV were assessed with the use of serial Doppler velocimetry, which also registered the presence of UV pulsations. The final examination before birth or fetal demise was the only one analyzed and was linked to the obstetric outcome (defined as gestational age at birth, birth weight, and perinatal mortality). The venous velocimetry of 15 nonsurviving fetuses with BFC III was compared with the results of the 22 survivors.

Results.—Forty-seven fetuses had UV pulsations; 18 were double and 27 were single. Correlations were noted between increased impedance in the umbilical artery and an increased pulsatility index (PI), bilateral notching in the uterine arteries, and a decrease in gestational age, which served as signs of early onset placental insufficiency, particularly in BFC III cases. Signs of increased brain sparing were found with increasing placental vascular resistance. The S and D peaks differed slightly on venous waveforms, but, at ES and A peak, a dramatic decline in blood velocity accompanied increased placental vascular resistance. Reversal of flow in late diastole and increased pulsatility in the HV and DV were closely correlated with increased placen-

FIGURE 2

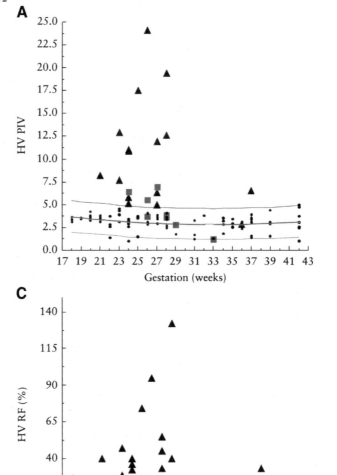

(*Continued*)

FIGURE 2 (cont.)

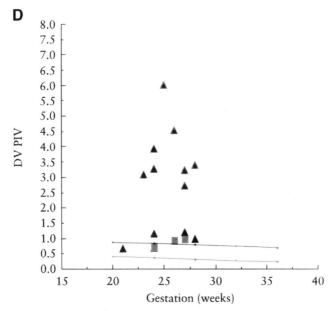

FIGURE 2.—Venous velocimetry values in cases of intrauterine death (*solid triangle*) and neonatal death (*solid square*) in relation to normal values of pulsatility index for veins (PIV) (A) and reversed flow (RF) in the right hepatic vein (HV) (C) and of PIV in the ductus venosus (DV) (D). *Small circles and triangles* represent values of normal fetuses. *Three horizontal lines* represent 5th, 50th, and 95th centiles, and 2 *horizontal lines* represent 5th and 95th centiles. (Courtesy of Hofstaetter C, Gudmundsson S, Hansmann M: Venous Doppler velocimetry in the surveillance of severely compromised fetuses. *Ultrasound Obstet Gynecol* 20:233-239, 2002. Reprinted by permission of Wiley-Liss, Inc., a subsidiary of John Wiley & Sons, Inc.)

tal vascular resistance, especially in fetuses less than 30 weeks of gestational age (Fig 2). The UV pulsation frequency exceeded the reversal of flow in the DV. An average of 2 days for infants in BFC II and III and 10 days in BFC I and 0 passed between the last US examination and delivery or fetal demise (Table 2). Of the fetuses with normal umbilical artery blood flow, 3 died perinatally; in addition, 3 fetuses in BFC I, 3 in BFC II, and 15 in BFC III died perinatally. In the BFC III class, nonsurvivors had a higher umbilical artery PI and change of A-velocity in the HV and DV than did survivors. The blood velocity pattern in the HV was slightly better at predicting impending death than was that in the DV.

Conclusions.—When placental insufficiency is severe, early and extreme growth restriction occurs, and most of these fetuses have pathologic venous velocimetry. Generally, the ES and A velocities are decreased and the pulsatility of the right HV and DV are increased, which indicates impaired myocardial functioning. Adverse outcomes were also highly likely in fetuses with double pulsations in the UV. Thus, monitoring of high-risk pregnancies may benefit from the use of venous Doppler evaluation.

TABLE 2.—Perinatal Outcome of Pregnancies With Growth Restriction and Different Grade of Placental Impedance

Outcome	Umbilical Artery Blood Flow Class (BFC)			
	0	I	II	III
Number	50	55	12	37
GA at birth (weeks) (range)	36 ± 3 (28-41)	34 ± 4* (26-41)	32 ± 4* (24-38)	28 ± 2† (23-33)
Birth weight (g)	2064 ± 539	1572 ± 759*	1225 ± 543*	641 ± 299†
VSGA (< 3rd centile)	20	32*	5	27†
Apgar at 5 min = 7	6	7	5	23†
Umbilical artery pH = 7.35	44	45	8	17
Cesarean section	28	37	9	23
ODFD	22	27	6	22
NICU admission	25	37*	10*	23
Stay at NICU (days)	18	34	32*	49†
Perinatal mortality	3	3	3	15†
Intrauterine fetal death	1	1	2	12

* P < .05.
† P < .01.
Abbreviations: GA, Gestational age; *VSGA,* very small for gestational age; *ODFD,* operative delivery for fetal distress; *NICU,* neonatal intensive care unit.
(Courtesy of Hofstaetter C, Gudmundsson S, Hansmann M: Venous Doppler velocimetry in the surveillance of severely compromised fetuses. *Ultrasound Obstet Gynecol* 20:233-239, 2002. Reprinted by permission of Wiley-Liss, Inc., a subsidiary of John Wiley & Sons, Inc.)

▶ Pulsations in the UV and the fetal inferior vena cava are reliable signs of impending fetal cardiac failure as shown in work reviewed early.[1,2] Further, their interpretation does not require the flawed assumptions associated with the evaluation of umbilical or uterine artery velocimetric signals, that is, that they are directly related to bulk blood flow and vascular resistance. These authors expand on those venous Doppler US findings by evaluating a series of 154 pregnancies exhibiting intrauterine growth retardation. Pulsations are defined here as rhythmic blood velocity reductions equal to or greater than 15% as defined by venous Doppler. The pulsations appear to reflect increased systolic and diastolic pressure in the right atrium and ventricle, compounded by decreased myocardial compliance as the ventricles begin to decrease stroke volume. The result is an increase in UV blood flow diverted through the DV to the left ventricle and carotid arteries, away from the right ventricle and ductus arteriosus, which is the conduit that would normally convey 70% to 80% of oxygenated blood from the placenta. The authors wisely avoid the use of quantitative measurements, which are nearly always impossible to obtain, and categorize umbilical arterial blood flow after Lauren, using classes 2 and 3 to represent absent end diastolic flow velocity and reverse umbilical artery blood flow, respectively.

Perinatal mortality was 15.6%, and 16 cases of intrauterine death occurred. As expected, both Lauren's BFCs applied to umbilical arteries correlated inversely with measured PI values. At the time of maximum atrial systole and the peak of end systolic pressure, venous inflow of blood from the placenta virtually ceased in many fetuses. In general, UV pulsations occurred far more often than the reverse flow in the DV. Pulsations in the HV were slightly better indicators of fetal compromise than were DV pulses. Reverse flow in the DV had the lowest sensitivity for perinatal mortality as shown in Figure 2, A, C, and D. Although perinatal mortality was related to absent or reverse diastolic velocity in the umbilical artery, the relationship is complicated by the ability of very premature fetuses to tolerate Lauren umbilical artery BFC II and III for long periods. Their nonquantitative nature and uncertain evidence of the duration of that tolerance are severe handicaps in the use of umbilical artery data clinically. This work strongly supports the use of the PI based on the pulsatility noted in the HV or DV as signs of fetal jeopardy and suggests that they are superior to arterial Doppler signals used by others.

T. H. Kirschbaum, MD

References

1. 1991 Year Book of Obstetrics, Gynecology, and Women's Health, pp 101-102.
2. 2001 Year Book of Obstetrics, Gynecology, and Women's Health, pp 147-149.

Fetal Nasal Bone Length: Reference Range and Clinical Application in Ultrasound Screening for Trisomy 21

Bunduki V, Ruano R, Miguelez J, et al (Univ of Sao Paulo, Brazil)

Ultrasound Obstet Gynecol 21:156-160, 2003   5–2

Background.—Down syndrome is the most common chromosomal abnormality in newborns. Invasive diagnostic procedures, such as chorionic villus sampling and amniocentesis, are proposed for women considered at high risk for delivery of Down syndrome infants, and these procedures have a procedure-related fetal loss rate of 0.5% to 1%. Increasingly, patients at risk would prefer a screening program based on US screening before deciding whether to undergo invasive screening. Fetuses with trisomy 21 are typically seen with subtle facial abnormalities, including a hypoplastic nasal bone. This study provided a reference range for the length of the fetal nasal bone and an evaluation of its value for use in US screening for trisomy 21 in the second trimester.

Methods.—Cross-sectional data from 1923 consecutive singleton pregnancies were used to establish a reference range of fetal nasal bone length. The fetuses were scanned at 16 to 24 weeks' gestation in women over age 35 years. In addition, screening for trisomy 21 was prospectively studied using nasal bone lengths smaller than the fifth percentile as a cutoff value.

Results.—Of the 1923 cases studied, follow-up data were available in 1631 cases (84.4%). Trisomy 21 was identified in 22 cases (1.35%). Nasal

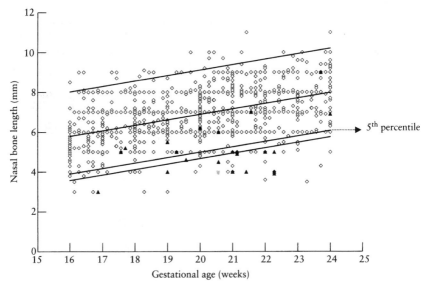

FIGURE 2.—Reference ranges of nasal bone length from 16 to 24 weeks' gestation. The 95% confidence interval is given and the fifth percentile line is indicated. *White diamonds* indicate normal cases and *black triangles* indicate trisomy 21 cases. (Courtesy of Bunduki V, Ruano R, Miguelez J, et al: Fetal nasal bone length: Reference range and clinical application in ultrasound screening for trisomy 21. *Ultrasound Obstet Gynecol* 21:156-160, 2003. Reprinted by permission of Wiley-Liss, Inc., a subsidiary of John Wiley & Sons, Inc.)

bone length increased as a function of gestational age in a linear relationship. Use of the fifth percentile as a cutoff value for screening for trisomy 21 resulted in a sensitivity of 59.1% for a 5.1% false-positive rate (Fig 2). The likelihood ratio was 11.6.

Conclusion.—The use of fetal nasal bone length measurement for screening for trisomy 21 provided a sensitivity comparable to that obtained from maternal biochemistry for a given false-positive length of 5%. The association of nasal bone lengths with other sonographic markers, with consideration of the background risk for maternal and gestational age, may provide additional improvements in sensitivity and reduce false positive findings.

▶ This evaluation of US measurements of nasal bone length as predictors of Down syndrome is an apparently unbiased attempt to evaluate measurements done between 16 and 24 weeks' gestational age in 1609 normal pregnancies and 22 instances of in utero Down syndrome—all with successful follow-up and complete data. Unlike some authors who report nasal bones absent in 27% of fetuses with proven Down syndrome (see Abstract 4–2), they report no failures of visualization and describe their care in establishing a sagittal plane US image and positioning the transducer at a 45° angle with the long axis of the nose. Using linear correlation with gestational age, they define the fifth percentile of nasal bone length as a function of gestational age, and using values equal or less than that value, test its predictive strength.

Their data reveal a 59% sensitivity with a false-positive rate of 75%. These results agree with earlier workers (see Abstract 4–2) who showed similarly low sensitivity, a high false-positive rate, and a somewhat lower false-negative rate, probably a result of fewer cases. Neither results approach the predictability reported in the earlier study by Cicero et al (see Abstract 4–2), but instead report false-positive rates prohibitively high in terms of clinical applicability.

T. H. Kirschbaum, MD

Nasal Bone Evaluation in Fetuses With Down Syndrome During the Second and Third Trimesters of Pregnancy
Lee W, DeVore GR, Comstock CH, et al (William Beaumont Hosp, Royal Oak, Mich; Natl Inst of Child Health and Human Development, Bethesda, Md; Wayne State Univ, Detroit)
J Ultrasound Med 22:55-60, 2003   5–3

Background.—Individuals with Down syndrome often have accompanying abnormalities in skeletal growth and development, and these may be evaluated with the use of US. It has been suggested that a nonvisualized nasal bone may indicate the presence of Down syndrome during the first trimester of pregnancy. Three-dimensional US was used to standardize multiplanar views of the fetal nasal bone and to investigate the significance of its presence or absence in relation to Down syndrome.

Methods.—Twenty fetuses with trisomy 21 and 20 fetuses without this aberration were scanned by three-dimensional US during the second and

Nasal Bone Visualization

(N = 40)

Examiner 1	Down Syndrome	Normal
Nonvisualized Nasal Bone	8	4
Visualized Nasal Bone	12	16

(N = 40)

Examiner 2	Down Syndrome	Normal
Nonvisualized Nasal Bone	9	2
Visualized Nasal Bone	11	18

FIGURE 5.—Nonvisualization of the nasal bone and Down syndrome. Two independent examiners showed significant agreement in scoring which fetuses had US visualized nasal bones. Approximately 40% to 45% of fetuses with a nonvisualized nasal bone were identified as having Down syndrome. (Courtesy of Lee W, DeVore GR, Comstock CH, et al: Nasal bone evaluation in fetuses with Down syndrome during the second and third trimesters of pregnancy. *J Ultrasound Med* 22:55-60, 2003.)

early third trimesters of pregnancy. The volume data were analyzed with the use of a midline sagittal view of the facial profile, and masked and randomly allocated volume data sets were reviewed by independent examiners; interobserver reliability was calculated with regard to the presence or absence of the nasal bone on these sonograms. Logistic regression was used to link this finding to the presence of Down syndrome.

Results.—The maternal age was slightly older for pregnancies with trisomy 21 (35.0 years) than for pregnancies without this disorder (30.7 years). With respect to finding the nasal bone on sonograms, the examiners showed substantial qualitative agreement. Technical factors were responsible for disagreements between the observers in 3 cases. Overall, 1 examiner identified 8 fetuses with abnormalities, and the other found 9 (Fig 5). For the first examiner, a nonvisualized nasal bone was not a statistically significant predictor of Down syndrome; for the second, who identified 1 additional case, statistical significance was achieved. In the fetuses who lacked trisomy 21, the first examiner found a nasal bone in 80% of cases, and the second found one in 90%.

Conclusions.—The use of three-dimensional multiplanar views can help to detect whether the nasal bone is present in fetuses with and without trisomy 21. However, because a substantial number of affected fetuses had the nasal bone present, its absence cannot be viewed as an accurate predictor of the presence of Down syndrome.

▶ Recently, a Kings College School of Medicine group[1] reported success in using the US absence of the fetal nasal bone at 11 to 14 weeks' gestation in identification of fetuses with trisomy 21. The authors' intent was that this observation be used in combination with other US data to increase the precision of the fetal diagnosis of Down syndrome. In brief, they found nasal bones to be present in 99.5% of healthy fetuses and in 27% of fetuses with trisomy 21. Because other investigators[2] have failed to confirm the results published by this group, it's helpful to have this attempt at confirmation by a group of 11 well-known American ultrasonographers.

Forty fetuses with Down syndrome proven by amniocentesis were scanned in blinded fashion by groups of 2 ultrasonographers using three-dimensional US. In 82% of the pregnancies less than 24 weeks' gestational age, they found nasal bones present in 80% to 90% of healthy fetuses and in 55% to 60% of fetuses with Down syndrome. Their results showed low sensitivity (40%-45%) and high false-negative rates (38%-43%) together with 29% to 33% false-positive rates. Although the data from Cicero et al[1] did not include false-positive rates, they indicated that adding their new data to that from a 1998 study would have reduced the resultant false-positive rate from 8.28% to 3.02% at a risk cutoff level of 1 to 300. It's not possible to evaluate this statement. The work of the American authors indicates that nasal bone imaging is unlikely to carry any merit for clinical application.

T. H. Kirschbaum, MD

References

1. Cicero S, Curcio P, Papageorghiou A, et al: Absence of nasal bone in fetuses with trisomy 21 at 11-14 weeks' gestation: An observational study. *Lancet* 358:1665-1667, 2001.
2. 2000 YEAR BOOK OF OBSTETRICS, GYNECOLOGY, AND WOMEN'S HEALTH, pp 158-160.

Changes in Fetoplacental Vessel Flow Velocity Waveforms Following Maternal Administration of Betamethasone
Edwards A, Baker LS, Wallace EM (Monash Univ, Clayton, Australia)
Ultrasound Obstet Gynecol 20:240-244, 2002   5–4

Introduction.—The maternal administration of betamethasone in pregnancies complicated by absent end-diastolic flow in the umbilical artery (UA AEDF) has recently been shown to be linked with a transient return of end-diastolic flow in most pregnancies. A prospective investigation of pregnancies complicated by UA AEDF was performed to further explore the timing of the effects of betamethasone administration on the umbilical artery and to evaluate its effects in other fetoplacental vessels.

Methods.—Flow velocity waveforms were recorded from the umbilical artery, fetal middle cerebral artery, renal artery, aorta, and ductus venosus before and after maternal betamethasone administration using real-time pulsed wave Doppler in 12 women with pregnancies complicated by UA AEDF.

Results.—The administration of maternal betamethasone was followed by the return of end-diastolic flow within 24 hours in all 12 pregnant women. The end-diastolic flow was initially observed at 4 hours and was present in all women at 8 hours. Additionally, there was a significant reduction in the pulsatility index in the fetal aorta at 8 hours and the middle cerebral artery at 24 hours (Fig 1). No change was seen in the ductus venosus or the renal artery flow velocity waveforms.

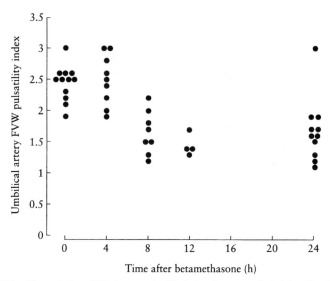

FIGURE 1.—Change in the umbilical artery pulsatility index after maternal administration of betamethasone in 12 fetuses with umbilical artery absent end-diastolic flow. *Abbreviation: FVW,* Flow velocity waveform. (Courtesy of Edwards A, Baker LS, Wallace EM: Changes in fetoplacental vessel flow velocity waveforms following maternal administration of betamethasone. *Ultrasound Obstet Gynecol* 20:240-244, 2002. Reprinted by permission of Wiley-Liss, Inc., a subsidiary of John Wiley & Sons, Inc.)

Conclusion.—Maternally administered betamethasone produces a return in umbilical artery end-diastolic flow in as early as 4 hours, along with widespread vasodilation throughout the fetoplacental vasculature in pregnancies complicated by UA AEDF.

▶ In 1999, Professor EM Wallace[1] reported a series of retrospective observations in 28 women at a median gestational age of 27 weeks with UA AEDF given betamethasone prior to attempts at delivery. In two thirds of those cases, the fetuses showed disappearance of AEDF—usually assumed to be evidence of placental structural abnormality and possible fetal jeopardy—for a period of 24 hours. The observations were associated with a decrease in Doppler pulsativity index in the umbilical arteries.

Though presumed to be a result of decreased placental vascular resistance after steroid administration—since placental bulk blood flow and pressure measurements are needed to measure vascular resistance and were not performed—that interpretation is arguable. Changes in the pulsatility index, ratios of blood velocities during fetal systole and diastole, were presumed, without rigorous proof, to be inversely related to bulk umbilical blood flow.

No placebo observations were included and the women, many with pregnancy hypertension, were receiving a variety of antihypertensive and vasoactive agents in irregular patterns. Nonetheless, since AEDF is presumed to result from faulty placental development and reduction in the number of placental stem arterioles and terminal placental villi, the disappearance of

AEDF was puzzling and an unexplainable indication of umbilical vascular plasticity in a circulation presumed to be structurally underdeveloped.

This prospective study, representing 51 sets of Doppler US measurements in 12 women, was designed to clarify the earlier observations. The women had a median gestational age of 28.5 weeks, all had fetal growth retardation, and some pregnancies were complicated by hypertension and diabetes mellitus. Doppler measurements of umbilical artery, middle cerebral artery 1 cm from the circle of Willis, descending aorta, ductus venosus, and renal arteries are made prior to a maternal dose of 11.4 milligrams of betamethasone and Doppler measurements are repeated at 4,8,12 and 24 hours thereafter. A reduction in umbilical artery and aortic pulsativity index was present within 8 hours, and the middle cerebral artery pulsativity index was decreased 24 hours after corticoid dosage. No other US velocity patterns were altered. Fetal cardiac output, a critical factor in umbilical artery bulk blood flow velocity, was not measured but fetal heart rate was unchanged.

There is considerable doubt as to the reality of fixed structural change in placental umbilical artery morphology in growth retardation and particularly in preeclampsia.[2-4] A placental morphometric study, including among its investigators Professor Peter Kaufman of the Technical University of Aachen, a pioneering figure in the placental development of the fetal vasculature, found no difference in the prevalence of stem and intermediate placental vessels in fetuses with AEDF compared with normals.[5] Although this is a work in progress, it certainly strongly suggests that AEDF patterns do not reflect fixed structural placental vascular pathology as commonly assumed, but rather the presence of a reversible vasoconstrictive process in the umbilical circulation to which Professor Wallace's observations were an important clue.

T. H. Kirschbaum, MD

References

1. 2000 YEAR BOOK OF OBSTETRICS, GYNECOLOGY, AND WOMEN'S HEALTH, pp 169-170.
2. 1997 YEAR BOOK OF OBSTETRICS, GYNECOLOGY, AND WOMEN'S HEALTH, pp 134-138.
3. 1998 YEAR BOOK OF OBSTETRICS, GYNECOLOGY, AND WOMEN'S HEALTH, pp 91-94.
4. 2000 YEAR BOOK OF OBSTETRICS, GYNECOLOGY, AND WOMEN'S HEALTH, pp 101-102.
5. 1997 YEAR BOOK OF OBSTETRICS, GYNECOLOGY, AND WOMEN'S HEALTH, pp 156-158.

The Amniotic Fluid Index in Late Pregnancy
Stigter RH, Mulder EJH, Bruinse HW, et al (Univ Med Ctr Utrecht, The Netherlands)
J Matern Fetal Neonatal Med 12:291-297, 2002   5–5

Background.—Several studies have used US techniques to measure the quantity of amniotic fluid during pregnancy, including the use of the amniotic fluid index (AFI) as a practical semiquantitative assessment. Reports suggest that AFI declines gradually during the final weeks of pregnancy but with significant variation between individuals. Changes in AFI were assessed in relation to the accurately calculated gestational age and to the onset of spontaneous labor.

Methods.—The prospective study included 137 women with uneventful term pregnancies, recruited at a mean gestational age of 275 days. All women underwent at least 1 AFI measurement, while 51 underwent more than 1 measurement. The analysis included a total of 220 AFI measure-

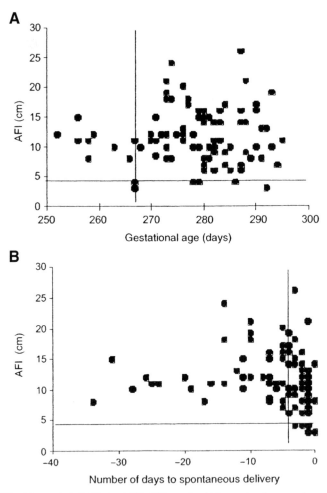

FIGURE 3.—The amniotic fluid index (*AFI*) of 88 cases in which gestational age was determined on the basis of a first-trimester US scan and labor onset was also spontaneous. *Horizontal lines* indicate the commonly defined level of oligohydramnios; *vertical lines* indicate the time by which the first abnormal measurement occurred. A, AFI measurements in relation to gestational age. B, The same measurements in relation to the time of onset of labor. (Courtesy of Stigter RH, Mulder EJH, Bruinse HW, et al: The amniotic fluid index in late pregnancy. *J Matern Fetal Neonatal Med* 12:291-297, 2002.)

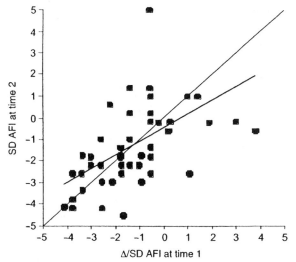

FIGURE 4.—Relationship between pairs of amniotic fluid index (*AFI*) measurements obtained at a mean interval of 8 days (range, 1-22 days) from each other. The AFT is shown as the Δ/SD on the basis of the normal values of Nwosu and colleagues (Nwosu EC, Welch CR, Manasse PR, et al: Longitudinal assessment of amniotic fluid index. *Br J Obstet Gynaecol* 100:816-819, 1993.). The *regression line* and the *line of equality* are shown. (Courtesy of Stigter RH, Mulder EJH, Bruinse HW, et al: The amniotic fluid index in late pregnancy. *J Matern Fetal Neonatal Med* 12:291-297, 2002.)

ments. Changes in the AFI were determined in relation to gestational age, assessed using a first-trimester crown-rump length measurement. The association between AFI and time to onset of spontaneous labor was analyzed as well.

Results.—No significant change in the AFI was apparent from week 37 to week 42 of gestation. However, over the last 11 days before spontaneous labor occurred, there was a significant reduction in the AFI (Fig 3). With correction for gestational age, the AFI of individual patients remained stable for periods as long as 2 weeks (Fig 4). Meconium staining was significantly related to gestational age but not to the AFI nor to fetal distress at birth. Fetal distress was unrelated to the AFI and to the measured reduction in AFI on the last 2 measurements before labor.

Conclusion.—In term pregnancies, the observed reduction in the AFI in the final weeks before the onset of labor does not reflect increasing gestational age, even in the postterm period. Rather, the decline in the AFI appears to be related to the process of labor itself. Amniotic fluid volume reduction appears to occur via circulatory redistribution and reduced production of fetal urine, and to be followed by spontaneous onset of labor.

▶ This is an attempt to define the presence or size of the decrease in amniotic fluid after 37 weeks' gestation reported by several investigators using unblinded observations and cross-sectional data. These authors made use of longitudinal observations of 137 pregnancies. It's a difficult task and their results are not wholly satisfactory. When amniotic fluid volume is studied longitudinally through gestation, the number of subjects decreases with time as delivery removes data sources, producing serious problems in statistical evaluation.

Relatively few women reach or exceed 42 weeks' gestational age. Original estimates of 8.5% to 10% of all pregnancies reaching that duration include poorly dated pregnancies, as the work of ML Reuss et al proved. Using first-trimester US dating of patients, they found the incidence of women exceeding 41 completed weeks of pregnancy was 2.5% to 3%.[1] Further, those women whose pregnancies reached 42 weeks' gestational age may represent a subset with qualitative differences still undefined from women delivering closer to term. Previously reported results suggest any decrease in AFI past 40 weeks' gestational age is small and possibly exhibited by only a few gravidas who reach that gestational age.

Using only 88 of the women for whom early US dating was available, no relationship of AFI to gestational age could be demonstrated (see Fig 3), but when the independent variable was changed to the number of days prior to spontaneous delivery (excluding those whose labors were induced), the only 5 women whose AFIs reached levels of oligohydramnios were confined to the last 4 days prior to delivery. The coefficient of linear correlation of AFI with time determined at 2 intervals 8 days apart in the same women range from 0.57 to 0.73, showing most women had relatively constant AFIs through the intervals from 37 to 42 weeks' gestational age (see Fig 4).

The incidence of fetal distress based on perinatal data was not significantly reflected by decreased AFI, though uncertainty about both dependent and independent variables, as discussed above, makes that an arguable conclusion. This work confirms that oligohydramnios in late pregnancy is minor in amount and confined to a minority of women, occurring shortly before onset of labor.

T. H. Kirschbaum, MD

Reference

1. Reuss ML, Hatch MC, Sasser M: Early US dating of pregnancy. *J Clin Epidemiol* 48:667, 1995.

Uterine Artery Doppler Patterns in Abdominal Pregnancy
Acácio GL (Universidade de Taubaté, Brazil)
Ultrasound Obstet Gynecol 20:194-196, 2002   5–6

Introduction.—Changes in the uterine artery blood flow waveform during pregnancy are usually attributed to trophoblastic invasion of the myometrium. Described was a case report of a third trimester abdominal pregnancy in which Doppler velocimetry of the uterine artery was performed.

Case Report.—Woman with 2 previous uncomplicated pregnancies was referred with a diagnosis of third trimester abdominal pregnancy. US showed a singleton fetus at 26 weeks' gestation situated transversely in the upper abdomen and an empty uterus. The placenta was situated behind and below the fetus and there was a vertical pocket of amniotic fluid measuring 1.5 cm between the fetus and the placenta.

Fetal assessment demonstrated a reactive non-stress test. Doppler velocimetry of the umbilical and middle cerebral arteries revealed a normal pattern. Doppler assessment of the uterine arteries showed low-resistance flow and absence of notching bilaterally (left uterine artery pulsatility index [PI] = 0.78, resistance index [RI] = 0.51; right uterine artery PI = 1.16, RI = 0.65). These values continued to be similar in all assessments performed at 26 to 29 weeks' gestation.

The patient was hospitalized for rest and monitoring. She reported mild diffuse abdominal pain. Sonographic examinations revealed normal fetal growth up to 28 weeks' gestation. At 29 weeks' gestation, there was an increase in resistance to flow in the umbilical artery and a reduction in the PI of the middle cerebral artery. The infant was delivered by a median abdominal incision from the xiphisternum to the suprapubic region at 29 weeks' gestation. The placenta was over the intestinal rings and slightly adherent to them and firmly attached to the left ovary. The placenta and left ovary were removed.

The neonate weighed 1340 g, had no breathing distress, and was discharged from the hospital after gaining the necessary weight. The mother's recovery was uncomplicated and she was discharged home after 7 days. At-9 month follow-up, a transvaginal sonogram was performed. Doppler velocimetry of the uterine arteries revealed high resistance with bilateral notching (left uterine artery PI = 2.49, RI = 0.88; right uterine artery PI = 2.00, RI = 0.83).

Conclusion.—Modification of the uterine artery waveform may occur independently of trophoblastic invasion of the spiral arteries. Systemic factors, including hematologic modifications and local regulation may interfere with the flow of the uterine arteries and thus be cofactors in the modification of the Doppler pattern in such arteries.

▶ Those who feel Doppler US of the uterine arteries in pregnancies is useful in predicting and detecting preeclampsia[1] and fetal growth retardation[2] and that it should therefore be used routinely in asymptomatic gravidas,[3] rely on an hypothesis explaining the changes they see in Doppler analysis done on preeclamptics. With interaction between material decidual spiral arterioles and wandering placental trophoblast, normal maternal arteries entering the intravillous space become dilated and function as low resistance high flow rate conduits during the first trimester of pregnancy. Further, a notch occurring in diastole in the Doppler velocity flow profile of the uterine artery appearing in the first trimester of pregnancy disappears normally at 24 to 26 weeks.

An important additional assumption, difficult to prove, is that such Doppler-based variables as the pulsativity index can be used to represent bulk blood flow volume based on the Doppler signal which itself depicts only blood flow velocity. Failure of the progressive decrease in pulsativity index and persistence of the diastolic notch past 26 weeks of pregnancy suggest to believers abnormal placentation and the possibility of growth retardation and/or eventual preeclampsia.

This is a case report of an abdominal pregnancy terminated at 29 weeks on clinical grounds with birth of a normal 1340-g newborn in which there was no uterine placentation, yet uterine artery Doppler changes as customarily seen proceeded apparently normally along the uterine arteries supplying an empty uterus and perfusing no placenta. As the authors point out, there's something incomplete about the assumptions inherent in normal uterine artery Doppler US evaluation in addition to the serious problems involved in the analysis of their clinical usefulness in preeclampsia.[4]

T. H. Kirschbaum, MD

References

1. 1998 YEAR BOOK OF OBSTETRICS, GYNECOLOGY, AND WOMEN'S HEALTH, pp 153-155.
2. 1998 YEAR BOOK OF OBSTETRICS, GYNECOLOGY, AND WOMEN'S HEALTH, pp 89-91.
3. 1998 YEAR BOOK OF OBSTETRICS, GYNECOLOGY, AND WOMEN'S HEALTH, pp 143-147.
4. 2001 YEAR BOOK OF OBSTETRICS, GYNECOLOGY, AND WOMEN'S HEALTH, pp 160-162, 166-167.

A Long-term Transdermal Nitric Oxide Donor Improves Uteroplacental Circulation in Women With Preeclampsia
Nakatsuka M, Takata M, Tada K, et al (Okayama Univ, Japan)
J Ultrasound Med 21:831-836, 2002   5–7

Background.—Nitric oxide (NO) is an important regulator of vascular tone. NO deficiency may be a cause of preeclampsia. The effect of long-term transdermal administration of the NO donor isosorbide dinitrate (ISDN) on maternal and fetoplacental circulation in patients with preeclampsia was examined.

Study Design.—The study group consisted of 12 women with preeclampsia and oligohydramnios. Preeclampsia was defined as blood pressure greater than 190/90 mm Hg and proteinuria of 1+ by dipstick. Arterial pressures were assessed by color image pulsed Doppler ultrasonograhy. Amniotic fluid volume was evaluated by measuring the largest amniotic fluid pocket. The average patient age was 30.4 years. Of the 12 women in the study group, 8 were nulliparous and 4 were multiparous. Ten of the women had severe preeclampsia. Patients were treated with ISDN until delivery, from 4 to 30 days.

Findings.—Transdermal application of a long-term ISDN patch significantly suppressed patient blood pressure. ISDN also significantly reduced the average pulsatility index (PI) in the uterine and umbilical arteries. The amniotic fluid pocket size also increased several-fold after treatment (Fig 2). The only side effects were mild and temporary headache in 2 of 12 women.

Conclusions.—Transdermal administration of low-dose ISDN to preeclamptic women improved maternal blood pressure and fetoplacental cir-

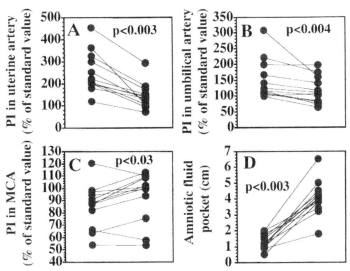

FIGURE 2.—Effects of transdermal ISDN on PI in the uterine arteries, umbilical arteries, and fetal middle cerebral arteries (MCAs) and volume of amniotic fluid. **A**, PI in the uterine arteries. The average PI was significantly decreased by treatment with ISDN ($P < .003$, Wilcoxon signed rank test). **B**, PI index in the UA. The average PI was significantly decreased by treatment with ISDN ($P < .004$, Wilcoxon signed rank test). **C**, PI in the fetal MCA. The average PI was not significantly elevated by treatment with ISDN ($P < .003$, Wilcoxon signed rank test after Bonferroni correction). **D**, Volume of amniotic fluid. The size of the amniotic pocket was significantly increased by treatment with ISDN ($P < .003$, Wilcoxon signed rank test). (Courtesy of Nakatsuka M, Takata M, Tada K, et al: A long-term transdermal nitric oxide donor improves uteroplacental circulation in women with preeclampsia. *J Ultrasound Med* 21: 831-836, 2002.)

culation and was associated with increases in amniotic fluid. This treatment was not associated with any serious side effects. A lower rate of cesarean delivery was also associated with treatment. A controlled, clinical trial is warranted to investigate the clinical effect of the treatment of preeclamptic women with long-term ISDN on pregnancy outcome.

▶ These investigators have provided some interesting findings in 12 women with severe pregnancy-induced hypertension, 8 of them nulliparous and probably preeclamptic, which makes more extended clinical trials appropriate. NO, administered acutely, has the ability to induce vasodilation and reduce blood pressure in hypertensive gravidas.[1,2] In experimental animals it also shows the capacity to inhibit aggregation of platelets and white blood cells on endothelial surfaces. Despite earlier claims to the contrary, hypertensive pregnancies are associated not with reduced concentrations of NO but, rather, with increased evidence of NO production compared with normal pregnant women, making it likely that NO deficiency does not exist in acutely hypertensive women.[3,4] These investigators, using transdermal tape applications of ISDN, a NO donor proven in acute experiments employing both the sublingual and transdermal routes to increase NO absorption, administered 20 mg over 24 hours daily in hypertensive women for a mean of 11 days beginning at an average gestational age of 30.2 weeks until they delivered.

The authors observed, during the course of treatment, a significant decrease in mean systolic and diastolic blood pressure, decreased PI in uterine and umbilical arteries, but no significant change in fetal MCA PI. Average amniotic fluid index was said to increase from a mean of 1.4 cm to 4.0 cm, but the absence of observer blinding in this often subjective measurement makes this a questionable finding. Clinical outcome was uncontrolled in this experience, and nothing for certain can be inferred about it.

Ultrasonically derived blood velocity measurements and their arithmetic permutations bear only a remote relationship to blood flow volume and no clear relationship to vascular resistance, the ratio of blood pressure to blood bulk flow rate. Nonetheless, the ultrasonic PI of uterine and UA blood signals are currently in clinical use, and observations of this sort provide support for prospective controlled blinded experiments designed to explore the clinical significance of the use of chronic NO administration in pregnancy hypertension.

T. H. Kirschbaum, MD

References

1. 1998 YEAR BOOK OF OBSTETRICS, GYNECOLOGY, AND WOMEN'S HEALTH, pp 23-25,
2. 2001 YEAR BOOK OF OBSTETRICS, GYNECOLOGY, AND WOMEN'S HEALTH, pp 6-8.
3. 2000 YEAR BOOK OF OBSTETRICS, GYNECOLOGY, AND WOMEN'S HEALTH, pp 28-31.
4. 2002 YEAR BOOK OF OBSTETRICS, GYNECOLOGY, AND WOMEN'S HEALTH, pp 128-131.

Umbilical Artery Doppler Waveform Notching: Is It a Marker for Cord and Placental Abnormalities?

Abuhamad A, Sclater AJ, Carlson EJ, et al (Eastern Virginia Med School, Norfolk)

J Ultrasound Med 21:857-860, 2002   5–8

Background.—Umbilical cord abnormalities are associated with fetal morbidity and mortality. A notch in the umbilical artery Doppler waveform has been associated with cord abnormalities. The prevalence of umbilical artery waveform notching and its association with cord and placental abnormalities were examined.

Study Design.—During a 6-month period, pregnant patients undergoing sonographic evaluation at a single institution, who had singleton pregnancies, gestational age greater than 27 weeks, normal fetal growth and anatomy, and absence of maternal metabolic or vascular disease could participate in this study. Umbilical artery velocity waveforms were obtained in 1857 pregnancies. The cases included all patients with a fetal umbilical artery waveform notch. Two controls, with normal umbilical artery waveforms and matched for gestational age, were selected for each case. Obstetric and neonatal outcome data were prospectively collected. Outcome data included gestational age at delivery, delivery method, indications for surgical delivery, birth weight, and umbilical artery pH. Two pathologists, who were blinded to the prenatal Doppler results, examined all umbilical cords and placentas.

Findings.—Overall, an umbilical artery waveform notch was detected in 1.6% of these pregnancies. Postnatal placental examination revealed an accessory placental lobe in 17% of the patients compared with 1.8% of the controls. There were umbilical cord abnormalities in 72% of the cases and in 14% of the controls.

Conclusions.—This prospective, controlled study indicated that umbilical artery waveform notching was associated with cord and placental abnormalities. The presence of umbilical artery waveform notching should suggest a need for increased fetal surveillance in these pregnancies.

▶ This small study of 1857 pregnancies in which Doppler umbilical artery US was performed says something important about the origin of notching of the umbilical artery signal, often interpreted as a sign of a compromised fetus.[1-3] Among women with singlet pregnancies in the third trimester with no evidence of US abnormalities and normal fetal growth, a 1.6% incidence (29 cases) of umbilical artery Doppler notching was seen. Compared with a control group of 54 normal controls, there was no significant difference in gestational age or weight at birth or in umbilical artery pH at the time of delivery between those with or without this finding. Although the cesarean section incidence was greater than in those with notching than in controls (31% vs 18%), the difference was not statistically significant. The diagnosis of nonreassuring fetal heart rate patterns as an indication for cesarean section was significantly more common among those with umbilical artery notching (78%) than in controls (20%). Nearly one fourth of those with umbilical artery notching showed marginal or velamentous cord insertion, cord strictures (2 cases), or true or false cord knots. Fairly clearly, these generally harmless anomalous cord variations gave umbilical Doppler signals which were misinterpreted as reflecting fetuses in potential in utero jeopardy. It's hard to know how often this misinterpretation is made. Clearly, in this experience, it was an important consideration in obstetric management.

T. H. Kirschbaum, MD

References

1. 1998 Year Book of Obstetrics, Gynecology, and Women's Health, pp 53-55.
2. 2000 Year Book of Obstetrics, Gynecology, and Women's Health, pp 166-167.
3. 2001 Year Book of Obstetrics, Gynecology, and Women's Health, pp 163-164.

Intrapartum Fetal Heart Rate Patterns in the Prediction of Neonatal Acidemia
Williams KP, Galerneau F (Yale Univ, New Haven, Conn)
Am J Obstet Gynecol 188:820-823, 2003   5–9

Background.—Severe fetal metabolic acidemia at birth is defined as an umbilical artery pH of 7.0 or less. This condition occurs in approximately 20 to 25 infants per 1000 births, and long-term neurologic damage and damage to other fetal organ systems results in 10% to 30% of these infants. Continuous intrapartum electronic fetal monitoring was introduced to provide a screening test to predict the development of fetal asphyxia. Evaluation of fetal heart rate (FHR) was expected to identify fetuses at risk for asphyxia and allow early intervention before the development of intrapartum asphyxia. However, FHR monitoring has a low sensitivity for prediction of asphyxia due to variability in the interpretation of FHR patterns and a lack of standardization in the definition of electronic fetal monitoring parameters. The purpose of this study was to correlate changes in the intrapartum electronic FHR patterns with the development of significant neonatal acidemia.

Methods.—The study group included 488 fetuses at a gestational age of more than 37 weeks who had continuous electronic fetal monitoring during the last 2 hours of labor. Umbilical artery cord gas analysis was performed at delivery. An investigator blinded to the cord gas analysis findings reviewed all 488 tracings, using the National Institute of Child Health and Human Development guidelines for fetal heart rate monitoring. FHR tracings with bradycardia were removed for additional analysis.

The patients were assigned to 1 of 6 groups on the basis of the presence or absence of normal variability during the last hour of monitoring, combined with the absence of decelerations or the presence of variable or late decelerations. The relationship between changes in variability and the outcome variables of pH and base deficit in the various groups were assessed by means of analysis of variance and χ^2 test, with significance at the $P < .05$ level.

Results.—Patients with normal variability and accelerations maintained an umbilical artery pH of 7.0 or greater in over 97% of cases, even in the presence of late or variable decelerations. In patients with minimal or absent variability (amplitude less than 5) for at least 1 hour, the incidence of significant acidemia (pH less than 7.0) ranged from 12% to 31%.

Conclusion.—In intrapartum fetal heart rate monitoring for prediction of the development of significant acidemia, the most significant finding is the presence of minimal or absent variability for at least 1 hour as a solitary abnormal finding or in conjunction with late decelerations in the absence of accelerations. Urgent delivery should be considered in these cases.

▶ In 1999, Dr James Low and colleagues from Ontario's Queens University in a very important study clarified the reasons for the high false-positive rates for prediction of fetal asphyxia and acidemia from FHR tracings.[1] It is useful to have this similar confirmatory effort to support those earlier findings. In both cases, the studies were similarly structured.

In 488 cases, interpretable FHR tracings done at least 2 hours antepartum and subsequent cord blood values were available, excluding multiple pregnancies, anomalous fetuses, and cases of prolonged bradycardia. The results were studied against evidence of neonatal acidemia (umbilical artery pH, 7.0 or less; BE, −17 mL or greater). The Canadian study added clinical neonatal evidence of asphyxia as a criterion for newborn acidosis.

In both cases, since transient FHR abnormalities are very common before normal births, only FHR records obtained within 1 hour prior to birth proved useful in establishing generalizations. Low's group found absent short-term baseline variability associated with late decelerations had a significant relationship to the occurrence of neonatal acidemia. The New Haven group noted prolonged bradycardia important as well, but those cases were exempted from their study. Applying those variables as predictive criteria to the entire population of 488 cases and observing newborn outcome allowed an estimate of prospective positive value.

In this study, false-positive rates ranged from 50% to 69%. Criteria of absent baseline variability, late decelerations, and prolonged bradycardia studied in the Canadian series yielded sensitivity values of 17%, with false-positive values of 82% being noted. Using all FHR abnormalities as predictors yielded a sensitivity of 93% with a false-positive rate of 97.4%. Clearly, there are definable relationships between common patterns of FHR abnormalities and newborn acidosis, but they lack sufficient strength in predicting newborn fetal acidemia for clinical usefulness without additional evidence of pathology in labor.

T. H. Kirschbaum, MD

Reference

1. 2000 Year Book of Obstetrics, Gynecology, and Women's Health, pp 153-155.

Antepartum Fetal Asphyxia in the Preterm Pregnancy

Low JA, Killen H, Derrick EJ (Queen's Univ, Kingston, Ont, Canada)
Am J Obstet Gynecol 188:461-465, 2003   5–10

Introduction.—An important gap in the current knowledge concerning fetal asphyxia is the prevalence of antepartum fetal asphyxia and its significance as a cause of brain and other organ system dysfunction and damage. More than 1 decade of experience in a single tertiary care obstetric unit was reviewed to provide insight into the frequency and characteristics of antepartum fetal asphyxia in pregnancies delivered preterm.

Methods.—A total of 1182 pregnancies were delivered preterm between May 1984 and May 1996 and underwent clinical blood gas and acid-base evaluation at delivery. Of these, 30 preterm pregnancies had biochemically proven antepartum fetal asphyxia, defined as an umbilical artery base deficit of more than 12 mmol/L. Antepartum clinical characteristics, fetal assessment tests, and neonatal complications were recorded. Fetal asphyxia was classified as either mild, moderate, or severe on the basis of umbilical artery deficit and newborn encephalopathy and other organ system complications.

Results.—Antepartum fetal asphyxia made up at least 34% of the fetal asphyxia in the pregnancies delivered preterm. Predictive criteria that prompted intervention and diagnosis included clinical risk factors and abnormal fetal assessment tests. There were 50% and 15% incidences of moderate or severe asphyxia in antepartum preterm pregnancies and in

TABLE 3.—The Clinical Complications and Treatment of the
Preterm Pregnancies

	Preterm Pregnancy (No.)	
Clinical Complication	< 32 Weeks	32-36 Weeks
Previous stillbirth	0	1
Hypertension	2	3
Diabetes mellitus	1	4
Antepartum hemorrhage	3	8
Preeclampsia	4	6
Premature rupture of membranes	0	1
Small-for-gestational age	2	6
Hydramnios	0	1
Oligohydramnios	4	2
Treatment		
Early intervention	4	16
Delayed intervention	5	5

(Reprinted by permission of the publisher courtesy of Low JA, Killen H, Derrick EJ: Antepartum fetal asphyxia in the preterm pregnancy. *Am J Obstet Gynecol* 188:461-465. Copyright 2003 by Elsevier.)

term pregnancies, respectively. Moderate or severe asphyxia occurred at equal rates with early and delayed intervention (Table 3).

Conclusion.—Fetal asphyxia in pregnancies delivered preterm is often present before the onset of labor. Abnormal fetal assessment tests are important predictors of antepartum fetal asphyxia. The increased incidence of moderate and severe fetal asphyxia in pregnancies delivered preterm implies a greater likelihood of long-term morbidity and death.

▶ This investigator, experienced in the diagnosis and significance of fetal asphyxia,[1,2] addresses himself here to a small—but important—question: How often is fetal asphyxia present prior to labor? *Asphyxia* is defined here as the presence of sufficient metabolic acidosis in umbilical artery blood to result in a base deficit greater than 12 mmol/L. In a collection of 1182 preterm deliveries at Queen's University, Dr Low reports on 30 fetuses delivered abdominally prior to labor. Including all 1182 pregnancies, the incidence of asphyxia was 7.2%, and of those 9 pregnancies delivering prior to 32 weeks and the 21 delivering between 32 and 36 weeks, 50% showed moderate to severe asphyxia immediately after cesarean section. Only 8 of the 30 infants delivered abdominally had normal antenatal tests. The obstetric problems requiring abdominal birth are listed in Table 3. Because false-positive antenatal tests are not included, one cannot estimate the predictivity of antenatal testing in this unit. What is clear is that in preterm infants with a compelling clinical indication for early intervention, the chances of predelivery asphyxia as reflected in cord blood studies are in the range of 1:2 to 1:3 in this obstetric practice.

T. H. Kirschbaum, MD

References

1. 1991 YEAR BOOK OF OBSTETRICS AND GYNECOLOGY, pp 174-176.
2. 2000 YEAR BOOK OF OBSTETRICS, GYNECOLOGY, AND WOMEN'S HEALTH, pp 153-155.

How Well Does Reflectance Pulse Oximetry Reflect Intrapartum Fetal Acidosis?

Stiller R, von Mering R, König V, et al (Univ Hosp, Zurich, Switzerland)
Am J Obstet Gynecol 186:1351-1357, 2002   5–11

Background.—The sensitivity of cardiotocography is good, but its specificity is poor, which has led to unneeded obstetric interventions. Fetal scalp blood gas measurements accurately indicate intrapartum fetal acid–base balance, but the technique is invasive and shows only the condition at the time of measurement and not the fluctuations that occur constantly. Transmission pulse oximetry is a continuous noninvasive measure of fetal oxygen saturation (SpO_2) but is impractical for the presenting fetal head. Reflectance pulse oximetry incorporates light-emitting and light-receiving diodes on the same side of the tissue, which allows continuous intrapartum monitoring. The clinical utility of intrapartum reflectance pulse oximetry as demonstrated by its sensitivity and specificity for measuring fetal SpO_2 to determine if acidosis is present was assessed.

Methods.—One hundred seven sets of measures were evaluated. Correlations were made between intrapartum fetal SpO_2 in relation to labor stage and umbilical artery pH, base excess, and partial pressure of carbon dioxide (PCO_2). With the use of historic umbilical arterial cutoff values, a receiver operating characteristic curves analysis was performed. Calculations were carried out to determine the fetal SpO_2 cutoff range and optimal sensitivity and specificity.

Results.—The values for the umbilical artery were generally less favorable when the SpO_2 level was less than 40%, but none of those greater than 40% were unfavorable. The values for pH and PCO_2 followed a similar pattern. Base excess values at about –10 mmol/L were found when the SpO_2 levels were about 60%, but no clear pattern emerged for these values. Fetal SpO_2 levels were both sensitive and specific with respect to pH values for the first stage of labor, but a decline was seen in area under the curve value as birth approached. The values were 0.77 for the first stage, 0.71 for the second, and 0.54 for the third. PCO_2 values followed the same pattern; area under the curve values were 0.8, 0.68, and 0.58 for the 3 stages. Base excess showed poor sensitivity and specificity overall and for each stage and was excluded from further analysis. The fetal SpO_2 cutoff values were determined for pH to be 33.3% for the total monitoring period, 33.2% for the first and second stages, and 36.2% for the third stage; for PCO_2, the cutoff values were 33.3% overall, 35.5% for the first stage, 33.2% for the second stage, and 36.2% for the third stage. Positive predictive values were poor and decreased steadily as birth approached, but negative predictive values were satisfactory at 96% to 98% in all stages.

Conclusions.—Reflectance pulse oximetry should not be needed routinely to monitor for fetal acidosis during labor and delivery.

► The use of reflectance pulse oximetry has been discussed here previously,[1,2] both times unfavorably. The method rests on a fetal scalp sensor and light source. Reflected light from the scalp is collected, split, and transmitted through filters appropriate for the optical absorption maxima of oxidized and reduced hemoglobin. Photometry transforms each of the 2 light intensities to an electrical potential, and the ratio of those voltages can be used to estimate oxyhemoglobin saturation and, in turn, PO_2. All 3 respiratory blood variables, PO_2, PCO_2, and pH, vary constantly during labor as changes in intrauterine pressure change blood flow rates through the skin of the scalp. During high pressure, exchanges between blood and tissue are impeded, PO_2 and pH decline because of prolonged extraction of nutrients, and PCO_2 increases. With uterine diastole, the pressure and blood gas variables reverse. No one of these variables may be used to define fetal hypoxia, for example, only fetal hypoxemia. Hypoxemia is a regular occurrence in fetal life, but fetal hypoxia can be defined only if one knows blood flow rates and arterial and venous blood oxygen contents, as the Fick equation requires. What these authors demonstrate quite nicely is that metabolic acidosis, that is, a significant reduction in fetal blood base excess, is not altered by fluctuations of PO_2, PCO_2, and pH in these cases but only by hypoxia and the resultant accumulation of lactate and pyruvate, which reflect reduced aerobic fetal metabolism. That is why judgments of fetal compromise based on reflectance oximetry measurements have a false-positive rate ranging from 72.7% to 89.9%, which is, clearly, too imprecise for clinical use.

T. H. Kirschbaum, MD

References

1. 1999 Year Book of Obstetrics, Gynecology, and Women's Health, pp 147-149.
2. 2002 Year Book of Obstetrics, Gynecology, and Women's Health, pp 171-174.

Accuracy of Fetal Pulse Oximetry
Luttkus AK, Lübke M, Büscher U, et al (Humboldt-Universität Berlin)
Acta Obstet Gynecol Scand 81:417-423, 2002   5–12

Background.—Some authors have reported that pulse oximetry inadequately detects fetal compromise. The correlation of fetal pulse oximetry and saturation readings from hemoximetry at low oxygen saturation was determined in a prospective observational study.

Methods.—The study included fetuses with nonreassuring fetal heart rate tracings suggesting hypoxia and necessitating fetal scalp blood samples. Fetal oxygen saturation measures obtained by pulse oximetry were compared with those acquired by the use of hemoximetry in fetal scalp blood samplings. A blinded pulse oximeter was used to determine arterial oxygen saturation values, which were stored continuously on a computer. Data were obtained on 42 neonates with normal outcomes and on 18 with combined respiratory and metabolic acidemia at birth.

Findings.—Hemoximetry and pulse oximetry measures had a correlation coefficient of 0.72. The median absolute difference in saturation was +5.2% saturation, with a range of −21% to +36% saturation. The median of relative differences was 23%, with a range of −30% to +217%. The saturation distribution between the 2 groups was a median hemoximetry (pulse oximetry) of 38% (42%) in the normal group and 26% (39%) in the acidemic group. The correlation coefficient was 0.19 between pH and saturation from pulse oximetry in fetal scalp blood from the samplings.

Conclusions.—Compared with hemoximeter values, fetal pulse oximetry measurements tend to overestimate arterial oxygen saturation levels. Further research is warranted.

▶ There are some serious theoretical problems in the use of fetal reflectance pulse oximetry in evaluation of fetal oxygenation (Abstract 9–12), which may by themselves explain the failure of benefit disclosed by a recent prospective randomized trial.[1] This study raises the additional prospect of technical inaccuracy in the resultant data. Here, comparisons of oxyhemoglobin saturation values were made on 170 women felt to be at risk for fetal hypoxemia based on fetal heart rate analysis. Forty-two had vaginal deliveries of infants with normal cord blood values, but 18 were born with umbilical blood acidosis (pH < 7.16; BE < 9.4 mmol/L). Comparisons were made between saturation values determined in vitro on umbilical artery blood, using a standard reflectance oximeter. Here, linear correlation coefficients for the 2 techniques were significant (r = 0.72) but the difference in values determined by the 2 modalities was plus or minus 6.4% oxyhemoglobin saturation over a total range of approximately 40% saturation. The absolute differences ranged from −21% to +36% and pulse oximetry values tended to be false high in the critical range of umbilical artery blood saturation less than 30%. The problems with pulse oximetry rest with changes in transducer positioning, subcutaneous edema formation, and changes in cutaneous blood flow and blood oxygen extraction with and following uterine contractions. Enthusiasm for fetal pulse oximetry is hard to justify at this point.

T. H. Kirschbaum, MD

Reference

1. 2002 Year Book of Obstetrics, Gynecology, and Women's Health, pp 170-174.

Doppler Assessment of the Uterine Circulation in the Second Trimester in Twin Pregnancies: Prediction of Pre-Eclampsia, Fetal Growth Restriction and Birth Weight Discordance
Geipel A, Berg C, Germer U, et al (Univ Med School Bonn, Germany; Med Univ of Lübeck, Germany; Inst of Cancer Epidemiology and Inst of Social Medicine Lübeck, Germany)
Ultrasound Obstet Gynecol 20:541-545, 2002   5–13

Background.—Compared with singleton pregnancies, twin pregnancies show increased rates of fetal and maternal morbidity and mortality and, thus, are considered high risk, requiring careful antenatal management.

From 9% to 26% of twin pregnancies involve fetal growth restriction (FGR) (depending on the definition used), and antenatal care may be improved if cases of FGR or significant growth discordance are identified early. Whether uterine artery Doppler investigations have predictive value in cases of pre-eclampsia, FGR, or birth weight discordance of 20% or greater among twin or singleton pregnancies was evaluated.

Methods.—The maternal and perinatal data gleaned from 256 dichorionic twin pregnancies were reviewed retrospectively. Documented findings included the mean uterine artery resistance index from both sides and the presence or absence of notching. The 95th centile of reference ranges for singleton or twin nomograms was chosen as the cutoff level for abnormal flow variables.

Results.—In 14% of patients, the Doppler findings were abnormal when the twin reference values were used; abnormal findings were found in 3.1% of patients when the singleton reference values were used. Forty-two patients had persistent unilateral or bilateral notching, and 14 had bilateral notches. Combining the resistance indices (RIs) over the 95th centile with unilateral or bilateral notching yielded a reduced screen positive rate of 9% when twin reference values were used. Growth restriction was found in 45 fetuses (8.9%), and discordant growth of 20% or greater was present in 38 pairs (14.8%). Pre-eclampsia developed in 22 patients (8.6%). When twin reference values were used, significantly earlier delivery occurred in patients with abnormal uterine artery RIs, along with a lower mean birth weight, a higher rate of discordance of 20% or greater, and significantly more instances of pre-eclampsia. When singleton reference values were used, only pre-eclampsia was statistically significant. Patients whose RI was greater than the 95th centile and who had unilateral or bilateral notching had the highest rate of adverse outcomes of pregnancy. The overall sensitivity of pathologic Doppler results for the main outcome variables was low, and the use of twin reference values yielded a higher sensitivity and negative predictive value but a lower specificity and positive predictive value. The combination of RIs greater than the 95th centile and notching proved to have a higher specificity and positive predictive value. The highest sensitivity for predicting adverse outcomes accompanied unilateral or bilateral uterine artery notching. Focusing solely on cases with bilateral notching yielded lower predictive values. In twin pregnancies, bilateral notching did not achieve the high negative predictive value it had with singleton gestations.

Conclusions.—Applying adapted twin nomograms to find pregnancies with complications had higher sensitivity than using singleton nomograms. Compared with unselected singleton pregnancies, however, the negative predictive values for adverse pregnancy outcomes were lower. A higher rate of complications occurred even when the uterine artery Doppler results were normal. Bilateral and unilateral notching in the uterine artery waveform had the highest sensitivity for predicting a complicated pregnancy.

▶ A series of negative findings should lead to a lack of enthusiasm for uterine artery Doppler US in early and mid pregnancy as a predictor of fetal growth retardation or maternal pre-eclampsia in either unselected or high-risk pregnancies.[1-5] Because the incidences of pregnancy hypertension, birth rate discordance, and growth retardation are higher in multiple than singlet pregnancies, there is still some justification for investigating the predictive strength of Doppler uterine velocimetry in twin pregnancies, and this retrospective cohort study of 256 dichorionic twin pregnancies with Doppler uterine artery evaluations at 18 to 24 weeks' gestation provides the necessary data. The patients were seen during 1998-2001, so the study had the advantages of color flow Doppler technology, evaluation of unilateral or bilateral Doppler systolic notching, and complete pregnancy outcome data. Confidence limits for normality were defined with the use of nomograms obtained from twin pregnancies.[6] The incidence of hypertensive pregnancy was 8.6%, and birth weights discordant by at least 20% occurred in 14.8%. Growth retardation occurred in 8.9%, which was a consequence of the use of birth weight equal to or less than 10% to define growth retardation.

Indices of predictability (ie, sensitivity, 29%-35%; false-positive rates, 54%-78%; false-negative rates, 7%-15%) among a variety of outcome permutations were, if anything, less hopeful than in similar studies of singlets. Uterine artery Doppler US clearly seems a forlorn hope in terms or predicting fetal growth retardation in multiple pregnancies.

T. H. Kirschbaum, MD

References

1. 1991 Year Book of Obstetrics and Gynecology, pp 116-117.
2. 1998 Year Book of Obstetrics, Gynecology, and Women's Health, pp 51-53.
3. 1998 Year Book of Obstetrics, Gynecology, and Women's Health, pp 153-155.
4. 2001 Year Book of Obstetrics, Gynecology, and Women's Health, pp 165-167.
5. 2002 Year Book of Obstetrics, Gynecology, and Women's Health, pp 174-175.
6. Rizzo G, Arduini D, Romanini C: Uterine artery Doppler velocity waveforms in twin pregnancies. *Obstet Gynecol* 82:978-983, 1993.

6 Labor, Operative Obstetrics, and Anesthesiology

Caesarean Delivery and Outcome in Very Low Birthweight Infants
Paul DA, Sciscione A, Leef KH, et al (Christiana Care Health System, Newark, Del; Thomas Jefferson Med College, Philadelphia)
Aust N Z J Obstet Gynaecol 42:41-45, 2002   6–1

Background.—Intraventricular hemorrhage (IVH) is a problem in very low birth weight infants (<1500 g). The relation between delivery mode and both IVH and death were evaluated.

Study Design.—The study group included 400 very low birth weight infants born by cesarean delivery and 305 very low birth weight infants born by vaginal delivery from 1993 to 1998. Univariate and multivariate analyses were performed comparing delivery mode to outcome.

Findings.—After controlling for gestational age, fetal presentation, and multiple birth, cesarean delivery was not associated with decreased risk of IVH, severe IVH, or death among very low birth weight infants (Table 6).

TABLE 6.—Results of Multivariate Analysis, Unadjusted and Adjusted Odds Ratio for IVH and Death

	Unadjusted Odds Ratio (95% CI)	Adjusted Odds Ratio (95% CI)*
Caesarean compared to vaginal delivery		
IVH	0.6 (0.4-0.9)	1.2 (0.7-2.0)
Severe IVH (grade III-IV)	0.8 (0.5-1.3)	1.9 (0.9-4.0)
Mortality	0.7 (0.5-1.1)	1.2 (0.6-2.4)
Vaginal breech versus caesarean breech delivery		
IVH	2.3 (1.1-4.9)	1.2 (0.5-3.1)
Severe IVH (grade III-IV)	2.9 (1.0-7.9)	2.4 (0.7-7.8)
Mortality	1.5 (0.6-3.6)	0.5 (0.2-1.7)

Abbreviation: CI, Confidence interval.
*Variables adjusted for in multivariate model: race, gestational age, small for gestational age, maternal age, prolonged and preterm rupture of membranes, oligohydramnios, multiple gestation, preeclampsia, fetal presentation, and inborn status.
(Courtesy of Paul DA, Sciscione A, Leef KH, et al: Caesarean delivery and outcome in very low birthweight infants. *Aust N Z J Obstet Gynaecol* 42:41-45, 2002.)

Conclusions.—In this population of very low birth weight infants, cesarean delivery was not associated with a decreased risk of intraventricular hemorrhage or death. The decision to perform cesarean delivery should be based on obstetric factors.

▶ Several older studies that have failed to support the value of abdominal birth for low birth weight and very low birth weight fetuses have been reviewed here earlier,[1-4] but this report of 705 very low birth weight infants delivered over a 5-year period in the Christiana Health Care System is noteworthy for the regular use of predelivery steroids, neonatal, exogenous surfactant, and high-frequency ventilation techniques, all part of modern neonatal care. As a retrospective cohort study, it was designed to evaluate the impact of the route of delivery on perinatal mortality rate and IVH for very low birth weight infants. Cranial ultrasounds were done on day 4 of life and every month thereafter to the time of discharge. The population consisted of 400 infants, the majority delivered abdominally, two thirds after the onset of labor. Of 126 fetuses presenting by the breech, only 40 were delivered vaginally, which complicates evaluation of that variable considerably. Inevitably, the 2 groups differ in some regards—more growth retardation, preeclampsia, and multiple pregnancy among breech presentations in the cesarean section group and more prolonged ruptured membranes and prolonged labor in women delivered vaginally. Some of these differences are evaluated by logistic regression multivariate analysis.

Univariate analysis showed a significantly larger incidence of grade 1 to 2 IVH among vaginal births but no significant difference in the incidence of more severe IVH grades 3 and 4 or perinatal mortality following vaginal delivery. Abdominal breech delivery was less likely to result in grade 3 to 4 IVH, but mortality rates did not differ between those delivered abdominally and vaginally. When multivariate analysis was used to adjust for group differences in gestational age, race, gravidity, maternal age, and several other obstetric abnormalities, no significant differences in the chances of IVH, severe IVH, or perinatal mortality as a result of cesarean section in either vertex or breech presentations could be proven. This conclusion is concordant with and therefore enforces earlier studies regarding the failure of benefit of abdominal compared with vaginal delivery for very low birth weight infants.

T. H. Kirschbaum, MD

References

1. 1991 YEAR BOOK OF OBSTETRICS, GYNECOLOGY, AND WOMEN'S HEALTH, pp 146-148.
2. 1991 YEAR BOOK OF OBSTETRICS, GYNECOLOGY, AND WOMEN'S HEALTH, pp 179-180.
3. 1992 YEAR BOOK OF OBSTETRICS, GYNECOLOGY, AND WOMEN'S HEALTH, pp 166-167.
4. 2000 YEAR BOOK OF OBSTETRICS, GYNECOLOGY, AND WOMEN'S HEALTH, pp 83-84.

Factors That Are Associated With Cesarean Delivery in a Large Private Practice: The Importance of Prepregnancy Body Mass Index and Weight Gain
Young TK, Woodmansee B (Gainesville, Fla)
Am J Obstet Gynecol 187:312-320, 2002   6–2

Background.—The incidence of cesarean delivery is increasing, as is the incidence of obesity. The relationship between maternal body mass index (BMI), maternal weight gain, cesarean delivery, and diagnosis of cephalopelvic disproportion (CPD) was examined with the use of data from a large private obstetric practice.

Study Design.—The study group consisted of 3375 primiparous deliveries from February 1993 to June 2001 from a large private obstetric practice. Maternal height was self-reported. The initial weight or a self-reported prepregnancy weight was used to calculate BMI. Weight gain was the difference between the first recorded weight and the last recorded weight in women initially seen before 20 weeks' gestation. CPD was defined as little to no labor progress over a 2- to 4-hour period, adequate contractions, and cervix dilated to at least 3 cm. Z statistics were used to determine the significance of BMI and maternal weight gain on cesarean delivery.

Findings.—The overall cesarean rate for the primiparous women in this group was 21.76%. The risk of cesarean delivery increased significantly with increasing BMI. This was primarily due to an increase in cesarean delivery for CPD/failure to progress. In this large private practice, a woman with a BMI of more than 30 kg/m² was 6 times more likely to have a cesarean delivery for a diagnosis of CPD/failure to progress than a woman with a BMI

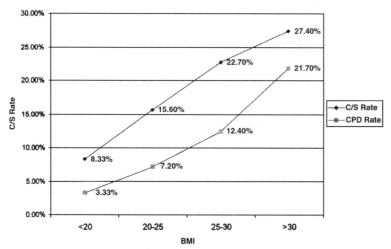

FIGURE 1.—BMI versus cesarean delivery (*C/S*) and CPD rate-controlled gestational age (38-40 weeks) and birth weight (3250-3750 g). The *closed diamonds* denote C/S, and the *closed squares* denote the CPD rate. (Reprinted by permission of the publisher courtesy of Young TK, Woodmansee B: Factors that are associated with cesarean delivery in a large private practice: The importance of prepregnancy body mass index and weight gain. *Am J Obstet Gynecol* 187:312-320. Copyright 2002 by Elsevier.)

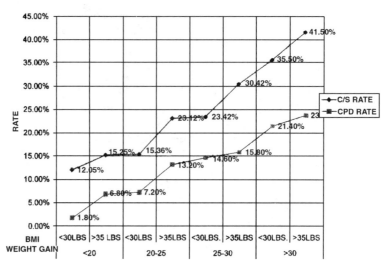

FIGURE 2.—The cesarean delivery (*C/S*) and CPD rate versus excessive weight gain (<30 pounds vs >35 pounds of weight gain). The *closed diamonds* denote C/S, and the *closed squares* denote the CPD rate. (Reprinted by permission of the publisher courtesy of Young TK, Woodmansee B: Factors that are associated with cesarean delivery in a large private practice: The importance of prepregnancy body mass index and weight gain. *Am J Obstet Gynecol* 187:312-320. Copyright 2002 by Elsevier.)

of less than 20 kg/m² (Fig 1). This difference persisted after controlling for birth weight, gestational age, maternal age, and maternal height. Excessive pregnancy weight gain also had a significant effect on cesarean delivery rate (Fig 2). This effect was also primarily related to CPD/failure to progress.

Conclusions.—This retrospective study of 1 large obstetrical private practice found an association between cesarean delivery rate, especially for CPD/failure to progress, and both maternal BMI and weight gain during pregnancy. The strong statistical relationship suggests a causative role. A rethinking of maternal diet, weight, and weight gain may be necessary to increase labor performance and reduce the cesarean delivery rate.

▶ This study demonstrates a direct relationship between BMI of primigravid women at the beginning of prenatal care and the occurrence of abdominal delivery in a population of 3383 primigravida women delivered over 8 years by a single large practice group. The authors suggest that the relationship is causal. The overall section rate was 21.8%, 11.7% or 54% of the total attributed to CPD. It's the use of this latter term, stemming from 19th century obstetrics when it frequently meant that pelvic inlet contraction in growing female children altered the pelvis weakened by osteomalacia secondary to rickets, that is problematic.[1] Currently CPD is a rare cause of dystocia and is difficult but possible to diagnosis objectively. Inefficient uterine contractions and fetal malpresentation, more common causes of dystocia in modern obstetrics, must be ruled out in the process. The diagnosis of CPD must be made after full or at least advanced cervical dilation is attained. Observations of women with proven pelvic abnormality in good labor demonstrate arrest of progress with inlet abnormality with the cervix 8 to 10 cm dilated and the presenting vertex

0 to −1 station. For midplane contraction in normal labor, progress usually ceases with the cervix fully dilated and the vertex at +3 station in OA or OP position. Pelvic examination and x-ray examination or MRI can be used to prove the absence of pelvic bony abnormality and extension or asynclitism of the vertex to assist in the diagnosis.

The 1980 NICHD Consensus Statement on Caesarean Childbirth[2] handled these uncertainties by grouping diagnoses of fetopelvic disproportion, abnormal pelvis, and prolonged labor under the term *dystocia* and found it to occur in 2.5% of pregnancies in 1970 and 4.6% in 1980. A more recent 1990 report based on American data showed the incidence of dystocia to be 12%, considerably less than the 45% reported by these authors. Factors leading to the overdiagnosis of CPD include inadequate diagnosis, epidural analgesia, fear of litigation, and doctor convenience.[3] The ability of 60% to 80% of secundigravidas attempting vaginal birth after a cesarean section because of dystocia in a preceding first pregnancy to deliver vaginally supports that opinion.[4,5] At least during the years 1963 to 1976, the use of active management of labor at Dublin's Royal Maternity Hospital, employing individual nursing care and labor induction in 12% to 36% of cases, decreased the incidence of cesarean section for absolute dystocia to approximately 3% to 4%, and reduced the mean duration of labor for primigravida patients to approximately 6 hours. They used oxytosis supplementation when cervical dilatation occurred at the rate of less than 1 cm per hour.[6]

The present authors made the diagnosis of CPD with no progress of cervical dilatation for 2 to 4 hours, "adequate" uterine contractions, and a cervix dilated 3 cm or more. The adequacy of uterine contractions can be judged objectively by progressive cervical dilatation or measurement of intrauterine pressure during uterine contractions. The use of an intrauterine pressure catheter is not reported here. The Committee on Obstetrics of the ACOG has recommended that the diagnosis of latent arrest disorder not be made until the cervix is at least 4 cm dilated. This suggests that many of the primigravidas studied here were not in active labor at the time of the decision for abdominal birth. It seems fair to conclude that, for many of the women described, the diagnosis of CPD/failure to progress was made without objective evidence of dystocia. It reasonably follows that those decisions were based at least in part on subjective evaluations and that the BMI of the women was a strong continuous monotonic factor in supporting the judgment for abdominal birth. Granted that obesity is a serious risk to women's health, this study fails to provide objective evidence that it predisposes to dystocia and cesarean section independent of obstetricians' subjective judgment.

T. H. Kirschbaum, MD

References

1. Olah KS, Nielson J: Failure to progress in the management of labor. *Br J Obstet Gynaecol* 101:1,1994.
2. US Department of Health & Human Services. Public Health Service, NIH publication No 82-2067, October 1981.
3. Cunningham FG, Grant NF, Levno KJ, et al (eds): *Williams Obstetrics*, ed 21. New York, McGraw-Hill, 2002, pp 426-427.

4. Wing DA, Paul RH: Vaginal birth after cesarean section: Selection and management. *Clin Obstet Gynecol* 42:835, 1999.
5. Haskins IH, Gomez JL: Correlation between maximum cervical dilatation and cesarean section in subsequent vaginal delivery. *Obstet Gynecol* 89:591, 1997.
6. O'Driscoll K, Meagher D: *Active Management of Labor.* London, WB Saunders, Ltd, 1980.

The Effects of Labor on Infant Mortality Among Small-for-Gestational-Age Infants in the USA

Kinzler WL, Ananth CV, Smulian JC, et al (UMDNJ-Robert Wood Johnson Med School, New Brunswick, NJ)
J Matern Fetal Neonatal Med 12:201-206, 2002   6–3

Background.—For certain high-risk situations, the mode of delivery has been claimed to bear less impact on the outcome of the newborn than the presence of labor. In one study, a 2.5-fold increased risk of neonatal death was present among low birth weight newborns delivered after labor began as compared with those delivered before the onset of labor. It is believed that the intrauterine stress of labor may contribute to poor neonatal outcomes, especially among infants with impaired oxygen reserves, without regard for the mode of delivery. Whether the presence of labor is detrimental to small-for-gestational-age (SGA) infants was evaluated.

Methods.—The data were gleaned from the United States national linked birth/infant death data sets for 1995 through 1997 and included 986,405 singleton SGA live births in cephalic presentation who were delivered at age 24 to 42 weeks of gestation. Measurements included mortality rates for SGA infants who were and were not exposed to labor and relative risks derived from multivariable logistic regression analysis, after adjustments for a long list of confounding factors.

Results.—More than 87% of the infants were exposed to labor (862,156 infants). The SGA infants had an 11.4 per 1000 mortality rate overall, and early neonatal deaths constituted 41% of the deaths (Table 2). The relative risk was 1.15 for risk of early neonatal death among SGA infants exposed to labor, but these infants had decreased rates of late and postneonatal death, even when fetal distress was not present. Early neonatal death rates were higher among infants aged 24 to 31 weeks of gestation, but after 34 weeks of gestation, the rates of overall infant death and early neonatal death for those exposed to labor declined. Late and postneonatal deaths among infants exposed to labor showed similar trends, regardless of the gestational age category. The infant death risk increased for each gestational age week under 32 weeks (Fig 1).

Conclusions.—The risk of early neonatal death was increased among SGA infants exposed to labor, especially if they were younger than 32 weeks' gestational age. Further study is recommended to determine the optimal obstetric management of SGA infants who are born when they are younger than 33 weeks' gestation.

TABLE 2.—Risks and Relative Risks for Infant Death Based on the Presence of Labor Among Small-for-Gestational-Age Infants: USA 1995-1997

	Overall		Labor Present		Absent		Relative Risk			
	n	Rate/1000	n	Rate/1000	n	Rate/1000	Unadjusted	95% CI	Adjusted	95% CI
ID	11 126	11.4	8238	9.7	2888	23.8	0.41	0.39, 0.43	0.91	0.87, 0.96
END	4563	4.7	3340	3.9	1223	10.1	0.39	0.36, 0.42	1.15	1.06, 1.25
LND	1683	1.7	1114	1.3	569	4.7	0.28	0.25, 0.31	0.66	0.58, 0.74
PND	4880	5.0	3784	4.4	1096	9.0	0.49	0.46, 0.53	0.83	0.87, 0.96

Note: Relative risks were adjusted for maternal age, gravidity, maternal race, marital status, gestational age, birth weight, intrapartum fever, placental abruption, chronic hypertension, pregnancy-induced hypertension, and fetal distress.

Abbreviations: ID, Infant death; *END,* early neonatal death; *LND,* late neonatal death; *PND,* postneonatal death.

(Courtesy of Kinzler WL, Ananth CV, Smulian JC, et al: The effects of labor on infant mortality among small-for-gestational-age infants in the USA. *J Matern Fetal Neonatal Med* 12:201-206, 2002.)

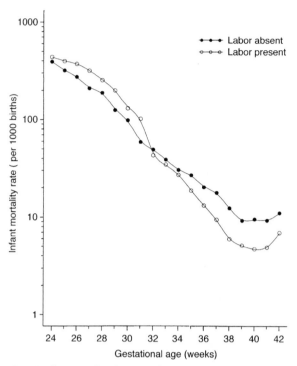

FIGURE 1.—Gestational age-specific infant mortality rates among small-for-gestational-age infants based on the presence and absence of labor: US 1995-1997. (Courtesy of Kinzler WL, Ananth CV, Smulian JC, et al: The effects of labor on infant mortality among small-for-gestational-age infants in the USA. *J Matern Fetal Neonatal Med* 12:201-206, 2002.)

▶ This review of data from the National Center for Health Statistics Infant Birth & Death Registry for United States for 1995-1997 is focused on infants born at the lowest 10 percentile of weight for gestational age delivering by the vertex at 24 to 42 weeks. Risk ratios comparing infants delivered after the onset of labor with those delivered before labor served as derived outcome variables. The results showed that labor was associated with a small but significant increase in total infant death and early neonatal death during the interval from 24 to 31 weeks of gestational age. Otherwise, for all gestational age groupings, labor was associated with decreased early and late neonatal death. The diagnosis of fetal distress seemed to have no impact on these results.

What obscures the authors' conclusions are the usual problems in dealing with massive cohort data necessitated by issues of low prevalence. With heterogeneity in confounding variables and the lack of a uniform protocol, management decisions about vaginal versus abdominal birth vary uncontrollably. Here, logistic regression is the multivariate technique used to correct for 22 independent variables. As Table 2 reveals, the resultant adjustments were massive, largely peripheral changes, except for the conclusions pertaining to neonatal deaths, in which the adjustment factors were 3-fold. As the authors point out, whether the diagnosis of SGA was made antepartum and influenced the management decision was unrecorded and, in addition, the causes of death were unknown, so the incidence of genital anomalies could not be evaluated. There's not much that can be concluded from this analysis.

T. H. Kirschbaum, MD

The Prognostic Impact of a Prolonged Second Stage of Labor on Maternal and Fetal Outcome
Janni W, Schiessl B, Peschers U, et al (Ludwig-Maximilians-Univ, Munich)
Acta Obstet Gynecol Scand 81:214-221, 2002   6–4

Background.—The normal duration of second-stage labor is considered to be 2 hours or less. If second-stage labor is prolonged beyond this point, it is believed that maternal and fetal risk increases, but intervention usually involves operative delivery. There is little evidence to support the 2-hour limit for second-stage labor. A detailed, contemporaneous analysis was conducted on the effect of second-stage labor duration on fetal and maternal morbidity in 1200 consecutive vaginal deliveries.

Study Design.—The study group included 1200 vaginal deliveries of a singleton fetus in cephalic presentation beyond the thirty-fourth week of gestation between May 1999 and June 2000 at a single institution. Of these deliveries, 1017 were spontaneous and 183 were instrumentally assisted. All patients had continuous fetal heart rate and uterine contraction monitoring. Labor was induced in 239 patients. Epidural analgesia was administered in 364 patients. Data collection was contemporaneous and included 128 parameters per patient.

Findings.—The average duration of second-stage labor was 70 minutes. For 79.3% of the patients in this study group, it was less than 2 hours. For 3.9%, it exceeded 4 hours. Prolonged duration of second-stage labor was not associated with low Apgar scores at 5 and 10 minutes, higher incidence of umbilical artery pH less than 7.2, or increased admission to the neonatal ICU. There was a significant increase in maternal blood loss associated with prolonged second-stage labor. The incidence of third-degree anal sphincter tears was also significantly increased by prolonged second-stage labor by univariate analysis, but not by corrected multivariate analysis.

Conclusions.—In the absence of fetal distress, there is no fetal indication to terminate labor after an arbitrary time in second-stage labor. Although increased maternal blood loss is associated with prolonged second-stage labor, this appears to be attributable, at least in part, to increased surgical interventions in these patients. Interventions should not be performed in these patients based only on the elapsed time from cervical dilatation.

▶ This is a second attack on the 2-hour limit for normal second-stage of labor,[1] if anything more convincing than the study earlier reviewed. In this case, 2000 women with singlet cephalic presentations past 34 weeks' gestation were studied after admission for uterine contractions, premature rupture of membranes (20.3%), or other clinical indications for fetal and uterine monitoring.

With a mean age of 31 years, 53% were primigravid, admitted on average at 39.7 weeks' gestational age. Electronic fetal heart rate monitoring bolstered by fetal blood analysis was regularly used. Those 17.6% of women who delivered abdominally were excluded, leaving 1457 pregnancies available for study of second-stage events. Spontaneous vaginal births occurred in 84.8%, forceps delivery in 0.7%, and vacuum extraction in 14.3%. About 20% of the women had induced labor, 30% receiving epidurals, and oxytocin augmentation was used in 42%. In true Bavarian fashion, 128 patient-independent variables were subjected to logistic regression analysis and dependent variables pertaining to labor; maternal and fetal welfare were studied as outcome measures.

The average duration of the second stage was 70 minutes, but 9.8% of cases had second stages from 2 to 3 hours long, with 69% (83 patients) from 3 to 4 hours and 3.9% in 47 patients greater than 4 hours. Though Apgar scores were significantly lower for those whose second stages were greater than 2 hours compared with those with shorter second stages, 5-minute Apgar scores were independent of second-stage duration. Cord blood acidosis occurred in 6.7% in infants born following second stages less than 2 hours and 7.7% in those with second stages greater than 2 hours. Acidosis was not statistically significantly increased as a function of second-stage length. Those with prolonged second stages had no significant increase in newborn neonatal ICU admission, mechanical ventilation, or continuous positive airway pressure resuscitation. Oxygen by mask was more commonly elected by health attendants in groups with prolonged second stages. Though newborn effects of second stage longer than 2 hours were minor, maternal morbidity was greater after a long second stage, with an increased risk of postpartum hemorrhage stage independent of operative delivery, surgery, lacerations of the perineum, and postpartum fever occurring more commonly.

In the earlier study referenced above, findings were similar and the principal finding was that given a woman with uterine contraction intensity at least 200 Montevideo units undelivered at the end of 2 hours of second stage, the chance for ultimate vaginal delivery was 60%. These authors, convinced that there are no measurable adverse consequences to the fetus, only to the mother in such a case, did not analyze their data in that way. Both studies presume and likely benefit from experienced careful obstetric care. Given that assumption, their evidence concerning the benign status of second stage longer than 2 hours seems quite convincing.

T. H. Kirschbaum, MD

Reference

1. 2003 Year Book of Obstetrics, Gynecology, and Women's Health, pp 100-102.

Risk Factors and Outcome of Failure to Progress During the First Stage of Labor: A Population-Based Study
Sheiner E, Levy A, Feinstein U, et al (Ben Gurion Univ of the Negev, Beer-Sheva, Israel)
Acta Obstet Gynecol Scand 81:222-226, 2002   6–5

Background.—Cesarean section (CS) is the most commonly performed major operation in the United States. The primary indication for a CS is a previous CS, but the primary indication for a primary CS is nonprogressive labor (NPL). The obstetric risk factors for NPL during the first stage of labor requiring cesarean section and outcome were investigated.

Study Design.—The study group included 92,918 singleton, vertex, term deliveries with an unscarred uterus complicated by NPL during the first stage. The definition of failure to progress was based on Friedman's plots. Multiple logistic regression analysis was performed to identify independent obstetric risk factors associated with NPL.

Findings.—Failure of labor to progress during the first stage resulting in CS complicated 1.3% (n = 1197) of all deliveries included in this study. Multivariate analysis indicated that independent risk factors for NPL during the first stage of labor were premature rupture of membranes, nulliparity, labor induction, maternal age greater than 35 years, birth weight, hypertensive disorders, hydramnios, fertility treatment, epidural analgesia, and gestational diabetes. Although newborns delivered after NPL during the first labor stage had significantly lower Apgar scores at both 1 and 5 minutes, there were no significant differences in perinatal mortality rate between those with NPL and those whose labor progressed normally. Maternal anemia and packed cells transfusion were also more common among pregnancies complicated with NPL.

Conclusions.—The major independent risk factors for failure of labor to progress during the first stage were premature membrane rupture, nulliparity, labor induction, and older maternal age. The indications for labor induction should be scrutinized to decrease the number of CSs.

▶ This is a conceptually simple broadsided application of a statistical package to a large database of 92,918 gravidas delivered over 11 years at this hospital in southern Israel. The aim is, by exploring definable risk factors, to understand the dynamics of prolonged first stage of labor as defined by the norms provided by Friedman, the third most common cause of dystocia and primary CS.[1] Continuous variables were investigated by Student's *t* tests and discrete variables by X^2 tests. Variables showing strong relationships to CS were selected for correlation and multiple logistic regression to construct a polynomial from which prediction of CS occurrence may be estimated and risk ratios and confidence intervals defined by coefficients of the several terms in the polynomial. The evaluation of this approach requires a certain amount of common sense.

Here, primigravidity, infertility therapy, and maternal age greater than 40 years defined a subset of patients with a 71.4% CS rate, all other things being equal. Clearly this is evidence of perception of a highly prized fetus and a certain amount of obstetrician anxiety. Epidural analgesia is strongly associated with prolonged labor here, but factors of technical competence in anesthesia and obstetric management are important and not available as variables in this data collection. The analysis has some merit in showing that gestational diabetes mellitus, both class A1 and A2, when controlled by multivariate analysis for fetal weight, hydramnios, and pregnancy hypertension, still carries a significantly increased risk of CS and may constitute an independent variable in failure to progress in the first stage. The major conclusion here is that the sequence of labor induction in a primigravid patient with premature rupture of membranes combines the 3 dependent variables most strikingly associated with primary CS. It is well to bear that in mind as you weigh the merits of induction of labor in such women.

T. H. Kirschbaum, MD

Reference

1. Friedman EA: *Labor: Clinical evaluation and management.* Appleton Century, Crofts, 1978.

The Impact of a Single-Layer or Double-Layer Closure On Uterine Rupture

Bujold E, Bujold C, Hamilton EF, et al (Université de Montréal; McGill Univ, Montreal)

Am J Obstet Gynecol 186:1326-1330, 2002   6–6

Background.—Uterine rupture and its associated morbidity are important considerations when deciding whether to attempt a trial of labor in women who have had previous cesarean deliveries. The effect of single-layer closure and that of double-layer closure on uterine rupture at subsequent deliveries were compared.

Methods and Findings.—An observational cohort of 2142 women undergoing a trial of labor between 1988 and 2000 after a single low transverse cesarean delivery was studied. The records and original operative reports of 92.4% could be reviewed. In a multivariate logistic regression analysis adjusted for selected confounding variables, the odds ratio for uterine rupture in women undergoing single-layer closure was 3.95.

Conclusions.—These data suggest that the most influential factor in uterine rupture in women undergoing a trial of labor after a previous cesarean delivery was single-layer closure of the previous lower segment incision. Compared with double-layer closure, single-layer closure increased the risk of uterine rupture 4-fold.

▶ This is a surprising and somewhat disturbing observation that certainly requires confirmation. Data collection from Montreal's Ste-Justine Hospital ran from 1988 to 2000, beginning with the general introduction of single-layer myometrial closure of low transverse cesarean sections at that facility. Prior to that time, a 2-layer myometrial closure with peritonealization was the norm. Only women with a single prior low transverse cesarean section were studied, and of 4627 such gravidas, 46% had a trial of labor, which was successful in 76%. The incidence of asymptomatic dehiscence was 0.1%, but of uterine rupture, defined as full-thickness uterine separation including peritoneum with fetal extrusion and the need for emergency surgery, the incidence was 1.07%. Uterine rupture occurred in 3.1% of 489 women with single-layer closures and 0.5% of those with a double-layer closure. The latter is roughly the incidence figure reported for uterine rupture in a trial of labor after a prior section by others. Perhaps some local management practices are important here and unspecified, but certainly this study makes it appropriate for us to look to our data experience to justify continued use of the single-layer closure.

T. H. Kirschbaum, MD

Maternal and Perinatal Morbidity Associated With Classic and Inverted T Cesarean Incisions
Patterson LS, O'Connell CM, Baskett TF (Dalhousie Univ, Halifax, NS, Canada)
Obstet Gynecol 100:633-637, 2002   6–7

Introduction.—Trials comparing the low transverse cesarean delivery with classic cesarean delivery have shown an increase in maternal puerperal infection, hemorrhage, blood transfusion, and hysterectomy in the former delivery approach. The maternal and perinatal morbidities associated with cesarean delivery involving the upper uterine segment versus low transverse cesarean delivery were estimated. A large provincial database was reviewed to evaluate the maternal and perinatal morbidity linked with upper uterine segment incisions compared with low transverse cesarean.

Methods.—A 19-year (1980-1998) review of a perinatal database and relevant medical records was performed to ascertain the maternal and perinatal morbidity associated with low transverse cesarean, classic cesarean, and inverted "T" cesarean deliveries. Because the number of low vertical cesarean deliveries was so low, this subgroup was excluded from analysis. Medical records were reviewed concerning indications for cesarean delivery and type of uterine incision.

Results.—There were 19,726 cesarean deliveries during the evaluation period. Of these, 19,422 (98.5%) were low transverse cesarean, 221 (1.1%) were classic cesarean, and 83 (0.4%) were inverted "T" cesarean deliveries. The rates of inverted "T" cesarean and classic cesarean deliveries remained stable; the rate of inverted "T" cesarean deliveries rose from 0.2% to 0.9%. Maternal morbidity (puerperal infection, blood transfusion, hysterectomy, ICU admission, death) and perinatal morbidity (stillborn fetus, neonatal death, 5-minute Apgar less than 7, ICU) were significantly higher in patients who underwent classic cesarean compared with low transverse cesarean. Some maternal morbidity (puerperal infection, blood transfusion) and perinatal morbidity (5-minute Apgar less than 7, ICU) were also significantly higher in the inverted "T" group compared with the low transverse cesarean group.

Conclusion.—Classic cesarean section has a higher maternal and perinatal morbidity compared with inverted "T" cesarean and low transverse cesarean. There is no increase in maternal or perinatal morbidity when an attempted low transverse incision needs to be converted to an inverted "T" incision compared with performing a classic cesarean section.

▶ It has long been clear that the low transverse uterine incision of Kerr and Pfaneuf is associated with fewer incidents of excessive maternal blood loss, parametrial hematoma, transfusion, and emergency hysterectomy than the classical fundal incision. Part of the difference comes from the tendency for classic incisions to be motivated preferentially by premature birth, antepartum hemorrhage, fetal malpresentation, and other urgent obstetric problems such as cord prolapse and severe acute hypertension. The impact of what begins as a Kerr incision but is compounded by performance of an upward inverted T extension to gain space has never been clear for want of sufficient reported cases. This review of data from the Grace Maternity Hospital of Halifax, Nova Scotia, from 19,726 deliveries—including 221 classic and 83 inverted T incisions—was used for that purpose.

Like the classic uterine incision, T incisions are reported more often in women of advanced parity and age and earlier gestational age than those with a Kerr incision, but differences between classic and inverted T incisions are minor both in that regard and with respect to obstetric indication. The women with an inverted T incision shared most of the puerperal problems of those with classic incisions compared to those with Kerr incisions. There is, however, no clear added jeopardy of inverted T incisions compared to classic incisions except for a slightly longer mean length of hospital stay. Perinatal morbidity and mortality rates were improved among women with an inverted T incision compared to the classic incision, primarily because their mean gestational ages were greater. In brief, vertical extension confers most of the disadvantage of the classic incision with respect to the lower transverse incision in women, but results were not incrementally worse. Since only 20 simple vertical incisions were reported, no comparisons are possible with respect to that group.

T. H. Kirschbaum, MD

Expectant Management Versus Labor Induction for Suspected Fetal Macrosomia: A Systematic Review
Sanchez-Ramos L, Bernstein S, Kaunitz AM (Univ of Florida, Jacksonville)
Obstet Gynecol 100:997-1002, 2002   6–8

Background.—Fetal macrosomia is associated with increased maternal and perinatal morbidity, but its management remains controversial. A systematic review and meta-analysis was performed to compare the effects of expectant management and labor induction on mode of delivery and perinatal morbidity in term patients with suspected fetal macrosomia.

Methods.—Computerized databases, published article references, textbook chapters, and meeting abstracts published from 1996 to June 2002 were searched for studies that compared expectant management and labor induction for suspected fetal macrosomia. Mode of delivery and perinatal outcome were evaluated.

Results.—Nine observational studies and 2 randomized clinical trials met the inclusion criteria for this systematic review. These studies included 2700 patients with suspected macrosomia who were managed expectantly and 1051 who were managed by labor induction. Summary statistics for the 9 observational studies revealed that women with spontaneous onset of labor had a lower incidence of cesarean delivery and higher rates of spontaneous vaginal delivery. There were no significant differences between the 2 types of management when the 2 randomized trials were examined. There were no differences in rates of operative vaginal deliveries, shoulder dystocia incidence, or abnormal Apgar scores between the 2 types of management.

Conclusions.—The results of this meta-analysis suggest that expectant management of suspected fetal macrosomia leads to a lower rate of cesarean delivery than labor induction, without sacrificing perinatal outcome.

▶ Whenever a clinician recognizes a large fetus by Leopold's maneuvers, with or without confirmation by US weight estimates, the possibility of avoiding birth trauma by labor induction to prevent further growth in utero or a cesarean section arises. Fairly clearly, estimated fetal weight in the range of approximately 4K is often inaccurate by either method, and it's not surprising that a decision for cesarean section based solely on this indication is not often pursued.[1] Labor induction in such women, however, remains a viable option for many obstetricians. A single prospective randomized study led to the conclusion that induction of labor decreased neither cesarean section rate nor neonatal morbidity.[2] After surveying 4 computer-based data collections bearing on this issue, the authors found 11 acceptable studies, 9 of them observational in form, and offer their meta-analysis of the 3751 macrosomic newborns, with birth weight greater than 4 kg, 2700 managed expectantly and 105 by labor induction, and offer an analysis of the relationship between the mode of delivery and perinatal outcome.

There are inevitable problems in the analysis. The basis for choosing either of the 2 alternative approaches was not a structured part of the observational studies and constitutes an important uncontrolled variable in the results. The definition of macrosomia varies within the range of 3.6 to 5 kg. The failure to use a rigorous definition (for instance, weight equal to or greater than 4.5 kg, my personal choice) is a problem, but the relationship between birth weight and reported birth dystocia is not a simple one. Approximately 40% of reported cases of shoulder dystocia occur with fetal weight less than 4 kg.[3] Further, coexisting diabetes mellitus increases the risk of shoulder dystocia at birth weight less than 4 to 4.5 kg anywhere from 2- to 4½-fold.[4] One reason for the uncertainty of the definition of macrosomia likely rests with the tendency of inexperienced obstetricians, once they have delivered a large fetal head, not to await the next uterine contraction to facilitate shoulder delivery. Another problem is the heterogeneity seen on analysis of the observational studies for which adjustments of the results of meta-anaylsis are difficult. To resolve this in part, the authors analyzed the randomized clinical trials separately from the aggregated observational studies. For the latter, the expectantly managed cases had a lower cesarean section rate (8.4% vs 16.6%), higher rates of spontaneous vaginal birth rate (82.8% vs 72.8%), and no significant difference in operative vaginal birth compared with the women with induced labors. Adding the randomized clinical trials published only in abstract form[5] abolishes the difference in cesarean section rates between the 2 subsets. Inclusion of data reported only in abstract was probably an error in the meta-analysis, however. In aggregate, there is no significant difference in the incidence of shoulder dystocia (6% vs 7.1%) or Apgar scores of less than 7 (1.8% vs 1.7%) in the 2 groups.

With the reservations cited here, this analysis offers no support for elective labor induction based on suspected macrosomia and helps confirm the conclusion stemming from the single published prospective randomized trial referenced.

T. H. Kirschbaum, MD

References

1. Rouse DJ, Owen J, Goldenberg RL, et al: The effectiveness and costs of elective cesarean delivery for fetal macrosomia diagnosed by ultrasound. *JAMA* 276:1480,1996.
2. Gonen O, Rosen DJ, Dolfin Z, et al: Induction of labor versus expectant management in macrosomia: A randomized study. *Obstet Gynecol* 89:913,1997.
3. Langer O, Berkus MD, Huff RW, et al: Shoulder dystocia: Should the fetus weighing greater than or equal to 4000 grams be delivered by cesarean section? *Am J Obstet Gynecol* 165:831, 1991.
4. Dildy GA, Clark SL: Shoulder dystocia: Risk identification. *Clin Obstet Gynecol* 43:265, 2000.
5. Tey A, Eriksen N, Blanco JD: A prospective randomized trial of induction versus expectant management in nondiabetic pregnancies with fetal macrosomia. *J Am Obstet Gynecol* 172:293,1995.

Cesarean Delivery for Twins: A Systematic Review and Meta-analysis
Hogle KL, Hutton EK, McBrien KA, et al (Univ of Toronto)
Am J Obstet Gynecol 188:220-227, 2003   6–9

Introduction.—Twin gestations make up approximately 1% of all pregnancies and account for nearly 10% of all perinatal mortalities. Vaginal birth is considered appropriate for vertex/vertex twins born after 33 weeks or weighing a minimum of 1500 to 2000 g. There is less agreement regarding the optimal mode of delivery for infants weighing less than 1500 g or born before 33 weeks' gestation. A systematic review and meta-analysis were performed to ascertain whether a policy of planned cesarean section or vaginal delivery is better for twin births.

Methods.—MEDLINE and EMBASE were searched from 1980 through May 2001 to identify trials that compared planned cesarean section with planned vaginal birth for infants weighing at least 1500 g or reaching a mini-

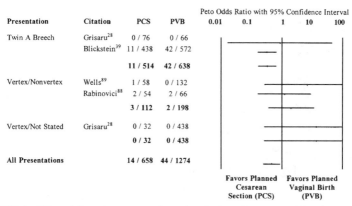

FIGURE 1.—Effect of planned cesarean section on low 5-minute Apgar score. A low Apgar score was defined as <8 in the study by Rabinovici et al, whereas in the other 3 studies, it was defined as <7. (Reprinted by permission of the publisher courtesy of Hogle KL, Hutton EK, McBrien KA, et al: Cesarean delivery for twins: A systematic review and meta-analysis. *Am J Obstet Gynecol* 188:220-227. Copyright 2003 by Elsevier.)

mum of 32 weeks' gestation. Pooled odds ratios (ORs) for perinatal or neo-natal mortality, the low 5-minute Apgar score, neonatal morbidity, and maternal morbidity were determined.

Results.—Of 67 articles retrieved, 63 were excluded. Four trials with 1932 infants were analyzed. A low 5-minute Apgar score was observed less often in twins delivered by planned cesarean section (OR, 0.47; 95% confidence interval [CI], 0.26-0.88) principally because of a decrease among twins if twin A was in a breech position (OR, 0.33; 95% CI, 0.17-0.65) (Fig 1). Twins delivered by planned cesarean section had a significantly longer hospital stay (mean difference, 4.01 days; 95% CI, 0.73-7.28 days). There were no significant between-group differences in perinatal or neonatal mortality or maternal morbidity (Figs 2 and 3).

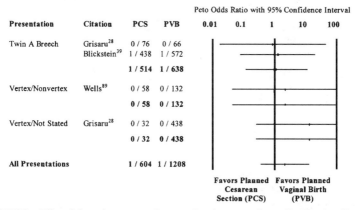

FIGURE 2.—Effect of planned cesarean section on perinatal or neonatal mortality. (Reprinted by permission of the publisher courtesy of Hogle KL, Hutton EK, McBrien KA, et al: Cesarean delivery for twins: A systematic review and meta-analysis. *Am J Obstet Gynecol* 188:220-227. Copyright 2003 by Elsevier.)

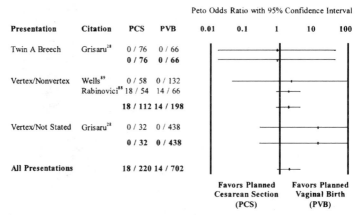

FIGURE 3.—Effect of planned cesarean section on neonatal morbidity. *Morbidity* was defined as birth trauma or neurologic complications in the study by Grisaru et al, as birth trauma in the study by Wells et al, and as birth trauma, hyperbilirubinemia, hypoglycemia, transient tachypnea, or secondary apnea in the study by Rabinovici et al. *Note:* See original journal article for references. (Reprinted by permission of the publisher courtesy of Hogle KL, Hutton EK, McBrien KA, et al: Cesarean delivery for twins: A systematic review and meta-analysis. *Am J Obstet Gynecol* 188:220-227. Copyright 2003 by Elsevier.)

Conclusion.—Planned cesarean section may reduce the risk of a low 5-minute Apgar score, especially if twin A is breech. Otherwise, there is no evidence to support planned cesarean section for twin births.

▶ In a multicenter randomized prospective study, this University of Toronto group has, in the Term Breech Trial, shown some evidence that newborn outcome is better with planned caesarean section for singlet fetuses than is a trial of vaginal birth.[1] The high crossover range, which found 45% of those women randomized to vaginal birth delivering abdominally, and the probable heterogeneity in management among the participant centers in 36 countries provided serious reservations to that conclusion. Subsequently, the authors were able to refute the claim of increased maternal morbidity associated with cesarean section for breech pregnancies based on 3 months' follow-up data from the same participants.[2] Here the issue is optimal delivery strategy for twin pregnancies at or less than 32 weeks' gestational age or with birth weight less than 1.5 kg using meta-analysis based on data published from 1980 to 2001. The authors report that only 4 studies—only 1 a prospective randomized, controlled trial of 120 twin pregnancies (authors' reference 88)—were selected from the 67 publications indexed. The large number of rejected data aggregates without description of their results and the evidence of heterogeneity, the bête noire of meta-analysis, among the 3 retrospective cohort studies included in this study are serious problems. Nonetheless, this is likely to be a work often cited by others.

The data from 1932 infants and 966 pregnancies were used to construct ORs and CIs comparing the results of abdominal versus vaginal births with respect to neonatal and prenatal mortality, the incidence of Apgar scores of less than 7 in 5 minutes, and neonatal and maternal morbidity.

Only the probability of low 5-minute Apgar scores were altered and apparently decreased in infants delivered abdominally in those twin pregnancies with first fetuses presented by the breech and in pooled data from all 4 studies. The pooled data showed significant evidence of heterogeneity. No significant difference appeared in comparing vaginal versus breech delivery with the first twin presenting by the vertex, nor in neonatal or maternal morbidity. Though the conclusions are not statistically very robust, they at least fail to show evidence favoring routine cesarean section for delivery of twins in this gestational age range. Others have reported the same finding for singlet pregnancies.[3-8]

T. H. Kirschbaum, MD

References

1. 2002 YEAR BOOK OF OBSTETRICS, GYNECOLOGY, AND WOMEN'S HEALTH, pp 81-85.
2. 2003 YEAR BOOK OF OBSTETRICS, GYNECOLOGY, AND WOMEN'S HEALTH, pp 167-168.
3. 1987 YEAR BOOK OF OBSTETRICS AND GYNECOLOGY, pp 183-185.
4. 1991 YEAR BOOK OF OBSTETRICS AND GYNECOLOGY, pp 146-148.
5. 1992 YEAR BOOK OF OBSTETRICS AND GYNECOLOGY, pp 166-167.
6. 1993 YEAR BOOK OF OBSTETRICS AND GYNECOLOGY, pp 164-166.
7. 1995 YEAR BOOK OF OBSTETRICS, GYNECOLOGY, AND WOMEN'S HEALTH, pp 202-204.
8. 1998 YEAR BOOK OF OBSTETRICS, GYNECOLOGY, AND WOMEN'S HEALTH, pp 192-196.

Delivery of the Second Twin: Comparison of Two Approaches

Pons J-C, Dommergues M, Ayoubi J-M, et al (CHU Grenoble, France; Necker-Enfants Malades Hosp, Paris; Hosp Cochin, Paris)
Eur J Obstet Gynecol Reprod Biol 104:32-39, 2002   6–10

Background.—Uterine delivery of the second twin is controversial. Some use expectant management based on respect for the natural mechanism of twin delivery and avoidance of traumatizing maneuvers, whereas others prefer to use obstetric maneuvers to decrease the interbirth interval. These 2 approaches were compared.

Study Design.—The study group consisted of 191 twin births occurring in 2 hospitals in Paris, Antione Beclere (AB) and Port-Royal (PR). Outcomes were compared between expectant management and active reduction of birth interval.

Findings.—The average interbirth interval was 9 minutes at AB and 5 minutes at PR (Fig 6). Intrauterine manipulation of the second twin occurred for 2% of the births at AB and 43% of the births at PR. There were 5 cesarean births in this study group at AB and none at PR. Apgar scores were identical at 1 and 5 minutes for births at the 2 hospitals. The rate at which second twins went to the neonatal care unit was the same for both hospitals.

Conclusions.—This retrospective study compared expectant management with active reduction of birth interval for deliveries of second twins. There were no significant differences in neonatal results between these 2 approaches. There was a reduction in the rate of cesarean births with an active management approach. Therefore, this suggests that an active approach to

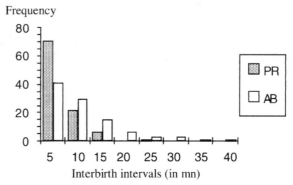

FIGURE 6.—Distribution of interbirth intervals (PR and AB). (Reprinted from Pons J-C, Dommergues M, Ayoubi J-M, et al: Delivery of the second twin: Comparison of two approaches. *Eur J Obstet Gynecol Reprod Biol* 104:32-39. Copyright 2002 with permission from the American Society for Reproductive Medicine.)

the delivery of a second twin reduces the cesarean delivery rate without increasing neonatal risk.

▶ This retrospective cohort study attempts to judge the relative merits, after delivery of a first twin, of allowing sufficient time for the uterus spontaneously to return to labor, aiming for spontaneous delivery or of promptly rupturing membranes and using intrauterine maneuvers if necessary to effect delivery from a possibly temporarily hostile uterine environment.[1] The latter is probably currently more often employed in this country, but it's been difficult to mount supportive proof. That's a reflection of the multitude of uncontrollable variables, as is this study comparing time to deliveries of second twin in 111 births in a Parisian hospital that allows the return of spontaneous labor (hospital A) and 68 births in hospital B, which effects delivery promptly. The skill with which decisions are made and the maneuvers performed are important complicating and uncontrollable variables here.

In hospital A, 51% of second twins delivered spontaneously compared with 27% in hospital B, where general anesthesia was used 3 times more often (9% of cases) for uterine relaxation for intrauterine manipulations such as internal and external version, total breech extraction, and the like. The difference in time between births at the 2 hospitals was not large, with 40% delivering within 5 minutes of the first birth in hospital A and 70% in hospital B. Mean interbirth delivery intervals were 9 minutes in hospital A and 5 minutes in hospital B. The authors found that, past 32 weeks, newborn well-being was independent of which option was pursued. Perinatal death of first twins occurred in 2.7% cases in hospital A versus 4.4% in hospital B. Corresponding rates for second twins in hospital A was 0.9% versus 2.9% in hospital B. Deaths at both hospitals were largely confined to preterm births complicated by infectious disease and respiratory complications. Since betamethazone was underused and given to only 20% of the patients in hospital A and 5% in hospital B, it's difficult to evaluate the role of delivery techniques per se in these cases. In only 1 of the 9 neonatal deaths reported had intrauterine betamethazone been given.

CNS injury was part of 3 of 5 neonatal deaths, all of them in premature infants in hospital B. Cesarean section for a second twin was confined to hospital A, in 1 case for placental abruption, in a second for brow presentation, and in 3 cases for inability to convert malpositioned fetuses to longitudinal lies. Newborn trauma was noted in 2.6% of the deliveries at hospital A, but these were largely trivial clavicular fractures. It was difficult to estimate intrauterine hypoxia in the second twin or reduced Apgar scores as a result of delay in delivery of second twins in hospital A.

In brief, skill in management, especially in intrauterine manipulations, appears to be more important than the issue of intertwin time interval. Prompt delivery of twin No. 2 makes it incumbent on the obstetric staff to possess the practice skills in managing abnormalities of fetal lie at the time of membrane rupture.

T. H. Kirschbaum, MD

Reference

1. 2002 YEAR BOOK OF OBSTETRICS, GYNECOLOGY, AND WOMEN'S HEALTH, pp 260-262.

Perinatal Outcome After Preterm Premature Rupture of Membranes With In Situ Cervical Cerclage
McElrath TF, Norwitz ER, Lieberman ES, et al (Harvard Med School, Boston)
Am J Obstet Gynecol 187:1147-1152, 2002   6–11

Introduction.—The presence of a cervical cerclage at the time of premature rupture of the membranes (pPROM) could foster clinically evident infection and adverse pregnancy outcome. The presence of cerclage at the time of pPROM was evaluated to determine whether it is associated with increased maternal or neonatal inflammatory morbidity.

Methods.—All singleton pregnancies with cerclage and pPROM between 24.0 and 33.9 weeks' gestation seen between January 1985 and December 1997 were evaluated. Control subjects (pPROM without cerclage) were matched 2.5:1 by year they were seen. Outcome measures that indicated clinical evidence of an infectious response were assessed, including maternal admission white blood count, time to onset of preterm labor, clinical chorioamnionitis, postpartum fever, neonatal white-matter disease (intraventricular hemorrhage or periventricular leukomalacia) at less than 33 weeks, neonatal sepsis, and neonatal death.

Results.—There were 114 cases of pPROM and cerclage that were matched with 288 controls. The study had power to identify a 2-fold difference in the incidence of adverse neonatal outcome ($\alpha = 0.05$, power = 0.8). Among mothers, the incidence of clinical chorioamnionitis (14.0% vs 18.8%; $P = .26$), uterine activity at admission (33.3% vs 32.2%; $P = .44$), and maternal postpartum fever (7.9% vs 7.6%; $P = .93$) were equivalent for those who did and did not have cerclage. Among infants, the incidence of latency duration to the onset of labor (Fig 1), white-matter disease (15.3% vs

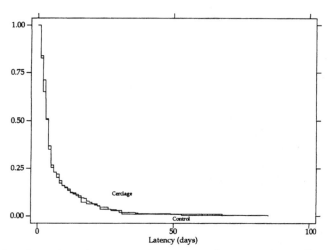

FIGURE 1.—Latency by cerclage status (Kaplan-Meier survival estimates). (Reprinted by permission of the publisher courtesy of McElrath TF, Norwitz ER, Lieberman ES, et al: Perinatal outcome after preterm premature rupture of membranes with in situ cervical cerclage. *Am J Obstet Gynecol* 187:1147-1152. Copyright 2002 by Elsevier.)

13.7%; $P = .75$), neonatal sepsis (9.1% vs 6.0%; $P = .21$), and neonatal death were similar with and without cerclage.

Conclusion.—Rates of maternal and neonatal morbidity were equivalent with and without cerclage. The close overall similarity indicates clinically insignificant differences between the 2 groups. Cervical cerclage at the time of pPROM under 34 weeks' gestation does not adversely impact pregnancy outcome.

▶ This well-conducted study deals with the management of women with cervical cerclage in place for whatever reason who subsequently develop pPROM. Guided by a fear of neonatal sepsis, many of us opt to remove the cerclage promptly, despite the lack of evidence in support of that position.[1] Using a 12-year experience with women with pPROM occurring between 24 and 35 weeks' gestational age, this study addresses the wisdom of removing the cerclage, comparing results of 114 women with ruptured membranes with a cerclage already in place, in more than half of cases after 15 weeks' gestational age.

The control group of 228 women was computer-selected with matching for year of service to control for possible changes in trends of practice. There were no significant differences in antibiotic, tocolytic, and steroid use among patients, nor differences in maternal peripheral blood white cell count or the incidence of uterine contractions greater than 6 per hour between the 2 groups. Women were accepted into the study only if, 48 hours after premature rupture of membranes, they were afebrile and presumed free of chorioamnionitis. Whether or not the cerclage was in place made no significant difference either in the latency duration to the onset of labor, the incidence of newborn intraventricular hemorrhage (23.9% in controls), or white brain matter lesions

(15.3% vs 13.7%); no significant differences were noted in analysis by year of service between the first half of the study compared with the second. There was no significant difference in neonatal outcome noted as a function of gestational age between cerclage and noncerclage groups. Significantly, cervical lacerations occurred in 3.5% of women allowed to labor inadvertently with a cerclage in place. Though this cohort study fails to settle the issue, it at least suggests that removal of a cervical cerclage is not mandatory following pPROM and that management might well be individualized, based on close observation thereafter.

T. H. Kirschbaum, MD

Reference

1. American College of Obstetricians and Gynecologists Practice Bulletin No. 1, 1998, p 443.

Emergency Peripartum Hysterectomy: Experience at a Community Teaching Hospital

Kastner ES, Figueroa R, Garry D, et al (Winthrop-Univ Hosp, Mineola, NY)
Obstet Gynecol 99:971-975, 2002   6–12

Background.—The most common indications for emergency peripartum hysterectomy have been uterine atony and uterine rupture. More recently, placenta accreta appears to be the most common indication. The incidence, indications, risk factors, and complications associated with emergency peripartum hysterectomy at a community-based, academic medical center were studied.

Study Design.—The study group included 47 emergency peripartum hysterectomies performed at 1 institution from 1991 through 1997. Emergency peripartum hysterectomy was defined as hysterectomy performed for hemorrhage unresponsive to other treatment within 24 hours of delivery. Maternal and surgical factors were recorded for each hysterectomy. The population was subdivided based on parity and type of hysterectomy.

Findings.—The rate of emergency peripartum hysterectomy at this institution was 1.4 per 1000. The most common indications were placenta accreta, uterine atony, and uterine laceration. Placenta accreta was the most common indication in multiparous women, and uterine atony was the most common indication in primiparas. Of the women with placenta accreta, 95.6% had a previous cesarean delivery or curettage. Risk of placenta accreta increased with number of cesarean deliveries or curettages. Of all the hysterectomies in this series, 80.9% were subtotal. There were no differences in morbidity between total and subtotal hysterectomy (Table 3). Postoperative total febrile morbidity occurred in 34% of the study group and other morbidity occurred in 26.3%.

Conclusions.—Placenta accreta has become the primary indication for emergency peripartum hysterectomy. This may be because of the increase in cesarean deliveries and uterine curettages as well as better treatment of uter-

TABLE 3.—Comparison of Total Abdominal and Subtotal Emergency
Peripartum Hysterectomy

	Total	Subtotal	P
Number	9	38	
Indication (%)			<.01
Placenta accreta	5 (55.6)	18 (47.4)	
Uterine atony only	0	14 (36.8)	
Previa without accreta	3 (33.3)	1 (2.6)	
Other	1 (11.1)	5 (13.2)	
Hemoglobin (g/dL)			
Preoperative	10.9 ± 1.7	11.8 ± 1.4	.18
Postoperative	8.5 ± 1.7	8.3 ± 1.6	.73
Operating time (min)	130.3 ± 53.6	135.3 ± 44.1	.64
Blood transfusions (%)	8 (88.9)	34 (89.5)	.99
SICU admissions (%)	4 (44.4)	6 (15.8)	.08
Postoperative (%)			
Febrile morbidity	3 (33.3)	13 (34.2)	.99
Other complications	5 (55.5)	10 (26.3)	.12

Results are expressed as mean ± standard deviation unless specified.
Abbreviation: SICU, Surgical ICU.
(Courtesy of Kastner ES, Figueroa R, Garry D, et al: Emergency peripartum hysterectomy: Experience at a community teaching hospital. *Obstet Gynecol* 99:971-975, 2002. Reprinted with permission from The American College of Obstetricians and Gynecologists.)

ine atony. Subtotal hysterectomy does not appear to be associated with increased morbidity and should be considered when emergency peripartum hysterectomy is required.

▶ It's easy to see parts of the history of operative delivery in this retrospective case-control study of 47 cases collected over 7 years. Studies of peripartum hysterectomies treated in 1970 and 1980 showed a preponderance of indications for procedures done within 24 hours of delivery for uterine atony and uterine lacerations, often from internal version or operative forceps procedures. As the number of available effective uterotonic agents for treatment has increased, the impact of the increased likelihood of abdominal birth has reflected indications primarily based on ruptured uterine scars, placenta previa, and placenta accreta. The latter accounted for about half the cases reported here, uterine atony and placenta previa 30%, usually bleeding from a poorly contracted lower uterine segment, 8.5%. Two thirds of women with accreta had prior cesarean sections and all but 1 case had either a prior cesarean section or a curettage.

The customary problems in reporting abdominal hysterectomies are all here, and unlike some purists, both those confirmed pathologically and not were reported as showing placenta accreta.[1] Twenty-two percent of women with preoperative diagnosis of placenta previa had placenta accreta. Evaluation of the prospective risks of accreta, such as from parity and number of prior cesarean sections, becomes difficult because of inadequate numbers. In 80% of these cases, subtotal hysterectomy was carried out though operating times and blood replacement needs were no different than in those with total hysterectomy. Time in the ICU and postoperative complications were said to be greater with removal of the cervix, but I have found it hard to rein in an enthusiastic resident physician short of removal of the cervix, as have those authors, I presume, who usually report that at least 50% of total hysterectomies were done for placenta accreta.

T. H. Kirschbaum, MD

Reference

1. 1994 YEAR BOOK OF OBSTETRICS, GYNECOLOGY, AND WOMEN'S HEALTH, pp 198-199.

▶ Though medical management of uterine atony has improved, specific antepartum counseling is prudent for women with 1 or more risk factors for peripartum hysterectomy. This uncommon but potentially morbid procedure will predictably occur more often in women with a previous cesarean birth and a placenta previa. Transfusion risk could be decreased if the operating surgeon moved more quickly to hysterectomy having previously discussed the patient's preference for future fertility. As the proportion of cesarean deliveries increases, complications associated with subsequent gestations will necessarily increase. Preoperative discussion of associated risks should be noted in the medical record, along with patient preference regarding emergency interventions such as hysterectomy.

R. D. Arias, MD

Outpatient Cervical Ripening With Prostaglandin E₂ and Estradiol

Larmon JE, Magann EF, Dickerson GA, et al (Univ of Mississippi, Jackson; Univ of Western Australia, Perth)
J Matern Fetal Neonatal Med 11:113-117, 2002   6–13

Background.—An unfavorable cervix is common in women who reach the forty-second week of pregnancy. At 42 weeks, perinatal mortality rate is increased, which leads physicians to induce labor even in women with an unfavorable cervix. Improving the cervical condition with ripening agents could reduce rates of operative delivery and maternal morbidity. Prostaglandin and estradiol are the most common ripening agents. Cervical ripening with prostaglandin, estradiol, or placebo in patients with an unripe cervix was studied.

Study Design.—The study group included 128 patients with an uncomplicated pregnancy of at least 37 weeks' gestation who were candidates for a vaginal delivery with a Bishop score of no more than 6. Patients were randomly assigned to receive prostaglandin E_2, estradiol, or an inert lubricant jelly in the posterior fornix each week until the onset of spontaneous labor, membrane rupture, or an indication for delivery occurred. A Bishop score was calculated at each visit. Detailed information was collected on outcome.

Findings.—There were no significant differences in maternal age, gestational age, gravidity, parity, ethnicity, or Bishop score at entry among these 3 groups. There were no differences in weekly Bishop scores, cervical dilatation, gestational age at admission (Table 2), the percentage of patients pre-

TABLE 2.—Data on Admission of Women in the 3 Groups to the Labor and Delivery Suite

	Prostaglandin E$_2$ (n = 41)	Estradiol (n = 44)	Control (n = 43)	P Value
Estimated gestational age (weeks)	39.7 ± 1.2	39.7 ± 1.2	39.8 ± 1.0	0.96
Bishop score	7.9 ± 3.0	8.0 ± 2.6	7.21 ± 2.8	0.34
Change in Bishop score	4.5 ± 2.4	5.4 ± 2.5	4.8 ± 2.4	0.22
Days to admission	16.8	15.4	15.4	0.71
Spontaneous labor*	33 (80%)	32 (73%)	32 (74%)	0.87
Cesarean section without labor	1 (2%)	2 (5%)	1 (2%)	0.59
Induction of labor	7 (17%)	7 (16%)	10 (23%)	0.83

*With and without spontaneous rupture of the membranes.
(Courtesy of Larmon JE, Magann EF, Dickerson GA, et al: Outpatient cervical ripening with prostaglandin E$_2$ and estradiol. *J Matern Fetal Neonatal Med* 11:113-117, 2002.)

senting with spontaneous labor or ruptured membranes, the number of inductions, or neonatal outcome among these 3 groups.

Conclusions.—Weekly placement of the cervical ripening agents, prostaglandin, or estradiol, on an outpatient basis was no more effective than placebo in women with an unfavorable cervix at 37 weeks' gestation. Studies are underway to determine whether more frequent treatment may help to ripen an unfavorable cervix.

▶ Prostaglandin E$_2$ is in wide use for cervical ripening when labor induction with an unfavorable cervix is deemed appropriate. Even though it is the only agent with Food and Drug Administration approval for this indication and numerous small studies support its usefulness, it has been difficult to prove its effectiveness in randomized, placebo-controlled studies. Most notably, the Maternal Fetal Medicine Network study of the treatment of postdatism[1] failed to show benefit from its use in cervical ripening in that part of the study aimed at its evaluation, somewhat to the surprise of the investigators. Here, though the primary purpose is to explore its effectiveness on cervical ripening in a group of 128 normal pregnancies past 37 weeks' gestational age (mean age, 37.1 weeks), a related observation is somewhat more interesting. Women were randomly divided into 3 subsets. One consisted of use of prostaglandin E$_2$ (Prepidil 5 mg intracervically every week), vaginal estrogen cream (4 mg in the posterior fornix every week), and a vaginal placebo until, in 18.8% of ruptured membranes, uterine contractions or bleeding intervened and provided an indication for induction.

Vaginal estrogen has a long history of use in the United Kingdom for cervical ripening, similarly without strong evidentiary support. Women delivered on average at 39.7 weeks' gestational age and the incidence of postdatism is not provided. There were few significant differences in entry variables, intrapartum outcome, or neonatal outcome among the 3 subclasses. The estrogen group had more labor complications and fetal heart rate abnormalities than did the others. As other investigators have noted, prostaglandin E$_2$ improves the gravidas' Bishop score but does not seem to alter inducibility or the resultant rate of abdominal delivery. Surely if it were effective in that regard, it might be expected to show some evidence of effectiveness in a study like this. As the authors point out, neither prostaglandin E₂ nor vaginal estrogen result in greater inducibility in such patients than does placebo administration.

T. H. Kirschbaum, MD

Reference

1. 1995 Year Book of Obstetrics, Gynecology, and Women's Health, pp 74-76.

A Comparison of Vaginally Administered Misoprostol With Extra-amniotic Saline Solution Infusion for Cervical Ripening and Labor Induction
Mullin PM, House M, Paul RH, et al (Univ of Southern California, Los Angeles)
Am J Obstet Gynecol 187:847-852, 2002   6–14

Background.—There are many options for cervical ripening and labor induction. This prospective, randomized study compared intravaginal misoprostol (prostagladin E_1) administration and Foley balloon catheter dilation with extra-amniotic saline solution infusion (EASI) with oxytocin administration for cervical ripening and labor induction.

Study Design.—The study group included 200 women who required labor induction at a single institution from February 1999 to July 2001. Inclusion criteria were singleton pregnancy, cephalic presentation, intact membranes, Bishop score of no more than 4, fewer than 8 uterine contractions per hour, and a reactive fetal heart rate (FHR) tracing. Women were randomly assigned to either misoprostol or EASI. The 2 groups were similar with respect to average age, gravidity, parity, height, weight, reasons for induction, and gestational age. Continuous FHR and uterine activity monitoring was performed. Frequency and duration of tachysystole, hypertonus, and hyperstimulation syndrome were assessed. The primary outcome was the average time from the start of induction to delivery. Other outcome variables included delivery route and induction success.

Findings.—No women withdrew from either study group. The average interval from induction to vaginal delivery was longer in the misoprostol group than in the EASI group. Abnormal fetal heart rate tracings occurred in 30% of patients in the misoprostol group and 19% of the EASI group. There was also more tachysystole in the misoprostol group. There were no differences in the routes of delivery or neonatal outcomes between the 2 groups.

Conclusions.—EASI appears to be more effective and associated with fewer fetal heart rate tracing and uterine abnormalities than misoprostol when used for cervical ripening and labor induction.

▶ This is a well-conducted prospective randomly allocated but unblinded study to compare the merits of 2 commonly employed methods of labor induction. Two hundred women were enrolled in this study, which was conducted at the LAC-USC Medical Center over 2½ years. About 38% of the inductions were done because of oligohydramnios, 21% because of pregnancy hypertension, and 17% because of postdate pregnancies. Enrollment requirements were for pregnancies with singlet cephalic presentation, Bishop score of 4 kg or less with intact membranes, and normal fetal heart rate tracings. Exclusions included birth weight greater than 4.5 kg or less than 1.8 kg, abnormal placental implantation, prior cesarean section, advanced parity, and medical complications precluding the use of prostaglandins. Misoprostol, 25 µg every 4 hours, was placed in the posterior vagina, a dose found to minimize uterine tachysystole by this experienced group. The EASI procedure involved extra-chorionic placement of a 30 mL Foley catheter followed by 30 mL per hour infusion of sterile saline solution and intravenous oxytocin beginning at a rate of 1 mU/min. In both cases artificial rupture of membranes was done with the cervix 3 cm or more dilated, Bishop's score of 8 or greater, and at least 3 uterine contractions every 10 minutes.

The EASI procedure proved to be significantly more efficacious, with a shorter interval between the onset of induction and delivery (a mean of 16⅛ hours) and with significantly less common tachysystole and transient abnormality in fetal heart rate patterns. Effectiveness was measured by delivery in 24 hours and occurred in 79% of those receiving EASI and 52% of those receiving misoprostol. Presumably, many of these 69 women (34.5%) underwent abdominal birth, although the cesarean section incidence is not provided. That omission begs the question of whether induction because of an amniotic fluid index of less than 5 cm[1-3] or postdatism[4] in more than half the cases studied here is warranted in view of the lack of evidence of benefit of induction for such indications.

T. H. Kirschbaum, MD

References

1. 2001 YEAR BOOK OF OBSTETRICS, GYNECOLOGY, AND WOMEN'S HEALTH, pp 35-36.
2. 2003 YEAR BOOK OF OBSTETRICS, GYNECOLOGY, AND WOMEN'S HEALTH, pp 57-59.
3. 2000 YEAR BOOK OF OBSTETRICS, GYNECOLOGY, AND WOMEN'S HEALTH, pp 35-38.
4. 2002 YEAR BOOK OF OBSTETRICS, GYNECOLOGY, AND WOMEN'S HEALTH, pp 192-197.

Ambulatory Epidural Anesthesia and the Duration of Labor
Karraz MA (Hôpital Louise Michel, Evry, France)
Int J Gynaecol Obstet 80:117-122, 2003   6–15

Background.—Epidural analgesia is usually administered in the supine position, preventing women in labor from walking around. Ambulatory epidural analgesia has become common at the Beauvais Central Hospital in France. The effect of ambulatory epidural analgesia on delivery mode, oxytocin dosage, and labor duration was evaluated in this prospective study.

Study Design.—The study group consisted of 221 women in labor at 36 to 42 weeks of gestation, with a singleton pregnancy and cephalic presentation. These women were randomly assigned to either ambulatory epidural analgesia or supine epidural analgesia. Use of oxytocin, amount of local anesthetic utilized, labor duration, and mode of delivery were recorded. This

TABLE 4.—Mode of Delivery

	Ambulatory Group (n = 141)	Non-Ambulatory Group (n = 74)	P-Value
Spontaneous vaginal delivery	117 (82.98%)	56 (75.67%)	0.45
Cesarean delivery	13 (9.2%)	12 (16.2%)	0.15
Forceps	11 (7.8%)	6 (8.1%)	0.93

(Reprinted by permission of the publisher from Karraz MA: Ambulatory epidural anesthesia and the duration of labor. *Int J Gynaecol Obstet* 80:117-122. Copyright 2003 International Federation of Gynecology and Obstetrics with permission from Elsevier.)

study was conducted only for daytime deliveries, as women in labor at night are less inclined to walk.

Findings.—There were no significant differences between these 2 groups in mode of delivery or use of local anesthetic or oxytocin. There was a significant difference in labor duration (Table 4).

Conclusion.—Ambulatory epidural analgesia shortens labor duration when compared with supine epidural analgesia but has no other effect on labor progress or outcome.

▶ Modifications of the techniques for epidural analgesia so as to allow women in labor to remain ambulant have, as at this French hospital, gained in popularity over the past 4 to 5 years.[1,2] This prospective, randomized unblinded study of 215 women, two thirds proscribed to an ambulant technique and one third serving as nonambulant controls, was designed to investigate the effects of ambulation on the course of labor and neonatal outcome.

Entry was limited to women between 36 and 42 weeks' gestational age—either in spontaneous labor or candidates for labor induction—without pregnancy abnormality, hypertensive disease, or prior cesarean sections. Intermittent dosages of an analgesic agent at a concentration less than the usual 0.25% bupivacaine were employed. Patients did not choose to ambulate at night and such women were excluded from the study. Ambulant patients demonstrated a systolic blood pressure of at least a 100 mm Hg, satisfactory pain relief, and the ability to stand without aid on 1 leg.

The 2 groups were indistinguishable in terms of mean age, parity, height and weight, and cervical dilation at onset of analgesia. Epidural analgesia was begun with mean cervical dilation 3 to 4 cm, and the length of labor was defined by the time from the onset of the epidural technique to delivery. No statistically significant differences were noted in cesarean section rate, though the incidence rates were 9.2% for the ambulant and 16.2% for the nonambulant group.

Labor duration was shorter among the ambulant women (mean, 173 vs 236 minutes), and the forceps rate was the same in both groups. No fetal effects expressed by mean Apgar scores were noted. Though the mean anesthetic dosages were not significantly different between the 2 groups; the nonambulant group requested repeat dosage more often than average. Certainly one can conclude that there were no adverse consequences as a result of ambulation in labor. Labor appeared shortened and a trend toward a decrease in cesarean section likelihood was noted.

T. H. Kirschbaum, MD

References

1. 2001 YEAR BOOK OF OBSTETRICS, GYNECOLOGY, AND WOMEN'S HEALTH, pp 195-196.
2. 2003 YEAR BOOK OF OBSTETRICS, GYNECOLOGY, AND WOMEN'S HEALTH, pp 187-189.

Intrathecal Versus Intravenous Fentanyl for Supplementation of Subarachnoid Block During Cesarean Delivery
Siddik-Sayyid SM, Aouad MT, Jalbout MI, et al (American Univ of Beirut, Lebanon)
Anesth Analg 95:209-213, 2002   6–16

Introduction.—Although intrathecal (IT) opioids supplement spinal anesthesia, it does not mean that the drug site of analgesic action resides in the spinal cord. It has been shown that a significant amount of an IT-administered lipophilic opioid, such as fentanyl, is lost by diffusion into the epidural space and subsequently into the plasma. This suggests that IT-administered fentanyl can induce analgesia by a systemic rather than a spinal action. The effect of IT fentanyl was compared with that of the same dose of IV fentanyl on the amount of intraoperative analgesic supplementation required by women undergoing elective cesarean delivery.

Methods.—Forty-eight healthy parturients scheduled for elective cesarean delivery were randomly assigned to IT administration of 12 mg of hyperbaric bupivacaine 0.75% plus 12.5 µg of fentanyl or IT administration of bupivacaine 0.75% alone. The latter group received 12.5 µg of fentanyl IV immediately after spinal anesthesia. The amount of IV fentanyl needed for supplementation of spinal anesthesia during surgery, the intraoperative visual analogue scale, the time to the first request for postoperative analgesia, and the incidence of adverse effects were compared.

Results.—A mean of 32 µg of additional IV fentanyl supplementation was needed in the IV fentanyl group compared with no need for supplementation in the IT fentanyl group ($P = .009$). The mean time to initial request for postoperative analgesia was significantly longer in the IT fentanyl than in the IV fentanyl group (159 minutes vs 119 minutes, $P = .003$). The incidence of systolic blood pressure less than 90 mm Hg and the ephedrine requirements were significantly higher in the IV fentanyl group compared with the IT fentanyl group ($P = .01$). Intraoperative nausea and vomiting were less common in the IT fentanyl group than in the IV fentanyl group.

Conclusion.—During cesarean delivery, supplementation of bupivacaine spinal block with 12.5 µg of IT fentanyl offers a better quality of IT spinal anesthesia than supplementation with the same dose of IV fentanyl. Patients in the IT fentanyl group did not need additional intraoperative analgesia, had a lower visual analogue scale before delivery, and had a longer time to first request for analgesia. In addition, the IT fentanyl group had a lower rate of side effects, including severe hypotension, nausea, and vomiting.

▶ Clearly supplementation of subarachnoid analgesia with an opioid improves the effectiveness of the clinical result. Since the lipid soluble opioid diffuses through the epidural space and enters the maternal circulation, it's never been entirely clear whether the IT opioid might not be equally effective when given IV, avoiding the pruritus and delayed respiratory depression seen with its IT route. In a randomized, double-blind prospective study of 48 women undergoing elective cesarean section, this group explores that question.

Both experimental subsets received a subarachnoid dose of 12.0 mg of hyperbaric bupivacaine. The IT opioid group also received 12.5 µg of fentanyl while the second group received IV fentanyl sufficient for adequate analgesia. Though no difference in anesthetic efficacy or motor blockade was noted in the 2 groups, 8 of 24 women in the IV opioid group required IV supplementation and the mean IV dose of fentanyl was 42 µg for all 24 patients. A significantly greater occurrence of hypotension, nausea, and vomiting was noted in the IV opioid group. Clearly, opioid IT administration is superior to its IV use, and whatever systematic absorption from the intrathecal route is clinical unimportant.

T. H. Kirschbaum

Elevated Maternal and Fetal Serum Interleukin-6 Levels Are Associated With Epidural Fever
Goetzl L, Evans T, Rivers J, et al (Baylor College of Medicine, Houston; Harvard Med School, Boston)
Am J Obstet Gynecol 187:834-838, 2002   6–17

Background.—Approximately 24% of nulliparous women who receive epidural anesthesia develop epidural fever. The mechanism of this fever is not understood. A secondary analysis of data from a randomized, double-blind, placebo-controlled study was performed to examine inflammatory causes of epidural fever.

Study Design.—The original prospective trial was performed to evaluate the efficacy of acetaminophen in the prevention of epidural fever. After epidural placement, maternal temperatures were obtained every hour until delivery by means of a tympanic membrane thermometer. Maternal blood samples were obtained every 4 hours, and cord blood was obtained at delivery. A blood culture was also drawn from the infant 2 hours after birth. Maternal and fetal blood samples were analyzed for interleukin-1 (IL-1), interleukin-6 (IL-6), interleukin-8 (IL-8), and tumor necrosis factor-α (TNF-α) by ELISA.

Findings.—The rate of fever was identical between the acetaminophen and placebo groups. Maternal IL-6 levels before delivery were significantly higher in mothers who had epidural fever (Fig 1). Cord blood levels of IL-6 were also higher in their infants. Linear regression analysis demonstrated

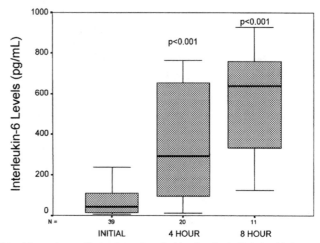

FIGURE 1.—Maternal serum IL-6 and duration of epidural analgesia. Relationship between duration of epidural anesthesia and IL-6 levels was evaluated with the use of repeated ANOVA ($P < .0001$). P values above represent post hoc comparisons between initial and 4-hour levels and between initial 8-hour levels. (Reprinted by permission of the publisher courtesy of Goetzl L, Evans T, Rivers J, et al: Elevated maternal and fetal serum interleukin-6 levels are associated with epidural fever. *Am J Obstet Gynecol* 187:834-838. Copyright 2002 by Elsevier.)

that initial maternal serum IL-6 level, fever, and duration of epidural anesthesia were significantly associated with final maternal serum IL-6 levels. Length of rupture of membranes and number of vaginal examinations were not associated with maternal IL-6. All neonatal blood cultures were negative.

Conclusions.—Epidural fever was associated with elevated IL-6 levels in maternal and fetal serum, suggesting an inflammatory basis for epidural fever. Further research is necessary to understand the inflammatory process associated with epidural analgesia to prevent epidural fever.

▶ About 25% of primigravid women experience temperature elevation greater than 100.4°F shortly after the placement of an epidural line for analgesia. Generally modest in intensity, it tends to appear within 4 to 6 hours after placement of the line and is not clearly associated with increased perinatal morbidity in either mother or infant. Here is a study designed to test the value of acetaminophen as pharmacologic prophylaxis for this purpose. Forty two afebrile primigravidas requesting epidural analgesic were studied through maternal and newborn blood culture and analysis of cytokines IL-6, IL-8, and TNF-α. The 23.8% of women who had experienced fever after an epidural analgesic showed no effect of acetaminophen but a significant increase in maternal IL-6 concentration in both maternal and fetal cord blood. No other measured cytokine concentrations were increased, and blood cultures were sterile. No neonatal consequences of the maternal fever were seen. IL-6 concentration increased with prolongation and duration of the epidural analgesic but was uncorrelated with the duration of labor, rupture of membranes, or the number of vaginal examinations conducted during labor. Clearly, the procedure itself, requiring separation and introduction of foreign material into the areolar connective tissue, lymphatics and venous plexes in the potential space between the spinal dura and the ligamentum flavum produces an inflammatory reaction that is, with care, usually not infectious and generally harmless.

T. H. Kirschbaum, MD

The Relative Motor Blocking Potencies of Epidural Bupivacaine and Ropivacaine in Labor

Lacassie HJ, Columb MO, Lacassie HP, et al (Pontificia Universidad Católica de Chile, Santiago; Clínica Alemana, Santiago, Chile; South Manchester Univ, Withington, England)
Anesth Analg 95:204-208, 2002   6–18

Introduction.—Minimal local analgesia concentrations (MLACs) are used to determine the pharmacodynamic contribution of various epidural drugs during the first stage of labor. The MLAC is considered to be the median effective concentration (EC_{50}) for epidural analgesia in the first stage of labor. No trials address the motor-blocking potencies of bupivacaine and ropivacaine. The motor block MLACs of bupivacaine and ropivacaine were examined, along with their relative potency ratio.

Methods.—Sixty ASA physical status I and II parturients were randomly assigned to a 20-mL bolus of either epidural bupivacaine or ropivacaine. The first patient in each group received 0.35%. Up-down sequential allocation was used to ascertain subsequent concentrations at a testing interval of 0.025% (Fig 1). Effective motor block was considered a Bromage score of less than 4 within 30 minutes.

Results.—The motor block MLAC for bupivacaine was 0.326% (95% confidence interval [CI], 0.285-0.367]); for ropivacaine, it was 0.497%

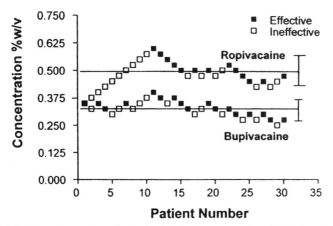

FIGURE 1.—The motor median effective local analgesic concentrations (EC_{50}) of bupivacaine and ropivacaine as determined by the technique of up-down sequential allocation. *Error bars* represent 95% confidence interval. (Courtesy of Lacassie HJ, Columb MO, Lacassie HP, et al: The relative motor blocking potencies of epidural bupivacaine and ropivacaine in labor. *Anesth Analg* 95:204-208, 2002.)

(95% CI, 0.431-0.563) (*P* = .0008). Thus, ropivacaine was significantly less potent than bupivacaine, with a potency ratio of 0.66 (95% CI, 0.52-0.82).

Conclusion.—The motor block EC_{50} for bupivacaine and ropivacaine during the first stage of labor revealed that ropivacaine was significantly less potent for motor block, at 66% of bupivacaine.

▶ Ropivacaine, stereoisomer of bupivacaine, has been shown to have lesser toxic effects than bupivacaine and less motor impairment, therefore offering some possible benefits in the reduction of cardiac irritability well known with bupivacaine. In this study, 60 parturients are studied in a randomized double-blinded prospective study, which both clarifies the differences between the drugs and illustrates an effective statistical device described by the renowned biostatistical unit at UCLA.[1] Dose effectiveness with respect to reported pain relief and observed motor impairment by Bromage score were independent variables as a function of the dosage of each of the 2 agents with a 20-mL epidural bolus. Initial drug concentration was 0.35% in units of weight per unit volume of each drug, and the dose was increased or decreased in units of concentration of .025% with the next ordinal patient, depending on the previous effectiveness of pain relief. The ultimate median values for concentrations yielding effective analgesic and the inability to perform leg raising were used for comparisons between the 2 drugs. The dosage of ropivacaine required for pain relief comparable to that of bupivacaine was 50% larger, yielding a potency ratio of 0.67. Since the potency ratio with respect to motor blockade was also 0.66, it's clear that ropivacaine does not have a broader separation of motor to sensory function than does bupivacaine; it is simply less potent, and the apparent sparing of motor blocking is simply an effect of the larger dose of ropivacaine required for pain relief.

T. H. Kirschbaum, MD

Reference

1. Dixon WJ, Massey FJ: *Introduction to Statistic Analysis*, ed 4. New York, McGraw-Hill, 1983, pp 426-441.

7 Genetics and Tratology

RNA Interference: A New Weapon Against HIV and Beyond
Kitabwalla M, Ruprecht RM (Dana-Farber Cancer Inst, Boston)
N Engl J Med 347:1364-1367, 2002   7–1

Background.—The reports of an increase in North America of infections with drug-resistant HIV underscores the need for development of inhibitors of HIV molecules other than reverse transcriptase and protease. The potential of RNA interference for use not only against HIV but also against other viruses was explored. The mechanism of action of RNA interference and the implications of this exciting research were described.

Overview.—Work has focused on HIV messenger RNAs (mRNAs) and the viral genome itself, which can be degraded by RNA interference. RNA interference is a mechanism for silencing the transcript of an active gene, mRNA, a process that is initiated by small interfering RNA (siRNA). In plant and drosophila cells, siRNAs are generated by dicer, an endonuclease that cleaves long, double-stranded RNA molecules into fragments of 21 to 23 base pairs (bp). Dicer has not been identified in differentiated mammalian cells. However, it was discovered recently that transfection of differentiated mammalian cells with synthetic siRNA resulted in highly sequence-specific RNA interference, indicating that dicer-mediated mechanisms are not essential to the formation of RNA-induced silencing complexes. Important problems must be solved before siRNA can be used clinically. First, a change in even 1 bp will drastically lower the potency of siRNA. Thus, so-called siRNA escape mutants could emerge quickly. In addition, the enormous sequence diversity of HIV between and within infected persons creates difficult problems in designing highly specific siRNAs. In addition, delivery of siRNA to cells is inefficient. Finally, the stability of siRNA is a critical concern.

Conclusions.—RNA interference is a promising therapeutic technique that has the potential to revolutionize biology. This therapy has implications beyond the treatment of HIV infection, as siRNA can degrade RNA produced by other viruses, such as poliovirus and respiratory syncytial virus.

Other potential applications of this technology exist in cancer therapy and in functional genomics.

▶ For decades, RNA has been viewed in the central dogma of genetics as an important but highly constrained component of molecular genetics, bridging the gap between gene activation and production of mRNA, a single-stranded complementary copy of genic DNA (the product of transcription) and, after transport of mRNA to a ribosome, of production of the protein encoded in the message (translation). The past year has seen evidence derived from research in plants and animals that small 21- to 28-nucleotide double-stranded segments of RNA can play a number of important roles in command, control, and regulation of gene expression. This area of investigation has become important enough so that it has been labeled "Breakthrough of the Year" for 2002 in the biological sciences. Among the roles for what has come to be called small interferine RNAs (siRNAs) have the capacities to block or alter levels of gene expression, to remodel DNA by discarding segments, to regulate developmental sequences, to shape chromatin through regulation of heterochromatin at centromeres, to regulate stem cell differentiation (in plants), and to alter genetic expression past the level of gene transcription. This article reviews and provides references for earlier work and describes ongoing and future research applying the capacity of siRNAs to block gene expression in HIV and infected cells, certainly an important application

In some species, siRNAs are produced by an endonuclease dicer, which produces 21- to 23-bp double-stranded RNAs with highly specific nucleotide sequences, as well as micro RNA capable of shifting matching segments of RNA in the genome. These strands, together with helicase and nuclease enzymes, form RNA-inducing silencing complex (RISC), including a blocking protein component that is capable of specific mRNA interference and inactivation without destroying the cells of residence. This approach to blocking gene expression is far simpler and less time-consuming than is the production of gene knockout transgenic animals, which may take months of labor to prepare.

So far, siRNAs have been designed to block the HIV *gag* gene, which expresses p24 and Gag protein, responsible for uncoating and packaging viral RNA from the HIV virus, essential for HIV replication. Another is dedicated to blocking CD4 protein expression, the principle HIV receptor, inactivation of which results in decreased HIV protein production. In development is an siRNA directed at the chemokine cytoreceptor 5 (CCR 5), homozygous mutational inactivation of which results in human resistance to HIV infection despite repeated contacts.[1]

There are problems in terms of loss of specificity through siRNA production, still inefficient means of cell insertion, and instability in storage. This is, however, an important new chapter in research in cell biology, applied first to the control of HIV infection. You'll be reading much more about it.

T. H. Kirschbaum, MD

Reference

1. 2003 Year Book of Ostetrics, Gynecology, and Women's Health, pp 63-65.

Cell-Free Fetal DNA in the Plasma of Pregnant Women With Severe Fetal Growth Restriction

Sekizawa A, Jimbo M, Saito H, et al (Showa Univ, Tokyo; Univ of Bologna, Italy)
Am J Obstet Gynecol 188:480-484, 2003   7–2

Background.—Fetal DNA has been demonstrated to circulate in maternal plasma. It is increased in the plasma of women with preeclampsia. It has also been reported to be increased in cases of fetal growth restriction (FGR). The fetal DNA concentration in plasma was quantified in pregnant women with preeclampsia, with FGR, and in healthy control subjects.

Study Design.—The study group consisted of 9 pregnant women with FGR; 9 with preeclampsia; and 20 healthy, pregnant, gestational-matched control subjects. Five of the 9 women with preeclampsia also had FGR. All fetuses were male. Maternal blood samples were collected and processed for quantitative polymerase chain reaction with a Y chromosome–specific probe to assess the amount of fetal DNA in the maternal circulation.

Findings.—The concentration of fetal DNA in the maternal circulation was significantly higher in those with preeclampsia than in healthy controls. The concentration of fetal DNA was not significantly higher in pregnancies with FGR (Fig 1).

Conclusion.—Fetal DNA was not increased in the plasma of pregnant women with FGR pregnancies. FGR does not appear to be associated with trophoblast damage.

▶ Though it has been claimed by others that fetal erythroblasts are increased in number in the blood of women with growth-retarded pregnancies,[1] this study refutes that claim. Maternal blood was obtained from gravidas at 29 to 36 weeks' gestational age, 9 of them with preeclampsia and 9 with growth-retarded fetuses at or below the 2.5 percentile at specified gestational age. Plasma was centrifuged and DNA extracted and subject to polymerase chain reaction using primers specific to the DYS 14 gene on the Y chromosome and the gene for β-globin as an internal control. Fluorescent DNA probes specific for male and female gender were used to identify male DNA.

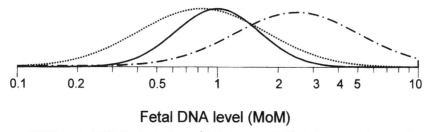

Fetal DNA level (MoM)

FIGURE 1.—Fetal DNA distribution (log scale) in the 3 groups. *Solid line* indicates control subjects; *dotted line*, subjects with FGR; *broken line*, subjects with preeclampsia. *Abbreviation: MoM*, Multiples of the median. (Reprinted by permission of the publisher courtesy of Sekizawa A, Jimbo M, Saito H, et al: Cell-free fetal DNA in the plasma of pregnant women with severe fetal growth restriction. *Am J Obstet Gynecol* 188:480-484. Copyright 2003 by Elsevier.)

Though pregnancies from 33 to 36 weeks had larger concentrations of DYS DNA than those at 29 to 32 weeks, the difference was not statistically significant. Though median free DNA in women with preeclampsia was greater than that in normals (486 vs 191 genome eq/mL), no increase was seen in plasma from growth-retarded pregnancies compared to those with normally grown fetuses. Total DNA, including that contained in intact fetal cells in maternal plasma, was elevated in cases of preeclampsia but unchanged from normotensive women with or without growth retardation. Since free DNA in plasma from growth-retarded pregnancies did not increase as it did in preeclamptics where increased numbers of red blood cells did increase the fetal DNA load, the frequency of fetal red blood cells was not increased in growth-retarded pregnancies either.

T. H. Kirschbaum, MD

Reference

1. 2002 YEAR BOOK OF OBSTETRICS, GYNECOLOGY, AND WOMEN'S HEALTH, pp 131-132.

Fetal DNA Clearance From Maternal Plasma Is Impaired in Preeclampsia

Lau T-W, Leung TN, Chan LYS, et al (Chinese Univ of Hong Kong, Shatin, New Territories, SAR)

Clin Chem 48:2141-2146, 2002   7–3

Background.—Preeclampsia is a leading cause of maternal and fetal mortality and morbidity in the developed world. The pathogenesis of this condition is unclear despite numerous studies. However, increased fetal DNA in maternal plasma/serum has been reported in pregnancies complicated by preeclampsia. It was hypothesized that impaired clearance of fetal DNA might be a contributing factor to the development of preeclampsia.

Methods.—A group of 7 women with preeclampsia were compared with a group of 10 control pregnant women. All the women had male fetuses. Serial blood samples were obtained from predelivery to 6 hours' postpartum. Male fetal DNA in plasma was measured by real-time quantitative polymerase chain reaction for the *SRY* gene on the Y chromosome.

Results.—Median concentrations of fetal DNA were significantly higher in the preeclamptic women than in the control women before delivery (521 vs 227 genome-equivalents/mL) (Fig 1). The median fetal DNA concentrations at 6 hours after delivery were also significantly different between the preeclamptic and control women (208 vs 0 genome-equivalents/mL, respectively.) A first-order clearance model was determined to best describe the kinetics of maternal plasma fetal DNA clearance. In addition, a significant difference was noted in the median apparent clearance half-lives of fetal DNA between the preeclamptic women (114 minutes) and the control women (28 minutes).

Conclusions.—These findings provide the first documentation of impaired fetal DNA clearance from maternal plasma in women with pre-

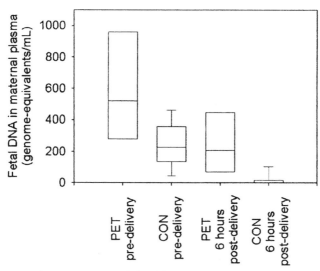

FIGURE 1.—Fetal DNA concentrations before delivery and at 6 h postpartum. The *y axis* represents the concentrations of fetal DNA in maternal plasma (genome-equivalents/mL). The *lines inside the boxes* denote the medians. The *boxes* mark the interval between the 25th and 75th percentiles. The *whiskers* denote the interval between the 10th and the 90th percentiles for the control cases. The whiskers are not marked for the preeclamptic cases because of the small number of cases. The predelivery data point from preeclamptic case 355M (see Fig 2A) was not plotted because it was above the 75th percentile. *Abbreviations:* PET, Preeclamptic cases; CON, control, non-preeclamptic cases. (Courtesy of Lau T-W, Leung TN, Chan LYS, et al: Fetal DNA clearance from maternal plasma is impaired in preeclampsia. *Clin Chem* 48:2141-2146, 2002. Copyright 2002, The American Association for Clinical Chemistry [1-800-892-1400].)

eclampsia. This abnormality may also be present in other conditions associated with quantitative aberrations in circulating DNA concentrations.

▶ The search for fetal DNA in maternal serum as a substrate for fetal genetic analysis has led to some interesting observations concerning the dynamics of its concentration in preeclampsia. Fetal DNA concentration increases with increasing gestational age,[1-3] has a rapid rate of disappearance, averaging a disappearance rate of 16.3 minutes,[4] and exists in larger concentrations in the serum of preeclamptic women than in normal pregnant women.[5] This study attempts to determine whether the increased concentration in preeclampsia is caused by faster rates of shedding of placenta cells into the maternal circulation or by slower rates of clearance. Surprisingly, the latter appears to be the case.

Sera from 7 preeclamptic women, 5 of them severe, were compared with those from 10 controls, all with normal male neonates, using samples drawn just before and at increasing intervals up to 360 minutes after cesarean section. This approach resulted in a difference in gestational age between preeclamptic women (median, 32 weeks) and controls (median, 38 weeks), the latter sectioned largely electively at term. This may well have reduced the median fetal DNA serum concentration in these preeclamptic women compared with the results of other studies. After DNA extraction in both patient groups, the TAQ man polymerase system directed at the *SRY* gene on the Y chromosome and using the betaglobin gene on chromosomel 11 to control the amplification was carried out.[6]

The results confirm the increase in fetal DNA concentration in preeclamptic sera compared with control sera (521 genome equivalents/mL vs 227), but less so than the 5-fold increase reported earlier in preeclamptic women, presumably because of the differing ranges of gestational ages. Calculation of concentration half-time assumes first-order kinetics in which the rate of disappearance of cells is proportional to their concentration at any time. This proved to be a better model for the data generated than did zero-order kinetics in which the rate of change of concentration is independent of DNA concentration and related only to time. The half-time was calculated by dividing the negative logarithm of the slope of the time-concentration plot, both expressed in the Naperian system. The results showed median half-times of 208 minutes for the preeclamptic women and zero (in 7 of 10 cases) for controls. At 6 hours' postpartum, the median DNA concentration in preeclamptic women was 208 genome equivalents/mL versus zero for controls. These observations need to be repeated in women delivering vaginally and in serum samples with gestational age controlled. As before, the mechanisms involved here are obscure but may well prove important in understanding the pathophysiology of pregnancy-induced hypertension, and certainly need to be studied further.

T. H. Kirschbaum, MD

References

1. 2000 YEAR BOOK OF OBSTETRICS, GYNECOLOGY, AND WOMEN'S HEALTH, pp 210-211, 219-220.
2. 2003 YEAR BOOK OF OBSTETRICS, GYNECOLOGY, AND WOMEN'S HEALTH, pp 197-199, 206-209, and 210-212.
3. 2000 YEAR BOOK OF OBSTETRICS, GYNECOLOGY, AND WOMEN'S HEALTH, pp 210-211.
4. 2000 YEAR BOOK OF OBSTETRICS, GYNECOLOGY, AND WOMEN'S HEALTH, pp 207-208.
5. 2000 YEAR BOOK OF OBSTETRICS, GYNECOLOGY, AND WOMEN'S HEALTH, pp 103-104.
6. 1999 YEAR BOOK OF OBSTETRICS, GYNECOLOGY, AND WOMEN'S HEALTH, pp 193-196.

Down Syndrome and Cell-Free Fetal DNA in Archived Maternal Serum
Lee T, LeShane ES, Messerlian GM, et al (Brown Univ, Providence, RI; Tufts Univ, Boston)
Am J Obstet Gynecol 187:1217-1221, 2002   7–4

Introduction.—Increased levels of cell-free fetal DNA (f-DNA) in the maternal circulation are a possible noninvasive marker for fetal Down syndrome. Archived serum specimens from 11 pregnant women and amniotic fluid from 6 women verified as carrying a singleton male fetus with Down syndrome (47,XY,+21) were examined to determine: (1) whether f-DNA could be quantified in the archived serum and amniotic fluid; (2) whether serum f-DNA levels are increased in Down syndrome pregnancies in a case-control series matched for gestational age and duration of sample storage; and (3) whether f-DNA levels are increased in the amniotic fluid of Down syndrome fetuses.

TABLE 1.—Adjusted Means of Fetal DNA Concentrations from Mixed Model Analysis of Variance

| | Serum | | Amniotic Fluid | |
Group	Trisomy 21 (n = 11)	Euploid (n = 55)	Trisomy 21 (n = 6)	Euploid (n = 30)
Adjusted mean	41.2	24.2	12,052	19,426
(GE/mL) (95% CI)	(31.6-50.7)	(20.0-28.4)	(5338-27,214)	(13,395-28,172)
P value		.002		.28

(Reprinted by permission of the publisher courtesy of Lee T, LeShane ES, Messerlian GM, et al: Down syndrome and cell-free fetal DNA in archived maternal serum. *Am J Obstet Gynecol* 187:1217-1221. Copyright 2002 by Elsevier.)

Methods.—All serum and amniotic fluid samples had been collected and stored at $-20°C$ from gravid women carrying a $47,XY,+21$ fetus. Each sample was paired with 5 matched control samples of identical specimen type from gravid women carrying a presumed euploid male fetus. The f-DNA concentration was quantified blindly by real-time polymerase chain reaction amplification for a Y-chromosome sequence.

Results.—The mean observed rank of 5.0 in the Down syndrome group was significantly higher than what was expected ($P \le .005$). The adjusted mean serum f-DNA concentrations were 41.2 genomic equivalents (GE)/mL for the Down syndrome specimens and 24.2 GE/mL for euploid control specimens ($P = .002$) (Table 1). Differences among amniotic fluid samples were not significant. There was an indication of a sample storage effect on f-DNA concentration on the order of -0.66 GE/month ($P = .071$).

Conclusion.—Down syndrome pregnancies demonstrated 1.7-fold higher levels of maternal serum cell-free f-DNA versus those of controls. No such correlation was seen in the amniotic fluid. Archived serum seems to be a useful source of clinical material for retrospective examinations, yet it may necessitate controlling for the duration of sample storage.

▶ From the time of demonstration of f-DNA in maternal plasma and serum,[1] the potential for cell-free DNA use in noninvasive fetal genetic analysis has stimulated many investigators. Maternal blood cell-free f-DNA is seen as early as 7 weeks of pregnancy, increases progressively with gestation, and has a rapid rate of disappearance from the maternal circulation.[2] An increased concentration of f-DNA has been reported in preeclampsia[3] and in fetal aneuploidy, especially Down syndrome.[4,5]

In this blinded case control study comparing archival maternal serum and amniotic fluid samples obtained at 15 to 19 weeks' gestational age during years 1999 through 2000, the authors seek to compare f-DNA concentrations in women with Down syndrome (11 cases) with that in women with euploidy pregnancies (55 cases). Their hope is to evaluate amniotic fluid f-DNA concentration with gestation age to determine whether pre-assay storage affects concentration in predictable form and to affirm that archival samples may be employed in this way. DNA was extracted from samples and quantified by real time polymerase chain reaction[6] and its concentration expressed in genome equivalents per milliliter.[7] Only women with male fetuses were studied since oligonucleotide probes for Y-chromosomal DNA are needed to differentiate f-DNA from maternal DNA in the maternal circulation.

The results confirm cell-free f-DNA in maternal serum with Down syndrome pregnancies at a greater mean concentration than in controls, while cell-free DNA in amniotic fluid concentrations showed no such difference from controls. Deterioration with time between sampling and DNA concentration measurements was noted at the rate of −0.66 GE/mL/mo, a new finding. Clearly, these archival samples nevertheless yielded some interesting results in this ongoing story of fetal genetic analysis.

T. H. Kirschbaum, MD

References

1. 1999 YEAR BOOK OF OBSTETRICS, GYNECOLOGY, AND WOMEN'S HEALTH, pp 193-196.
2. 2000 YEAR BOOK OF OBSTETRICS, GYNECOLOGY, AND WOMEN'S HEALTH, pp 207-208.
3. 2000 YEAR BOOK OF OBSTETRICS, GYNECOLOGY, AND WOMEN'S HEALTH, pp 103-104, 207-208.
4. 1999 YEAR BOOK OF OBSTETRICS, GYNECOLOGY, AND WOMEN'S HEALTH, pp 191-193.
5. 2001 YEAR BOOK OF OBSTETRICS, GYNECOLOGY, AND WOMEN'S HEALTH, pp 217-218.
6. 1999 YEAR BOOK OF OBSTETRICS, GYNECOLOGY, AND WOMEN'S HEALTH, pp 193-196.
7. 1999 YEAR BOOK OF OBSTETRICS, GYNECOLOGY, AND WOMEN'S HEALTH, pp 191-193.

Prediction of Fetal D Status From Maternal Plasma: Introduction of a New Noninvasive Fetal *RHD* Genotyping Service

Finning KM, Martin PG, Soothill PW, et al (Natl Blood Service, Bristol, England; Univ of Bristol, England; Univ of the West of England, Bristol)

Transfusion 42:1079-1085, 2002　　　　　　　　　　　　　　　　　7–5

Introduction.—The prenatal determination of fetal D blood group is greatly beneficial in the management of pregnancies at risk for *RHD* because of maternal anti-D. Invasive procedures performed to obtain fetal DNA for prenatal blood grouping may place the fetus at risk. During pregnancy, cell-free DNA can be observed in maternal blood. Identification of *RHD* sequences in maternal plasma has been used to predict fetal D status based on the assumption that *RHD* is absent in D-genomes.

Methods.—Real-time polymerase chain reaction (PCR) assays were created to distinguish *RHD* from *RHD*Ψ (possessed by most of D− African Americans). Plasma derived DNA from 137 D− women underwent real-time PCR to identify fetal *RHD* and Y chromosome-related *SRY* sequences. The accuracy of *RHD* genotyping from maternal plasma was assessed by comparing findings with those seen on conventional *RHD* genotyping from fetal tissue or serologic tests of the infant's red blood cells. The quantity of fetal DNA in maternal plasma was assessed in 94 pregnancies.

Results.—Fetal D status was predicted with 100% accuracy with maternal plasma. The number of copies of fetal DNA in maternal plasma increased with duration of gestation. At 23 weeks' gestation, the mean number of copies of fetal DNA present in maternal plasma was significantly higher in female versus male fetuses ($P = .01$).

Conclusion.—Combination of the sensitivity of real-time PCR with an improved *RHD* typing assay to differentiate *RHD* from *RHD*Ψ enables highly accurate prediction of fetal D status from maternal plasma.

▶ Noninvasive testing for fetal DNA status is important in the management of pregnancies sired by heterozygous *RHD+* fathers but analysis of fetal blood, placental villi, or amniotic fluid to establish fetal Rh positivity involves risk to the pregnancy and the possibility of increased fetal-to-maternal RHD antigen transfer, which may induce or heighten sensitization. These authors, in response to the demonstration that DNA exists in maternal plasma with far more prevalence than fetal normoblast,[1,2] provide some simultaneous comparative data from 30 *RHD−* women from a Bristol hospital together with 107 samples submitted to the Fetal Genotypic Service located in Western England. A further refinement is offered by their exclusion of intact but nonfunctioning D antigen (*RHD*Ψ) found in more than 50% of blacks based on point mutations in *RHD* exons 4, 5, and 6, and a 15% incidence of a hybrid CE-D gene, both of which yield false-positive D antigen testing.

Fetal DNA was extracted from maternal plasma in test subjects, all of whom had *RHD* fetal antigen testing done on amniotic fluid or chorion villus sampling. Real-time PCR was done by a Taq man polymerase and oligonucleotide probes bearing a fluorescent reporter and a quencher dye allowing DNA quantitation.[3] Primers were also chosen appropriate to the CCR5 receptor important in HIV infectivity in an effort to provide accurate quantitation of fetal DNA in 94 women.[4] A second set of primers was used to detect by PCR the *SRY* gene on the Y chromosome useful in detecting fetal male gender. The results of gender identification with maternal plasma were compared with the results of older, more classic invasive techniques.

The accuracy of D antigen testing with these techniques was 100% with fetal DNA concentration converted to call copy number by Lo's identity, 6.6 pg of DNA equivalent to 1 cell.[5,6] The results are reported in Table 4 in the original journal article, in which the increasing transfer of fetal DNA during pregnancy was again demonstrated. In a new finding, fetal DNA was found to be present in greater concentration in the presence of a female fetus than in a male fetus judged by the results of CCR5 quantitation. This is a fine demonstration of the precision that these investigators bring to this undertaking. The reader may wish to compare their work with that earlier review here.[7]

T. H. Kirschbaum, MD

References

1. 1999 Year Book of Obstetrics, Gynecology, and Women's Health, pp 191-196.
2. 2003 Year Book of Obstetrics, Gynecology, and Women's Health, p 20b9.
3. 1999 Year Book of Obstetrics, Gynecology, and Women's Health, pp 193-196.
4. 1999 Year Book of Obstetrics, Gynecology, and Women's Health, pp 77-78.
5. 1999 Year Book of Obstetrics, Gynecology, and Women's Health, pp 191-196.
6. 2003 Year Book of Obstetrics, Gynecology, and Women's Health, pp 197-199.
7. 2003 Year Book of Obstetrics, Gynecology, and Women's Health, pp 203-204.

Long-term Persistence of Donor Nuclei in a Duchenne Muscular Dystrophy Patient Receiving Bone Marrow Transplantation
Gussoni E, Bennett RR, Muskiewicz KR, et al (Children's Hosp, Boston; Children's Hosp, Los Angeles; Rancho Los Amigos Med Ctr, Downey, Calif; et al)
J Clin Invest 110:807-814, 2002   7–6

Introduction.—Duchenne muscular dystrophy (DMD) is a severe progressive muscle-wasting disease caused by mutations in the *dystrophin* gene. Loss of dystrophin protein has also been seen in the *mdx* mouse model of DMD. Bone marrow cells transplanted into lethally irradiated *mdx* mice can become part of skeletal muscle myofibers. It is not known if human marrow cells also have this ability. Reported is the analysis of muscle biopsies from a 15-year-old male diagnosed with DMD at age 6 months who received bone marrow transplantation at age 1 year for X-linked severe combined immune deficiency and who was diagnosed with DMD at age 12 years.

Findings.—Analysis of muscle biopsies from the young man showed the presence of donor nuclei within a small number of muscle myofibers (0.5%-0.9%). Most of the myofibrils produced a truncated, in-frame isoform of dystrophin lacking exons 44 and 45 (not wild-type). The patient's mother was apparently homozygous for G; the father and the patient had an A in this position (Fig 1).

Conclusion.—The presence of bone marrow–derived donor nuclei in the muscle of this patient substantiates the ability of exogenous human bone marrow cells to fuse into skeletal muscle and persist up to 13 years after transplantation.

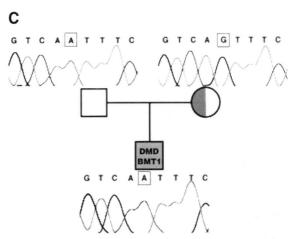

FIGURE 1C.—Chromatograms of DNA sequence analyses performed on *dystrophin* exon 45 band amplified by PCR from the young man and his parents. He and his father are homozygous for A at nucleotide 143 upstream of exon 45, whereas mother has a G in this position. (Courtesy of Gussoni E, Bennett RR, Muskiewicz KR, et al: Long-term persistence of donor nuclei in a Duchenne muscular dystrophy patient receiving bone marrow transplantation. *J Clin Invest* 110:807-814, 2002. Republished with permission of the *Journal of Clinical Investigation*. Reproduced by permission of the publisher via Copyright Clearance Center, Inc.)

▶ Interest in microchimerisms derived from fetal-to-maternal cell transfers in pregnancy as a cause of primary biliary cirrhosis, systemic sclerosis, and autoimmune thyroiditis presumes the ability of allogenic cells to reside for long periods of time in host tissues.[1-6] Strong evidence for persistence of fetal cells identified by Y chromosomal DNA in parous women for 27 years has been established,[7] but it's comforting to receive confirmatory evidence of 13 years of survival in this complex case.

The subject is a 15-year-old male in whom the diagnosis of X-linked severe combined immune deficiency was made at 6 months of age and a series of bone marrow transfusions given at 1 year of age from his donor father. His therapy was successful, though he lacks humoral immunity and requires monthly IgG infusions.

At age 12 years, the diagnosis of DMD, a sex-linked recessive disorder, was made and the diagnosis confirmed by polymerase chain reaction and probes for *dystrophin*, a gene with mutations known to be responsible for expression of the disease. A maternal mutation in exon 45 was noted, and immunohistochemistry done on muscle biopsy material from the young man demonstrated donor nuclei in 0.5% to 0.9% of his muscle myofibrils sampled. DNA sequence analysis on the exon 45 segment of the *dystrophin* gene demonstrated sequences characteristic of the father's DNA. Since DMD is x-linked, paternal DNA could only come from the transfusions for severe combined immunodeficiency syndrome and the mixture of mesenchymal, hepatic, and epithelial stem cells they are known to contain in procedures carried out 13 years earlier. It's convincing serendipitous evidence for the survival of chimeric cells and important reassuring confirmation of the prolonged persistence of microtransplants.

T. H. Kirschbaum, MD

References

1. 1997 YEAR BOOK OF OBSTETRICS, GYNECOLOGY, AND WOMEN'S HEALTH, pp 202-203.
2. 1999 YEAR BOOK OF OBSTETRICS, GYNECOLOGY, AND WOMEN'S HEALTH, pp 189-91.
3. 2000 YEAR BOOK OF OBSTETRICS, GYNECOLOGY, AND WOMEN'S HEALTH, pp 99-100.
4. 2001 YEAR BOOK OF OBSTETRICS, GYNECOLOGY, AND WOMEN'S HEALTH, pp 219-220.
5. 2003 YEAR BOOK OF OBSTETRICS, GYNECOLOGY, AND WOMEN'S HEALTH, pp 197-199.
6. 2003 YEAR BOOK OF OBSTETRICS, GYNECOLOGY, AND WOMEN'S HEALTH, pp 143-144.
7. 2001 YEAR BOOK OF OBSTETRICS, GYNECOLOGY, AND WOMEN'S HEALTH, pp 219-220.

Fetal Gender and Aneuploidy Detection Using Fetal Cells in Maternal Blood: Analysis of NIFTY I Data
Bianchi DW, Simpson JL, Jackson LG, et al (Tufts Univ, Boston; Baylor College of Medicine, Houston; Jefferson Med College, Philadelphia; et al)
Prenat Diagn 22:609-615, 2002   7–7

Background.—Currently, only invasive procedures can be used to obtain fetal karyotype. The National Institute of Child Health and Human Development (NICHD) Fetal Cell Isolation Study (NIFTY) was performed to examine the use of fetal cells isolated from maternal blood to detect fetal male sex and fetal chromosome abnormalities. This analysis was performed after the first 5 years of data collection.

Study Design.—This multicenter study was performed at 9 academic medical centers and 1 biotechnology company from January 1995 through November 1999. Pregnant women at least 16 years of age, with an assigned gestational age between 10 and 24 weeks and considered at high risk for fetal aneuploidy, were eligible to participate in this study. Blood samples were processed and fetal cells separated according to protocols that varied between the centers, introducing potentially confounding variables. Separated fetal cells were analyzed by fluorescence in situ hybridization (FISH). The results of FISH were compared with those of invasive procedures (amniocentesis and chorionic villi sampling) and to pregnancy outcome.

Results.—As of November 1999, 3658 women were enrolled in the study group. The average age of the women enrolled was 36.3 years, 86% were white, 95.6% were married, and the average gestational age was 13.9 weeks. Of 3302 samples processed, 2744 were available for analysis. Inability to detect target cells was a bigger problem for centers using flow-sorting rather than magnetic-based separation systems. Blinded FISH evaluation of blood samples from women carrying singleton male fetuses detected at least 1 cell with an XY signal in 41.4%. The false-positive rate was 11.1%. The detection rate for fetal aneuploidy was 74.4%, with a false-positive rate of 0.6% to 4.1%.

Conclusions.—Fetal cells can be detected in maternal blood and used for analysis of sex and aneuploidy, but the process is not yet ready for clinical application in low-risk women. Ongoing research will use information from these data to optimize procedures with the ultimate goal of developing a technique to allow routine noninvasive detection of fetal abnormalities.

▶ This international multicenter, prospective, 5-year clinical study on 2744 cases is an attempt to evaluate the clinical test effectiveness of the isolation, separation, and characterization of fetal cells, usually normoblasts, from maternal blood samples without fetal perturbation.[1-5] The performance characteristics of such methodology in determination of fetal gender and chromosomal abnormalities are compared with results from more conventional invasive fetal methodology, such as amniocentesis and chorion villus sampling, and ultimate pregnancy outcome. The effort suffered from a failure of definition of uniform management protocols among the 9 participating academic centers. Specifically, cell separation and selection techniques differed in using hemoglobin F as identification or immunoidentification with antibodies to CD45 or CD4 epitopes. Magnetic and flow separation with antibodies to HbF-positive fetal normoblasts were variously used. Details of cell straining and FISH protocols varied among centers, as did methods and timing for sample handling and transfer. In comparing results among centers and using the ability to find fetal X or Y signals, the best results were obtained with maternal samples obtained at or past 14 weeks' gestational age and processed within 18 to 24 hours of blood sampling. Magnetic cell sorters were used more often (81%) than antibody-labeled flow sorting (19%). Of 3658 maternal samples, 10% were lost and 17%

failed to yield targeted fetal cells. No significant differences in results based on maternal blood type, Rh type, or race were noted. Fetal gender was identified, after removing data from 1 center with outlying data, in 35.6% cases, with a false-positive rate of 5%. In 108 cases, fetal aneuploidy, usually an autosomal abnormality, was identified with a sensitivity of 74.4% and a false-positive rate of 4.1%. These latter estimates are based on only 43 cases. Though this study failed to prove clinical performance more efficient than that reported with invasive methods, the interaction among centers associated will have an impact on their future performances and will likely lead to improvements and subsequently aggregated results. This is a very important first step in evaluating the long-awaited general use of noninvasive techniques in clinical genetic testing.

T. H. Kirschbaum, MD

References

1. 1999 YEAR BOOK OF OBSTETRICS, GYNECOLOGY, AND WOMEN'S HEALTH, pp 191-193.
2. 2000 YEAR BOOK OF OBSTETRICS, GYNECOLOGY, AND WOMEN'S HEALTH, pp 57-59.
3. 2000 YEAR BOOK OF OBSTETRICS, GYNECOLOGY, AND WOMEN'S HEALTH, pp 219-220.
4. 2001 YEAR BOOK OF OBSTETRICS, GYNECOLOGY, AND WOMEN'S HEALTH, pp 219-220.
5. 2003 YEAR BOOK OF OBSTETRICS, GYNECOLOGY, AND WOMEN'S HEALTH, pp 197-199.

Intrathyroidal Fetal Microchimerism in Graves' Disease

Ando T, Imaizumi M, Graves PN, et al (Mount Sinai School of Medicine, New York)
J Clin Endocrinol Metab 87:3315-3320, 2002
7–8

Introduction.—During pregnancy, fetal cells reach the maternal circulation and infiltrate a variety of tissues (fetal microchimerism). The presence of these cells has the potential to modulate the maternal immune response to both self-antigens and fetal alloantigens. The degree of their influence has not been determined. Hyperthyroidism frequently abates in patients with Graves' disease during pregnancy and exacerbates after childbearing. It may be that fetal cells in the maternal circulation and tissues affect this decrescendo-to-crescendo pattern in autoimmune thyroid disease. An animal model of experimental autoimmune thyroiditis was used to assess the influence of pregnancy on autoimmune thyroid disease.

Methods.—Forty-seven samples of peripheral blood from pregnant women with Graves' disease were compared with those of female nonpregnant patients with Graves' disease. Enzyme-linked immunosorbent assay–polymerase chain reaction was used for the detection of DNA for a male-specific gene, sex-determining region Y. The sensitivity of this assay was comparable to about 1 male cell among 10^5 female cells.

Results.—Examination of paraffin-embedded thyroid tissues showed male cells in 4 of 20 female Graves' thyroid specimens; none were detected in 6 of 6 female adenoma specimens. An additional 6 of 7 Graves' disease samples showed intrathyroidal fetal microchimerism; 1 of 4 female samples with thyroid nodules demonstrated male cells. The greater detection of the

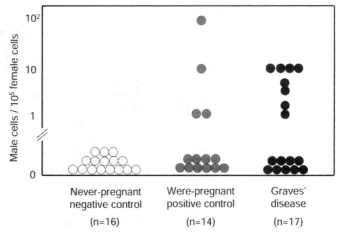

FIGURE 3.—Identification of peripheral blood fetal microchimerism. The enzyme-linked immunosorbent assay–polymerase chain reaction format for SRY detection was applied to genomic DNA taken from peripheral blood mononuclear cells. Male cells were detected in 4 of 14 previously pregnant (were pregnant) positive controls (*shaded circles*) and in 8 of 17 anonymous female Grave's samples (*solid circles*). SRY was not detected in any never-pregnant control subjects (*open circles*). (Courtesy of Ando T, Imaizumi M, Graves PN, et al: Intrathyroidal fetal microchimerism in Graves' disease. *J Clin Endocrinol* 87:3315-3320, 2002. Copyright The Endocrine Society.)

sex-determining region Y gene in frozen female thyroid tissues was probably the result of DNA fragmentation in the paraffin-derived samples. In peripheral blood samples, none of the 16 never-pregnant women had male cells. By contrast, in previously pregnant positive control subjects, male cells were

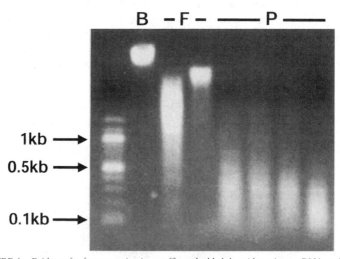

FIGURE 4.—Evidence for fragmentation in paraffin-embedded thyroid specimens. DNA purified from peripheral blood mononuclear cells (*B*), frozen thyroid (*F*), and paraffin-embedded thyroid (*P*) specimens was analyzed by agarose gel electrophoresis. Marked fragmentation was observed in DNA specimens prepared from paraffin-embedded sections, and less fragmentation was present in frozen specimens. (Courtesy of Ando T, Imaizumi M, Graves PN, et al: Intrathyroidal fetal microchimerism in Graves' disease. *J Clin Endocrinol* 87:3315-3320, 2002. Copyright The Endocrine Society.)

identified in 4 of 14 blood samples and 8 of 17 anonymous female Graves' blood specimens (Fig 3). The DNA prepared from paraffin-embedded tissues was severely fragmented to sizes below 500 bp (Fig 4).
Conclusion.—Intrathyroidal fetal microchimerism was common and profound in women with Graves' disease. Fetal male cells are valid candidates for modulating autoimmune thyroid disease during pregnancy and in the postpartum period.

▶ Pregnancy is associated with bidirectional transfers between mother and fetus of DNA either contained within monocytic cells or in soluble form.[1] Transfers from fetal to maternal circulation are most numerous and easiest to demonstrate through identification, as these authors have, of DNA containing the SRY gene, characteristic of the sex-determining segment of the Y chromosome. Identification of this gene in a phenotypic woman is proof of microchimerism, that is, the presence of more than 1 genome existing in a single host. Fetal microchimerism has been identified in human scleroderma, primary biliary sclerosis, and autoimmune thyroid disease.[2-5] In late pregnancy, DNA corresponding to 1550 male cells per milliliter of maternal blood or anywhere between 2 to 6 male fetal cells per milliliter of maternal blood have been identified and similar quantities noted in the pregnancy duration up to 23 weeks' gestation.[6] (There is good support for the hypothesis that these fetal cells, known to be discernable for intervals up to 27 years after pregnancy may, by provoking maternal immunoreactivity and the production of antibody reacting with maternal epitopes, result in autoimmune disturbances.[5]

The immune tolerance of pregnancy facilitates relatively asymptomatic fetal to maternal transfer of DNA, but with placental delivery, the effects of antigen antibody reactivity begin to manifest in women in the form of lymphocytic thyroiditis and hypothyroidism. Such a sequence has been demonstrated in experimental animals.[7] These authors sought to identify the SRY gene employing polymerase chain reaction on DNA isolated from 17 nonpregnant women with Graves' disease, 14 healthy pregnancy donors with male offspring, 16 women who had never been pregnant, and surgical specimens from thyroid adenomas (n = 6), and thyroid biopsy from women with Graves' disease (n = 20). Some of the specimens were paraffin embedded and some were studied in the form of frozen tissue. No male DNA was seen in the peripheral blood of 16 nulligravidas but was seen in about 30% (4 of 14) of women with prior delivery of male infants and in 50% (8 of 17) of women with Graves' disease who bore male children. SRY sequences were more readily seen in frozen than in fixed thyroid tissue. With the Taq polymerase method for real-time quantitation,[8] evidence of a male genome was found in 1 of 4 thyroid adenomas in the amount of 17 cells per 100,000 female cells and in Graves thyroid tissue in 6 of 7 cases with between 14 to 295 male cell equivalents per 100,000 female cells.

This ease of demonstration of thyroidal fetal microchimerism has been reported by others. The clinical pattern of quiescence of Graves' disease during pregnancy and exacerbation after delivery as immune tolerance is diminished is a familiar one,[9-11] and this work goes a long way to make its basis clear.

T. H. Kirschbaum, MD

References

1. 2003 YEAR BOOK OF OBSTETRICS, GYNECOLOGY, AND WOMEN'S HEALTH, p 209.
2. 1997 YEAR BOOK OF OBSTETRICS, GYNECOLOGY, AND WOMEN'S HEALTH, pp 202-203.
3. 1999 YEAR BOOK OF OBSTETRICS, GYNECOLOGY, AND WOMEN'S HEALTH, pp 189-191.
4. 2000 YEAR BOOK OF OBSTETRICS, GYNECOLOGY, AND WOMEN'S HEALTH, pp 99-100.
5. 2001 YEAR BOOK OF OBSTETRICS, GYNECOLOGY, AND WOMEN'S HEALTH, pp 219-220.
6. 2002 YEAR BOOK OF OBSTETRICS, GYNECOLOGY, AND WOMEN'S HEALTH, pp 221-222.
7. Imaizumi M, Pritsker A, Kita M, et al: Intrathyroidal fetal microchimerism in pregnancy and postpartum. *Endocrinology* 143:247-253, 2002.
8. 1999 YEAR BOOK OF OBSTETRICS, GYNECOLOGY, AND WOMEN'S HEALTH, pp 193-196.
9. 1987 YEAR BOOK OF OBSTETRICS, GYNECOLOGY, AND WOMEN'S HEALTH, pp 70-72.
10. 1988 YEAR BOOK OF OBSTETRICS, GYNECOLOGY, AND WOMEN'S HEALTH, pp 189-191.
11. 1989 YEAR BOOK OF OBSTETRICS, GYNECOLOGY, AND WOMEN'S HEALTH, pp 77-78.

Lack of Evidence for Involvement of Fetal Microchimerism in Pathogenesis of Primary Biliary Cirrhosis

Schöniger-Hekele M, Müller C, Ackermann J, et al (Univ of Vienna)
Dig Dis Sci 47:1909-1914, 2002 7–9

Introduction.—Microchimerism may be involved in the etiopathogenesis of autoimmune diseases, including scleroderma. Primary biliary cirrhosis (PBC) has some of the same characteristics of scleroderma, including a female predominance and a histologic pattern similar to that of chronic graft-versus-host disease. Liver biopsy specimens of women with PBC and various other liver diseases were examined, irrespective of a history of a male pregnancy, for the presence of Y chromosomal sequences by both polymerase chain reaction (PCR) and fluorescence in situ hybridization (FISH) techniques.

Methods.—Liver biopsies of 105 women were assessed: 28 had PBC, 25 had chronic hepatitis C, 6 had chronic hepatitis, 9 had autoimmune hepatitis, and 37 had other liver diseases. All patients were evaluated by a sensitive Y-chromosome-specific PCR and/or FISH for identification of the Y chromosome on a single cell level.

Results.—In the liver of 9 (8.6%) female patients, Y-chromosome-specific sequences were identified by PCR. Of these, 5 had PBC as underlying disease, 2 had chronic hepatitis C, and the remaining 2 had other liver diseases. No significant difference was observed in the positivity rate for Y-specific sequences in patients with PBC or those with other liver diseases ($P > .05$). Single cells with 1 Y chromosome were identified in other liver diseases.

Conclusion.—Microchimerism can be identified in the livers of patients with hepatic diseases. No evidence was found in the livers of patients with PBC. Microchimerism does not have a significant role in the development of PBC.

▶ PBC, a form of chronic liver disease focused around intrahepatic biliary conduits, has many of the clinical concomitants of autoimmune disease. It occurs preferentially in women with a sex ratio of 10:1, and its incidence is associated with increasing age and its regular covariant, parity. The disease tends to occur late in the reproductive epoch and is not seen in children. It shares with autoimmune thyroiditis a strong relationship to the presence of anti-mitochondrial antibody and occasionally coexists with systemic sclerosis, a skin disease known to be marked by dermal microchimeric deposits of fetal cells deposited after fetal-to-maternal transfer during pregnancy.[1] With the demonstration of chimeric fetal cells in the livers of women with primary biliary cirrhosis, several investigators have come to consider an autoimmune mechanism likely in this disease.

This group offers data that they feel refutes that conclusion, largely on the basis of the identification of an 8.6% incidence of microchimerism among a total of 28 women with biliary cirrhosis, 74 with other forms of chronic liver disease, and 3 normal women. Identification of fetal cells was done by PCR on 90 fresh liver biopsy specimens with primers chosen to bridge DNA segments of the Y chromosome and FISH orange and green fluours tagging probes for X and Y chromosomes. Five (17.9%) of 28 women with PBC exhibited microchimerism either by PCR or by FISH or both, but 4 women (5.2%) of 77 with other forms of hepatic disease, 2 of them with chronic hepatitis C infections, were also positive. The authors' claim that they fail to prove involvement of PBC with microchimerism is correct but ignores the effect of grouping small numbers of patients in each of the more than 12 other diagnostic entities to compare with biliary cirrhotics. Comparison is possible with chi-square with 4 of 25 women with hepatitis C, the result of which fails to demonstrate a significant difference from the cirrhotic group. The authors provide an interesting set of observations but they fail to prove the negative hypothesis that primary biliary cirrhosis is not an autoimmune disease.

T. H. Kirschbaum, MD

Reference

1. 1999 Year Book of Obstetrics, Gynecology, and Women's Health, pp 189-191.

Detection of Maternal–Fetal Microchimerism in the Inflammatory Lesions of Patients With Sjögren's Syndrome
Kuroki M, Okayama A, Nakamura S, et al (Miyazaki Med College, Japan; Kyushu Univ, Fukuoka, Japan; Kumamoto Univ, Japan)
Ann Rheum Dis 61:1041-1046, 2002   7–10

Background.—Fetal cells have been detected in a woman's circulation up to 27 years after giving birth. The concentration of male DNA in the peripheral blood was greater in patients with systemic sclerosis (SSc) than in healthy women, and cells with male DNA were also found in the skin lesions of female patients with SSc and in pregnant women with polymorphic eruptions. Thus, maternal–fetal microchimerism may play a role in the pathogenesis of certain diseases, such as juvenile idiopathic inflammatory myopathy and juvenile dermatomyositis. Sjögren's syndrome (SS) is an autoimmune disease

TABLE 2.—Positive Rates of the Y Chromosome–Specific Sequence in Patients With and Without Sjögren's Syndrome

| | | Samples | |
	PBMC	LSG	BALF
SS	0/22	10/28 (35.7%)*†	2/9 (22.2%)
Without SS	NT	0/10	0/15

*P = .0013, LSG of patients with SS versus PBMC of patients with SS.
†P = .028, LSG of patients with SS versus without SS.
Abbreviations: PBMC, Peripheral blood mononuclear cells; *LSG,* labial salivary gland; *BALF,* bronchoalveolar lavage fluid; *SS,* patients with Sjögren's syndrome who have at least 1 male child; *without SS,* patients with other diseases not due to Sjögren's syndrome; *NT,* not tested.
(Courtesy of Kuroki M, Okayama A, Nakamura S, et al: Detection of maternal–fetal microchimerism in the inflammatory lesions of patients with Sjögren's syndrome. *Ann Rheum Dis* 61:1041-1046, 2002, with permission from the BMJ Publishing Group.)

with chronic inflammatory lesions that principally affect the excretion glands. Whether female patients with SS have cells with male DNA and the possible role of microchimerism in the pathogenesis of SS were investigated.

Methods.—Extraction of DNA was performed on 27 samples of peripheral blood mononuclear cells (PBMC), 42 biopsy samples of labial salivary glands (LSG), and 9 samples of bronchoalveolar lavage fluid cells taken from 56 women (mean age, 51.7 years; age range, 17-74 years) with SS. Nested polymerase chain reaction (PCR) and fluorescence in situ hybridization (FISH) were used to detect male DNA.

Results.—Forty-two of the 56 patients had given birth to at least 1 male child. None of the 22 PBMC samples from these women were positive for the sex-determining region Y chromosome (SRY), but 10 of the 28 LSG samples were. The incidence of SRY detection did not differ between those with primary and secondary SS. None of the PBMC samples from women who had not been pregnant or the LSG samples from women who did not have SS were positive for SRY. None of the patients with lung disease but no SS had positive findings for SRY (Table 2). Of the bronchoalveolar lavage fluid samples, 2 of 9 patients with SS and at least 1 male child had positive findings for SRY. Two patients who did not have a male child tested positive for SRY; 1 had received a blood transfusion, and the other had a history of abortion. The LSG biopsy specimens were tested with the use of FISH to detect cells containing the Y chromosome: none were found in a female control patient, who served as a negative control subject, but test results were positive in a male patient, who served as a positive control subject. FISH detected the Y chromosome in cells from all the LSG specimens from 3 female patients with SS.

Conclusions.—Cells of the salivary glands and lungs were shown to have maternal–fetal microchimerism in patients with SS. Because non–host cells were found in the inflammatory lesions but not in the peripheral blood, non–host cells may be active in the pathogenesis of SS in these patients. How microchimerism contributes to the pathogenesis of SS was not determined.

▶ This study of 56 women with SS suffices to add it to a list of other chronic progressive (autoimmune) diseases for which there is evidence of long-term microchimerism based on presumed fetal–maternal cell traffic during pregnancy. Specifically, these diseases include SSC, Hashimoto's thyroiditis, and primary biliary cirrhosis.[1-5] Women selected for study had a mean age of 51.7 years, and each had delivered a male newborn, which is essential because the determination of chimerism is based on identification of Y chromosome–specific DNA sequences in female host tissues. SS is expressed as xerostomia and deficient lacrimal secretion, apparently on the basis of lymphocytic infiltration of exocrine glands (ie, salivary, lacrimal, respiratory, gastric, and pancreatic). B-lymphocyte activation is often present, and the syndrome is often associated with other rheumatoid diseases, especially rheumatoid arthritis and lupus erythematosus, as well as those diseases listed above. Microchimerism is identified in DNA from peripheral blood monocytes with the use of nested PCR that uses the TAQ polymerase and primers appropriate to the SRY. In addition, 28 women and 10 control subjects were studied by FISH applied to salivary gland biopsy samples and, in 9 cases of interstitial pneumonia, cellular pellets derived from bronchial washings. FISH was performed with the use of X and Y chromosome probes labeled with rhodamine for X and fluorescein for Y chromosomal material.

In none of the 26 cases tested was SRY DNA identified in peripheral blood monocytes, but in 10 of 28 salivary gland biopsy samples and in 2 of 9 bronchial washings, the Y chromosomal probe showed positive results. In 2 patients who had not delivered male infants (patients 47 and 49), PBMC, salivary biopsy samples, or both showed positive results for microchimerism. One of those women had a history of abortion, and the other had received blood transfusions. The presence of chimerism in 4 women older than 60 years attests to the prolonged survival of the Y chromosomal clones. The presence of male cells primarily in sites of active chronic inflammatory change suggests that the chimeric cells may well be etiologic, but it does not conclusively prove it.

T. H. Kirschbaum, MD

References

1. 1997 Year Book of Obstetrics, Gynecology, and Women's Health, pp 202-203.
2. 1999 Year Book of Obstetrics, Gynecology, and Women's Health, pp 189-191.
3. 2000 Year Book of Obstetrics, Gynecology, and Women's Health, pp 99-100.
4. 2001 Year Book of Obstetrics, Gynecology, and Women's Health, pp 219-220.
5. 2003 Year Book of Obstetrics, Gynecology, and Women's Health, pp 197-199 and 143-145.

Maternal Cell Microchimerism in Newborn Tissues

Srivatsa B, Srivatsa S, Johnson KL, et al (Tufts Univ, Boston)
J Pediatr 142:31-35, 2003   7–11

Introduction.—Fetal cell microchimerism indicates the presence of fetal cells in the mother. Persistent fetal hematologic progenitor cells have been observed in maternal peripheral blood as long as 27 years after delivery. The reverse phenomenon, maternal cell microchimerism, has been seen with routine karyotyping of newborn males; sex chromosome mosaicisms have been

TABLE 1.—Clinical Histories and Fluorescence In situ Hybridization Results of Study Subjects

Case	Maternal Age (y)	Gestational Age (wk)	Age at Autopsy (d)	Clinical Summary and Diagnosis	Clinical Summary and Diagnosis Slide (by FISH)*				
					Liver	Spleen	Thymus	Thyroid	Skin
1	41	35-5/7	2	Trisomy 21, nonimmune hydrops	dense	dense	45	not available	3
2	30	34	2	multiple congenital anomalies, complex congenital heart disease, karyotype 46,XY 4q$^+$	dense	dense	dense	14	0
3	33	37	2	pulmonary insufficiency secondary to bilateral renal dysplasia	4	not available	3	not available	5
4	21	37	5	severe congenital ichthyosis	7	dense	dense	0	0

All tissue sections were approximately 1.5 × 2 cm in area.
*"Dense" refers to overlapping cells within the tissue section leading to inability to reliably detect female nuclei.
(Reproduced by permission of the publisher courtesy of Srivatsa B, Srivatsa S, Johnson KL, et al: Maternal cell microchimerism in newborn tissues. *J Pediatr* 142:31-35. Copyright 2003 by Elsevier.)

observed. The migration of maternal cells out of the circulation into newborn tissues was examined to ascertain whether there is an association between maternal cell microchimerisms and neonatal pathophysiology.

Methods.—Autopsy materials from 4 singleton newborn male infants who never received a blood transfusion and died during the first week of life were examined. Female infants were excluded because the study design involved the use of sex chromosome–specific probes to identify female maternal cells. Of 28 male infants who died between January 1988 and December 1999, only 4 met all inclusion criteria. Diagnoses of autopsied infants were trisomy 21 with nonimmune hydrops, 46,XY,4q+ with multiple congenital anomalies, Potter syndrome, and congenital ichthyosis. These paraffin-embedded tissues were examined: liver, spleen, thymus, thyroid, and skin. Paraffin-embedded tissues underwent fluorescence in situ hybridization.

Results.—Female cells, as defined by the presence of intact nuclei with 2 X chromosome signals, were identified in multiple tissue types from all 4 male infants. The number of female cells ranged from 3 to 45/slide (Table 1).

Conclusion.—Maternal cells enter the fetal circulation and are able to migrate to fetal and neonatal organs. This is of importance concerning the potential consequences of umbilical cord blood transplantation and postnatal development of autoimmune disease.

▶ Bilateral blood cell trafficking occurs across the placenta and is associated with the occasional development of chimerism: that is, the presence of more than 1 genome in a single phenome. It has been demonstrated in newborn karyotypes and polymerase chain reaction of umbilical blood and experimental human adult blood studies (see authors' references 2 through 10 and 12). Chronic residence of maternal cells in fetal tissue, however, has only been identified in mice (authors' reference 11), a species that shares the hemochorial placenta with the human. This pilot study done on archival autopsy material from 28 male newborns who died within the first 7 days of life provides evidence of passage of presumed maternal DNA material into the fetal umbilical circulation and into fetal parenchymal organs. Twenty-four of the cases were excluded based on the presence of blood transfusion and multiple pregnancies. From the 4 remaining cases, tissue blocks were re-cut and exposed to fluorescence in situ hybridization using DNA probes complementary to the tandem repeat sequences in the X and Y chromosomes, labeled by red and green fluors, respectively. In all 4 cases, female DNA sequences, chimeric in normal males, were found in a variety of fetal organs, as seen in the table. It's interesting that maternal cell chimerism was most intense in the 1 case with trisomy 21, suggesting that the increase in fetal DNA in maternal blood seen in aneuploidies may also be true for maternal-to-fetal trafficking. Whether this is a general phenomenon unrelated to the causes of fetal death, the cohort identifier here, and whether maternal cell chimerism is responsible for pathologic change in fetal tissues are clearly goals for future studies by these productive investigators.

T. H. Kirschbaum, MD

Decidual Relaxins: Gene and Protein Up-Regulation in Preterm Premature Rupture of the Membranes by Complementary DNA Arrays and Quantitative Immunocytochemistry
Tashima LS, Yamamoto SY, Yasuda M, et al (Univ of Hawaii, Honolulu)
Am J Obstet Gynecol 187:785-797, 2002   7–12

Introduction.—Preterm premature rupture of the fetal membranes has been evaluated in many laboratories with a focused single gene/protein approach. This has provided a significant generation of new data. Integration of these data is challenging because the tissues used for analysis are particularly difficult to obtain; all patients who are delivered preterm have significant maternal or fetal medical conditions that result in preterm birth. Two commercially available arrays that contain a total of 488 genes were used to examine relaxin and a range of cytokine and cell/matrix interaction gene expression. The expression of the 2 relaxin proteins in the decidual cells was quantified. Only highly selected fetal membranes were used to eliminate as many confounding variables as possible.

Methods.—Membranes after preterm rupture were matched in pairs with preterm intact membranes (4 in each set, respectively). Tissues were obtained from patients without infection, labor, preeclampsia, or intrauterine

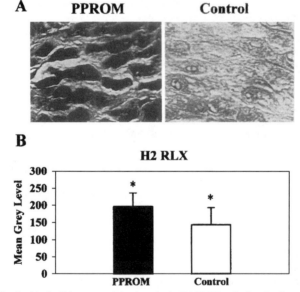

FIGURE 5.—Decidual cell immunostaining for relaxin (*RLX*) H2 and microdensitometric quantification. **A,** Decidual cells that were immunostained with antiserum to relaxin H2 from a patient with preterm premature rupture of membranes (*PPROM*) compared with lighter staining of decidual cells in tissue from a control patient (original magnification, ×400). **B,** Microdensitometry with sections from 3 preterm ruptured membranes and 5 controls showed significantly more relaxin H2 (*P* < .0001) in those tissues with rupture. (Reprinted by permission of the publisher courtesy of Tashima LS, Yamamoto SY, Yasuda M, et al: Decidual relaxins: Gene and protein up-regulation in preterm rupture of the membranes by complementary DNA arrays and quantitative immunocytochemistry. *Am J Obstet Gynecol* 187:785-797. Copyright 2002 by Elsevier.)

growth restriction, and none of the patients had a latency period of more than 8 hours. Messenger RNA from these tissues was used on complementary DNA expression arrays; 488 genes were evaluated. Relaxin gene expression was quantified from the arrays and in additional tissues by Northern analysis.

Results.—Relaxin gene expression was upregulated 3.4-fold on the complementary DNA arrays; this was not verified on Northern analysis. Protein analysis for relaxin H1 and H2 in the decidual cells revealed that they were significantly upregulated ($P < .0001$ for both proteins) in patients with preterm premature rupture of the membranes compared with control subjects (Fig 5). The 20 most highly expressed genes at preterm in tissues without rupture were identified. Additionally, analysis of the genes that were upregulated with preterm rupture of the membranes revealed 30 differentially expressed genes. Seventeen genes were significantly upregulated and 13 were downregulated (Table 4).

Conclusion.—Relaxin gene expression in the decidua is upregulated. Its protein expression is significantly increased with preterm rupture of the fetal membranes. Although there are likely many causes of preterm premature membrane rupture, it may be that the primary cause of preterm membrane rupture is present from early gestation or may occur close to the time of rupture (Fig 7).

▶ This group of University of Hawaii investigators is approaching an old problem, premature rupture of membranes, with a set of new techniques that use complementary DNA macroarrays. It's important not only to understand their conclusion, that relaxin proteins H1 and H2 are overexpressed in premature rupture of membranes, but also to understand their experimental approach.

Messenger RNA, the product of gene transcription, was obtained from placental membranes from 8 selected patients, matched for gestational age, absence of growth retardation, preeclampsia, infection, and chorioamnionitis, 1 from a woman with spontaneous premature rupture of membranes and its pair after cesarean section either indicated or elective with membranes intact. Rupture of membranes had to have occurred less than 8 hours prior to delivery and membranes obtained less than 30 minutes after birth, all requirements designed to reduce confounding variables. Messenger RNA was extracted from each specimen, and a portion prepared for Northern blotting, a process that identifies without cloning the number and sizes of RNA segments that are complementary to probes of known composition. A probe is a segment of RNA or DNA, often tagged with a radioisotope for identification and quantification, that can anneal to another segment based on the cohesion of base segments. Guanine anneals to cytosine, and adenine to thymine (uracil for RNA) to form double-stranded structures. These samples were used to confirm the presence of relaxin by a secondary chemical method. Another portion of each RNA sample was treated with DNAase to destroy DNA and the product used to prepare genic cDNA by allowing complementary bases to anneal in the presence of a ^{32}P label. Those samples were applied to cDNA macroarrays, which consist of a collection of hundreds of known cDNAs, prepared by polymerase chain reaction and mounted on templates. Material prepared from membrane

TABLE 4.—Genes* Upregulated or Downregulated More Than 2-Fold in Preterm Rupture Compared With Preterm Cesarean Delivery Tissues

Account	Name of Gene Encoding mRNA	Up- or Down-Regulated	Fold Change†
Growth and proliferation			
L38518	Sonic hedgehog	Up	+7.1
U84401	Smoothened homolog	Up	+3.4
X00588	Epidermal growth factor receptor	Up	+2.6
U36223	Fibroblast growth factor-8	Down	−2.5‡
J05081	Endothelin 3	Down	−2.5
M31159	Insulin-like growth factor binding protein 3	Down	−2.0
Cell survival			
D38122	Fas ligand	Down	−2.5
M36375	Ephrin receptor A2	Down	−2.0
Cell secretion			
M31470	Ras-like protein	Down	−2.0
M29870	Ras-related protein	Down	−2.0
Inflammatory mediators			
M23452	MIP-1α	Up	+4.0
M57765	IL-11	Up	+3.0
X02851	IL-1 precursor	Up	+3.0
X01394	Tumor necrosis factor-α precursor	Up	+2.6
M37476	LERK 1	Up	+4.3
Anti-inflammatory/host defense			
L06801	IL-13	Up	+3.0
L11015	Tumor necrosis factor C	Down	−3.3
M83941	Tyrosine-protein kinase receptor human embryo kinase	Down	−5.0‡

Tissue injury			
M6599	Endothelin-2	Up	+4.4
D14012	Hepatocyte growth factor activator	Up	+3.2
X04429	PAI-1	Up	+2.3
J03040	SPARC	Up	+2.2
Extracellular matrix remodeling			
A06925	Relaxin	Up	+3.
J04599	Biglycan	Up	+3.8
D49742	Hyaluronan-binding protein	Up	+3.1
X57766	MMP-11 (stromelysin 3)	Up	+2.0
M73780	Integrin β 8	Down	−2.0
Unknown function			
J03634	Inhibin β A	Down	−2.5
U14722	Activin type 1 receptor	Down	−2.5
M95489	Follicle-stimulating hormone receptor	Down	−3.3

*Genes are grouped according to probable function.

†Average fold change from 4 tissue pairs.

‡Average fold change from 3 tissue pairs.

(Reprinted by permission of the publisher courtesy of Tashima LS, Yamamoto SY, Yasuda M, et al: Decidual relaxins: Gene and protein up-regulation in preterm rupture of the membranes by complementary DNA arrays and quantitative immunocytochemistry. *Am J Obstet Gynecol* 187:785-797. Copyright 2002 by Elsevier.)

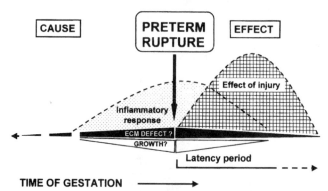

TIME OF GESTATION ⟶

FIGURE 7.—Hypothesis of preterm premature rupture of membranes shows possible separation between its causes and effects. The primary cause of rupture may be present from early gestation and may involve genes whose products can modify its growth or the structure of the extracellular matrix (*ECM*). An inflammatory response may be a consequence of these changes in extracellular matrix. A rapid effect of the injury is shown, which increases over latency period and is of unknown duration. Evidence of this was shown by increased expression of genes that are known to be involved in response to tissue injury. (Reprinted by permission of the publisher courtesy of Tashima LS, Yamamoto SY, Yasuda M, et al: Decidual relaxins: Gene and protein up-regulation in preterm rupture of the membranes by complementary DNA arrays and quantitative immunocytochemistry. *Am J Obstet Gynecol* 187:785-797. Copyright 2002 by Elsevier.)

RNA was added to each of the wells of the template and a match with known cDNA proven by isotope localization. The technique allows simultaneous identification of genes with known and unknown functions, grouped in clusters defined by function, and allows the identification of genes expressed or suppressed, in this case by rupture of membranes.

In comparison to controls, 3 arrays were used, 1 for gene identity and sensitivity, the second to explore genes associated with growth and differentiation; the third was used to explore cell interaction genes (membrane receptors, matrix proteins, protease, cytoskeleton, etc). The identity and quantification were estimated by the presence and concentration of the probe radioisotope annealed to its known complementary RNA on the template.

Most highly expressed genes in normal membranes were insulin-like growth factor binding protein with a role in growth stimulation and regulation, metalloproteinase (MMP) tissue inhibitors active in mitogen control, and plasminogen activator inhibitor, which is responsible for collagenase activity and matrix remodeling. In cases of rupture of membranes, genes involved in growth and differentiation were highly regulated. Proinflammatory mediators were upregulated probably as an expression of inflammatory changes, tissue injury genes were upregulated in response to the disruption of membranes or labor, and genes responsible for matrix remodeling were all upregulated. Fas ligand was downregulated, suggesting apoptosis is not a prominent factor in premature rupture of membranes. Significantly, relaxin was moderately strongly upregulated and its abundance in decidua proven by the immunocytochemistry with monoclonal-antibody raised to relaxin. The classical MMPs were not altered 8 hours after premature rupture of membranes, suggesting their role is more related to wound healing than to rupture of membranes.

Since relaxin H2 stimulates the production of MMP-1, it is possible this is a response that begins more than 8 hours after rupture of membranes.

The authors point out these demanding techniques are semiquantitative with 10% to 20% false-positive rates or more, and that patient variables are not fully controlled. It would be reassuring if the RNA expression for relaxin were more than 3.4 times increased, but mRNA has a short half-life and its relaxin protein in decidua that likely plays the more important role. This is an important paper and an important general approach to the innumerable biologic processes involved in obstetric events. Hopefully there will be other investigators who apply these methods to genetic expression in reproductive biology.

T. H. Kirschbaum, MD

Placental Apoptosis in Discordant Twins
Almog B, Fainaru O, Gamzu R, et al (Tel Aviv Univ, Israel; Weizmann Inst of Science, Rehovot, Israel)
Placenta 23:331-336, 2002   7–13

Background.—Perinatal mortality generally increases proportionately with increased discordancy between weights in twin pairs. The pathophysiology of intrauterine growth restriction in singletons appears comparable to that in twin discordancy. Thus, the current authors hypothesized that placental apoptosis would be increased in the smaller twin of a pair with discordancy.

Methods.—Placental samples from 7 twin pairs were obtained in the third trimester. Discordancy was defined as a newborn weight difference exceeding 25%. The incidence of apoptosis was confirmed by light microscopy with hematoxylin and eosin–stained paraffin slides and terminal deoxynucleotidyl transferase–mediated deoxyuridine triphosphate nick end–labeling (TUNEL) methods.

Findings.—Both techniques exhibited a significantly greater incidence of apoptosis in the placentas of the smaller fetuses than in the placentas of the larger fetuses. The incidence of TUNEL-positive cells was 1.4% in the smaller twins, compared with 0.9% in the larger twins. The hematoxylin and eosin findings also revealed a significantly greater incidence of apoptosis in the smaller than in the larger twins, with values of 1.07% and 0.72%, respectively.

Conclusions.—Placental apoptosis is increased in the smaller fetus of twin pairs with discordancy. Thus, placental apoptosis may play a role in twin discordancy. These data support the hypothesis that the smaller twin in a twin pair with discordancy is selectively growth-restricted.

▶ This placental study uses an increasingly common method (TUNEL) for the investigation of the occurrence of apoptosis in growth retardation and discordant twin pregnancy. Apoptosis is a safe, selective, and noninflammatory genetic mechanism for the removal of unnecessary cells, an essential part of embryonic and adult growth and development, and the maintenance of stable cell numbers and composition in tissue and organ populations. Apoptosis removes billions of cells from the intestinal tract and bone marrow each hour in order to balance high rates of new cell production at those sites. Apoptotic cells are destroyed by shrinkage of the cytoskeleton, disruption of the nuclear envelope, and lysis and shrinkage of DNA content without necrosis, which, in contrast, releases cell contents locally and affects neighboring cells. A signal that initiates apoptosis, as, for instance, from Fas protein (CD95) or from monitors of mitochondrial function, from DNA damage, or from T-cell injury such as that occurring with p53 results in the synthesis of proteases acting on cysteine components of aspartic acid (caspases), often resulting from binding of Fas protein (*fas*) to its membrane-bound receptor. Caspase precursors (procaspases) are activated by adaptor proteins that aggregate Fas ligand–receptor complexes, allowing formation of a death-inducing signal complex that starts a cascade of caspase production. Caspases, in turn, produce nuclear laminases that free DNA from the nucleus and DNAase, which cleaves DNA, often in lengths of about 180 base-pairs. Apoptosis may be detected and quantified by using microscopic recognition of its nuclear changes; DNA chromatography, which yields typical stepladder patterns representing regular integral multiples of 180 base-pair fragments; or monoclonal antibodies specific to many of the protein intermediates listed earlier.

This study used placental biopsies from 7 dichorionic twin pregnancies discordant by virtue of a difference in birth weight of at least 25%. Complicated pregnancies (anomalous development, pregnancy hypertension, illicit drug use, etc) were excluded. Biopsies of placentas were exposed both through light microscopic morphologic review and the TUNEL procedure. Deoxyuridine triphosphate (dUTP) is capable of binding its fluorescein label to apoptotic breaks in DNA strands induced by DNAase, and immunohistochemistry is used to demonstrate the location and frequency of apoptotic DNA lysis. Compared with the larger of the 2 twins, the smaller twins showed a significant increase in the incidence of such apoptotic DNA—both by TUNEL and light microscopy. This difference occurred despite similar environments and without the vascular abnormalities seen in, for instance, monoamniotic twins. This means that the smaller of such twins are likely undergoing greater degrees of placental remodeling than are their larger siblings. What remains is to increase the number of experimental subjects and to seek evidence of subsets with particularly high rates of apoptosis, to shed light on specific etiology. You will be reading a great deal more about the use of the maternal methodology and studies of cell biology.

T. H. Kirschbaum, MD

Antiphospholipid Syndrome in Pregnancy: A Randomized, Controlled Trial of Treatment

Farquharson RG, Quenby S, Greaves M (Liverpool Women's Hosp, England; Univ of Liverpool, England; Univ of Aberdeen, Scotland)

Obstet Gynecol 100:408-413, 2002   7–14

Background.—Antiphospholipid syndrome in pregnant women correlates strongly with recurrent miscarriage and, less often, maternal thrombosis. The efficacy of low-dose aspirin alone compared with low-dose aspirin combined with low-molecular weight heparin as prophylaxis against pregnancy loss in women with antiphospholipid syndrome was investigated.

Methods.—The study included 98 women in the first 12 weeks of pregnancy with persistently positive tests for lupus anticoagulant and/or anticardiolipin IgG and IgM antibodies who were recruited from a regional miscarriage clinic between 1997 and 2000. Forty-seven women were assigned to low-dose aspirin, 75 mg daily (group A), and 51 were assigned to low-dose aspirin plus low-molecular weight heparin, 5000 U, subcutaneously daily (group B). Treatments were continued for the entire pregnancy.

Findings.—Groups A and B had 13 and 11 pregnancy losses, respectively. The live birth rate was 72% in group A and 78% in group B, equivalent to an odds ratio of 1.39 in the latter. None of the women developed thrombosis.

Conclusions.—Low-dose-aspirin therapy for antiphospholipid syndrome in pregnant women yields highly successful outcomes. Adding low-molecular weight heparin does not appear to significantly improve these outcomes.

▶ These Liverpool investigators provide us a blinded prospective randomized study of 98 women designed to test whether subcutaneous daily heparin has adjunctive value to low-dose aspirin therapy of antiphospholipid syndrome.[1,2] Entry criteria required either 3 consecutive pregnancy losses without US evidence of a fetus or 2 pregnancy losses plus 1 fetal death in which fetal heart activity was discerned prior to demise. Laboratory confirmation used Russell Viper Venom prolongation for lupus anticoagulant and ELISA positivity for IgM and IgG anticardiolipin. Exclusion criteria included parental aneuploidy, uterine anomaly, prior thromboembolus or evidence of genetic thrombophilia, lupus nephritis, or steroid use. Women, 18 to 41 years old, were recruited over 3 years and randomized at 12 weeks' gestational age to aspirin 75 mg every day with or without low-dose heparin in dosages of 5000 U subcutaneously daily.

The results showed no significant difference in the incidence of live births between the 2 groups nor of pregnancy losses (28% and 22%). The fetal loss rate was, as others have pointed out, larger in the heparin receiving subset (10.2% vs 8.5%), but the difference was not statistically significant. Although it's difficult to prove a negative hypothesis, there seems little positive evidence that the use of daily heparin improves the 80% success rate usually associated with low-dose aspirin in these diseases, and there is some suggestion of possible increased fetal loss.

T. H. Kirschbaum, MD

References

1. 1995 YEAR BOOK OF OBSTETRICS, GYNECOLOGY, AND WOMEN'S HEALTH, pp 99-104.
2. 2000 YEAR BOOK OF OBSTETRICS, GYNECOLOGY, AND WOMEN'S HEALTH, pp 367-368.

8 The Puerperium

Perinatal Outcomes in Preeclampsia That Is Complicated by Massive Proteinuria
Newman MG, Robichaux AG, Stedman CM, et al (Woman's Hosp, Baton Rouge, La; Univ of Kentucky, Lexington)
Am J Obstet Gynecol 188:264-268, 2003   8–1

Introduction.—The management of severe preeclampsia in women well before term is a topic of ongoing debate. Despite disagreement over the use of "expectant" versus "aggressive" treatment in this situation, both sides agree that severe proteinuria (>5 g/24 h) is no longer an indication for immediate delivery. The impact of delayed delivery for preeclampsia with massive proteinuria (>10 g/24 h) was evaluated in a retrospective study.

Methods.—Over a 4.5-year period, 209 women with preeclampsia delivered before 37 weeks' gestation at 2 study hospitals. Patients with underlying kidney disease or multiple gestations were excluded. Proteinuria was classified as mild (<5 g/24 h) in 125 patients, severe (5 to 9.9 g/24 h) in 43, and massive (>10 g/24 h) in 41. Maternal and perinatal outcomes were compared for women with severe versus massive proteinuria.

Results.—The 3 groups were similar in terms of demographic characteristics and severity of preeclampsia. Women with mild proteinuria were more likely to achieve 37 weeks' gestation. None of the women died, and the rate of serious complications of preeclampsia was similar among groups. However, women with massive proteinuria had an earlier onset of preeclampsia. Massive proteinuria was also associated with higher rates of complications of prematurity, including neonatal ICU admission, respiratory distress syndrome, and intraventricular hemorrhage. However, with adjustment for prematurity, neonatal outcomes were not significantly affected by massive proteinuria per se.

Conclusion.—Among women with preeclampsia, the presence of massive proteinuria does not appear to lead to worse maternal outcomes compared with severe or mild proteinuria. Preeclamptic pregnancies with massive proteinuria are associated with early-onset disease and progression to severe preeclampsia. However, the increase in neonatal morbidity appears to reflect prematurity rather than the extreme level of proteinuria.

▶ This retrospective cohort study of women admitted with the diagnosis of preeclampsia consists of a series of comparisons of demographic, obstetric, maternal, and neonatal outcome data as a function of 3 levels of quantitative proteinuria measured within 24 hours of hospital admission. Patients were categorized as having mild (<5 g per 24 hours), severe (5-10 g per 24 hours), and massive (>10 g per 24 hours), and comparisons were made by analysis of variance among those 3 subsets. Most of the data are presented as means plus or minus what may be variances.

The 41 women with massive proteinuria were delivered somewhat earlier (mean, 30.6 weeks' gestational age) and delivered smaller infants who were more often admitted to the neonatal ICU with respiratory distress syndrome than the others. However, over a wide range of outcome variables, those pregnancies solely with massive proteinuria fared as well as those with lesser levels of proteinuria. The authors' implicit conclusion is that massive proteinuria alone does not suffice to define preeclamptics at high risk sufficient to require urgent or special management.

That's probably true but it's important to look for signs of chronic parenchymal renal disease during pregnancy in such women. Persistent, sometimes minor, hematuria may mean the presence of focal or general membranoproliferative glomerulonephritis. Signs of the nephrotic syndrome (proteinuria greater than 3.5 g per day, hyperlipidemia, edema not otherwise explained, and hypercoagulability) may coexist with only modest hypertension. Diabetic nephropathy needs to be excluded, as does lupus erythematosus.

An important obligation for the obstetrician is to be certain proteinuria relents during or after the puerperium. Such concerns, either prepartum or postpartum, should lead to consultation by a nephrologist who may well consider renal biopsy and glomerular immunofluorescent studies for IgG, complement C3, and the like. The possibility that massive albuminuria is a first sign of significant latent chronic renal disease must be excluded in the total care of such women.

T. H. Kirschbaum, MD

9 The Newborn

Immunoreactive Ghrelin in Human Cord Blood: Relation to Anthropometry, Leptin, and Growth Hormone
Chanoine J-P, Yeung LPK, Wong ACK, et al (British Columbia's Children's Hosp, Vancouver, Canada; St Paul's Hosp, Vancouver, BC, Canada)
J Pediatr Gastroenterol Nutr 35:282-286, 2002   9–1

Background.—Ghrelin is a peptide secreted by the hypothalamus, stomach, and placenta. Ghrelin stimulates growth hormone (GH) secretion and has orexigenic effects when injected. Leptin is secreted predominantly by adipocytes and has an important role in energy balance. Leptin decreases food intake when injected. The central, opposing effects of ghrelin and leptin are mediated through the neuropeptide Y/Y1 receptor pathway in the arcuate nucleus of the hypothalamus. The relationship between cord plasma concentrations of ghrelin, GH, leptin, and anthropomorphic measurements at birth was examined to determine whether ghrelin has a potential role in the initiation of feeding.

Study Design.—The study group consisted of 90 healthy, full term newborns born at Children's and Women's Health Center of British Columbia over a 2-month period. Birth weight and length were recorded at birth, and calf and abdominal circumference were measured within 24 hours of birth. Venous cord blood was collected for radioimmunoassay of ghrelin, leptin, and GH.

Findings.—Ghrelin was detected by immunoassay in all cord blood samples (range, 66-594 pmol/L). There was no significant difference between boys and girls. GH concentrations were also similar in boys and girls. Leptin concentrations were higher in female newborns. In female newborns, ghrelin was inversely correlated with anthropomorphic measurements, while in male newborns, ghrelin was positively correlated with leptin and negatively with GH.

Conclusion.—Ghrelin, a GH stimulant with orexigenic activity, is found in human cord plasma in widely varying amounts. Ghrelin may play a physiologic role in the initiation of feeding. The relationship between ghrelin and feeding behavior remains to be elucidated.

▶ With time and more information, hopes that leptin—a hormone product of adipocytes which decreases food intake on parenteral injection in leptin-deficient subjects—might join insulin as a major factor in weight regulation have diminished. Originally identified in a strain of obese mice genetically unable to produce leptin, the hormone concentration is positively correlated with body mass index in both human infants and adults but is of no value in the treatment of obesity, usually marked by high leptin blood levels and resistance to its additional administration. Leptin appears designed primarily to counteract and protect against weight loss in the face of inadequate nutrition, acting over periods of months to years in weight regulation and is of benefit only to those incapable of producing their own.

Ghrelin is a 28–amino acid peptide produced by the stomach, placenta, and hypothalamus which stimulates appetite, hyperglycemia, and GH production, acting through the GH receptor in a time span of minutes to a few hours. In this way ghrelin provides short-term appetite control of ingestion. It acts through the arcuate nucleus of the hypothalamus to activate peptide neurotransmitters of the neuropeptide Y class, which in turn serve to stimulate appetite and reduce metabolic activity. Its action produces the hunger before meals unrepresented by changes in leptin concentration. A peptide with opposing properties, PPY, acts through the same arcuate nucleus neurons to produce satiety and weight loss and is under further study.

These authors provide blood ghrelin concentrations and body measurements from the umbilical vein blood of 90 full-term normal infants. They find ghrelin values similar to those in normal adults who have mean concentrations of 234 pmol/L and fasting values at 179 pmol/L after breakfast. Newborn values averaged 187 pmol/L with a wide range (66 to 594 pmol/L) unrelated to body weight, length, body mass index, or gender. Ghrelin's origin in cord blood is uncertain, but it is unlikely to be placental since ghrelin mRNA becomes increasingly rare in late pregnancy. Its role in neonatal life is obscure though it may play some part in the initiation of newborn feeding. Its possible implications for the control of obesity are clear.

T. H. Kirschbaum, MD

Early Determinants of Childhood Overweight and Adiposity in a Birth Cohort Study: Role of Breast-Feeding
Bergmann KE, Bergmann RL, von Kries R, et al (Robert Koch Inst, Berlin)
Int J Obes 27:162-172, 2003   9–2

Background.—Childhood obesity is increasing. Cross-sectional studies have suggested a negative dose-effect relationship between breast-feeding and obesity. The German Multicenter Atopy Study followed its participants from birth and presents an opportunity to examine the relationship between breast-feeding and childhood obesity in a longitudinal, birth cohort, noninterventional setting.

Study Design.—The study group consisted of 1314 healthy singleton births taking place during 1990. To obtain sufficiently large groups for multivariate analysis, those who had been partially breast-fed for 2 months or less were combined with bottle-fed infants. Study participants were fol-

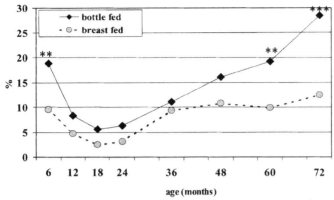

FIGURE 1.—Prevalence of overweight, according to body mass index. Proportion (percentage) of children exceeding the 90th percentile of the body mass index reference values, depending on feeding mode in infancy. The 480 cases used were those for whom complete data were still available at the age of 6 years. *Double asterisk* indicates $P < .01$; *triple asterisk*, $P < .001$. (Courtesy of Bergmann KE, Bergmann RL, von Kries R, et al: Early determinants of childhood overweight and adiposity in a birth cohort study: Role of breast feeding. *Int J Obes* 27:162-172, 2003, Nature Publishing Group.)

lowed up for 6 years. At each follow-up visit, physical examination, anthropometry, and feeding data were collected.

Findings.—There were no significant differences in body mass index at birth between these 2 groups. At the age of 1 month, breast-fed infants were lightly heavier. By the third month, bottle-fed infants had a higher body mass index (Figs 1 and 2) and thicker skin folds (Fig 3) than breast-fed babies. By 60 months, these differences became and remained significant. Logistic regression analysis indicated that maternal weight, maternal smoking, bottle feeding, and low social status were independent risk factors for overweight at 6 years of age.

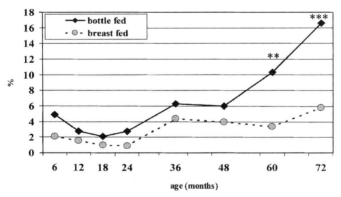

FIGURE 2.—Prevalence of overweight, according to body mass index. Proportion (percentage) of children exceeding the 97th percentile of the body mass index reference values, depending on feeding mode in infancy. The 480 cases used were those for whom complete data were still available at the age of 6 years. *Double asterisk* indicates $P < .01$; *triple asterisk*, $P < .001$. (Courtesy of Bergmann KE, Bergmann RL, von Kries R, et al: Early determinants of childhood overweight and adiposity in a birth cohort study: Role of breast feeding. *Int J Obes* 27:162-172, 2003, Nature Publishing Group.)

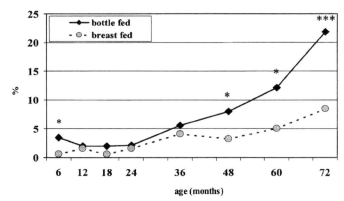

FIGURE 3.—Prevalence of adiposity, according to triceps skin-fold thickness. Proportion (percentage) of children exceeding the 97th percentile of the reference values, depending on feeding mode in infancy. The 480 cases used were those for whom complete data were still available at the age of 6 years. *Single asterisk* indicates $P < .05$; *triple asterisk*, $P < .001$. (Courtesy of Bergmann KE, Bergmann RL, von Kries R, et al: Early determinants of childhood overweight and adiposity in a birth cohort study: Role of breast feeding. *Int J Obes* 27:162-172, 2003, Nature Publishing Group.)

Conclusion.—This longitudinal birth cohort study demonstrates that bottle feeding is associated with increased childhood obesity. Other independent risk factors include maternal obesity, maternal smoking, and low social status.

▶ Though an inverse relationship between infant breast-feeding and childhood obesity was first described more than 20 years ago,[1] the nature of previous data has been unconvincing. Largely consisting of cross-sectional observations—complicated by faulty retrospective recall, lack of continuous individual observations, and inadequate definitions for obesity as well as inadequate attention to confounding variables—prior publications have led to persisting uncertainty. This study of data originally collected in a German multicenter atopy study during 1990 seems to answer many earlier objections.

Comparisons were made between 815 breast-fed infants fed only by breast for the first 3 months of life and 480 infants totally bottle-fed or only breast-fed less than 2 months of early life. Obesity was defined by skin-fold thickness using European norms[2] and by body mass indices greater than the 97th percentile of values reported for infants greater than 3 months of life.[3] Those with body mass index greater than the 90th percentile were termed overweight. A full range of confounders were considered in multivariant analyses. This is an important issue since breast-fed infants who were born to mothers of higher socioeconomic and educational strata and educational attainment, were decreasingly likely to be smokers and had with lower maternal body mass indexes than those receiving bottle feeding. Breast-fed infants were later in beginning solid foods as well. Complete data were available for infants through the first 72 months of age.

Measured either by the incidence of overweight as defined above or by skin-fold measurements, both breast- and bottle-fed infants showed reductions of obesity incidence to a nadir at 18 months, but between the ages of 3 and 4 years, bottle-fed infants were progressively and significantly more often obese than those who nursed. In view of the recent emergence of childhood obesity as a serious American health problem and the difficulty in achieving effective therapy, the possibility of prevention through nursing seems an important possibility.

In discussing mechanisms, the authors point to breast-feeding as a direct function of infant need as the infant controls milk production by the degree to which the infant drains the breast-collecting system. In contrast, the nutrient content and the amount of oral feeding are determined largely by parents, only indirectly a function of infant need. Women nursing do so as part of a life style (no smoking, higher educational and social attainment, personal health interest, etc) which constitutes environmental factors possibly important in obesity prevention. These are impressive data, well managed statistically and quite persuasive.

T. H. Kirschbaum, MD

References

1. Kramer MS: Do breast-feeding and delayed introduction of solid foods protect against subsequent obesity? *J Pediatr* 98:883, 1981.
2. Prader A, Largo RH, Molinari L, et al: Physical growth of Swiss children from birth to 20 years of age. *Helv Paediatr Acta* 52 (suppl):82-85, 1989.
3. Rolland-Cachera MF, Cole TJ, Sempé M, et al: Body mass index variations: Centiles from birth to 87 years. *Eur J Clin Nutr* 45:13-21, 1991.

Familial Aggregation of Fetal Growth Restriction in a French Cohort of 7,822 Term Births Between 1971 and 1985
La Batide-Alanore A, Trégouët D-A, Jaquet D, et al (INSERM U525, Paris; INSERM U457, Paris; INSERM U292, Villejuif, France)
Am J Epidemiol 156:180-187, 2002   9–3

Background.—Repeated small for gestational age (SGA) births in a large population of live infants born at term were studied, plus and minus adjustment for maternal characteristics and ponderal index, to look for potential genetic components.

Study Design.—The study group consisted of 7822 siblings in 3505 sibships born from 1971 to 1985 in the metropolitan Haguenau, France, area. To be included in the study group each birth had to be singleton; without infection, chromosomal abnormalities, or malformations; and term. SGA was defined by local standards as below the tenth percentile of sex-specific curve of birth weight by gestational age. Gestational age was defined by mother's last menstrual period. Ponderal index was calculated as birth weight divided by length. Maternal characteristics included age, weight, smoking status, marital status, and hypertension. Familial aggregation of SGA was expressed as the odds ratio.

Findings.—Of the 7822 live term births in the study, 751 were born SGA, 30.8% with a normal ponderal index and 39.8% with a low ponderal index.

Of the sibships, 13.6% had a single SGA and 3.6% had multiple SGA births. SGA births decreased with parity. Mothers in the SGA group were smaller and were more often primiparous, smokers, and unmarried than non-SGA mothers. As the number of SGA sibs increased, maternal factors became less favorable. Forty-one percent of mothers with multiple SGA births smoked during pregnancy, but only 14% of those with no SGA births smoked during pregnancy. Maternal hypertension was associated with single SGA births. Those born SGA and with a low ponderal index had a lower birth weight but a longer length than those who were born SGA with a normal ponderal index. SGA with a low ponderal index was associated with primiparity and pregnancy-associated hypertension. There was a strong family aggregation of SGA births, which was strengthened by stratification according to ponderal index and not influenced by maternal factors.

Conclusions.—This study demonstrated aggregation of SGA births within families. Although certain maternal factors, such as mother's size, primiparity, and smoking were associated with SGA births, additional factors, such as shared environmental or genetic traits, also appear to play a role. Family aggregation of SGA birth was strengthened by stratification by ponderal index, suggesting that proportional and disproportional intrauterine growth restriction may have different causes. A prospective follow-up study of those born SGA is currently underway to further explore these factors and their relation to health later in life.

▶ In calculating the odds ratio for growth retardation of newborns following the birth of an earlier growth-retarded sibling, these investigators provide strong support for common genetic factors predisposing both to growth retardation and adult cardiovascular disease, a conclusion that conflicts with the Barker hypothesis as frequently reviewed here.[1-5] The study population consisted of 20,000 singleton term live births without evidence of infection or anomalous development. Gestational age was determined by menstrual dates, physical examination, and ultrasound, and local standards for birth weight as a function of gestational age were employed because of the high frequency of births of Germanic origin in this eastern region of France. Odds ratios among the 3505 sibships with 751 growth-retarded newborns were constructed by dividing the ratio of prevalence of infants born SGA with growth-retarded siblings to a prevalence of SGA infants with siblings of normal birth weight. Data were adjusted for primigravidity since growth retardation is most common in primigravid women and becomes less common with advancing parity. Maternal smoking accounted for 41% of women with repeated growth-retarded infants but only 14% of women with only a singleton first growth-retarded birth. Maternal pregnancy hypertension proved not to be associated with the pattern of repeated newborn growth retardation. Growth-retarded infants delivered of smokers had normal ponderal indexes and tended to be longer, thinner infants of normal weight than those of hypertensive women whose infants had low ponderal indexes. Basing the definition of growth retardation on ponderal indexes of newborns rather than birth weight rate alone decreased the odds ratios for familial aggregation of fetal growth retardation with normal ponderal indices from 10.1 to 4.4, indicating the strong role of maternal environmental factors, especially smoking, in the history of repeated growth-retarded births. Adjusting for maternal factors in infants with low ponderal indexes, particularly primigravidity and maternal hypertension, failed to reduce the odds ratios for repeated growth-retarded newborns, changing the value from 8.0 to 7.7. This finding confirms the importance of genetic, nonenvironmental factors in determining this pattern of repeated growth retardation. These observations lead these investigators to the conclusion that common genetic factors, not maternal pregnancy-induced hypertension or other environmental factors, predispose infants both to growth retardation at birth and other genetically determined disease in later life, specifically hypertension, atherosclerosis, and coronary disease.

T. H. Kirschbaum, MD

References

1. 2002 YEAR BOOK OF OBSTETRICS, GYNECOLOGY, AND WOMEN'S HEALTH, pp 73-77.
2. 2002 YEAR BOOK OF OBSTETRICS, GYNECOLOGY, AND WOMEN'S HEALTH, pp 254-256.
3. 2003 YEAR BOOK OF OBSTETRICS, GYNECOLOGY, AND WOMEN'S HEALTH, pp 232-235.
4. 2003 YEAR BOOK OF OBSTETRICS, GYNECOLOGY, AND WOMEN'S HEALTH, pp 3-4.
5. 2003 YEAR BOOK OF OBSTETRICS, GYNECOLOGY, AND WOMEN'S HEALTH, pp 15-17.

High-Frequency Oscillatory Ventilation for the Prevention of Chronic Lung Disease of Prematurity

Calvert SA, for the United Kingdom Oscillation Study Group (St George's Hosp Med School, London, et al)

N Engl J Med 347:633-642, 2002   9–4

Background.—The safety and efficacy of high-frequency oscillatory ventilation are uncertain compared with those of conventional ventilation in very preterm infants needing respiratory support. Whether early intervention with high-frequency oscillatory ventilation can decrease mortality rates and the incidence of chronic lung disease in newborns, aged 28 weeks' gestation or less, was investigated in a multicenter randomized study.

Methods.—The study included 797 preterm infants whose gestational age ranged from 23 to 28 weeks. After stratification by center and gestational age, infants were randomly assigned to conventional ventilation or high-frequency oscillatory ventilation within 1 hour after birth.

Findings.—Death or chronic lung disease at 36 weeks postmenstrual age occurred in 66% of infants in the high-frequency oscillatory ventilation group and in 68% in the conventional ventilation group (Fig 2). Similar proportions in each gestational-age group died or had chronic lung disease. Treatment failure occurred in 10% of infants in both groups. The groups did not differ in secondary outcome measures, including serious brain injury and air leak.

Conclusions.—The outcomes of high-frequency oscillatory ventilation and conventional ventilation did not differ significantly in these very pre-

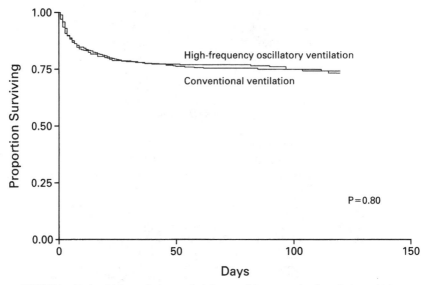

FIGURE 2.—Kaplan-Meier survival curves for infants receiving conventional ventilation and infants receiving high-frequency oscillatory ventilation. (Reprinted by permission of *The New England Journal of Medicine* from Calvert SA, for the United Kingdom Oscillation Study Group: High-frequency oscillatory ventilation for the prevention of chronic lung disease of prematurity. *N Engl J Med* 347:633-642, 2002. Copyright 2002, Massachusetts Medical Society. All rights reserved.)

term infants with respiratory disease. Additional follow-up is needed to establish whether long-term effects are different.

High-Frequency Oscillatory Ventilation Versus Conventional Mechanical Ventilation for Very-Low-Birth-Weight Infants

Courtney SE, for the Neonatal Ventilation Study Group (Cooper Hosp-Univ Med Ctr, Camden, NJ; et al)
N Engl J Med 347:643-652, 2002   9–5

Background.—The safety and efficacy of early high-frequency oscillatory ventilation compared with those of conventional synchronized intermittent mandatory ventilation in very-low-birth-weight infants remain unclear. Whether infants receiving early high-frequency oscillatory ventilation were more likely to be alive than those receiving synchronized intermittent mandatory ventilation and free of supplemental oxygen at 36 weeks' postmenstrual age was investigated in a multicenter study.

Methods.—The study included 500 infants weighing 601 to 1200 g at birth. All were less than 4 hours old, had received 1 dose of surfactant, and required ventilation with a mean airway pressure of 6 cm of water or more and a fraction of inspired oxygen of 0.25 or greater. After stratification by birth weight and prenatal corticosteroid exposure, infants were assigned to high-frequency oscillatory ventilation or synchronized intermittent mandatory ventilation.

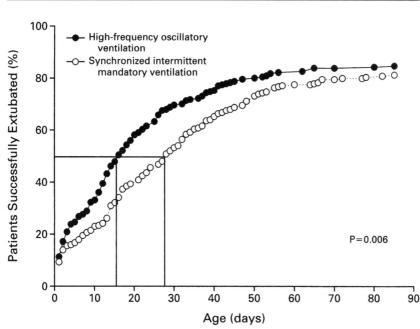

FIGURE 2.—Kaplan-Meier curves showing ages at which infants were successfully extubated. The curves are significantly different (*P* = .006 by the Cox proportional-hazards estimate; hazard ratio, 0.76 [95 percent confidence interval, 0.62 to 0.92]). The vertical lines show the age at which 50 percent of the infants assigned to each group were successfully extubated. (Reprinted by permission of *The New England Journal of Medicine* from Courtney SE, for the Neonatal Ventilation Study Group: High-frequency oscillatory ventilation versus conventional mechanical ventilation for very-low-birth-weight infants. *N Engl J Med* 347:643-652, 2002. Copyright 2002, Massachusetts Medical Society. All rights reserved.)

Findings.—Infants receiving high-frequency oscillatory ventilation were extubated successfully earlier than infants receiving synchronized intermittent mandatory ventilation (Fig 2). Fifty-six percent of infants receiving high-frequency oscillatory ventilation and 47% receiving synchronized intermittent mandatory ventilation were alive with no need for supplemental oxygen at 36 weeks' postmenstrual age (Fig 3). The 2 groups did not differ in their risk of intracranial bleeding, cystic periventricular leukomalacia, or other complications.

Conclusions.—Very-low-birth-weight infants receiving high-frequency oscillatory ventilation had a small but significant advantage in pulmonary outcomes than those receiving synchronized intermittent mandatory ventilation. The former group had no increase in the occurrence of other complications of premature birth.

▶ High-frequency oscillatory ventilation is a technique introduced into human use after extensive experimental animal experience showed it to improve substantially the results of ventilatory support of preterm newborn animals in short-term observations. The technique superimposes high frequency (300-900 cpm) low-volume pressure increments over a continuously inflating pressure usually initially in the range of 4 to 6 cm of water. This journal issue

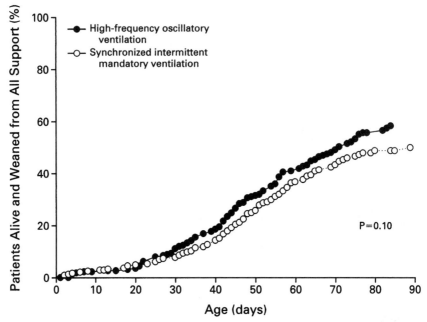

FIGURE 3.—Kaplan-Meier curves showing ages at which infants were successfully weaned from all support. *P* = .10 by the Cox proportional-hazards estimate; hazard ratio, 0.81 (95 percent confidence interval, 0.62 to 1.04). (Reprinted by permission of *The New England Journal of Medicine* from Courtney SE, for the Neonatal Ventilation Study Group: High-frequency oscillatory ventilation versus conventional mechanical ventilation for very-low-birth-weight infants. *N Engl J Med* 347:643-652, 2002. Copyright 2002, Massachusetts Medical Society. All rights reserved.)

provides accounts of the 2 largest randomized, multicenter, prospective, uncontrolled but blinded comparisons with conventional ventilation support in existence. Obstetricians should know about them I believe.

The first report of the United Kingdom Oscillatory Study Group, hereafter called the UK Study, and the second, of the Neonatal Ventilation Study Group, hereafter called the US Study, were similarly conducted but resulted in different conclusions.

The UK Study accepted infants requiring intubation and ventilation in the first 60 minutes of life, from 23 weeks to 28 weeks gestational age and with clinical evidence of need for continuing respiratory care. The US Study accepted neonates in the range of 0.6 to 1.2 kg birth weight and similar clinical predictive data as in the UK report. The UK Study was comprised of 797 cases and the US Study of 498. All conventionally ventilated infants, less than 1.5 kg birth weight requiring intubation, were exposed to 60 cps with an inflation interval of 0.4 second. The UK Study adjusted ventilation parameters to obtain acceptable blood gas values with a PaO_2 of 49-75 mm Hg and a $PaCO_2$ of 34-53 mm Hg. The US Study required arterial blood oxyhemoglobin saturations in the range of 88% to 96% with the same $PaCO_2$ as the UK Study and arterial pH = 7.2. Both newborn groups received surfactants, and ventilation strategies governing the innumerable ventilation variables based on clinical and laboratory observations were perhaps more rigorously formulated in the US Study than in its alternative. The UK Study demonstrated no significant difference in the number of infants alive and free of need for oxygen supplementation at 36 weeks between the 2 groups (34% vs 32%). Cranial US done 3, 7, and 28 days of life showed no significant difference in the incidence of intracranial hemorrhages, periventricular leucomalacia, pneumothorax, or interstitial emphysema in either study. The US Study showed 56% of those experiencing high frequency ventilation were alive and free of need for supplementary oxygen at 36 weeks compared with 47% of those treated with conventional ventilation support (relative risk, 1.2; confidence index, 1.0-1.5). Contrary to the suggestion of some prior investigators, there was no significant difference in occurrence of CNS complications and pulmonary hemorrhage was less common with high frequency ventilation, but the statistical support for that conclusion was not robust. The time of successful extubation was also earlier for those receiving high frequency oscillatory ventilation.

The differences between the study findings reflect the large number of uncontrolled variables that contribute to the severity of bronchopulmonary dysplasia and the outcome of the complex neonatal management of infants on ventilators. Bronchopulmonary dysplasia is caused by primary or secondary interference with alveolar development. Alveolar development begins at 24 weeks' gestational age and is impeded by pulmonary infection, oxygen toxicity, mechanical trauma due to over inflation, the degree of immaturity of lung tissue, and the nature of initial resuscitation and respiratory support. What can be said for certain is that high-frequency oscillatory ventilation can be done safely, and when performed by experienced pediatricians with rigorous uniform ventilation strategies, a small increase in the number of infants alive without chronic pulmonary disease may be attainable. Neither study should be used to support discontinuance of conventional ventilation support techniques that have evolved in the hands of experienced neonatal specialists.

T. H. Kirschbaum, MD

Neuroprotection by Selective Nitric Oxide Synthase Inhibition at 24 Hours After Perinatal Hypoxia-Ischemia
Peeters-Scholte C, Koster J, Veldhuis W, et al (Univ Med Ctr Utrecht, The Netherlands; Göteborg Univ, Sweden)
Stroke 33:2304-2310, 2002   9–6

Background.—Perinatal hypoxia-ischemia leads to neuronal injury and death. The mechanism of neuronal injury involves an increase in intracellular calcium elevation and generation of reactive oxygen species (ROS) and nitric oxide (NO). A piglet model of perinatal hypoxia-ischemia was used to test the protective role of inhibition of neuronal and inducible NO synthase (NOS) after hypoxia-ischemia.

Study Design.—Hypoxia-ischemia was induced in newborn piglets. With reperfusion, piglets received either the NOS inhibitor, 2-iminobiotin, or vehicle (control). Five piglets did not have hypoxia and served as sham-oper-

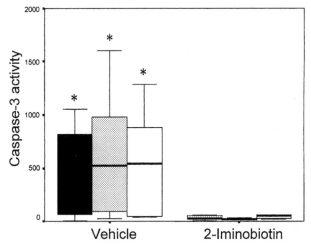

FIGURE 2.—Caspase-3 activity in parietal and temporal cortex and striatum. Box plots of caspase-3 activity (in picomoles of substrate per minute times milligrams of protein) as demonstrated in parietal cortex (*black*), temporal cortex (*gray*), and striatum (*white*). *P < .05. (Courtesy of Peeters-Scholte C, Koster J, Veldhuis W, et al: Neuroprotection by selective nitric oxide synthase inhibition at 24 hours after perinatal hypoxia-ischemia. *Stroke* 33:2304-2310, 2002.)

ated controls. Vasogenic edema was investigated by MRI. Brain sections were analyzed for caspase-3 activity, histology, and immunohistochemistry. DNA fragmentation was evaluated by terminal deoxynucleotidyl transferase–mediated dUTP-biotin in situ nick end labeling (TUNEL).

Findings.—At 24 hours after reperfusion, there was a 90% improvement in cerebral energy state, a 90% reduction in vasogenic edema, and a 60% to 80% reduction in neuronal cell death (Fig 2) in those piglets treated with 2-iminobiotin versus controls. There was also a significant reduction in tyrosine nitration in the cerebral cortex (Table 4), indicating decreased formation of reactive nitrogen species.

Conclusions.—Selective inhibition of neuronal and inducible nitric oxide synthase by 2-iminobiotin was neuroprotective after hypoxia-ischemia in a

TABLE 4.—Histology, TUNEL Labeling, and Tyrosine Nitration Immunohistochemistry

	Parietal Cortex			Striatum			Hippocampus		
	Vehicle	2-Iminobiotin	Sham	Vehicle	2-Iminobiotin	Sham	Vehicle	2-Iminobiotin	Sham
Cresyl violet	155±37	281±36*	349±71	222±60	376±42*	409±23	45±12	78±10*	101±17
TUNEL	2.2±0.2	1.5±0.2*	1.6±0.2	2.1±0.2	1.1±0.1*	1.2±0.2	1.9±0.2	1.2±0.1*	1.0±0.0
Tyrosine-nitration	2.4±0.2	1.7±0.2*	2.0±0.3	1.9±0.2	1.5±0.2	1.6±0.2	1.8±0.2	1.4±0.2	2.0±0.0

Histology and immunohistochemistry were performed at 24 hours after hypoxia-ischemia. Piglets were treated with vehicle (n = 12) or 2-iminobiotin (n = 11) or were sham-operated (n = 5). Sections were stained with cresyl violet, and the amount of apparently normal cells was counted in a grid consisting of 100 compartments. Hippocampus indicates the mean value from CA1 to CA4, plus dentate gyrus. TUNEL labeling and tyrosine nitration were scored on a 3-point scale. Although these data are original data, the mean ±SEM is reported for reasons of clarity.
*P <.05 compared with vehicle-treated piglets.
(Courtesy of Peeters-Scholte C, Koster J, Veldhuis W, et al: Neuroprotection by selective nitric oxide synthase inhibition at 24 hours after perinatal hypoxia-ischemia. *Stroke* 33:2304-2310, 2002.)

newborn pig model of neonatal hypoxia-ischemia. This may be a promising strategy for the prevention of neuronal damage after hypoxia-ischemia in neonates.

▶ In experimental work done of necessity in experimental animals, it's been possible to show that, immediately after severe ischemic-hypoxic brain injury, there's a 2- to 4-hour interval prior to the onset of irreversible neuronal injury.[1-3] This is 1 of several attempts to define treatment useful in that interval which might prevent or minimize long-term neural injury destined to ensue subsequently.[3] In the meanwhile, some conceptional changes and improved instrumentation have been applied to this quest.

The approach here is to explore the neuroprotective role of nitric oxide synthase (NOS) inhibitors as an intermediate step in preventing brain injury. Nitric oxide is generated by 3 isoforms of NOS—neuronal, endothelial, and inducible forms—designated by tissue locus and the capacity for local synthesis of nitric oxide. Endothelial based NOS is useful in providing vasodilatation through endothelial exposure to nitric oxide after an acute hypoxic-ischemia injury, and its inhibition increases risk of permanent brain injury.[4] Neuronal and inducible NOS produce nitric oxide, which, after combining with oxygen free radical donors like super oxide ion, produces peroxynitrite, which enhances neuronal injury. Peroxynitrite, stainable in fixed section, results in irreversible injury to DNA, lipids and proteins, and the oxidative enzymes housed predominantly in mitochondria. What then results is neuronal and glial apoptosis, evident by increased concentrations of caspase proteinases, increasing numbers of newly fragmented DNA segments evident with the TUNEL procedure[4] (Abstract 7–6) and by histologic evidence of nerve cell loss in tissue section.

Piglets, 1 to 3 days of age, were anesthetized, put on respiratory assist, and fitted with bilateral carotid occluders. The animals were subjected to baseline observations and then 1 hour of hypoxic-ischemia brain injury, monitored by magnetic resonance spectrography using ^{32}P. Following hypoxic injury, there is evidence of decreased ATP concentration and phosphocreatine and an increase in inorganic phosphate in brain tissue. These changes were followed through 2 hours of recovery during the latency period prior to the onset of irreversible neuronal cell loss. Eighteen piglets were treated either with an inhibitor of neuronal and inducible NOS (2-iminobiotin) or inert vehicle. Both groups shared the same degree of tachycardia, hypotension, and reduced pO2 during the early phase of hypoxic injury and the same evidence of degradation in cellular energy flow on ^{32}P magnetic resonance spectroscopy. The iminobiotin-treated animals showed little cellular brain edema and evidence of decreased apoptosis as measured by TUNEL, caspase activity, and histologic neuronal loss compared with controls. Nitrotyrosine, measured by immunohistochemistry, evidence of NO induced injury, was reduced in the iminobiotin-treated group. This is strong evidence that selected inhibition of specific NOS isoforms in non-intravascular sites in experimental animals given 24 hours after hypoxic-ischemic brain injury reduces the amount of resultant permanent brain injury ultimately found. In instances in which the hypoxic-ischemic injury is acute and occurs at a known time, this agent appears to be of potential clinical value, pending experimental confirmation in a human subject.

T. H. Kirschbaum, MD

References

1. 1992 YEAR BOOK OF OBSTETRICS, GYNECOLOGY, AND WOMEN'S HEALTH, pp 189-191.
2. 1996 YEAR BOOK OF OBSTETRICS, GYNECOLOGY, AND WOMEN'S HEALTH, pp 134-137.
3. 1998 YEAR BOOK OF OBSTETRICS, GYNECOLOGY, AND WOMEN'S HEALTH, pp 231-235.
4. 1998 YEAR BOOK OF OBSTETRICS, GYNECOLOGY, AND WOMEN'S HEALTH, pp 241-243.

Neonatal Organ System Injury in Acute Birth Asphyxia Sufficient to Result in Neonatal Encephalopathy
Hankins GDV, Koen S, Gei AF, et al (Univ of Texas, Galveston)
Obstet Gynecol 99:688-691, 2002   9–7

Background.—The diagnosis of acute birth asphyxia has an implication of mismanagement by the obstetric team and is often misapplied. The proportion of major organ system injuries sufficient to enable neonatal encephalopathy to more definitively diagnose this condition was examined.

Study Design.—All diagnoses of acute intrapartum asphyxia, acute birth asphyxia, and neonatal encephalopathy made from 1994 to 2000 were identified in a prospectively maintained database at a single institution. An acute intrapartum hypoxic event was defined as a sentinel hypoxic event occurring during or immediately preceding labor; sudden sustained deterioration of the fetal heart rate pattern or an acute catastrophic event; early onset of neonatal encephalopathy; and absence of a severe congenital abnormality that would impact transition from fetal to neonatal life.

Neonatal encephalopathy was defined as disturbed neurologic function during the first week after birth manifested as breathing difficulties, reflex depression, altered consciousness, and often seizures. Causes of injury prior to presentation were investigated. The injury pattern was investigated with laboratory and imaging tests.

Findings.—Over the 6 years of the study, 46 cases of acute peripartum asphyxia sufficient to result in a diagnosis of neonatal encephalopathy were identified within the database. Liver injury occurred in 80% of patients, heart injury in 78%, renal injury in 72%, and elevated red blood cell counts in 41%.

Conclusion.—When peripartum encephalopathy develops in an infant, it should not be termed "birth asphyxia" unless it is accompanied by significant multiple organ system injury.

▶ This is a retrospective cohort study of neonates of at least 32 weeks' gestational age with evidence of acute hypoxic-ischemic brain injury manifest in the first week of life, designed to explore the incidence and the possible diagnostic import of multiple organ system injury in establishing and/or confirming the diagnosis of CNS pathology. Forty-six cases were selected on the basis of all of the following: a signal perinatal event capable of inducing hypoxic-ischemic brain injury, an abrupt sustained fetal heart rate abnormality related in time to that event, the clinical diagnosis of neonatal encephalopathy, and the absence of congential fetal anomaly.

The diagnosis of CNS abnormality was made by neurologic exam, CNS imaging techniques, and electroencephalogram. Clinical findings of impaired initiation and maintenance of respiration, depression of neuromuscular reflex and tone, seizures, and altered states of consciousness were essential findings. Umbilical artery pH was less than 7.0 in 61% of the infants, base excess less than -18 mM/L in 38%, and 5-minute Apgar scores less than 6 in 76%. The incidence of evidence of neonatal cerebral vascular, CNS, hepatic, and renal injury varied from 70% to 80%. Least commonly occurring was evidence of hematologic injury such as thrombopenia and normoblastemia, present in only 54%.

The authors conclude that multiple organ system injury is common among early neonates in whom the diagnosis of brain injury using their criteria occurs, and that with evidence of neonatal brain injury without evidence of multiple organ system changes, the diagnosis of hypoxic-ischemic injury should at least be questioned. Exempting hematologic changes, somewhere about 20% of brain-injured infants failed to show evidence of injury in all 4 organ systems. Unfortunately, the data do not allow evaluation of the prognostic significant cases when only 1 or 2 organ systems were involved.

T. H. Kirschbaum, MD

Neurodevelopmental Outcome of Premature Infants After Antenatal Phenobarbital Exposure
Shankaran S, Papile L-A, Wright LL, et al (Wayne State Univ, Detroit; Univ of New Mexico, Albuquerque; Natl Inst of Child Health and Human Development, Bethesda, Md; et al)
Am J Obstet Gynecol 187:171-177, 2002   9–8

Background.—Previous research has shown that antenatal phenobarbital does not reduce the risk of intracranial bleeding or early death in premature infants. The impact of antenatal phenobarbital exposure on the neurodevelopmental outcome of premature infants born to participants in the randomized clinical trial of antenatal phenobarbital exposure was investigated.

Methods.—Of the 578 infants born before 34 weeks' gestation to participants in the original study, 436 (76%) were available for follow-up at 18 to 22 months of corrected age. Assessment included a standard neurologic examination and the Bayley scales of infant development measuring the mental developmental index (MDI) and psychomotor developmental index (PDI). The group exposed to antenatal phenobarbital and the placebo group were similar in mean birth weight and gestational age, maternal education, and frequency and distribution of intracranial bleeding.

Findings.—Eight percent of the infants in the antenatal phenobarbital group and 11% in the placebo group had cerebral palsy. The groups did not

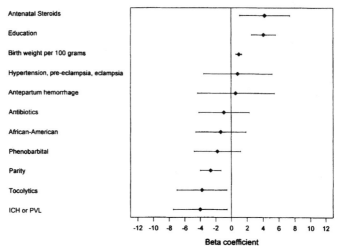

FIGURE 1.—Relationship of perinatal and neonatal characteristics and Bayley mental developmental index (MDI) scores. The relationship of perinatal and neonatal characteristics and antenatal phenobarbital exposure (linear regression estimates and 95% confidence intervals) on Bayley MDI is shown. The information to the right of the vertical line indicates higher MDI scores. *Abbreviations: ICH,* Intracranial hemorrhage; *PVL,* periventricular leukomalacia. (Reprinted by permission of the publisher courtesy of Shankaran S, Papile L-A, Wright LL, et al: Neurodevelopmental outcome of premature infants after antenatal phenobarbital exposure. *Am J Obstet Gynecol* 187:171-177. Copyright 2002 by Elsevier.)

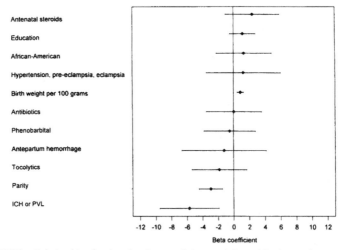

FIGURE 2.—Relationship of perinatal and neonatal characteristics and Bayley psychomotor developmental index (PDI) scores. The relationship of perinatal and neonatal characteristics and antenatal phenobarbital exposure (linear regression estimates and 95% confidence intervals) on Bayley PDI is shown. The information to the right of the vertical line indicates higher PDI scores. (Reprinted by permission of the publisher courtesy of Shankaran S, Papile L-A, Wright LL, et al: Neurodevelopmental outcome of premature infants after antenatal phenobarbital exposure. *Am J Obstet Gynecol* 187:171-177. Copyright 2002 by Elsevier.)

differ in terms of the median Bayley II MDI or the PDI (Figs 1 and 2). Independent of antenatal phenobarbital exposure, infants with intracranial hemorrhage had significantly lower MDI and PDI scores than infants without intracranial bleeding. Overall, the presence of intracranial bleeding or periventricular leukomalacia correlated with lower MDI and PDI scores. A higher MDI score correlated with increasing birth weight, maternal education, and a complete course of antenatal steroids.

Conclusions.—Antenatal phenobarbital exposure did not affect the neurodevelopmental outcomes—either favorably or adversely—in this population of premature infants followed up at 18 to 22 months of age. Preventing neonatal intracranial hemorrhage and reducing the rate of neurodevelopmental handicap are a continuing challenge.

▶ Use of prophylactic phenobarbital has been reported to prevent intracranial hemorrhage and early neonatal death in premature infants as a result of decreasing the tendency for intubated newborns to struggle with intubation and mechanical ventilation and thereby diminishing the surges of hypertension that occur during such incidents.[1,2] In a previous work this group demonstrated that phenobarbital administration in the dose of 10 mg/kg of maternal weight for greater than 2 hours prior to birth resulted in no reduction in the incidence of intracranial hemorrhage.[3] They had concerns that chronic exposure to phenobarbital in utero might negatively influence infant neurodevelopment, and this led to this prospective, randomly controlled multicenter study in which test women at 24 to 32 weeks' gestational age were given phenobarbital 10 mg/kg intravenously and 100 mg orally every day for 32 weeks' gestation while controls received placebo. Newborn cranial US scans were done on each of the 436 infants twice prior to 14 days of life for the detection of intracranial hemorrhage and periventricular leukomalacia. Certified neural examiners performed Bayley scale MDI and PDI testing, together with standard vision and hearing examinations, at 18 to 22 months of age.

The results again showed no significant difference in intracranial hemorrhage or early neonatal death, birth weight, gestational age at birth, ventriculomegaly, or periventricular leukomalacia between phenobarbital recipients and controls. As shown in Figures 1 and 2, there were no differences in MDI and PDI scores based on phenobarbital administration. Regrettably, but quite certainly, there seems no value in prophylactic phenobarbital in the prevention of intracranial hemorrhage in premature newborns.

T. H. Kirschbaum, MD

References

1. 1988 Year Book of Obstetrics and Gynecology, pp 209-210.
2. Volpe JJ: *Neurology of the Newborn.* Philadelphia, W. B. Saunders, 1995, pp 439-443.
3. 1999 Year Book of Obstetrics, Gynecology, and Women's Health, pp 215-216.

Central Nervous System Infection in Congenital Syphilis
Michelow IC, Wendel GD Jr, Norgard MV, et al (Univ of Texas, Dallas)
N Engl J Med 346:1792-1798, 2002   9–9

Background.—Identification of infants with *Treponema pallidum* infection of the CNS is still difficult. Rabbit-infectivity testing of the CSF was used to detect CNS *T pallidum* infection in infants born to mothers with syphilis.

Methods and Findings.—Rabbit-infectivity testing of 148 infants detected spirochetes in the CSF of 19. Antibiotic exposure of the infant before CSF was obtained was associated with a negative test finding. Spirochetes were identified in 22% of 76 infants with no previous antibiotic exposure. This group included the following: 41% of infants with some abnormality on clinical, laboratory, or radiographic assessment; 60% of infants with abnormal physical examination findings consistent with congenital syphilis; and 41% of infants with a positive finding on IgM immunoblotting or polymerase chain reaction (PCR) testing of serum, blood, or CSF, or a positive finding on rabbit-infectivity testing of serum or blood. Only 1 infant with normal results on clinical examination had positive CSF rabbit-infectivity

TABLE 3.—Comparison of Diagnostic Accuracy of Laboratory Tests and Cerebrospinal Fluid Rabbit-Infectivity Testing in 76 Infants Who Had No Antibiotic Exposure Before Cerebrospinal Fluid Was Obtained

Test	Sensitivity	Specificity	Positive Predictive Value	Negative Predictive Value	κ Value
			No./Total No. (%)		
Conventional tests					
Any abnormal result	16/17 (94)	36/59 (61)	16/39 (41)	36/37 (97)	0.38
Abnormal physical examination	15/17 (88)	49/59 (83)	15/25 (60)	49/51 (96)	0.61
Abnormality on bone radiograph	9/17 (53)	54/58 (93)	9/13 (69)	54/62 (87)	0.50
Anemia	4/16 (25)	57/59 (97)	4/6 (67)	57/69 (83)	0.28
Thrombocytopenia	8/16 (50)	56/58 (97)	8/10 (80)	56/64 (88)	0.54
CSF					
Reactive VDRL test	9/17 (53)	53/59 (90)	9/15 (60)	53/61 (87)	0.45
Elevated white-cell count	6/16 (38)	44/50 (88)	6/12 (50)	44/54 (81)	0.28
Elevated protein	9/16 (56)	39/50 (78)	9/20 (45)	39/46 (85)	0.32
Elevated white-cell count or protein	11/16 (69)	34/50 (68)	11/27 (41)	34/39 (87)	0.30
≥1 Abnormal CSF test	14/17 (82)	33/51 (65)	14/32 (44)	33/36 (92)	0.36
Other tests					
Any abnormal result	17/17 (100)	35/59 (59)	17/41 (41)	35/35 (100)	0.40
Positive serum or blood test					
Rabbit-infectivity test	13/14 (93)	40/49 (82)	13/22 (59)	40/41 (98)	0.62
IgM immunoblotting	17/17 (100)	39/59 (66)	17/37 (46)	39/39 (100)	0.47
PCR assay	16/17 (94)	53/59 (90)	16/22 (73)	53/54 (98)	0.76
Positive CSF					
IgM immunoblotting	8/17 (47)	54/58 (93)	8/12 (67)	54/63 (86)	0.45
PCR assay	11/17 (65)	57/59 (97)	11/13 (85)	57/63 (90)	0.67
IgM immunoblotting or PCR assay	13/17 (76)	53/59 (90)	13/19 (68)	53/57 (93)	0.64

Abbreviations: CSF, Cerebrospinal fluid; *VDRL,* Venereal Disease Research Laboratory; *PCR,* polymerase chain reaction.
(Reprinted by permission of *The New England Journal of Medicine* from Michelow IC, Wendel GD Jr, Norgard MV, et al: Central nervous system infection in congenital syphilis. *N Engl J Med* 346:1792-1798. Copyright 2002, Massachusetts Medical Society. All rights reserved.)

test findings. Overall, IgM immunoblotting of serum or PCR assay of serum or blood best predicted CNS infection (Table 3).

Conclusions.—Physical examination, conventional laboratory tests, and radiographic studies can identify most infants with *T pallidum* CNS infection. However, additional tests, such as IgM immunoblotting and PCR assay, are needed to identify all affected infants.

▶ Even when physical examination and x-ray findings make the presence of infant congenital syphilis clear, the diagnosis of congenital CNS infection is a problem, increasingly important as the incidence of congenital syphilis with and without HIV infection has become more common recently. Conventionally, the neonatal diagnosis is made by physical examination, presence of VDRL-positive CSF with greater than 25 white blood cells per cubic millimeter and protein concentration greater than 150 mg/dL. In newborn infants, both pleocytosis and increased protein concentrations are often less striking. This study provides comparison of the accuracy of these measures compared with PCR using primers for *T pallidum* DNA and immunoblotting for IgM antibody against *T pallidum*, conducted in newborn blood, serum, and CSF in 92% of the samples obtained on the first day of life. Comparisons were made by demonstrating rabbit infectivity, taking advantage of the exquisite sensitivity of the rabbit's immune reaction to treponemes injected in vivo. Of 148 infants born of the 146 women with early acute syphilis during pregnancy, 106 cases (93 with no antibiotic therapy and 29 treated less than 4 weeks before delivery) were studied. In 70 infants the diagnosis was made by conventional means, and in 65 by rabbit injection, IgM, and DNA analysis. Although any one positive conventional test had a 94% sensitivity, the false-positive rate was 59% and specificity rates were low. Conventional tests of CSF showed less sensitivity (82%) with similarly high false-positive rates. In 4 cases (2.7%) false-negative results of conventional tests were proven by rabbit IgM antibody positivity detected all cases of CNS infection, but the best results come from IgM or PCR (76% sensitivity, 32% false-positive). It's clear, though, that no combination of any of the elements of neonatal testing is perfect; the exclusion of the diagnosis and the best chance of detecting all cases requires search for IgM and treponemal DNA in the blood and CSF of suspect newborn.

T. H. Kirschbaum, MD

Fetal Lung Maturity Indices—A Plea for Gestational Age-Specific Interpretation: A Case Report and Discussion
Pinette MG, Blackstone J, Wax JR, et al (Maine Med Ctr, Portland)
Am J Obstet Gynecol 187:1721-1722, 2002   9–10

Background.—The maturity of the fetal lungs is linked to gestational age, but no single test is capable of absolutely predicting when a fetus is able to breathe independently without difficulty. Laboratory tests indicating that the lungs are mature can lead to the delivery of a newborn with respiratory distress. Thus, determining fetal lung maturity (FLM) should be regarded as a probability that relies on both gestational age and amniotic fluid analysis.

Case Report.—Woman, 35, gravida 4, para 0, was determined to a uterine size less than it should have been for the expected clinical date and underwent US at 28 weeks 4 days and 32 weeks 5 days. The fetus was at the 25th percentile for gestational age but had subjectively decreased amniotic fluid levels. At 35 weeks, the breech-presenting fetus was at the 15th percentile and had markedly decreased fluid. At 35 weeks 4 days, amniocentesis revealed a lecithin-to-sphingomyelin (L/S) ratio of 3.7, an FLM value of 23, and a negative phosphatidylglycerol value. FLM was determined on the basis of an L/S ratio of 2.5 or greater, so cesarean delivery was undertaken. Even with the mature L/S ratio, the newborn was given a diagnosis of mild respiratory distress syndrome (RDS) and required oxygen therapy.

Conclusions.—Based on gestational age alone or gestational age plus a laboratory test result, the probability of RDS may be inaccurate. FLM should be viewed as a determination of probability rather than a positive or negative result. The use of both gestational age and FLM to determine the risk of RDS provides a more accurate picture.

▶ The estimations of FLM have previously been based on assays of L/S ratios or of the phosphatidylglycerol level, but these assays are difficult to perform and are not amenable to automation. Further, use of a dichotomous readout (ie, mature or immature) leads to errors in which, for instance, as many as 12% of preterm infants judged mature by lipid analysis may subsequently develop RDS. An attempt to improve this system involves the introduction of an assay that measures the surfactant/albumin ratio; it uses a semiautomated fluorescent polarization method to determine the ratio of surfactant to albumin in amniotic fluid as an indicator of FLM. The results also independently depend on the concentration of phospholipids present in the amniotic fluid. Although not measured by the method, the saturated phospholipid concentration correlates with gestational age. It was for that reason that Tanasijevic and colleagues[1] suggested a series of calculations providing the probability of RDS as a function of FLM and gestational age as independent variables. A simple binary yes or no result requires an arbitrary limit to be set, usually chosen so as to exclude immaturity at the cost of poor specificity and false-positive indicators of immaturity. Adjusting the end point to reduce false-positive findings for immaturity increases the incidence of false-positive indicators of maturity.

Pinette et al, applying logistic regression to a series of 388 newborns with RDS, generated a table of probabilities of RDS based on gestational age and FLM, that is, the probability of disease, designed to rationalize the decision process with the use of the improved technology. In the same issue, Dr Phillip Stubblefield,[2] a distinguished Boston obstetrician–gynecologist, urges practicing obstetricians to heed the rediscovered wisdom present in both articles, which he fears may be overlooked as they decide about intentional preterm delivery. This article will be very useful for those physicians and laboratories who are in the process of making the change in instrumentation.

T. H. Kirschbaum, MD

References

1. Tanasijevic MJ, Wybenga DR, Richardson D, et al: A predictive model for fetal lung maturity employing gestational age and test results. *Am J Clin Pathol* 102:788-793, 1994.
2. Stubblefield PG: Using the TDx-FLM assay and gestational age together for more accurate production of risk for neonatal respiratory distress syndrome. *Am J Obstet Gynecol* 187:1429-1430, 2002.

Neonatal Brachial Plexus Palsy: An Unpredictable Injury
Donnelly V, Foran A, Murphy J, et al (Natl Maternity Hosp, Dublin; Univ College Dublin)
Am J Obstet Gynecol 187:1209-1212, 2002   9–11

Introduction.—Injury to the brachial plexus is a serious neonatal neurologic injury that usually resolves within the first months of life. The incidence and persistence of disability were examined, along with whether the occurrence could be predicted by maternal characteristics or partographic analysis.

Methods.—Between 1994 and 1998, all infants with neonatal evidence of obstetric brachial plexus injury were identified and followed up for 1 or more years. The obstetric details in these maternal-infant pairs were compared with those of 108 control pairs which were matched for maternal and gestational age, parity, and birth weight. Partographs of cases and controls were reviewed in a blinded fashion by 3 experienced obstetricians who were asked to identify likely cases of nerve injury. A risk score composed of 8 recognized associated clinical features was assigned.

Results.—There was evidence of brachial plexus injury in 45 of 35,796 infants (1.5/1000), 10 (19%) of whom had neurologic deficit that persisted to 1 year. The risk profile was relatively higher in patients than in control subjects. The highest score was 5 of 8 in 6 cases (2 cases, 4 controls). The obstetricians' partographic evaluation identified "likely brachial plexus injury" in 13 of 54 cases (24%) and 16 of 108 controls (15%). The assessors concurred in only 3 cases (6%). Ranges for positive predictive value, negative predictive value, sensitivity, and specificity, respectively, were 7% to 17%; 5% to 12%; 24% to 50%; and 66% to 68%. Risk scores were similar for persistently and transiently injured cases.

Conclusion.—Brachial plexus injury cannot be predicted before injury using either risk factor scoring or partographic analysis.

▶ Brachial plexus injury occurs in about 1 per 1000 deliveries, usually, but not always, conducted vaginally and may have tragic long-term consequences. It does not, however, follow that it can be effectively predicted or prevented.[1,2] This retrospective cohort analysis of 54 cases of brachial plexus injury encountered at Dublin's Royal Maternity Hospital over 5 years with an incidence of 1.5 per 1000 live births makes that point and obstetricians need to be cognizant of it. Controls were formed from the next delivery following that resulting in brachial plexus injury, matched for maternal age, parity, gestational age, and birth weight in a 2:1 frequency ratio. The primary variables, secondary arrest of labor, prolonged second stage, and instrumental vaginal birth were equally common in both groups.

No significant difference existed with respect to maternal weight greater than 100 K, pregnancy weight gain greater than 20 kg, maternal diabetes, a prior newborn weighing more than 4 kg at birth, or a history of previous shoulder dystocia. In 10 cases of brachial plexus injury with dysfunction persisting greater than 1 year, tendon transplant surgery was needed in 3 cases.[3] Of those cases, 6 resulted from apparently normal vaginal births and 1 of the infants, weighing 2.6 kg, was born by cesarean section. Best efforts aside, it appears we have no truly effective means of preventing this form of birth injury.

T. H. Kirschbaum, MD

References

1. 1991 Year Book of Obstetrics, Gynecology, and Women's Health, pp 97-98.
2. 1994 Year Book of Obstetrics, Gynecology, and Women's Health, pp 187-188.
3. 1990 Year Book of Obstetrics, Gynecology, and Women's Health, pp 203-204.

Cognitive and Behavioral Outcomes of School-Aged Children Who Were Born Preterm: A Meta-analysis
Bhutta AT, Cleves MA, Casey PH, et al (Univ of Arkansas, Little Rock)
JAMA 288:728-737, 2002   9–12

Background.—As infant mortality has decreased, an increasing percentage of children born preterm with low or very low birth weight (LBW) have survived. The effect of preterm birth on cognitive and behavioral outcomes in school-age children was explored.

Study Design.—A MEDLINE search was conducted for the period 1980 to November 2001 in English language publications. Studies were included with a case-control design, cognitive and/or behavioral data, evaluations after the fifth birthday, and an attrition rate of less than 30%. Only 15 studies that met these stringent criteria were included in this meta-analysis. Quality evaluation of these studies was performed with a 10-point scale.

Results.—There were 1556 cases and 1720 controls in these 15 studies. Controls had significantly higher cognitive scores. The mean cognitive scores of both cases and controls were directly proportional to birth weight. Age at evaluation was not correlated with cognitive score difference. Preterm children had increases in both externalizing and internalizing behaviors and had more than twice the relative risk of developing attention deficit–hyperactivity disorder.

Conclusions.—This meta-analysis demonstrated that preterm birth was associated with lower cognitive scores and increased risk for behaviors such as attention deficit–hyperactivity disorder among school-age children. Therapeutic interventions are necessary to prevent these long-term sequelae of preterm birth.

▶ The vast majority of studies of the infant consequences of preterm birth have been based on abnormalities of motor functions since those end points are relatively clear and objective.[1] This is a competently performed meta-analysis designed to explore the impact of preterm birth on "soft" neurologic outcomes—cognitive and behavioral functions. Case-control studies were selected where appropriate testing was done after the fifth birthday in work published in the last 20 years with attrition rates to follow-up less than 30%. Variation in quality was explored with the authors' novel 10-point scale and data heterogeneity with standard nonparametric tests. The 15 studies used in cognitive evaluation and 16 in behavioral analysis differed with respect to country of origin, presence and severity of physical disabilities of children, adequacy of neonatal history, differences among the 7 tests used for cognitive and behavioral appraisal, and demographic differences among infant populations. The cognitive data analysis showed excessive heterogeneity that stemmed from 2 studies (authors references 32 and 35) in which extreme physical disabilities interfered with test performance. Excluding 1 of those data aggregates removed the significance of testing for heterogeneity, but the problems persisted and weigh on the merits of the authors' conclusions.

Cognitive scores were positively correlated both with birth weight and gestational age. Comparisons with controls were done by calculating the mean differences, weighted for case numbers, between preterm and control groups and testing the weighted mean difference for significant difference from zero and evidence of no significant difference between premature infants and controls. Both measures showed a statistically significant decrease in cognitive ability and increase in behavior abnormalities, largely attention deficit–hyperactivity disorder among 5-year-olds born preterm compared with normal controls.

Whether a statistically significant difference is functionally significant in the lives of the infants is the crucial unevaluated issue here. In this connection, the recent work of Hack et al, where such infants were followed to age 20 years, is most important.[2] In that study, the malleability and ability to achieve shown by newborns at 1.5 kg or less at birth is demonstrated. These authors show with careful work that preterm infants may well suffer a statistically significant decrement in intellectual and social behavior capacity. Hack et al showed they often overcome them.

T. H. Kirschbaum, MD

References

1. 2002 YEAR BOOK OF OBSTETRICS, GYNECOLOGY, AND WOMEN'S HEALTH, p 85-89.
2. 2003 YEAR BOOK OF OBSTETRICS, GYNECOLOGY, AND WOMEN'S HEALTH, pp 225-229.

The Effect of Intrapartum Magnesium Sulfate Therapy on Fetal Cardiac Troponin I Levels at Delivery

Blackwell SC, Redman ME, Whitty JE, et al (Wayne State Univ, Detroit)
J Matern Fetal Neonatal Med 12:327-331, 2002   9–13

Background.—Pregnant women with preeclampsia-eclampsia receive magnesium sulfate therapy for seizure prophylaxis. At therapeutic concentrations, magnesium sulfate affects fetal heart rate parameters. Troponin I is a sensitive and specific serum marker of acute myocardial injury. Delivery umbilical troponin I levels were compared between term patients with preeclampsia who received magnesium sulfate therapy and term patients with normal pregnancies (control subjects) to assess whether maternal magnesium sulfate therapy was associated with fetal myocardial injury.

Study Design.—The study group consisted of 26 healthy term pregnancies and 13 term pregnancies with preeclampsia; the latter group received maternal magnesium sulfate antiseizure prophylaxis. In this cross-sectional–designed study, umbilical cord blood specimens were obtained at birth for troponin I concentration assays. Umbilical cord blood concentrations of troponin I were compared between these 2 groups; the groups were well matched for patient characteristics.

Findings.—There were no significant differences in troponin I umbilical blood concentrations between those who were exposed to magnesium sulfate therapy and those who were not exposed (Fig 1).

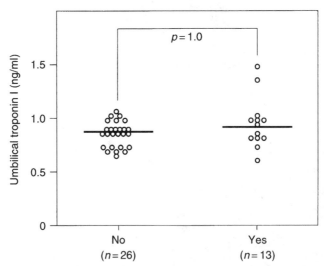

FIGURE 1.—Umbilical venous troponin I levels at delivery for patients who received intrapartum magnesium sulfate compared with controls without magnesium sulfate therapy. (Courtesy of Blackwell SC, Redman ME, Whitty JE, et al: The effect of intrapartum magnesium sulfate therapy on fetal cardiac troponin I levels at delivery. *J Matern Fetal Neonatal Med* 12:327-331, 2002.)

Conclusions.—Maternal magnesium sulfate anti-seizure therapy did not appear to have any effect on umbilical cord blood levels of troponin I, a marker of myocardial injury.

▶ Cardiac troponin I is a protein component of the myocardial tropomyosin complex important in regulating cardiac contractility. Its concentration is a sensitive measure of myocardial infarction, unmeasurable in normals and particularly useful to obstetricians since its concentration in human blood is independent of normal pregnancy, delivery, prolonged labor, cesarean section, operative vaginal birth, and anesthesia.[1] Concern for the effects of magnesium sulfate on fetal myocardium was raised by an earlier study in which troponin T concentration was found to be elevated in 12 of 191 cord blood samples, 10 of which were from preterm infants exposed to maternal magnesium sulfate administered for pregnancy hypertension.[2]

These authors provide data from 39 newborns, 13 of whom were exposed to maternal magnesium sulfate given for seizure prophylaxis for maternal hypertension. They chose to measure the troponin I isoform since it is specific to the myocardium, whereas troponin T is expressed in immature or diseased skeletal muscle. These authors showed no difference in troponin I concentration in term infants whether exposed or not to magnesium sulfate. Though the possibility of myocardial injury exists for preterm neonates, this study provides some reassurance regarding the fetal cardiac safety of this long-standing therapeutic for seizure prophylaxis.

T. H. Kirschbaum, MD

References

1. Shade GH Jr, Ross G, Bever FN, et al: Tropinin I in the diagnosis of acute myocardial infarction in pregnancy, labor and postpartum. *Am J Obstet Gynecol* 187:1719, 2002.
2. Shelton SD, Fause BL, Holleman CM, et al: Cardiac troponin T levels in umbilical cord blood. *Am J Obstet Gynecol* 181:1259, 1999.

Rate and Risk Factors of Hypoglycemia in Large-for-Gestational-Age Newborn Infants of Nondiabetic Mothers

Schaefer-Graf UM, Rossi R, Bührer C, et al (Vivantes Med Ctr Neukoelln, Charité, Germany; Humboldt-Univ, Berlin)
Am J Obstet Gynecol 187:913-917, 2002   9–14

Background.—Excessive intrauterine growth in the fetus of a mother with diabetes is associated with elevated risk of hypoglycemia in the newborn, which may cause brain damage. However, there is no consensus on whether to test large-for-gestational-age (LGA) neonates of nondiabetic mothers. The extent of neonatal hypoglycemia during the first 24 hours was investigated in a large population of LGA newborns of nondiabetic mothers to identify possible predictive factors.

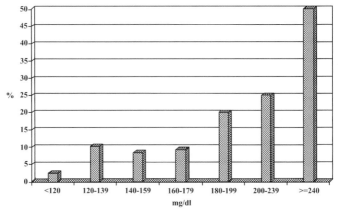

FIGURE 2.—Rate of severe hypoglycemia within the first 24 hours of life according to the 1-hour post-challenge glucose value of the maternal antenatal oGTT. There was a significant stepwise increase in the rate of hypoglycemia at 120, 180, and 240 mg/L. (Reprinted by permission of the publisher courtesy of Schaefer-Graf UM, Rossi R, Bührer C, et al: Rate and risk factors of hypoglycemia in large-for-gestational-age newborn infants of nondiabetic mothers. *Am J Obstet Gynecol* 187:913-917. Copyright 2002 by Elsevier.)

Study Design.—The study group consisted of 1210 LGA infants born to nondiabetic mothers at a single German institution from 1994 to 1998. Oral feeding was performed within 60 minutes for all LGA neonates; the first postnatal glucose test was performed 30 to 60 minutes after the first feeding and then every 4 to 6 hours for the first 24 hours. Maternal and neonatal information was retrospectively obtained from hospital charts and compared between neonates with and without hypoglycemia. Major outcome variables were hypoglycemia and the hour of life when it was diagnosed.

Findings.—Hypoglycemia occurred in 16% of LGA infants of nondiabetic mothers within the first 24 hours of life. The incidence of hypoglycemia decreased rapidly over time. Hypoglycemia was associated with a slightly lower gestational age. Increasing antenatal 1-hour oral glucose tolerance test (oGTT) values were the only predictive maternal factors (Fig 2) associated with hypoglycemia in LGA neonates.

Conclusions.—Routine glucose testing is indicated for all LGA neonates born to nondiabetic mothers. The maternal antenatal 1-hour glucose tolerance test appeared to be the only clinical factor that predicted risk of hypoglycemia among these neonates. Whether this risk also extends to non-LGA neonates remains to be investigated.

▶ The neonates of diabetic mothers, often having developed pancreatic islet cell hyperplasia from exposure to transplacental hyperglycemia in utero, are subject to reactive hyperinsulinism and hypoglycemia after initial neneonatal feedings. Some of the same clinical findings are found in LGA infants with or without maternal glucose tolerance testing, and the possibility of overt or subtle CNS injury from these undetected, possibly prolonged episodes of hypoglycemia is the motivation for this large retrospective cohort study of 887 pregnancies from a Berlin hospital for whom maternal and neonatal data were adequate for evaluation. The incidence of LGA newborns was 7.1%, using

German norms at or beyond the 90th percentile of weight and gestational age. Oral feedings were given within 1 hour of birth, and newborn blood glucose measurements were done 30 to 60 minutes later. The incidence of glucose concentration equal to or less than 30 mg/dL was 16%; for less than 15 mg/dL, it was 1%. In searching the prenatal labor and delivery neonatal records for indicators of neonatal hypoglycemia, the presence of an elevated glucose value in the maternal oral glucose tolerance test 1 hour after a 75-g glucose dose was, as Figure 2 shows, a reasonably good predictor of neonatal hypoglycemia. An obstetrician who wants to safeguard his LGA newborn from this hazard might, with a parturient who has a single elevated GTT value, check with the pediatric staff regarding the chance of possibly prolonged hyperglycemia during the early neonatal period.

T. H. Kirschbaum, MD

Influence of Twin-Twin Transfusion Syndrome on Fetal Cardiovascular Structure and Function: Prospective Case–Control Study of 136 Monochorionic Twin Pregnancies
Karatza AA, Wolfenden JL, Taylor MJO, et al (Imperial College, London; Royal Brompton and Harefield Hosp, London)
Heart 88:271-277, 2002   9–15

Background.—Twin-twin transfusion syndrome (TTTS) complications have been found in monochorionic diamniotic twin gestations. TTTS diagnosis is usually made by US in the second trimester. When left untreated, TTTS has an 80% perinatal mortality rate. However, there are management options available for improved overall perinatal survival. The results from small study series without controls may merely reflect the cardiovascular complications rather than the influence of TTTS. The influence of structural heart defects on TTTS in a larger series of subjects was assessed.

Methods.—One hundred thirty-six women with monochorionic diamniotic twin pregnancies had detailed fetal echocardiography of both fetuses performed at 24 weeks' gestation. Of these 136 women, 47 had TTTS. The fetal echocardiography was performed to detect structural abnormalities and to compare hemodynamic measurements between the twins. Color Doppler flow mapping was also used to assess whether arterio-arterial anastomoses were present.

Results.—TTTS complicated 47 of 136 pregnancies in the study. Forty-four (94%) had TTTS at the time of fetal echocardiography and 3 (6%) developed it later. Intervention was required for 34 (74%) of 46 pregnancies with TTTS at 20.4 weeks' gestation. There was a significant increase in the rate of congenital heart disease (11.9%) in the recipient twins compared with the donor twins (0.2%). However, in uncomplicated monochorionic diamniotic twin pregnancies, there were no hemodynamic differences.

Conclusion.—Monochorionic diamniotic twin pregnancy is associated with a 3.8% incidence of congenital heart disease. While uncomplicated monochorionic diamniotic twin pregnancy shows concordant hemodynamics, heart disease is usually seen in only 1 of a pair. TTTS increases the incidence of congenital heart disease in recipient twins.

▶ This is an account of 136 women with monochorionic diamniotic twin pregnancies, 47 of whom had TTTS and detailed fetal echocardiograms done at a median of 24 weeks' gestation. The diagnosis of TTTS was based on proof of monochorionicity with a diamniotic intervening septum, fetal weight discordance, and sharp differences in amniotic fluid indices. In comparison to those without TTTS, there were increased aortic and pulmonary vein velocities noted, together with biventricular hypertrophy and a few cases of functional right ventricular outflow obstruction.

Since the pathologic vascular anastomoses within the placenta in TTTS are dominantly unidirectional without adequate compensation in reverse flow direction, they constitute a decrease in umbilical vascular resistance, allowing rapid increase in the volume rate of blood flow through this organ, which normally consumes about 65% to 75% of fetal cardiac output. Increased venous return leads to increased functional ventricular output and cardiac hypertrophy.

But what's most interesting here is evidence of an increased risk of congenital heart disease overall (3.8%) in these fetuses, compared to the rate in normal singleton pregnancies of approximately 0.5% and a surplus of congenital heart disease among those with TTTS (6.9%) versus uncomplicated monochorionic twins (2.3%) which was not statistically significant. Recipient twins, however, had a significantly increased rate of congenital heart disease (11.9%) compared to donor twins (0.2%). The lesions noted in recipient twins included pulmonary vein stenosis, ventricular septal defects, and pulmonary atresia with an intact intraventricular septum. Surviving recipient twins in cases of TTTS deserve careful cardiac scrutiny as newborns and through infancy, looking for inapparent heart disease.

T. H. Kirschbaum, MD

10 Fetal Therapy

The EXIT Procedure: Experience and Outcome in 31 Cases
Bouchard S, Johnson MP, Flake AW, et al (Univ of Pennsylvania, Philadelphia)
J Pediatr Surg 37:418-426, 2002
10–1

Introduction.—The ex utero intrapartum treatment (EXIT) procedure, used initially for reversal of tracheal occlusion in fetuses with severe congenital diaphragmatic hernia (CDH), is also successful in the management of fetal neck masses. More recently, the EXIT procedure has been adapted to treat a variety of fetal conditions at delivery. A review was conducted of all cases of the EXIT procedure performed at Children's Hospital of Philadelphia since 1996.

Methods.—Data were collected of 31 women who underwent the EXIT procedure during the study period. The average maternal age was 29 years, and the mean gestational age at the time of surgery was 34.2 weeks. Each procedure used a multidisciplinary team consisting of 2 or 3 pediatric surgeons, an obstetrician, a neonatologist, an anesthesiologist, and 2 scrub nurses. The mother received general anesthesia, which also anesthetized the fetus. Fetal analgesia and paralysis were ensured with the administration of vecuronium, fentanyl, and atropine.

Results.—The most common indications for the EXIT procedure were airway obstruction from fetal neck mass (n = 13) and reversal or tracheal occlusion from in-utero clipping (n = 13). Singular indications were an EXIT-to-extracorporeal membrane oxygenation (ECMO) procedure for a fetus with CDH and a cardiac defect, congenital high airway obstruction syndrome, resection of a very large congenital cystic adenomatoid malformation of the lung on uteroplacental bypass, unilateral pulmonary agenesis, and thoraco-omphalopagus conjoined twins. The average time on placental bypass from uterine incision to umbilical cord clamping was 30.7 minutes. Hemodynamic instability in a fetus on uteroplacental gas exchange was recorded in only 1 of 31 cases. An airway was secured in 30 (97%) neonates, and 24 (77%) were successfully intubated endotracheally after direct laryngoscopy or rigid bronchoscopy. Four neonates required a formal surgical tracheostomy during the EXIT procedure. One neonate with a very large facial and neck lymphangioma died when the airway could not be secured. The average maternal blood loss was 848.3 mL. No maternal deaths occurred.

Conclusion.—The EXIT procedure can be used successfully in treating fetuses with a wide variety of pathologic disorders. Chances of survival are improved when there is a risk of cardiorespiratory instability when standard delivery techniques are used.

▶ Ex utero intrapartum therapy (EXIT) was first described in connection with the need to remove the occlusive tracheal clips used to treat the pulmonary hypoplasia associated with congenital diaphragmatic herniation.[1,2] The procedure was soon applied to fetuses with large occlusive neck masses[3] in an attempt to initiate tracheal intubation and respiratory stabilization prior to planned delivery. This report from the University of Pennsylvania Children's Hospital reports 31 such procedures for those indications and discusses the application of the technique to similar problems planned by this group of pediatric surgeons, obstetricians, neonatologist, and anesthesiologists. In addition to 13 cases of congenital diaphragmatic hernia, there were 13 cervical lymphangiomata, teratomas, and 1 gastrointestinal reduplication cyst. Other cases involved congenital heart disease and tetralogy of Fallot, congenital cystic adenomatous malformation, unilateral pulmonary agenesis, and thoracopagus twins. Procedures for CDH were done at a mean gestational age of 31.8 weeks, and for occlusive neck masses at an average of 36 weeks gestational age. The authors describe what they learned that enables the procedure to be done with safety and, in only 1 instance, tell of failure to achieve intubation in an infant whose parents declined to approve tracheostomy.

Tocolytic agents were used to prevent umbilical circuit compromise before intubation. Deep maternal anesthesia and fetal vecuronium, fentanyl, and atropine are useful to prevent fetal motion. Large cystic masses and ascites sometimes require aspiration, and intubation may require retrograde passage of a feeding tube via distal tracheostomy and pull-through of the endotracheal tube. In only 1 case did uterine atony require uterine stimulants, but blood transfusion was not needed. This appears to be a safe approach to avoiding fetal injury and death from a difficult intubation that begins only after occlusion of the umbilical circuit at delivery.

T. H. Kirschbaum, MD

References

1. Crombleholme TM, Albanese CT: *The Fetus With Airway Obstruction. The Unborn Patient,* ed 3. Philadelphia, PA, Saunders, 2001, pp 357-371.
2. 2000 YEAR BOOK OF OBSTETRICS, GYNECOLOGY, AND WOMEN'S HEALTH, pp 175-176.
3. 2003 YEAR BOOK OF OBSTETRICS, GYNECOLOGY, AND WOMEN'S HEALTH, pp 159-161.

Invasive Intrauterine Treatment of Pulmonary Atresia/Intact Ventricular Septum With Heart Failure

Arzt W, Tulzer G, Aigner M, et al (Maternity Hosp Linz, Austria; Children's Hosp of Linz, Austria; Donauspital, Vienna)
Ultrasound Obstet Gynecol 21:186-188, 2003   10–2

Background.—Pulmonary atresia with intact ventricular septum (PA/IVS) can result in underdevelopment of the tricuspid valve and right ventricle and sometimes abnormal coronary circulation. In utero death may result, and overall mortality in liveborn children is more than 50%. The mortality and morbidity in PA/IVS are linked to the degree of hypoplasia in the tricuspid valve and right ventricle and to the presence of large ventriculocoronary communications. It has been speculated that early in utero valvulotomy may lead to better growth of the right ventricle, making it more conducive to biventricular repair. This case study provided technical details and a description of the hemodynamic changes in a previously reported successful in utero pulmonary valvulotomy in a fetus with PA/IVS.

> *Case Report.*—Woman, 25, was referred for assessment and further management of a fetus with PA, which was detected on a 25-week routine US examination. Prenatal workup and amniocentesis revealed no additional remarkable findings. Fetal echocardiography at 26 weeks showed severe right ventricular hypoplasia, abnormal right ventricle filling, and holocystic tricuspid regurgitation leading to the diagnosis of PA/IVS with suprasystemic right ventricular pressures. No coronary fistulas were noted, but there were signs of impending congestive heart failure.
>
> General anesthesia was administered to avoid maternal movements and to provide fetal anesthesia. Under US guidance, a 16-gauge needle with a stylet and without sharpening at the end was advanced through the fetal chest wall in the right ventricle (Fig 2). After

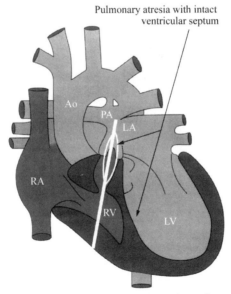

Pulmonary atresia with intact
ventricular septum

FIGURE 2.—Needle and balloon catheter in the right ventricular outflow tract. *Abbreviations: Ao,* Aorta; *LA,* left atrium; *LV,* left ventricle; *PA,* pulmonary artery; *RA,* right atrium; *RV,* right ventricle. (Courtesy of Arzt W, Tulzer G, Aigner M, et al: Invasive intrauterine treatment of pulmonary atresia/intact ventricular septum with heart failure. *Ultrasound Obstet Gynecol* 21:186-188, 2003. Reprinted by permission of Wiley-Liss, Inc., a subsidiary of John Wiley & Sons, Inc.)

the procedure, there was significant growth of the tricuspid valve and right ventricle. The neonate was delivered at 38 weeks with a right ventricle amenable to biventricular repair.

Conclusion.—This report provides technical details for in utero pulmonary valvulotomy in a fetus with PA/IVS. These findings demonstrate that this procedure is feasible and may favorably alter the natural history of this condition in affected fetuses.

▶ This case report of successful balloon valvuloplasty in a 26-week fetus with a dire congenital cardiac anomaly demonstrates feasibility and strongly suggests benefit. US examination at 25 weeks demonstrated a fetus with right ventricular hypoplasia and absent pulmonary artery blood flow, with the products of right ventricular systole passing in retrograde fashion through the tricuspid valve, unable to exit into the left heart through an intact interventricular septum. Cardiomegaly, marked umbilical vein pulsations, and reverse end–diastolic ductus arteriosus and ductus venosus blood flow denoting a high pulmonary artery and inferior vena cava pressure made congestive heart failure, nonimmune hydrops and fetal death apparently imminent.

Under US guidance, a 16-gauge needle was passed through the fetal chest into the ventral surface of the right atrium. A 4-mm–diameter balloon catheter was inserted into the atretic pulmonary valve and inflated 4 times. Immediately after the procedure, Doppler blood flow was noted in the pulmonary artery, tricuspid regurgitation disappeared, and a Doppler E-wave indicating normal right ventricular filling appeared. Later examination showed growth in the tricuspid valve diameter, absent umbilical vein pulsations, and progressive right ventricular growth but subsequent failure of pulmonary valve diameter and maximum blood velocity to increase normally.

Delivery was accomplished at 38 weeks and a 2.64-kg infant with normal Apgar scores was subsequently treated with balloon valvuloplasty. Ultimately, a Blalock-Taussig type shunt was performed. Though uncontrolled of course, this case report suggests this infant grew normally to term through the means of fetal endocardiac surgery, now a known feasibility.

T. H. Kirschbaum, MD

GYNECOLOGY

11 Urogynecology

Introduction

The field of female pelvic medicine and reconstructive surgery has matured in the last several years with the development of several 3-year fellowship programs and the training of subspecialists in this discipline. The current chapter includes several articles on the epidemiology and diagnosis of incontinence; considers irritative and infectious conditions, particularly relating to an increased knowledge of interstitial cystitis in women; considers some of the problems involved in detrusor instability; and addresses several aspects of the surgical treatment of incontinence, particularly the newer sling procedures.

Urinary incontinence has a high prevalence rate, particularly in older women, and older women are increasing in numbers in our population; therefore, it is important that practitioners identify and treat patients with incontinence in order to improve their quality of life. As women are often embarrassed to discuss a subject as sensitive as incontinence, physicians must take the initiative in asking about this condition and then offer appropriate diagnostic and treatment modalities. Diagnosis and treatment of urinary incontinence are major responsibilities of the specialty of obstetrics and gynecology.

Morton A. Stenchever, MD

Diagnosis/Epidemiology

Prevalence and Risk Factors of Urinary Incontinence in Young and Middle-Aged Women

Peyrat L, Haillot O, Bruyere F, et al (CHU Tenon, France; CHU Tours, France)

BJU Internatl 89:61-66, 2002   11–1

Introduction.—Epidemiologic studies have found high rates of urinary incontinence (UI) among women over 60 years of age, with reported prevalences of 4.5% to 44.0%. However, less is known about the rates of and risk factors for UI in younger women. Female hospital employees were surveyed regarding the presence of UI and associated factors.

Methods.—A questionnaire regarding UI was administered to 2800 women, aged 20 to 62 years, working at a French teaching hospital. The women received the questionnaire at their yearly occupational medicine interview. No clinical examination or urodynamic evaluation was performed. Stress UI was defined as involuntary urine loss associated with coughing, laughing, sneezing, or exercise; urge UI was defined as involuntary urine loss with urgency or sudden, uncontrollable voiding; and mixed UI was defined as a combination of these.

Results.—Responses were received from 1700 women, or 61% of the sample. The reported rate of UI was 27.5%, including stress UI in 12.4% of respondents, urge UI in 1.6%, and mixed UI in 13.5%. The UI rate was 38.5% for women over 40, compared to 18.2% for those aged 25 to 39 and 6.2% for those under 25. Leakage was rated frequent by 8.1% of women, including 0.5% with stress UI, 14.3% with urge UI, and 14.4% with mixed UI. Significant risk factors for UI included age 40 years or older, relative risk (RR), 2.16; pregnancy, RR 2.22; history of vaginal delivery, RR 2.15; postpartum incontinence, RR 2.57; and hysterectomy, RR 1.52. Obesity and cesarean delivery were not significant risk factors. The risk factors for stress UI were the same as for all UI.

Conclusion.—The survey results suggest a high rate of UI among young to middle-aged women working in a health care setting. Although stress UI is very common, it is an occasional problem in most cases; frequent stress UI was reported by just 8% of women in this study. In addition to age and hysterectomy, risk factors for UI in younger women include pregnancy, vaginal delivery, and postpartum incontinence.

▶ In this French study of 1700 female hospital workers, aged 20-62, who performed work that involved heavy lifting (37.5%) and light work (62.5%), an overall UI prevalence of 27.5% was noted. The authors found by questionnaire that 45% of the women who were incontinent apparently had stress UI; 6%, urge incontinence; and 49%, mixed stress and urge incontinence. These symptoms were self-reported by the patients and no clinical studies were performed. The prevalence of incontinence rose with age and increased with obesity, although the differences were not statistically significant. A history of previous pregnancies was a significant risk factor for incontinence, but no statistically significant differences were noted in incontinence or stress UI between the group with cesarean delivery and the group without children. A history of hysterectomy was also a significant risk factor in this study.

The current study comprised primarily young and middle-aged women. Although occasional leakage of urine was considered incontinence and therefore yielded a fairly high prevalence rate, frequent UI, mostly mixed, was observed in only 8.1% of women. The subjects in most studies of incontinence have been older postmenopausal women and a higher rate of incontinence has been observed. Whereas this study demonstrated that the problem should be considered in all women and certainly those with the risk factors that the authors have outlined, the major problem does appear to be among aging women.

M. A. Stenchever, MD

Effect of Adding Biofeedback to Pelvic Floor Muscle Training to Treat Urodynamic Stress Incontinence

Mørkved S, Bø K, Fjørtoft T (Norwegian Univ of Science and Technology, Trondheim, Norway; Norwegian Univ of Sport and Physical Education, Oslo, Norway; Univ Hosp, Trondheim, Norway)
Obstet Gynecol 100:730-739, 2002   11–2

Background.—Since the introduction of pelvic floor muscle training for female urinary incontinence by Kegel more than 50 years ago, several randomized, controlled studies have shown that the pelvic floor muscle training without biofeedback is more effective than no treatment for female stress and urinary incontinence. Biofeedback has been used in the area of pelvic floor muscle training by means of vaginal and anal surface electromyograms and urethral and vaginal squeeze pressure measurements with the goal of making the patient more aware of muscle function and of enhancing the patient's efforts and motivation during training. Several studies have examined the effects of pelvic floor muscle training with adjunctive biofeedback, and all but 1 failed to find an additional benefit. The effects of individual pelvic floor muscle training with and without biofeedback in women with urodynamic stress incontinence were compared.

Methods.—This single-blind randomized trial enrolled 103 women who were randomly assigned to 6 months of pelvic floor muscle contractions 3 times per day with or without the use of a biofeedback apparatus at home. The pelvic floor muscle contractions were performed under the supervision of a physical therapist. The primary outcome measures were pad test with standardized bladder volume and self-report of severity.

Results.—Data were analyzed from 94 of 103 women. The women ranged in age from 30 to 70 years, with a mean age of 46.6 years. The mean duration of symptoms was 9.7 years, with a range of 1 to 25 years. The majority of women (70) had urodynamic stress incontinence alone, and 24 women reported additional urge symptoms. Women in both groups showed a statistically significant reduction in leakage on the pad test after 6 months of pelvic floor training. Objective cure, which was defined as 2 g or less of leakage, was achieved in 58% of women training with biofeedback and in 46% of women training without biofeedback. In the subgroup of women with urinary stress incontinence alone, the objective cure rate was 69% in women training with biofeedback and 50% in women training without biofeedback. There were no statistically significant differences between the groups in any outcome measure after treatment.

Conclusions.—This study found high cure rates in women with urodynamic stress incontinence who trained with pelvic floor muscle exercises both with and without biofeedback. However, there was no statistically significant difference between the group of women who trained with adjunctive biofeedback and those who did not have adjunctive biofeedback as part of their training.

▶ This study demonstrated once again that pelvic floor muscle training was effective for a number of women with stress urinary incontinence and mixed incontinence. In this study, however, the authors demonstrated that biofeedback techniques did not enhance the improvement. Thus, it appears that muscle training procedures, if performed diligently by patients, can have a positive effect on reducing incontinence. Experience with this and many other studies indicates that physicians should seriously consider teaching these techniques to incontinent patients and encourage patients to continue using them. Because many patients and physicians alike consider stress urinary continence a condition that requires surgical intervention, muscle training programs have not been strongly advocated or used. Perhaps it is time to take another look at this approach, as it may reduce the need for surgical intervention in a number of women.

M. A. Stenchever, MD

Urinary Incontinence and Hysterectomy in a Large Prospective Cohort Study in American Women

Kjerulff KH, Langenberg PW, Greenaway L, et al (Univ of Maryland, Baltimore)
J Urol 167:2088-2092, 2002   11–3

Background.—The effects of a hysterectomy on urinary incontinence are unclear. Several factors that may influence the effect of a hysterectomy on urinary incontinence, such as preoperative incontinence severity and concomitant incontinence repair, have not been studied thoroughly. The effects of a hysterectomy with and without concomitant urinary incontinence repair on incontinence severity were studied in a large, prospective series.

Methods.—The Urinary Symptoms Scale for Women was administered to 1299 women before hysterectomies were performed for benign conditions. This instrument was then readministered at 6, 12, 18, and 24 months after surgery.

Findings.—Before hysterectomy, 29.5% of the women had severe urinary incontinence. This percentage declined to 10% at 12 and 24 months after hysterectomy. At 1 year after surgery, 89.1% of women with severe incontinence before hysterectomy had an improvement in incontinence. At 2 years, 86.5% were still improved. In addition, 62.4% of women with moderate incontinence before hysterectomy had improved symptoms 1 year postoperatively, and 61.2% still had improved symptoms at 2 years. However, 16.7% of women with mild or no incontinence before hysterectomy had new onset or worsened incontinence 1 year after surgery, and 14.4% had symptoms that remained worse at 2 years. Concomitant urinary incontinence repair significantly increased the probability of improvement in severe incontinence 1 year after hysterectomy and significantly reduced the probability of worsening of mild or no incontinence after 2 years.

Conclusions.—Most women undergoing hysterectomies for benign conditions will have an improvement in urinary incontinence in the first 2 years after the procedure. However, there is also a risk of about 10% of new onset or worsening urinary incontinence in the first 2 years after surgery.

▶ Although some studies have suggested that a hysterectomy increases a woman's chance of urinary incontinence, the current study, which was carried out in women undergoing hysterectomies for benign conditions, demonstrated that this is not always the case. In this series, 29.5% of the participants had severe urinary incontinence before the procedure, and a significant decrease to 10% was found 1 to 2 years after surgery. This decrease was also evident for women with moderate incontinence, but in women with mild incontinence or without incontinence before the hysterectomy, the onset of incontinence occurred and worsened in the 2 years after surgery. It is probable that the authors were measuring different factors. In women with moderate or severe incontinence before surgery who noted an improvement, conditions related to uterine pathologic features, such as large myomas, were probably responsible for the incontinence. In women with mild incontinence or without incontinence at the time of surgery, other factors, such as aging, lack of hormonal stimulation, or possibly surgical trauma, may have been responsible. Reasons for urinary incontinence are many, and must be sorted out for each woman. The findings of this study will help to reassure women who undergo a hysterectomy for benign conditions that incontinence, if it exists, may improve and that the risk of incontinence associated with surgery is relatively small and may be related to factors other than the surgical procedure.

M. A. Stenchever, MD

Prevalence of Urinary and Fecal Incontinence and Symptoms of Genital Prolapse in Women
Eva UF, Gun W, Preben K (Univ Hosp, Linköping, Sweden)
Acta Obstet Gynecol Scand 82:280-286, 2003   11–4

Background.—The prevalence and frequency of urinary and fecal incontinence and the prevalence of genital prolapse symptoms have not been established. These data were obtained in a Swedish population of 40- and 60-year-old women.

Methods.—One thousand 40-year-old women and one thousand 60-year-old women were selected randomly and given a questionnaire to elicit data on medical background, urinary and fecal incontinence, and genital prolapse symptoms. The response rate was 67%.

Findings.—Fifty-three percent of the women were continent for urine. Nine percent of the 40-year-old women and 19% of the 60-year-old women reported urinary incontinence weekly or more frequently. The older women had a significantly greater detrusor instability score than did the younger women. Nine percent of the 40-year-olds and 19% of the 60-year-olds reported incontinence of flatus weekly or more often. Five percent and 8% of the 40-year-olds and 60-year-olds, respectively, reported loose feces, and 0.3% and 1.7% reported solid feces. Fifteen percent of the women reported pelvic heaviness, 4% reported a genital bulge, and 12% reported use of fingers in the vagina or perineum by defecation.

Conclusions.—Urinary incontinence is a common problem among 40-year-old and 60-year-old women. The current authors found the International Continence Society's definition of urinary incontinence to be impractical for epidemiologic research and suggested leakage weekly or more often as a criterion for significant incontinence in such research.

▶ Although the information from this study pertains to a Swedish population, it probably applies to other white populations. The information is useful because it points out, once again, the relatively high prevalence of both urinary and fecal incontinence in older as well as in premenopausal women. This prevalence should remind us, as physicians, to inquire about symptoms of incontinence as part of the ongoing care of our patients. The study also demonstrated a moderately high incidence of pelvic prolapse symptoms, some of which were serious enough to require therapy. Clearly, these facts offer gynecologists an important challenge and responsibility. The population of the United States is aging, and the number of women with urinary and rectal incontinence, as well as pelvic prolapse problems, will increase. Because many women are embarrassed to discuss these issues until symptoms are severe, the physician should actively seek this information during routine health maintenance visits. Doing so should help to improve the quality of life in our older female population.

M. A. Stenchever, MD

Prevalence of Urinary Incontinence and Associated Risk Factors in a Cohort of Nuns

Buchsbaum GM, Chin M, Glantz C, et al (Univ of Rochester, NY)
Obstet Gynecol 100:226-229, 2002   11–5

Background.—The prevalence of urinary incontinence ranges from 35% to 45%. Vaginal birth with resultant injury to structures in the pelvic floor is thought to be a major risk factor for urinary incontinence. The prevalence of urinary incontinence and associated risk factors were investigated in a group of nulliparous nuns.

Methods.—One hundred forty-nine nuns, aged a mean 68 years, were included in the study. Data on symptoms of urinary incontinence, medical history, and demographics were obtained.

Findings.—Ninety-six percent of the participants were postmenopausal, and 25% were taking hormone replacement therapy. The mean body mass index (BMI) was 27.3. Based on self-reports, half the nuns had urinary incontinence. Thirty percent of these participants had stress incontinence, 24% had urge incontinence, 35% had mixed incontinence, and 11% had urine loss unrelated to stress and urge. More than half the participants with incontinence used sanitary pads. In a univariate analysis, significant risk factors for urinary incontinence were BMI, current hormone replacement therapy use, multiple urinary tract infections, hypertension, arthritis, depression, hysterectomy, and previous spinal surgery. In a multivariate logistic regression, the only significant variables were BMI, multiple urinary tract infections, and depression.

Conclusions.—The prevalence of incontinence in this group of nulliparous, mostly postmenopausal nuns was comparable to that in parous postmenopausal women. Urine loss correlates with symptoms of stress incontinence more often than with symptoms of urge incontinence, even in the absence of pelvic floor trauma from childbirth.

▶ The authors demonstrated that among older women the rates of incontinence in nulliparous, predominately postmenopausal nuns were similar to rates reported in parous, postmenopausal women. The average age of the women in this study was 68 years, and all but 1 were postmenopausal. Although pelvic floor trauma associated with childbirth has been addressed broadly in the literature as a cause of urinary incontinence, this group of women had never been pregnant or experienced childbirth, but half had urinary incontinence. Furthermore, 30% of the incontinent women had stress urinary incontinence, and 35% had mixed incontinence. Although these conditions are usually associated with pelvic floor damage, it is clear that they can also be related simply to the aging process.

Once again, as has been demonstrated by others, increasing BMI was strongly correlated with urinary incontinence. Urinary incontinence clearly has many causes, and age and obesity are 2 of the major ones. Half of the nuns who were incontinent used sanitary pads to maintain hygiene. It seems reasonable to assume that the prevalence of urinary incontinence is high, especially in older and more obese women, and these women should be carefully evaluated so appropriate therapy can be offered.

M. A. Stenchever, MD

Do Fertile Women Remember the Onset of Stress Incontinence?: Recall Bias 5 Years After 1st Delivery

Viktrup L, Lose G (Univ of Copenhagen)
Acta Obstet Gynecol Scand 80:952-955, 2001   11–6

Background.—Many studies have looked at the relationship between the onset of stress incontinence and pregnancy and delivery. However, few prospective studies have examined the onset of stress incontinence after delivery, raising the possibility that patient recall may be unreliable. This issue was addressed by 5-year follow-up of women participating in a prospective cohort study at the time of labor and delivery.

Methods.—The initial prospective cohort study included 305 consecutive women giving birth for the first time in 1989. The women were asked about the development of lower urinary tract symptoms and stress incontinence a few days after delivery and again 3 months later. At 5 years' follow-up, the questionnaire used in these interviews was mailed to the same group of women, of whom 278 responded. Responses were compared to assess the women's ability to remember the onset of stress incontinence.

Results.—At 5 years' follow-up, 68 women reported stress incontinence. Of these, just 26% correctly recalled the onset of stress incontinence accurately, in agreement with their answer of 5 years previously. Another 49% recalled the onset of this problem inaccurately. For the remaining 25%, recall could be interpreted as correct if the reference group was extended. Most women recalled the onset of stress incontinence as occurring after their first delivery; only 6 made no mention of pregnancy or delivery when recalling the onset of incontinence. Another 15 women misunderstood or did not respond to the question regarding onset of stress incontinence.

Conclusion.—Five years after delivery, women's recall of the onset of stress incontinence appears imprecise. Agreement among groups of women was poor. In clinical and research settings, women's reports of the onset of incontinence should be interpreted with caution.

▶ The authors have followed 305 women who were primipara in 1989—and at the time were between the ages of 17 and 41—in order to determine the onset of stress urinary incontinence. The authors originally interviewed the women just after their first delivery and 3 months later. In the current study, the authors followed the 83 women who became incontinent to determine when their incontinence began. As the reference was their first pregnancy, they were asked if incontinence occurred with their first pregnancy, during their pregnancy, during the period after their first pregnancy, or thereafter.

Five years after the first delivery, only 26% recalled the onset of stress incontinence correctly. The study may have been affected by several factors. Among them: incontinence inception was related to the first pregnancy by the questionnaire; many women may recall stress incontinence in relation to the latest episode they have experienced, assuming that there was a period when they were continent; and the interviewing technique used by the authors.

Nevertheless, it is interesting that with time confusion over the onset of incontinence may occur. Thus, the authors demonstrated that history-taking is not always an accurate science. As patients should be treated based on the problems with which they present, this factor may not be terribly important. However, confusion may be increased when other treatments and surgical procedures have been introduced along the way, making the interpretation of the patient's specific problem difficult at times.

M. A. Stenchever, MD

A Comparative Cross-Sectional Study of Lower Urinary Tract Symptoms in Both Sexes
Schatzl G, Temml C, Waldmüller J, et al (Univ of Vienna; City of Vienna)
Eur Urol 40:213-219, 2001   11–7

Purpose.—Older adults of both sexes are at risk for micturition disorders. Lower urinary tract symptoms (LUTS) may be classified as storage, or irritative, symptoms and voiding, or obstructive, symptoms. The effects of age on the risk of micturition symptoms among women and men were assessed, including evaluation of the daily-life impact of such symptoms.

Methods.—The analysis included 1191 women and 1211 men participating in voluntary, government-sponsored health examinations in Vienna. The presence and types of LUTS were evaluated by means of a German-language version of the Bristol female LUTS questionnaire. This 34-item instrument asks about a wide range of urinary symptoms and their perceived impact on quality of life.

Results.—The mean age of the female respondents was 49.8 years. The age ranges were 20 to 39 years in 19.8% of women, 40 to 49 years in 36.9%, 50 to 59 years in 23.9%, 60 to 69 years in 10.7%, and over 70 years in 8.7%. From the youngest to the oldest age group, LUTS increased by a mean of 43.7% for women, or 7.3% per decade. For men the increase was 23.6% or 3.9% per decade. In all age strata, storage symptoms—including frequency, urgency, and nocturia—were more frequent in women than in men. However, the discrepancy lessened after the age of 60 years.

The percentage of women reporting no "urgency" decreased from 39.2% in the youngest age group to 26.3% in the oldest, with a similar pattern in men. The percentage of women reporting no "frequency" was relatively stable, between about 30% and 35%, while for men frequency scores increased slightly after age 60. The percentage of women reporting no nocturia decreased from 66.9% in the youngest age group to 17.1% in the oldest, with an even wider spread for men. Symptoms of urgency and frequency were more bothersome to older than to younger respondents. However, nocturia and voiding symptoms were similarly bothersome for younger and older subjects.

Conclusion.—This cross-sectional study finds an age-related increase in LUTS among women as well as men. Storage symptoms are more of a problem for younger women than for younger men, whereas voiding symptoms are more of a problem for older men. Urinary symptoms are more bothersome for older than for younger patients, and this is especially so for the storage symptoms of urgency and frequency.

▶ This cross-sectional Austrian study of men and women was performed to determine the incidence of irritative and obstructive LUTS. As our interest is in gynecology, I will discuss the findings of the study in women. The authors studied 1191 women who were between 20 and 91 years of age, with an average age of 49.8 years. The subjects fell into the following groups by age: 20

to 39 years, 19.8%; 40 to 49 years, 36.9%; 50 to 59 years, 23.9%; 60 to 69 years, 10.7%; and over 70 years, 8.7%.

Symptoms of frequency, urgency, and nocturia were high among women, ranging from 61.8% in age group 20 to 39 to 73.7% in age group over 70 years for urgency; 67.2% in age group 20 to 39 to 69.6% in age group 60 to 69 for frequency; and 43.1% in age group 20 to 29 to 82.9% in age group over 70 for nocturia. Thus, the authors demonstrated that LUTS are prevalent and often bothersome for women in all age groups, with a greater incidence of more severe symptoms in the older age groups. They also noted that with respect to obstructive problems, women were fairly constant throughout all age groups, compared with men whose symptoms of obstruction increased with age. Even though incontinence may not be present in many individuals, LUTS are clearly commonplace and should be considered when discussing quality-of-life issues with patients.

M. A. Stenchever, MD

Perineal Ultrasound Evaluation of Urethral Angle and Bladder Neck Mobility in Women With Stress Urinary Incontinence
Pregazzi R, Sartore A, Bortoli P, et al (Univ of Trieste, Italy; IRCCS 'Burlo Garofolo,' Trieste, Italy)
Br J Obstet Gynaecol 109:821-827, 2002   11–8

Purpose.—Preoperative evaluation of urethrovesical mobility is recommended for women with stress urinary incontinence. One option is perineal US, which also permits visual assessment and measurement of the angle formed by the proximal, mobile part and the distal, fixed part of the urethra. The urethral angle may be a key indicator of functional integrity of the proximal and distal urethral supports. A perineal US technique for preoperative evaluation of the urethral angle and bladder neck mobility was assessed.

Methods.—The case-control study included 73 women (mean age, 49 years) undergoing urodynamic evaluation for lower urinary tract symptoms. Women over 70 years were excluded, as were those with a history of surgery for prolapse or urinary incontinence and those with anterior vaginal wall relaxation. Based on the urodynamic results, 23 of the women were classified as having genuine urinary stress incontinence; the remaining 50 had other urologic disorders but confirmed urethral sphincter competence.

Each woman underwent perineal US examination, including measurement of the distance from the bladder neck to the symphysis pubis, the "alpha angle" formed by the bladder neck/symphysis pubis line and the midline of the symphysis, and the "beta angle" formed by the proximal and distal urethra. The examination was performed with a full bladder at rest, during a Valsalva maneuver, and during maximal pelvic floor contraction. The relationship between the urethral angle and continence was assessed.

Findings.—The US examination technique showed good repeatability between 2 investigators, and the results were unaffected by bladder volume. In both incontinent patients and continent controls, the beta angle and ure-throvesical mobility were inversely related. The urethral angle was a strong predictor of the presence of genuine stress incontinence, with sensitivity of 96% and specificity of 92%. Urethrovesical mobility was less accurate, with sensitivity of 87% and specificity of 68%. Positive predictive values of the 2 techniques were 85% and 55%, respectively. All of the US measurements differed significantly between patients and controls.

Discussion.—This perineal US study suggests that the urethral angle plays an important role in female continence. In incontinent women, the urethral angle is reduced at rest and even lower during straining. Preoperative measurement of this angle, in addition to assessment of bladder neck mobility, improves the ability to differentiate between genuine stress incontinence and other urologic disorders.

▶ The authors studied 73 consecutive women aged 43 to 65 who were referred to their urodynamic clinic with complaints of lower urinary tract symptoms. All women underwent a full urodynamic evaluation. From this evaluation, the authors extracted 23 women with genuine stress incontinence and compared them with 50 women with other types of urologic problems, all of whom had urethral sphincter competence. Using perineal US, they investigated bladder neck mobility and the angle between the proximal and distal urethra, labeled beta angle. They demonstrated that whereas bladder neck mobility had reasonable sensitivity to identify genuine stress incontinence (87%), it had lesser specificity (68%) and poorer positive predictive value (55%).

The beta angle had excellent sensitivity (96%), specificity (92%), and positive predictive value (85%). The authors postulated that whereas bladder neck mobility was dependent on the anatomical and functional integrity of the supports of the proximal urethra, urethral angulation appeared to be dependent upon the anatomical and functional status of both the proximal and distal supports.

Years ago, it was believed that bladder neck mobility correlated with the diagnosis of stress incontinence, and several tests, including the Q-tip test and the chain urethrogram, were utilized. However, these tests proved to have poor sensitivity and specificity and were relegated to the status of useful observations that it was necessary to incorporate into the clinical picture in order to make a diagnosis. Therefore, most experts utilize urodynamic studies as more accurate tools.

Whereas the authors demonstrated that loss of supports of the distal urethra probably is involved in the development of stress urinary incontinence, the mere diagnosis of stress incontinence is not sufficient to identify mixed incontinence in women. Thus, whereas the use of the US-measured beta angle offers useful information in the workup of an incontinent patient, it does not replace the gold standard, namely, the multichannel urodynamic evaluation.

M. A. Stenchever, MD

Irritative and Infectious Conditions

Infections of the Urinary Tract in Women: A Prospective, Longitudinal Study of 235 Women Observed for 1-19 Years

Vosti KL (Stanford Univ, Calif)
Medicine 81:369-387, 2002   11–9

Introduction.—Despite the high frequency of urinary tract infections among women, there have been few long-term, prospective studies of this problem in otherwise healthy women. The long-term outcomes of urinary tract infections in a large group of young to middle-aged women were reported, including serologic studies for *Escherichia coli.*

Methods.—The study included 235 women with active or recent infections of the urinary tract. The women ranged in age from 16.5 to 64.2 years, with a mean age of 29.6 years. Follow-up included at least 2 yearly visits while the patients were asymptomatic. Total duration of follow-up ranged from 1.1 to 19.4 years, with a range of 7.4 years.

Findings.—During the study, 79.6% of women underwent IV pyelography, which showed structural abnormalities in 15.0% of cases. Infection was confirmed in 210 women, 19 of whom received antimicrobial prophylaxis (group 1) and 191 of whom did not receive prophylaxis (group 2). The remaining 25 women did not have confirmed infection (group 3). The mean infection rate was 3.1/y for women in group 1, compared of 0.8/y in group 2 and 0/y in group 3. The actual number of infections varied widely, from 0 to 42, with no predictable pattern of recurrence.

Clusters of infections, defined as 2 or more infections within 8 weeks, occurred in 45.7% of women. Some clusters consisted of as many as 12 infections. The infecting organisms and clinical syndromes were consistent with those in previous reports, with *E coli* accounting for about 70% of infections. Serogroups were identified for about 85% of *E coli* isolates; 3 O groups accounted for about half of the classifiable isolates. The same O groups were involved in the 4 clinical syndromes identified.

Conclusion.—The findings lend new insights into the characteristics of urinary tract infections among young to middle-aged women. Women vary significantly in terms of the frequency and timing of infections and other findings; there is no way to predict the future course of any individual patient. Antimicrobial prophylaxis may be beneficial for women with persistent recurrences or clusters of infections, although it is difficult to determine which patients should receive prophylaxis and for how long. Recurrent infections and clusters are thought to result from complex host-parasite interactions; sexual activity may be an important contributor.

▶ The authors followed a reasonably large group of young and middle-aged women (235) for 1 to 19 years who were ascertained to have urinary tract infection at entry into the study in order to analyze the experience of recurrence over a long period of time. They were unable to determine a means to identify which women would recur, how often they would recur, or whether they would recur in clusters of infections. However, they did observe that 69.3% of the infections were due to *E coli*, and an additional 2.4% that were mixed infections included *E coli*. They were able to identify serogroups of *E coli* in most of these isolates and demonstrated that no pattern existed with respect to recurrent infections with the same or different serotypes.

This finding is not particularly surprising as if the women were treated adequately for one infection, it is reasonable to assume that reinfection would be by an entirely different *E coli* serotype. The authors did point out the value of prophylaxis in some women, particularly single-dose antibiotic after intercourse, but were unable to identify which women would benefit from this particular therapy. They demonstrated that intercourse was a risk factor in younger women but that other risk factors probably occurred in older women as the pelvic anatomy changed.

In general, the information provided by the authors is interesting but difficult to apply clinically. It is common practice in women with recurrent infection to perform an IV pyelogram in search of an abnormality of the urinary tract. This test was performed in all patients in this series, and 15% were found to have abnormalities. This finding is in agreement with other studies that have been published. The take-home message from this study is that physicians have probably been managing women with urinary tract infection and recurrent infection in a reasonable fashion, and major changes in management strategies are not indicated.

M. A. Stenchever, MD

Diagnosing Interstitial Cystitis in Women With Chronic Pelvic Pain
Clemons JL, Arya LA, Myers DL (Brown Univ, Providence, RI; Univ of Pennsylvania, Philadelphia)
Obstet Gynecol 100:337-341, 2002   11–10

Background.—Chronic pelvic pain, which is pain persisting for more than 6 months, is a common disorder. The prevalence and risk factors for interstitial cystitis in women with chronic pelvic pain were determined.

Methods.—Forty-five women undergoing laparoscopy for chronic pelvic pain were included in the study. The Interstitial Cystitis Symptom Index and Problem Index were administered. At the time of laparoscopy, cystoscopy with hydrodistension and bladder biopsy were performed.

Findings.—Interstitial cystitis was diagnosed in 38% of the women. A symptom index score of 5 or more had a 94% sensitivity and a 93% negative predictive value for diagnosing interstitial cystitis. In a multivariate analysis, risk factors for interstitial cystitis were an increased symptom index score of 5 or more and an increased dyspareunia score of 7 or more.

Conclusions.—The prevalence of interstitial cystitis in this group of women with chronic pelvic pain was 38%. The Interstitial Cystitis Symptom

Index was useful as a screening tool for interstitial cystitis. Screening for interstitial cystitis is indicated in women with chronic pelvic pain.

▶ This study assessed the prevalence of interstitial cystitis among patients undergoing laparoscopy for chronic pelvic pain and demonstrated a correlation between the interstitial cystitis symptom index used by the authors, the incidence of dyspareunia, and the finding of interstitial cystitis. In their series of 45 patients, 17 (38%) had interstitial cystitis demonstrated by cystoscopic findings. All patients who received the diagnosis of interstitial cystitis had, in addition to the cystoscopic findings, the presence of urinary symptoms. Two patients in the series had positive cystoscopic findings but no urinary symptoms and were, therefore, not given a diagnosis of interstitial cystitis.

Laparoscopic correlation with gynecologic conditions was not found consistently; however, 7 patients found to have endometriosis on laparoscopy also had interstitial cystitis. I have had similar experiences when working up patients with endometriosis. The existence of a direct relationship between endometriosis and interstitial cystitis or the possibility that these are independent findings remains to be determined. However, the authors of this article are gynecologists and were investigating the possibility of the presence of interstitial cystitis in their patients with chronic pelvic pain. Therefore, they included cystoscopic evaluation as part of their workup. Evidence clearly indicates that this is a reasonable procedure to follow, particularly in women with urinary symptoms.

M. A. Stenchever, MD

Increased Prevalence of Interstitial Cystitis: Previously Unrecognized Urologic and Gynecologic Cases Identified Using a New Symptom Questionnaire and Intravesical Potassium Sensitivity
Parsons CL, Dell J, Stanford EJ, et al (Univ of California, San Diego; Knoxville, Tenn; St Mary's/Good Samaritan Med Ctrs, Centralia, Ill; et al)
Urology 60:573-578, 2002   11–11

Background.—Interstitial cystitis (IC), a clinical syndrome of urinary urgency/frequency, pelvic pain, or both, can be diagnosed with the intravesical potassium sensitivity test (PST). An IC symptom questionnaire, the pelvic pain and urgency/frequency (PUF) patient symptom scale, has now been developed as an aid to the diagnosis of IC. The PUF scale validation was described.

Study Design.—The PUF scale validation group consisted of 48 healthy controls, 213 patients with IC from several sites, and 121 patients from gynecologic clinics. These patients were administered the PUF scale. The scores were assessed as predictors of the PST to validate the PUF scale. Then 317 women from the general population were administered the PUF scale.

Findings.—The PST was positive in 74% of the patients with a PUF scale score of 10 to 15, 76% of those with a score of 15 to 19, and 91% of those who scored at least 20. All control PUF scale scores were less than 3. The rate of positive PST in healthy controls was 0%. The PUF scores of women from the general population suggested that approximately 22% have IC and that it is seriously underdiagnosed.

Conclusions.—The PUF scale was developed for the diagnosis of interstitial cystitis. This scale was validated by comparison with the diagnostic test, the PST. PUF scale scores in a general population sample suggest that about 22% of women may have IC. Use of the PUF appears to be an accurate method for the detection of interstitial cystitis.

▶ The authors of this study have had a long-time interest in IC and have written extensively on the topic. They have demonstrated that the intravesical potassium sensitivity test is accurate in diagnosing this condition, and in this study they used a questionnaire with both urologic and gynecologic questions to identify patients. With this questionnaire, they identified patients referred from both urologic and gynecologic clinics with bladder symptoms or symptoms of pelvic pain and discomfort and verified these findings with the potassium sensitivity test. They thus demonstrated that the prevalence of IC was high among patients presenting with gynecologic complaints. The authors estimated the incidence of IC among women to be 1 in 5 (20%) and administered the questionnaire to a sample of women attending lectures who were not seeking medical advice. According to the findings of the questionnaire, the incidence of IC in this sample was 22%.

The incidence of IC as judged by the authors seems quite high, and further investigation is necessary to verify these findings. However, gynecologists should keep the possibility of this diagnosis in mind when seeing patients who present with chronic pelvic pain or other pelvic discomfort, such as dyspareunia and backache.

M. A. Stenchever, MD

Detrusor Instability

Short-term Intravaginal Maximal Electrical Stimulation for Refractive Detrusor Instability

Yalcin OT, Hassa H, Sarac I (Osmangazi Univ, Eskisehir, Turkey)
Int J Gynaecol Obstet 79:241-244, 2002   11–12

Objective.—Maximal electric stimulation (MES) has been used in the treatment of lower urinary tract infection, but there are few data on how MES affects detrusor instability (DI). The outcomes of 35 patients undergoing intravaginal MES for refractive DI are reported.

Methods.—The patients all had pure DI that had failed to respond to conservative therapy. All underwent MES using an electrostimulation device and vaginal probe. Patients received two 30-minute treatments per day, with a duty cycle of 5 seconds of stimulation and 5 seconds of rest, for 7 days. Subjective and objective outcomes were assessed before and 1 week after MES.

Results.—The rate of subjective cure or improvement was 89%. On objective assessment, the success rate was 80% according to the 1-hour pad test and 74% according to subtracted cystometry. The only outcome that did not show improvement after MES was postvoid residual volume. Fourteen percent of patients experienced vaginal irritation; this was the only significant adverse effect.

Conclusion.—This experience supports the safety and efficacy of MES for women with treatment-refractory DI. Subjective and objective outcomes are good, but randomized trials are needed to establish the effect of MES on inhibition of detrusor contraction.

▶ In this relatively small study, the authors noted quite good results in treating 35 patients with refractive DI with MES. The study technique allowed for re-evaluation 1 week after treatment. Whereas the results were promising, longer-term follow-up and knowledge of the necessity for, and results of, retreatment, as well as final outcome are necessary to assess the overall value of this treatment. However, the authors' findings are interesting enough that a longer-term, larger study seems indicated as the therapy can be performed noninvasively, relatively easily, and inexpensively.

M. A. Stenchever, MD

Association of Smoking With Urgency in Older People
Nuotio M, Jylhä M, Koivisto A-M, et al (Univ of Tampere, Finland)
Eur Urol 40:206-212, 2001   11–13

Background.—An overactive bladder, characterized by urgency, frequency, and incontinence, has a negative impact on the quality of life of older persons. The association between smoking and urgency in older persons was examined in a cross-sectional study.

Study Design.—The study group consisted of 1059 persons, aged 60 to 89 years, who were participating in the Tampere Longitudinal Study of Aging. Participants were surveyed with respect to urinary symptoms, smoking, and alcohol and coffee drinking. Urgency prevalence was calculated according to gender in 15-year age groups. Logistic regression was used to analyze the association of urgency with smoking and with coffee and alcohol consumption.

Findings.—The prevalence of urgency was lowest among younger men and highest among older women, and it increased with age for both sexes. Current smokers were at the greatest risk of suffering from urgency in this study group. Alcohol and coffee drinking were not associated with urgency.

Conclusions.—The prevalence of urgency is higher among women and increases with age in both sexes. Smoking is associated with urgency in older persons. This finding provides yet another reason to avoid smoking.

▶ In this Finnish study, the authors defined overactive bladder as a condition involving symptoms of frequency, urgency, and urge or reflex incontinence, either singly or in combination, when appearing in the absence of local pathologic factors to explain these symptoms. Because urgency is a strong need to void, it is occasionally accompanied by urge incontinence. The authors evaluated the association of smoking with urgency in older persons, aged 60-89, and found a prevalence of urgency of 19.5% in older women. They found an increase in prevalence among current and past smokers, both men and women, but the prevalence in older female smokers, although elevated (odds ratio, 2.45), was not statistically significant. This finding could well be due to the fact that older women have multiple causes of urge incontinence, and many of these factors may have come into play in both smokers and non-smokers.

The authors noted that alcohol use and coffee drinking were not associated with urgency. This study apparently demonstrated another adverse effect of smoking. With respect to urgency, it may not have an effect on health directly, but it certainly has an effect on quality of life. Smoking may cause urgency in many ways, including the effect of a chronic cough on the bladder and bladder neck, which may lead to anatomic and neurologic damage over time. Nicotine may also have a direct effect on the muscular contraction of the bladder, as has been shown in animal models, and may affect circulation to the bladder and bladder neck. Thus, the findings from this and similar studies offer another reason for physicians to discourage smoking among their patients.

M. A. Stenchever, MD

Why Do Women Have Voiding Dysfunction and *De Novo* Detrusor Instability After Colposuspension?
Bombieri L, Freeman RM, Perkins EP, et al (Derriford Hosp, Plymouth, England; Univ of Plymouth, England)
Br J Obstet Gynaecol 109:402-412, 2002   11–14

Background.—Colposuspension has a high success rate and long-lasting benefits. However, complications can occur. The causes of voiding dysfunction and new detrusor instability after colposuspension were investigated.

Methods.—Seventy-seven women undergoing colposuspension for genuine stress incontinence were included in the prospective, observational study. Bladder neck elevation was investigated by MRI before and after surgery. Urethral compression was determined by measuring bladder neck approximation to the pubis with MRI after surgery (anterior compression) and the distance between the medial stitches during surgery (lateral compression). Clinical and urodynamic factors were also documented.

Findings.—The number of days of postoperative catheterization was associated with preoperative peak flow rate, straining during voiding, advancing age, operative election, and anterior urethral compression. Detrusor instability at 3 months correlated with increasing age, previous bladder neck surgery, surgical elevation, and anterior urethral compression.

Conclusions.—Operative factors such as bladder neck elevation and compression correlate with voiding dysfunction and detrusor instability after colposuspension. The current data have implications for preventing complications after this procedure.

▶ Two major complications of procedures designed to improve stress urinary incontinence are prolonged inability to void and the development of detrusor instability when it did not exist preoperatively. The authors attempted to evaluate the factors that might be responsible for these complications by investigating bladder neck elevation by MRI before and after surgery, urethral compression by measuring bladder neck approximation to the pubis with MRI after surgery (anterior compression), and the distance between the medial stitches during surgery (lateral compression), as well as clinical and urodynamic factors. The associations that they found to be significant with respect to these 2 fairly common complications are useful and of interest. Certainly, age seems to be a significant factor in each of these complications, as older women tend to experience these complications more often. Whether physicians will be able to use the information with respect to the positioning of the bladder neck to significantly decrease the complication rate remains to be seen, but it is worth trying.

M. A. Stenchever, MD

Surgical Treatment of Incontinence

Objective Assessment of Bladder Neck Elevation and Urethral Compression at Colposuspension

Bombieri L, Freeman RM, Perkins EP, et al (Derriford Hosp, Plymouth, England; Univ of Plymouth, England)

Br J Obstet Gynaecol 109:395-401, 2002   11–15

Background.—The colposuspension operation for genuine stress incontinence results in the repositioning of the bladder neck in a higher retropubic position. However, this can have an obstructing effect on the urethra. This procedure has a higher cure rate of 85% to 90%, but complications may adversely affect the quality of life. Voiding dysfunction and de novo detrusor instability have been reported to have a mean frequency of 12.5% and 9.6%, respectively.

The causes of these complications are unknown but are thought to result from excessive elevation and compression of the bladder neck and urethra. The purpose of this study was to determine whether MRI and intraoperative measurements are useful in the assessment of bladder neck elevation and urethral compression at colposuspension and to determine whether intraoperative measurements could be a substitute for MR scan measurements.

Methods.—This prospective observational study included 77 women undergoing colposuspension at the urogynecology unit of an NHS Trust hospital in England. Bladder neck elevation was assessed with MRI and measurement of the amount of suture bow-stringing intraoperatively. Urethral compression was assessed by means of MRI and measurement of the distance between the medial sutures (with a ruler) and the distance between the urethra and the pubic bone (using paired Hegar dilators).

Results.—Assessment of bladder neck elevation and compression against the pubic bone with MRI proved to be reliable. The intraoperative assessment of urethral compression with a ruler was also reproducible at both paravaginal and pectineal sites. However, intraoperative measurements of bladder neck elevation by the amount of suture bow-stringing and urethral compression by Hegar dilators did not correlate with equivalent MR scan measurements.

Conclusion.—This study presents objective assessments that can reliably indicate bladder neck elevation and urethral compression at colposuspension. These assessments should be useful for the investigation of morbidity after colposuspension.

▶ Using MRI pre- and post-Burch colposuspension procedure, the authors sought to correlate the findings from assessment of bladder neck elevation and urethral compression with intraoperative measurements. Lateral urethral compression was assessed by measuring the distance between the medial paraurethral sutures in millimeters, using a ruler while the sutures were held vertically. The authors assumed that a greater distance indicated less obstruction. This measurement did correlate with findings of MRI. Anterior urethral compression was measured objectively using Hegar dilators on each side of the urethra on the assumption that the greater the size of the Hegar dilator that fit into the urethropubic space after tying the sutures, the less the urethral compression. These findings did not correlate with the findings on MRI.

The authors concluded that MRI is the gold standard with respect to the position of the urethra and bladder neck behind the pubic symphysis following surgery, and was a worthwhile research tool to assess voiding problems following colposuspension procedures for incontinence. They also concluded that lateral urethral compression measurements were reliable for this purpose.

The Burch colposuspension procedure has proven to be a reliable approach to treating stress urinary incontinence, with success rates of 85% to 90%, and with lasting results. However, the complications of difficulty in voiding and detrusor instability, which are thought to be secondary to partial obstruction of the bladder neck, remain a concern in 10% to 15% of patients. If simple means of measuring suture placement during the operation help to prevent these complications, their utilization would be a welcome addition to the surgical management of these patients. The authors demonstrated that this is partially possible with their approach but is not entirely successful. Continued research in this area is a worthwhile endeavor.

M. A. Stenchever, MD

Short Term Complications of the Tension Free Vaginal Tape Operation for Stress Urinary Incontinence in Women

Bodelsson G, Henriksson L, Osser S, et al (Malmö Univ, Sweden)
Br J Obstet Gynaecol 109:566-569, 2002   11–16

Background.—The tension-free vaginal tape technique was introduced in 1995 for the treatment of stress urinary incontinence in women. In the same year, spinal anesthesia was introduced as an alternative to local anesthesia during this procedure. The technique is thought to have several advantages over the classic abdominal urethropexies, including minimal surgical trauma, a shorter postoperative hospital stay, and the ability to use a local anesthestic, which allows the patient to cough and thus facilitates proper adjustment of the tape. This report from the clinic that originated the tension-free vaginal tape technique was prompted by several cases of intraoperative bladder perforations and a higher rate of postoperative urinary retention. The focus of this study is the prevalence of complications with the tension-free vaginal tape procedure.

Methods.—The study population comprised 177 women with urodynamically confirmed genuine stress incontinence who underwent the tension-free vaginal tape procedure with local or spinal anesthesia. Twenty-six women (15%) also had symptomatic urge incontinence. The main outcome measures were intraoperative and postoperative complications in relation to individual surgeons and mode of anesthesia and continence at short-term follow-up.

Results.—Bladder or urethral perforation occurred in 26 women (15%), and 3 operations were abandoned because of these complications. Thirty-five women (20%) experienced a failure to void after the first 24 hours; 21 patients (12%) had to undergo urethral dilation, while 5 patients (2.8%) had persistent urinary retention that required excision of the sling. There was a significant association between these complications and the experience of the surgeon. In 7 patients (4%), hemorrhage required intravaginal tamponade. Three patients (1.7%) experienced postoperative sling rejection.

At 6 to 8 weeks postoperatively, 154 patients (88%) reported subjective cure, 21 (11%) reported significant improvement, and 2 (1%) reported no improvement. The use of spinal anesthesia increased the frequency of perioperative bladder perforation but did not affect the incidence of postoperative bladder obstruction nor the outcome of the tension-free vaginal tape procedure at follow-up.

Conclusion.—This retrospective investigation of the prevalence of complications with the tension-free vaginal tape procedure identified short-term complications that related in part to the experience of the individual surgeon. However, this review also found an 88% subjective cure rate, independent of these factors.

▶ The authors report on their series of 177 patients who underwent tension-free vaginal tape procedures for urodynamically proven stress urinary incontinence. Whereas their data are similar in many respects to other reports on the success and complications of this procedure, there were a few variations. They report a failure to void rate of 20% but this was measured 6 to 8 weeks postoperatively, and in several studies, surgeons have persisted with self-catheterization until this problem eased. Nevertheless, these authors demonstrated that this complication varied by surgeon and probably related to the amount of tension placed on the urethra at the time of surgery. Interestingly, they did not observe any variation associated with the type of anesthesia used, as has been reported in previous studies.

The authors reported only 7 cases (4%) of perioperative bleeding, and all but 1 responded to intravaginal tamponade. This incidence is an improvement over that reported by other researchers. The authors also noted, as have others, that 9 of their patients (6%) who had not experienced urgency before the procedure developed symptoms postoperatively. Some authors have suggested that this is related to excessive obstruction of the urethra at the time of surgery, but the authors of this study did not address this factor. Nevertheless, this bothersome symptom seems to respond well to medical management. The authors did demonstrate that the incidence of bladder perforation was higher in patients under spinal anesthesia than those under local anesthesia, but the reason for this finding is not readily apparent.

All in all, once again, the findings from a fairly large series of patients undergoing tension-free vaginal tape procedures appear to demonstrate that it is an effective means of treating stress urinary incontinence with a relatively small number of serious complications. Nevertheless, the authors only reviewed their 88% success rate 6 to 8 weeks postoperatively, and longer-term follow-up is necessary to determine the long-term benefits of this procedure.

M. A. Stenchever, MD

Urinary Stress Incontinence in Obese Women: Tension-free Vaginal Tape Is the Answer
Mukherjee K, Constantine G (Good Hope Hosp, Sutton Coldfield, England)
BJU Internatl 88:881-883, 2001   11–17

Background.—Body mass index (BMI) is positively associated with stress urinary incontinence (SUI). SUI is also more difficult to treat in obese patients. The use of tension-free vaginal tape (TVT) to treat SUI in obese women is described.

Study Design.—The study group consisted of 242 women, aged 34 to 79 years, with urodynamically confirmed SUI who underwent a TVT procedure under spinal anesthesia. The women were divided into 3 groups based on BMI: obese, overweight, and normal weight. The King's validated quality of life (QoL) assessment was completed before surgery and at 6-month follow-up. Results were described as cure, significant improvement, or failure. Relative cure rates were compared across the different weight groups with Fisher's exact test.

Findings.—There was no significant difference in cure rates among the 3 weight subgroups. The cure rate among the obese women was 90%, with the remaining 10% significantly improved. There were no treatment failures. There was a significant improvement in QoL in all 3 groups.

Conclusions.—TVT can be used successfully to treat stress urinary incontinence in obese women. This procedure is strongly recommended to treat SUI in this patient group.

▶ In this interesting study, the authors compared the cure and improvement rates in 242 women treated for stress urinary incontinence with TVT procedures. They compared the results in 87 women who were obese (body mass index [BMI] > 30) with 98 women who were overweight (BMI, 25-29), and 58 women of normal weight (BMI < 25). The cure rates were excellent in all groups, and the obese women did as well essentially as the nonobese women. The patients were evaluated both physically and by use of the King's validated QoL questionnaire (version 7). The evaluations occurred before the operative procedure and 6 months after surgery. Whereas these results are encouraging and it appears that this type of procedure may be the best choice for obese women, it would have been helpful if the follow-up had been longer. As with any procedure, the test of its value must be assessed over time.

The authors used spinal anesthesia to perform their operations. It has been demonstrated since that local anesthesia appears to be somewhat better in preventing postpartum voiding difficulties. It remains to be seen whether the use of local anesthesia in obese women will produce comparable results.

M. A. Stenchever, MD

Body Mass Index and Outcome of Tension-Free Vaginal Tape
Rafii A, Daraï E, Haab F, et al (Hôpital Beaujon, Clichy, France; Université Paris 7, Clichy, France)
Eur Urol 43:288-292, 2003   11–18

Objective.—Tension-free vaginal tape (TVT) has become a popular alternative to classic surgical techniques for the treatment of stress urinary incontinence. Little is known about the effectiveness of TVT in obese women, who may be at increased risk for stress urinary incontinence. The effects of body mass index (BMI) on the success rate of TVT were analyzed.

Methods and Findings.—The study included 2 groups of consecutive patients undergoing TVT treatment: 38 obese women (BMI 30 or over) and 149 normal-weight women (BMI, 20-25) or overweight women (BMI, 26-30). The 2 groups were otherwise similar, including age, parity, menopausal status, history of previous surgery, and type and severity of incontinence. Postoperatively, urge urinary incontinence was noted in 17.9% of obese women, compared with 3.4% of normal-weight women and 6.4% of overweight women. All 3 groups achieved high cure rates, both objective (82% to 93%) and subjective (72% to 74%).

Conclusion.—Obese women may have a higher rate of postoperative urge incontinence after TVT treatment, compared with women with lower BMIs. However, obesity is not a risk factor for TVT failure. More study of factors affecting the outcomes of the TVT technique is needed.

▶ The TVT procedure is a relatively new procedure for the treatment of genuine stress urinary incontinence. To date, it has been demonstrated to have many advantages over other procedures for this purpose, and although long-term follow-up is not available in most studies, the overall results are promising. Obese women pose an increased challenge, both because of a higher likelihood of morbidity related to their obesity and because of the possibility that a given procedure might not be as successful because of their obesity.

Happily, the authors discovered that the incidence of objective and subjective cures was similar for women of normal weight, overweight, and obesity. Also, the incidence of morbidity was similar in the 3 groups. The TVT procedure appears to be a useful procedure for treating stress urinary incontinence in women of all BMIs. Again, long-term follow-up is necessary to determine if these success rates continue in each of the weight groups.

M. A. Stenchever, MD

Intact Genetic Material Is Present in Commercially Processed Cadaver Allografts Used for Pubovaginal Slings
Hathaway JK, Choe JM (Univ of Cincinnati, Mount Vernon, Ohio)
J Urol 168:1040-1043, 2002   11–19

Background.—Human cadaver allograft donors are screened for various diseases. Donated tissue is processed to prevent disease transmission. Routine testing is done for the presence of DNA viruses, such as papillomavirus, polyomavirus, and herpes virus. However, DNA viruses that have incorporated into the host genome can be transmitted by allograft if the host DNA continues to be intact and functional. The presence, concentration, and length of DNA in 4 commercially available human cadaver allografts were determined.

Methods.—Ten tissue samples from each of 4 commercial sources of human allografts were analyzed for intact DNA segments. Samples were obtained from Mentor, Musculoskeletal Transplant Foundation, Regeneration Technologies, and Life Cell. A standard extraction technique was performed to isolate genetic material. Spectrophotometry was performed to quantify DNA concentrations, and polymerase chain reaction was used to amplify the retrieved DNA material. Agarose gel electrophoresis was also conducted to assess the DNA fragment size.

Findings.—Thirty-nine of the 40 samples tested (97.5%) contained DNA of 400- to 2000-base pair (bp) segments. A 400-bp DNA segment was present in 9 or 10 of the samples from all 4 commercial sources. A 700-bp DNA segment was documented in 10 samples from Musculoskeletal Transplant

Foundation, in 10 from Regeneration Technologies, and in 10 from Life Cell. In addition, 10 Life Cell allografts had a 2000-bp DNA segment.

Conclusions.—Commercially processed allografts from all 4 of these sources contained intact genetic material. The size of the intact DNA and the DNA concentration varied greatly by the processing method used.

▶ The authors studied 4 cadaver allografts, 10 each from 4 companies, intended for use in pubovaginal slings. Each company had stringently screened the donor tissue for various diseases and then processed the tissue to destroy any disease. Nevertheless, DNA fragments that replicated by polymerase chain reaction were found in 39 (97.5%) of the samples. Thus, foreign DNA capable of replication, which may have been of either host or viral source, was probably still viable in these tissues. In addition, there may have been several agents, such as viral prions for which screening was not possible, present in the tissue. Given the risk that DNA viruses may potentially infect the host and the risk of Creutzfeldt-Jacob disease, which is transmitted via prions, material from cadavers is probably inferior to other types of materials, such as the patient's own fascia or inert materials. Recently, a possible relation was demonstrated between the presence of cells, or perhaps DNA, introduced into a host and the development of autoimmune conditions. Until this risk is further understood, the use of allografts should also be withheld whenever possible.

M. A. Stenchever, MD

The Use of Porcine Dermal Implant in a Minimally Invasive Pubovaginal Sling Procedure for Genuine Stress Incontinence
Barrington JW, Edwards G, Arunkalaivanan AS, et al (Torbay Hosp, Torquay, England)
BJU Internatl 90:224-227, 2002   11–20

Background.—There has been a resurgence in the use of sling procedures for the surgical management of genuine stress incontinence. Synthetic sling materials have been introduced recently to reduce the potential complications associated with these procedures. These complications result from the need to harvest a strip of fascia through a large abdominal incision and the potentially weak quality of the connective tissue. Porcine dermis has been previously described as an allogenic graft material.

It was also shown that cross-linking protected the autografts from degradation, which prolonged their survival and permanence. However, the initial porcine grafts were cross-linked with the use of aldehyde, which was associated with a potential for development of foci of mineralization on the graft and possibly extensive calcification of the graft. The use of a porcine dermal implant (Pelvicol, Bard Urology, United Kingdom) that is cross-linked with diisocyanate in the surgical management of urinary stress incontinence was investigated.

Methods.—A total of 40 women with urodynamically confirmed genuine stress incontinence were enrolled in the study and followed up at 6 weeks and at least 6 months after the minimally invasive pubovaginal sling procedure. The minimal-access technique allowed 23 women to undergo the procedure on an outpatient basis. The main outcome measures included continence rates, voiding dysfunction, satisfaction scores, and whether or not the patients would recommend the procedure to a friend or relative.

Results.—The cure rate (sustained benefit) with this procedure was 85%. An additional 10% of patients were improved by surgery. Voiding dysfunction rates were low and patients' satisfaction scores were high. The majority of patients indicated that they would undergo the procedure again if necessary and would recommend the procedure to others.

Conclusion.—A porcine dermal implant cross-linked with diisocyanate and implanted by a minimally invasive approach is effective in treating stress incontinence. This treatment approach has a low rate of complications and for many patients can be performed as an outpatient procedure.

▶ In this British study, 40 women with a mean age of 56 years (42-79 years) who had urodynamically proven stress incontinence were treated with minimally invasive sling procedures utilizing a porcine dermal implant in which cross-linking was effected by using diisocyanate. This particular cross-linking agent is considered nontoxic, does not cause mineralization, and is believed to give permanence to the graft. The authors demonstrated that the procedure was effective (cure rate, 85% at 6 months) in treating women with stress incontinence. These grafts are anchored to the rectus sheath, and bleeding and voiding problems were comparable to those of other graft procedures.

The longest follow-up period in any of these patients was 18 months, and although the authors believe that long-term cure rates will be obtained, longer follow-up is necessary, both to ensure that patients remained dry and that no complications, such as urethral erosions, occur. Nevertheless, the authors demonstrated another type of sling material that can be used effectively in treating women with stress urinary incontinence. Its superiority to other techniques, such as the tension-free vaginal tape or autologous materials, remains to be ascertained.

M. A. Stenchever, MD

Determinants of Patient Dissatisfaction After a Tension-Free Vaginal Tape Procedure for Urinary Incontinence
Deval B, Jeffry L, Al Najjar F, et al (Hôpital Hôtel-Dieu de Paris)
J Urol 167:2093-2097, 2002   11–21

Background.—The tension-free vaginal tape procedure was first proposed for urinary stress incontinence in 1996. The goal of this procedure is to reinforce pubourethral ligaments, the suburethral vaginal hammock, and the connections of the suburethral vaginal hammock to the pubococcygeus muscles. Determinants of patient satisfaction after this procedure were reported.

Methods.—One hundred eighty-seven women with genuine stress or mixed incontinence were included in the retrospective analysis. The objective cure rate was assessed by clinical and urodynamic examinations. The subjective cure rate was determined by a visual analog scale and the Contilife questionnaire. Patients were followed up for a mean of 27 months.

Findings.—Overall, complications occurred in 35.3% of the women. Bladder injury was documented in 9.6%, urinary retention was present in 6.4%, difficult voiding was present in 10.7%, and new onset urge symptoms were present in 21.3%. Overall, the objective cure rate was 90.4%, and the subjective cure rate was 70.6%. Women undergoing the procedure with general or spinal anesthesia had a significantly lower subjective cure rate than those receiving local anesthesia. The subjective cure rate was unaffected by patient age, menopausal status, previous incontinence surgery, body mass index, additional procedures associated with tension-free vaginal tape surgery, and the Ingelman-Sundberg classification.

Conclusions.—The tension-free vaginal tape procedure is associated with a high objective cure rate. However, the subjective cure rate is lower. Using local anesthesia during the procedure seems to reduce the incidence of difficult voiding and new onset urge symptoms.

▶ In this French study of 187 women undergoing tension-free vaginal tape procedures for stress urinary incontinence (n = 133) and mixed incontinence (n = 54), the authors demonstrated an objective cure rate of 90.4%, which is similar to findings of previous studies. However, they noted a subjective cure rate of 70.6%. They measured subjective cure rates on an analog scale and were, therefore, assessing the patients' impression of their improvement.

Once again, differences between the physician's objective assessment and the patient's personal assessment of a cure were highlighted. No differences existed in the subjective cure rate by patient age, menopausal status, previous incontinence surgery, or body mass index. Because various degrees of urinary retention and urinary urgency are observed in women who have undergone this procedure (and in women who have had other procedures for stress urinary incontinence), patient dissatisfaction is probably partially related to these problems. The objective complications that the authors observed were similar to findings from other studies on the tension-free vaginal tape procedure. Therefore, it seems reasonable that the next step in managing such patients would be to determine the types of problems that lead to dissatisfaction and the means of correcting or preventing these problems.

M. A. Stenchever, MD

The Use of Intraoperative Cystoscopy in Major Vaginal and Urogynecologic Surgeries

Kwon CH, Goldberg RP, Koduri S, et al (Northwestern Univ, Evanston, Ill)
Am J Obstet Gynecol 187:1466-1472, 2002   11–22

Background.—During gynecologic procedures, it is easy to injure the urinary tract. Early recognition and repair of these injuries results in less patient morbidity and better outcome. For this reason, some recommend routine cystoscopy during all major gynecologic procedures. The occurrence of important intraoperative cystoscopic findings during major vaginal reconstructive and urogynecologic surgeries was reviewed in a large patient series.

Study Design.—The records of 526 women who had anti-incontinence or pelvic reconstructive surgery from January 1997 to April 2001 were reviewed. All patients underwent routine cystoscopy with intravenous indigo carmine after their procedures. The incidence of significant cystoscopic findings and their effects on management were recorded.

Findings.—Out of 526 operations in this series, there were 26 significant cystoscopic findings, of which 15 were operative injuries requiring intervention. Of these 15 cases, 7 were caused by anterior colporrhaphy sutures. There were no undetected injuries that caused morbidity after surgery. There were no significant demographic differences between those patients with normal and those with abnormal cystoscopic findings. Cystoscopy was not associated with any morbidity.

Conclusions.—Intraoperative cystoscopy is a safe and effective method for the detection of injury to the lower urinary tract after pelvic surgery. This allows for rapid detection and easier repair of intraoperative injuries, with a reduction in patient morbidity. Routine intraoperative cystoscopy should be considered after anti-incontinence and vaginal reconstructive surgery.

▶ Is it cost-effective and useful to perform intraoperative cystoscopy at the end of major vaginal and urogynecologic procedures? Some authors have suggested that intraoperative cystoscopy should be performed at the end of every pelvic procedure. In the current study, which involved major vaginal and urogynecologic surgery, a 4.9% incidence of unsuspected problems was noted; more than half of these problems required intervention. Of particular interest was the finding that problems were observed with anterior colporrhaphy and Burch procedures alike. Another important finding was that no complications or morbidity occurred as a direct result of the intraoperative cystoscopy. It appears that, on the basis of the authors' data, performing intraoperative cystoscopy and injection with indigo carmine is a prudent strategy when one is performing a major vaginal and urogynecologic procedure. Although the risk is relatively small, for the physician and patient involved, it would probably be quite chaotic if an injury went unnoticed.

M. A. Stenchever, MD

12 Menopause

Relationship of Changes in Physical Activity and Mortality Among Older Women
Gregg EW, for the Study of Osteoporotic Fractures Research Group (Ctrs for Disease Control and Prevention, Atlanta, Ga; et al)
JAMA 289:2379-2386, 2003   12–1

Background.—Physical activity has been associated with a decreased mortality rate. However, whether changes in physical activity affect mortality rate among older women is unclear.

Methods.—Four U.S. research centers enrolled 9518 community-dwelling white women aged 65 years or older in this prospective cohort study. The women were assessed at baseline between 1986 and 1988. A median 5.7 years later, 7553 were available for reassessment.

Findings.—Compared with women who remained sedentary during follow-up, women who increased their levels of physical activity had a lower mortality rate from all causes, with a hazard ratio (HR) of 0.52. This finding was independent of age, smoking, body mass index, comorbid conditions, and baseline physical activity level. Among women increasing their levels of physical activity, the HR for death from cardiovascular disease was 0.64 and 0.49 from cancer. The relation between changes in physical activity and decreased mortality rate were comparable in women with and without chronic diseases but tended to be weaker in women at least 75 years old and in women with a poor health status. Women who were physically active at both assessments also had a reduced all-cause and cardiovascular mortality rate when compared with sedentary women.

Conclusions.—Among elderly women, increasing and maintaining physical activity levels may prolong life. However, this appears less beneficial among women aged 75 years and older and in those with poor health status.

▶ This study provides objective evidence that physical activity is associated with a 50% significantly decreased risk of all-cause mortality as well as decreased mortality rate from cardiovascular disease and cancer in older white women. Changing from being sedentary to physically active also was associated with decreased mortality rate. All clinicians should encourage their elderly female patients to walk at least 2 miles each day as well as perform other physical activities.

D. R. Mishell, Jr, MD

Thyroid Stimulating Hormone (TSH) Concentrations and Menopausal Status in Women at the Mid-Life: SWAN

Sowers M, Luborsky J, Perdue C, et al (Univ of Michigan, Ann Arbor; Rush Univ, Chicago; New England Research Insts, Watertown, Mass)
Clin Endocrinol (Oxf) 58:340-347, 2003   12–2

Background.—Although the prevalence of thyroid disease increases with advancing age, few studies of thyroid status and menopausal transition have been published. The association of menopausal symptoms, menstrual cycle bleeding characteristics, and reproductive hormones to thyroid stimulating hormone (TSH) levels in middle-aged women from 5 ethnic groups was investigated.

Methods.—Data were obtained from the baseline evaluation of the Study of Women's Health Across the Nation (SWAN), a community-based multiethnic study of the natural history of menopausal transition. The 3242 participants were aged 42 and 52 years and included African American, European American, Chinese, Hispanic, and Japanese women. The participants were interviewed about diagnoses of hypothyroidism or hyperthyroidism, thyroid treatment, menopausal symptoms, and menstrual cycle bleeding. In addition, sera were obtained and assayed for TSH, estradiol, testosterone, follicle-stimulating hormone, and sex hormone–binding globulin.

Findings.—In 6.2% of the women, TSH exceeded 5 mIU/mL. In 3.2%, TSH was less than 0.5 mIU/mL; these cutoffs represented clinical and subclinical hypothyroidism and hyperthyroidism, respectively. Mean TSH levels were significantly lower in African American women than in the European American, Hispanic, and Chinese women. Fearfulness was the only menopausal symptom associated with a TSH value exceeding 5.0 mIU/mL or less than 0.5 mIU/mL. Women with abnormal TSH values were more likely to report shorter or longer menstrual periods. Levels of TSH were unrelated to follicle-stimulating hormone, sex hormone–binding globulin, dehydroepiandrosterone sulfate, testosterone, and estradiol.

Conclusions.—Among these middle-aged women, the prevalence of TSH values outside the euthyroid range was 9.6%. TSH levels were associated with length of menstrual bleeding and self-reported fearfulness but not with indicators of menopausal transition, such as menopausal stage defined by bleeding regularity, menopausal symptoms, or reproductive hormone levels.

▶ This report of TSH values in a large unscheduled group of premenopausal or perimenopausal women found there was a high prevalence of abnormal TSH levels (9.4%). Clinicians should therefore perform routine screening of TSH levels in women after age 40 years because TSH levels increase with age. Women with elevated TSH levels had an increased likelihood of prolonged bleeding episodes, so TSH should be measured in women with menses 8 or more days in duration. Finally, in the nearly 5% of women taking thyroid medications for hypothyroidism or hyperthyroidism, 42% had abnormal TSH levels. TSH should be measured at periodic intervals in individuals taking thyroid medication to determine whether the dosage should be changed.

D. R. Mishell, Jr, MD

Effects of Estrogen Plus Progestin on Health-Related Quality of Life
Hays J, for the Women's Health Initiative Investigators (Baylor College of Medicine, Houston; et al)
N Engl J Med 348:1839-1854, 2003   12–3

Background.—Recent studies have demonstrated increases in certain health risks among postmenopausal women using combination hormone replacement therapy (HRT). Studies of the effects of hormone therapy on health-related quality of life—especially among women taking hormones for disease prevention, rather than symptom relief—have yielded conflicting results. Data from a randomized controlled trial of estrogen plus progestin were used to investigate the effects of combination HRT on health-related quality of life.

Methods.—The analysis included 16,608 postmenopausal women, all 50 to 79 years of age and with an intact uterus. They were randomly assigned to receive combination hormone replacement therapy consisting of 0.625 mg conjugated equine estrogen plus 2.5 mg medroxyprogesterone acetate (Prempro) or placebo. The RAND 36-Item Health Survey was used to evaluate quality of life and functional status in the following areas: general health, physical functioning, limitations on usual role-related activities, social functioning, and emotional/mental health. A 1-year follow-up was available for the overall sample, and a 3-year follow-up was available for a subgroup of 1511 women.

Results.—The combination HRT and placebo groups had similar outcomes in general health, vitality, mental health, depression, and sexual satisfaction. At 1-year follow-up, hormone therapy had small but significant beneficial effects on sleep disturbance, physical functioning, and pain. However, the clinical significance of these gains was questionable. The 3-year follow-up found no significant improvements in any domain of quality of life. HRT was associated with improvement in vasomotor symptoms and sleep disturbance among 50- to 54-year-old women with initially moderate to severe vasomotor symptoms.

Conclusion.—Combination HRT appears to have little or no impact on health-related quality of life for postmenopausal women. Some statistically significant benefits were observed, but these were small and appeared to be offset by the increased risk of cardiovascular diseases and breast cancer with combination HRT. The findings may not be relevant to postmenopausal women who seek hormone treatment because of vasomotor or other troublesome menopausal symptoms.

▶ The Women's Health Initiative is a large, randomized trial that enrolled postmenopausal women and studied the effect of 1 oral estrogen-progestin preparation compared with a placebo on many parameters. In this report, it was found that the women who took hormones had significantly less severe hot flushes and night sweats and less sleep disturbance after 1 year but no benefit in other parameters affecting their quality of life. The Women's Health Initiative enrolled mainly asymptomatic women who had a mean age of 63 years. Only 17% of the women were within 5 years of menopause, and only 13% had moderate or severe vasomotor symptoms. Three fourths of the women enrolled had no history of prior hormone use. Thus, the findings of this study are not applicable to recently postmenopausal women with bothersome vasomotor symptoms who have been shown in other randomized studies to have a greater reduction in symptoms with estrogen than placebo.

D. R. Mishell, Jr, MD

Hormone Replacement Therapy and Incidence of Alzheimer Disease in Older Women: The Cache County Study
Breitner JCS, for the Cache County Memory Study Investigators (Johns Hopkins Univ, Baltimore, Md; et al)
JAMA 288:2123-2129, 2002   12–4

Background.—Women appear to be at increased risk for Alzheimer disease (AD) after the age of 80 compared with men. This may be due to estrogen depletion. A large Cache County (Utah) cohort was utilized to prospectively assess the relationship between hormone replacement therapy (HRT) and AD.

Study Design.—The study group consisted of 1357 elderly men and 1889 elderly women residing in Cache County, Utah. Participants were evaluated for dementia in 1995 to 1997 and then again in 1998 to 2000. The use of HRT, calcium, and multivitamin supplements was also recorded. Discrete-time survival analysis was used to compare risks of AD among HRT users, nonusers, and men.

Findings.—AD developed in 35 men and 88 women between their first and second evaluation. The incidence among women increased after age 80 and exceeded that for men of similar age. Women who had used HRT had a reduced risk of AD compared with nonusers. Risk decreased with the duration of HRT use, so that after 10 years of HRT, the incidence was similar to that of men. Neither calcium nor multivitamin use had any effect on AD incidence.

Conclusion.—Prior HRT therapy use was associated with a reduced incidence of AD years later among elderly women. This effect increased with the duration of HRT therapy. Long-term HRT therapy may be effective for the prevention of AD in women.

▶ The results of this well-done prospective study provide additional data indicating that use of estrogen postmenopausally significantly reduces the risk of women developing AD. The study found that AD developed after age 80 twice as frequently in women as in men. However, the use of estrogen for 10 or more years by women reduced their risk of developing AD by about 60% to about the same risk that occurred in men.

Prospective, randomized studies such as the Women's Health Initiative will be unable to assess the effect of estrogen upon AD because of the long latent period before benefit becomes apparent. Therefore, clinicians need to counsel patients about the beneficial effects of estrogen upon AD based upon observational studies such as this one. To have a benefit upon AD, women should start estrogen at the time of menopause and take it for long duration, at lease more than 10 years, to reduce their risk of developing AD. There are no good therapies for AD. Therefore, use of a safe agent that can prevent this relatively common disorder in elderly women should be encouraged.

D. R. Mishell, Jr, MD

The Influence of Hormone Replacement Therapy on the Aging-related Change in Cognitive Performance: Analysis Based on a Danish Cohort Study
Løkkegaard E, Pedersen AT, Laursen P, et al (Glostrup Univ Hosp, Denmark; Hvidovre Univ Hosp, Denmark)
Maturitas 42:209-218, 2002   12–5

Background.—Cognitive performance may be maintained or even improved with postmenopausal hormone replacement therapy (HRT). The impact of HRT on aging-related changes in cognitive performance was investigated.

Methods.—A subset of participants in the Danish MONICA Study of cardiovascular risk factors were included in the current study. Data were obtained from neuropsychological assessments, consisting of 28 cognitive parameters, performed from 1982 to 1983 and repeated from 1993 to 1994. The final analyses were of 126 women who had never used HRT, 40 current users, and 30 future users (those who began HRT during the study period).

Findings.—Current users of HRT had a less-pronounced decline in cognitive performance at follow-up than did women who had never used HRT in 1 of 6 parameters for ability to concentrate and 2 of 8 parameters for visuomotor function. Future HRT users had a better cognitive performance at baseline than did never-users in long-term visual memory, concentration, and reaction time. Future HRT users were also more precise but spent more time on the visuomotor function tests than did never-users.

Conclusions.—Aging-related cognitive decline in concentration and visuomotor function appears to be delayed in women taking HRT. However, women treated with HRT perform better on cognitive tests before starting treatment.

▶ The results of this prospective cohort study found that among healthy postmenopausal women, use of estrogen with or without a progestin enhanced cognitive performance regarding concentration and visuomotor function, but not memory function, compared with non–hormone users during an 11-year follow-up.

Women considering whether or not to take hormones postmenopausally should be informed about the beneficial effects of estrogen upon cognitive function reported in this and other studies of healthy women.

D. R. Mishell, Jr, MD

Estrogen Plus Progestin and the Incidence of Dementia and Mild Cognitive Impairment in Postmenopausal Women: The Women's Health Initiative Memory Study: A Randomized Controlled Trial
Shumaker SA, for the WHIMS Investigators (Wake Forest Univ, Winston-Salem, NC; et al)
JAMA 289:2651-2662, 2003   12–6

Background.—The risk of Alzheimer disease (AD) is greater in postmenopausal women than men. However, studies of the effects of estrogen therapy on AD have been inconsistent. The effects of estrogen plus progestin on the incidence of dementia and mild cognitive impairment were compared with those of placebo in data from the Women's Health Initiative trial.

Methods.—A total of 4532 postmenopausal women free of probable dementia, aged 65 years and older, were studied. Participants were given conjugated equine estrogen, 0.625 mg, plus medroxyprogesterone acetate, 2.5 mg, or matching placebo. The mean time between randomization and the last Modified Mini-Mental State Examination was 4.05 years.

Findings.—Overall, 61 women received a diagnosis of probable dementia, including 40 in the estrogen plus progestin group (66%) and 21 in the placebo group (34%). The former had a 2.05 hazard ratio for probable dementia. This increased risk would produce an additional 23 cases of dementia per 10,000 women per year. In both groups, AD was the most common classification of dementia. The 2 groups did not differ in treatment effects on mild cognitive impairment.

Conclusions.—Estrogen plus progestin treatment appears to increase the risk for probable dementia in postmenopausal women aged 65 years or older. Active treatment did not prevent mild cognitive impairment. These findings provide more evidence that the risks of estrogen plus progestin outweigh the benefits.

▶ The results of this randomized trial, which was a subset of women enrolled in the Women's Health Initiative, indicate that when estrogen plus progestin therapy is initiated in women aged 65 or older, there is a 2-fold increased risk of developing dementia compared with women randomized to placebo treatment. These findings differ from the majority of observational studies, which have reported that estrogen therapy reduces the risk of developing AD by about one third. Perhaps when estrogen is initiated soon after the menopause and is given for 10 years or more, there is a reduction in AD, but when estrogen is initiated after the age of 65, there is accelerated progression of early undiagnosed AD so that its diagnosis is made earlier. In this study, the increased risk of dementia in women receiving hormones occurred after 1 year of therapy. This finding supports the concept of accelerated progression, not initiation, of dementia when estrogen-progestin therapy is first given to elderly women.

D. R. Mishell, Jr, MD

Effect of Estrogen Plus Progestin on Global Cognitive Function in Postmenopausal Women: The Women's Health Initiative Memory Study: A Randomized Controlled Trial
Rapp SR, for the WHIMS Investigators (Wake Forest Univ, Winston-Salem, NC; et al)
JAMA 289:2663-2672, 2003   12–7

Background.—Observational studies suggest that hormone treatment may improve cognitive function in postmenopausal women, but randomized clinical studies have yielded inconclusive results. Whether estrogen plus progestin protects global cognitive function in older postmenopausal women was investigated in an ancillary study of the Women's Health Initiative.

Methods.—The 4381 participants received either conjugated equine estrogen, 0.625 mg, plus medroxyprogesterone acetate, 2.5 mg, or placebo. The Modified Mini-Mental State Examination was administered annually to determine global cognitive function.

Findings.—Total scores in both groups increased slightly during a mean follow-up of 4.2 years. Women receiving active treatment had smaller mean increases in total scores than did women receiving placebo. Previous hormone use, duration of previous use, and timing of previous use did not affect the findings. More women receiving estrogen plus progestin had a substantial, clinically important decrease in total score than did those receiving placebo (6.7% vs 4.8%).

Conclusions.—Estrogen plus progestin did not improve cognitive function in postmenopausal women aged 65 years or older compared with placebo. Most women receiving estrogen plus progestin did not have clinically relevant adverse effects on cognition compared with those receiving placebo. However, the former group had a small increased risk of clinically meaningful cognitive decline.

▶ The results of this study indicate that clinicians should not initiate estrogen plus progestin to women aged 65 or older to prevent a decline in cognition. Although some other observational studies suggest that elderly women taking estrogen have better scores on tests of memory, the results of this randomized trial do not indicate that estrogen improves cognition. One must remember that this study did not address the effect of estrogen on memory when estrogen or estrogen-progestin therapy is initiated before the age of 65.

D. R. Mishell, Jr, MD

Effect of Estrogen Plus Progestin on Stroke in Postmenopausal Women: The Women's Health Initiative: A Randomized Trial

Wassertheil-Smoller S, for the WHI Investigators (Albert Einstein College of Medicine, Bronx, NY; et al)

JAMA 289:2673-2684, 2003   12–8

Background.—Cerebrovascular disease is the third-leading cause of death in the United States and the leading cause of disability in adults. The Women's Health Initiative (WHI) began in the 1990s and was intended to evaluate a number of factors affecting the health of postmenopausal women. The arm of the WHI that involved a clinical trial of estrogen plus progestin was terminated 3 years early because the harmful effects of the trial outweighed its benefits. The overall results of this trial showed that women in the estrogen-plus-progestin group experienced a 41% increase in strokes over 5.2 years compared with women in the placebo group. The effect of estrogen-plus-progestin on ischemic and hemorrhagic stroke was assessed, and whether the effect of estrogen-plus-progestin was modified by baseline levels of blood biomarkers was determined.

Methods.—This multicenter, double-blind, placebo-controlled, randomized clinical trial involved 16,608 women aged 50 through 79 years, with an average follow-up of 5.6 years. The study participants received either 0.625 mg/day of conjugated equine estrogen plus 2.5 mg/d of medroxyprogesterone acetate or placebo. Baseline levels of blood-based markers of inflammation, thrombosis, and lipid levels were measured in the first 140 confirmed stroke cases and in 513 control participants. The main outcome measures were overall strokes and stroke subtype and severity.

Results.—Strokes occurred in 1.8% of patients in the estrogen-plus-progestin group and in 1.3% of patients in the placebo group. Overall, 79.8% of strokes were ischemic. Point estimates of the intention-to-treat hazard ratio for estrogen-plus-progestin showed an excess risk of all strokes (hemorrhagic or ischemic) in all age groups, in all categories of baseline stroke risk, and in women with and without hypertension; a prior history of cardiovascular disease; and the use of hormones, statins, or aspirin. The effect of estrogen-plus-progestin on stroke risk was not modified by other risk factors for stroke, including smoking, high blood pressure, diabetes, lower use of vitamin C supplements, blood-based biomarkers of inflammation, higher white blood cell count, and higher hematocrit levels.

Conclusion.—The risk of ischemic stroke is increased by estrogen-plus-progestin in generally healthy postmenopausal women. The excess risk of stroke associated with estrogen-plus-progestin was present in all subgroups of women in this study.

▶ This report provides additional analysis of data regarding stroke among women enrolled in the randomized WHI who received either an oral estrogen-progestin pill or placebo. The data show that 1 year after women with a mean age of 63 initiated estrogen-plus-progestin therapy they had an increased relative risk of developing an ischemic stroke, which after an average follow-up of

5.6 years reached a 1.44 increased relative risk. There was no increased risk of having a hemorrhagic stroke. These data do not necessarily apply to younger recently postmenopausal healthy women, as two thirds of the women in the WHI were older than age 60 at the time they were enrolled in the study.

D. R. Mishell, Jr, MD

Association Between Reproductive and Hormonal Factors and Age-Related Maculopathy in Postmenopausal Women
Snow KK, Cote J, Yang W, et al (Massachusetts Eye and Ear Infirmary, Boston; Harvard School of Public Health, Boston; Harvard Med School, Boston)
Am J Ophthalmol 134:842-848, 2002   12–9

Introduction.—Age-related maculopathy (ARM) is the most frequent cause of irreversible vision loss and legal blindness in the United States in persons aged 65 years or older. There are few therapeutic or preventive measures for ARM. The association between several reproductive risk factors, including the use of hormone replacement therapy (HRT) and oral contraceptives, and the severity of ARM were examined in the Registry Study of Macular Degeneration and the Progression of Macular Degeneration Study, a longitudinal investigation designed to measure various risk factors for the onset and progression of maculopathy.

Methods.—A total of 237 participants in the Progression Study and 333 in the Registry Study were female. Of these, 394 were postmenopausal women with ARM. Logistic regression analyses were used to compare the effects of various reproductive factors across 2 groups: 193 patients with nonadvanced ARM and 201 with advanced ARM. Multivariate model building was used to evaluate the relation between reproductive, hormonal variables and level of ARM.

Results.—Mean patient age was 69.8 years (range, 50-78 years). Women with ARM who had used postmenopausal estrogen therapy had significantly lower odds of advanced ARM compared with nonusers after controlling for other known and potential risk factors (odds ratio, 0.05; 95% confidence interval, 0.30-0.98). Older age at menarche was linked with increased odds of advanced ARM (odds ratio, 1.16; 95% confidence interval, 1.00-1.35). Women with advanced ARM were roughly twice as likely to have been heavy smokers as women with nonadvanced ARM (35.3% vs 17.7%).

Conclusion.—The use of postmenopausal estrogen therapy seems to decrease the odds of advanced ARM in postmenopausal women with ARM. Women who had received postmenopausal estrogen therapy had 54% lower odds of advanced ARM compared with estrogen nonusers after adjusting for other factors.

▶ ARM is the most common cause of vision loss and blindness among people in the United States older than 65 years. Some, but not all, previous observational studies have suggested that postmenopausal estrogen use is associated with a reduced incidence of ARM as well as cataracts in women. The results of this cross-sectional study of women with ARM suggest that use of postmenopausal estrogen is associated with a 50% reduction in the risk of developing advanced ARM. If these results are confirmed by prospective randomized trials, women need to be informed about this benefit of estrogen together with the other benefits and risks when they decide whether to take estrogen for long periods of time after menopause.

D. R. Mishell, Jr, MD

Influence of Estrogen Plus Progestin on Breast Cancer and Mammography in Healthy Postmenopausal Women: The Women's Health Initiative Randomized Trial
Chlebowski RT, for the WHI Investigators (Harbor-Univ of California, Torrance; et al)
JAMA 289:3243-3253, 2003   12–10

Background.—The Women's Health Initiative (WHI), a trial of combined estrogen and progestin, was terminated early because overall health risks, including invasive breast cancer, were found to exceed benefits. The relationship among estrogen plus progestin use, breast cancer characteristics, and mammography recommendations was investigated.

Methods.—Between 1993 and 1998, 16,608 postmenopausal women, aged 50 to 79 years, underwent a comprehensive breast cancer risk assessment at 40 centers and were randomly assigned to receive combined conjugated equine estrogens, 0.625 mg/d, plus medroxyprogesterone acetate, 2.5 mg/d, or placebo. All women had an intact uterus. Screening mammography and clinical breast examinations were done at baseline and annually thereafter.

Findings.—Intent-to-treat analyses demonstrated that, compared with placebo, estrogen plus progestin increased total and invasive breast cancers, the hazard ratios being 1.24 and 1.24, respectively. Compared with invasive breast cancers diagnosed in the placebo group, those diagnosed in the estrogen plus progestin group were larger and at a more advanced stage. The invasive breast cancers in the 2 groups were similar in histology and grade. After 1 year, the proportion of women with abnormal mammographic findings was markedly higher in the estrogen plus progestin group than in the placebo group, a pattern that continued throughout the study.

Conclusions.—Relatively short-term combined estrogen plus progestin use increased incident breast cancers. These cancers were diagnosed at a more advanced stage than those diagnosed in the placebo recipients. The percentage of women with abnormal mammograms was also substantially increased by short-term combined estrogen plus progestin use. Thus, estrogen plus progestin may stimulate the growth of breast cancer while hindering its diagnosis.

▶ The results of this analysis of breast cancer in the large randomized trial called the WHI are somewhat surprising because the increased risk of diagnosis in the women taking estrogen plus progestin became evident after 4 years in the trial, and the breast cancers in the group receiving hormone were more advanced than the breast cancers in the placebo group. Several observational studies have shown an increased risk of breast cancer diagnosis mainly in women who took estrogen plus progestin for periods longer than 5 years, and also showed that the cancers in hormone users were less advanced than women of similar age who had not taken hormones. Perhaps the combination of estrogen plus progestin increases the risk of diagnosis of breast cancer earlier in older than younger women. The median age of enrollment in the WHI was 63. Estrogen plus progestin appears to promote the growth of preexisting breast cancers and does not initiate breast cancer, as the risk of diagnosis is not increased in former users. Older women are more likely to have preexisting breast cancer than younger women. One must remember that the estrogen-only arm of the WHI showed no increase in risk of breast cancer diagnosis compared with placebo after 5 years of the trial, in contrast to the findings of estrogen plus progestin. Short-term use of estrogen alone for symptom relief should not alter the risk of breast cancer.

D. R. Mishell, Jr, MD

▶ This is a follow-up article from the original WHI report providing some more detail on the incident breast cancers that developed.[1] The follow-up data appear to show a more significant increase in total breast cancers and invasive breast cancers in the patients treated with estrogen and progestin. Most previous studies have shown that cancers occurring in patients on hormone replacement therapy tend to be smaller, better differentiated, and have a better prognosis.[2] Unfortunately, in this group, tumors were found to be slightly larger and a few more of them were at a more advanced stage than the patients in the control group. The effect on breast cancer mortality by these worse prognostic factors is not stated. The previous report had shown no increase in breast cancer mortality or in total mortality for the patients on estrogen and progestin.

D. S. Miller, MD

References

1. 2003 YEAR BOOK OF OBSTETRICS, GYNECOLOGY, AND WOMEN'S HEALTH, p 326.
2. Cheek J, Lacy J, Toth-Fejel S, et al: The impact of hormone replacement therapy on the detection and stage of breast cancer. *Arch Surg* 137:1015, 2002.

Relation of Regimens of Combined Hormone Replacement Therapy to Lobular, Ductal, and Other Histologic Types of Breast Carcinoma

Daling JR, Malone KE, Doody DR, et al (Fred Hutchinson Cancer Research Ctr, Seattle; Univ of Washington, Seattle; Univ of Southern California, Los Angeles; et al)

Cancer 95:2455-2464, 2002   12–11

Background.—The incidence of invasive lobular carcinoma among postmenopausal women has been increasing. This increase may be occurring partly because of changes in lesion classification over time, but the increase in combined hormone replacement therapy (CHRT) may also be partly responsible. Whether the CHRT played a role in the increased incidence of invasive lobular carcinoma was investigated.

Methods.—The current multicenter case-control study included 1749 postmenopausal women diagnosed with a first invasive breast tumor between 1994 and 1998 in addition to 1953 postmenopausal women without cancer identified through random-digit dialing. All cancer patients were younger than 65 years at diagnosis. Data were collected in in-person interviews.

Findings.—The use of unopposed estrogen replacement therapy (ERT) did not correlate with an increase in risk of any histologic type of breast cancer, and the risk did not increase with duration of use. However, the risks of invasive lobular breast carcinoma and of breast carcinoma of other histologic types was increased among women who were currently using CHRT, with odds ratios (ORs) of 2.2 (95% confidence interval [CI], 1.4-3.3) and 1.9 (95% CI, 1.0-3.4), respectively. The risk for the mixed lobular-ductal type was greater than that for the pure lobular type of breast cancer, though the difference was nonsignificant. Continuous CHRT use for 5 years or longer seemed to correlate with a greater risk of lobular breast carcinoma compared with that of sequential CHRT. Current continuous CHRT use correlated only moderately with risk of ductal breast carcinoma.

Conclusions.—Postmenopausal women who use CHRT seem to be at increased risk of developing lobular breast carcinoma. Neither ERT nor CHRT markedly increased the risk of ductal breast carcinoma in women younger than 65 years.

▶ Women with breast cancer of the lobular type have a better prognosis than women whose cancer has ductal histologic finding. Several studies, including this, indicate that postmenopausal hormone use is only associated with an increased risk of the less common more benign lobular type of breast cancer and not the more common ductal type. Several other studies have reported that the prognosis for survival among postmenopausal women whose breast cancer is diagnosed while they are taking hormones is significantly better than women of similar age who are not taking hormones at the time of breast cancer diagnosis. The better prognosis in hormone users may be related to an increased incidence of lobular cancer among hormone users. The results of this study, as well as the Women's Health Initiative, found an increased risk of breast cancer diagnosis to be present only among women who took estrogen plus a progestin, not estrogen alone. It appears that progestins, not estrogen, may stimulate the growth of lobular breast cancers and not ductal breast cancers, and thus, only increase the risk of diagnosis of breast cancers with a more favorable prognosis.

D. R. Mishell, Jr, MD

Relationship Between Long Durations and Different Regimens of Hormone Therapy and Risk of Breast Cancer

Li CI, Malone KE, Porter PI, et al (Fred Hutchinson Cancer Research Ctr, Seattle; Univ of Washington, Seattle)

JAMA 289:3254-3263, 2003   12–12

Background.—Women taking combined estrogen and progestin hormone replacement therapy (CHRT) are known to be at increased risk for breast cancer. However, few data are available on longer durations and risks associated with patterns of use. The relationships between durations and patterns of CHRT use and breast cancer risk by histologic type and hormone receptor status were investigated.

Methods.—This population-based, case-control study included 975 women, aged 65 to 69 years, diagnosed as having invasive breast cancer from 1997 to 1999 and 1007 population controls. One hundred ninety-six cancers were lobular; 656, ductal; 114, other histologic type; and 9, unspecified. Six hundred forty-six cancers were estrogen receptor (ER) and progesterone receptor (PR) positive (ER+/PR+); 147, ER+/PR−; and 101, ER−/PR−.

Findings.—Women taking unopposed estrogen replacement therapy, even for 25 years or more, did not have an appreciably increased risk of breast cancer, although the odds ratios were consistent with a possible small effect. Women who had ever used CHRT had a 1.7-fold increase in their risk of breast cancer, including a 2.7-fold increase in the risk of invasive lobular carcinoma, a 1.5-fold increase in the risk of invasive ductal carcinoma, and a 2-fold increase in the risk of ER+/PR+ breast cancers. This increase was highest among women using CHRT for longer durations. Users for 5 to 14.9 years and for 15 years or longer had increases of 1.5-fold and 1.6-fold, respectively, in the risk of invasive ductal carcinoma, along with a 3.7-fold and 2.6-fold increase in the risk of invasive lobular carcinoma, respectively.

Conclusions.—The use of CHRT appears to be associated with an increased risk of breast cancer, especially invasive lobular tumors. This risk is apparent whether the progestin is taken in a sequential or continuous fashion.

▶ There are now more than 5 observational studies, including this one, that have reported no increase in the risk of breast cancer diagnosis among postmenopausal women taking estrogen alone, and a significant increase in breast cancer diagnosis in women taking a combination of estrogen and progestin. These findings are in agreement with those of the large randomized trial called the Women's Health Initiative, which has also found an increased risk of breast cancer among women taking an estrogen-progestin combination, compared with placebo, but after a mean of 5 years, no increased risk of breast cancer in women taking estrogen alone. The only reason to give a progestin with estrogen postmenopausally is to reduce the risk of the estrogen-related increase in adenocarcinoma of the endometrium. Since this estrogen-related cancer is nearly always preceded by endometrial hyperplasia, perhaps women with a uterus should be treated with estrogen alone in low doses and have the endometrial thickness monitored periodically by sonography. If the endometrial echo complex exceeds 4 mm, a biopsy can be performed to determine the histology, followed by appropriate therapy.

D. R. Mishell, Jr, MD

Effects of Hormone Replacement Therapy on C-Reactive Protein Levels in Healthy Postmenopausal Women: Comparison Between Oral and Transdermal Administration of Estrogen
Modena MG, Bursi F, Fantini G, et al (Univ of Modena, Italy)
Am J Med 113:331-333, 2002   12–13

Background.—An elevated plasma level of C-reactive protein (CRP) is considered to be a risk factor associated with myocardial infarction and strokes and is found to be useful in cardiovascular risk stratification. Studies have shown that hormone replacement therapy (HRT) seems to increase CRP levels. Because the effects of different hormonal preparations and their methods of administration are unknown, the effects of oral estrogen and transdermal estradiol on CRP levels in postmenopausal women were compared.

Methods.—Eighty-two healthy postmenopausal women who had not undergone hysterectomy were enrolled in the study and divided into 3 groups that were based on HRT status: 29 women using oral conjugated equine estrogen (0.625 mg daily) plus medroxyprogesterone acetate (2.5 mg daily), 33 women using transdermal 17 β-estradiol (50 μg daily) plus medroxyprogesterone acetate (2.5 mg daily), and 20 women who were receiving no HRT.

Results.—No significant differences were found in age, heart rate, blood pressure, body mass index, exercise frequency, or time from menopause among the 3 groups of women. When compared with women not receiving HRT, women taking oral estrogen had median CRP levels that were 40% higher ($P < .05$) and women who were using transdermal estradiol had median CRP levels that were 35% lower ($P < .05$). When the oral estrogen group and the transdermal estradiol group were compared, the women taking oral estrogen had median CRP levels more than twice as high.

Conclusions.—The possibility exists that synthesis of CRP, which occurs exclusively in the liver, is induced by estrogen. It has been hypothesized that estrogen has 2 effects on hepatic cells, a direct effect and an indirect effect. The direct effect is when a large amount of the hormone reaches the hepatocyte as a result of the first-pass effect, and the indirect effect is one mediated by a reduction in circulating proinflammatory cytokines.

Effect of Transdermal Estradiol and Oral Conjugated Estrogen on C-Reactive Protein in Retinoid-Placebo Trial in Healthy Women

Decensi A, Omodei U, Robertson C, et al (European Inst of Oncology, Milan, Italy; Univ of Brescia, Italy; Univ of Varese, Italy)
Circulation 106:1224-1228, 2002   12–14

Background.—C-reactive protein (CRP) levels increase during oral conjugated equine estrogen (CEE) treatment and may explain the initial excess of cardiovascular disease that has been observed in clinical studies. The effects of oral CEE, transdermal estradiol (transdermal E2), fenretinide, and placebo on the 6- and 12-month changes in CRP levels in a biomarker trial of breast cancer and coronary heart disease risk were compared.

Methods.—A total of 226 research subjects were randomly selected from September 1, 1998, through October 1, 2000 (114 taking transdermal E2 and 112 taking oral CEE). Thirty-three participants had dropped out because of adverse events or voluntary withdrawal, and 4 participants had insufficient serum available. A total of 189 participants were randomly assigned for 1 year to 1 of 3 groups: (1) transdermal E2 weekly patch (50 µg/d) and fenretinide capsules (100 mg twice daily), (2) transdermal E2 and placebo capsules, oral CEE (0.625 mg/d) and fenretinide, or (3) oral CEE and placebo. Sequential medroxyprogesterone acetate (10 mg/d orally) was added to continuous estrogen replacement therapy for the first 12 days of each month.

Results.—All the variables were evenly distributed among the groups. Among women taking oral CEE, relative to baseline, CRP levels increased at 6 and 12 months; however, CRP levels did not increase among the women taking transdermal E2, as shown by repeated-measures analysis of covariance models. No change was found in CRP levels from 6 to 12 months ($P = .87$). The model predicted a 10% increase in the CRP level at 6 months compared with baseline for a woman with a median CRP level and median body mass index if she had been given transdermal E2 and a 48% increase if she had been given oral CEE. At 12 months, the corresponding figures were 3% and 64% for transdermal E2 and oral CEE, respectively. Transdermal E2 induced a mean percentage change in CRP levels at 6 months of –38% relative to oral CEE ($P = .004$) as indicated by analysis results, and at 12 months, the percentage change associated with transdermal E2 was –48% relative to oral CEE ($P = .012$).

Conclusions.—No significant changes were found in CRP levels for up to 12 months of treatment with transdermal E2, whereas oral CEE increased CRP levels by 48% and 64% at 6 and 12 months of treatment, respectively, relative to baseline. During the initial 12 months of estrogen replacement therapy, transdermal E2 may be associated with a safer effect on coronary heart disease. In contrast to CEE, transdermal E2 does not increase CRP levels in healthy women. However, women who are heavier and have a high body mass index showed high end point CRP values significantly above the effect of oral CEE.

▶ These 2 studies (Abstracts 12–13 and 12–14), one a prospective randomized controlled trial and the other an observational study, found that oral CEE was associated with an increase in CRP levels and transdermal E2 was not associated with such an increase. The CRP level is an index of low-grade inflammation associated with endothelial dysfunction. Elevated levels of CRP are a risk factor for myocardial infarction and strokes. The increase in CRP level associated with oral but not transdermal estrogen may be caused by the high hepatic concentrations of estrogen with oral administration due to the first-pass effect of the steroid and not due to inflammatory changes in the arteries. Whether the increase in CRP levels associated with oral estrogen is due to vascular inflammation and atherogenesis or only the metabolic effect of increased liver synthesis of this protein remains to be determined.

Until additional studies are performed to determine the cause of increased CRP levels with administration of oral estrogens, clinicians may prefer to prescribe transdermal E2 instead of oral estrogen to women with cardiovascular risk factors, including obesity.

D. R. Mishell, Jr, MD

Twice-Weekly Transdermal Estradiol and Vaginal Progesterone as Continuous Combined Hormone Replacement Therapy in Postmenopausal Women: A 1-Year Prospective Study
Cicinelli E, de Ziegler D, Galantino P, et al (Univ of Bari, Italy; Nyon Med Ctr, Switzerland)
Am J Obstet Gynecol 187:556-560, 2002   12–15

Introduction.—One of the major reasons women interrupt hormone replacement therapy (HRT) is uterine bleeding. Selecting the optimal progestational agent in HRT regimens is challenging and the subject of much debate. Examined was the acceptability and endometrial safety of twice-weekly transdermal estradiol 0.05 mg systems and Crinone 4% vaginal progesterone gel 45 mg/d as a continuous combined nonoral HRT regimen.

Methods.—Thirty-five postmenopausal women participated in a 1-year prospective, observational trial. Participants underwent evaluations of blood pressure, weight, endometrial thickness, and endometrial histologic characteristics. Mean values were compared before and after treatment. Patients made daily recordings of vaginal bleeding and spotting episodes and medications taken or omitted.

Results.—Twenty-six (74.3%) women completed the 1-year investigation. Of 350 menstrual cycles in the cohort, 287 (82%) were amenorrheic and 63 (18%) were associated with some bleeding or spotting. Twenty-three (88.5%) patients were amenorrheic after 6 months of therapy, as were all 26 by 12 months of treatment (Fig 1). At 3-month follow-up, blood pressure

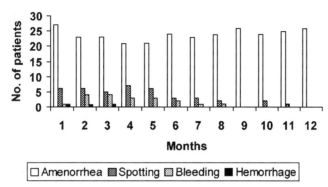

FIGURE 1.—Bleeding pattern as assessed by daily self-reporting diary card during 1-year study of 35 postmenopausal women treated with twice-weekly transdermal estradiol and vaginal progesterone (Crinone 4%). (Reprinted by permission of the publisher courtesy of Cicinelli E, de Ziegler D, Galantino P, et al: Twice-weekly transdermal estradiol and vaginal progesterone as continuous combined hormone replacement therapy in postmenopausal women: A 1-year prospective study. *Am J Obstet Gynecol* 187:556-560, 2002. Copyright 2002 by Elsevier.)

and weight were significantly reduced. These effects persisted through the 12-month follow-up. At the 12-month evaluation, endometrial thickness was significantly greater compared with baseline (4.6 mm vs 3.6 mm; $P <$ .0005). Histologic examination showed endometrial atrophy in 24 (92.3%) women and signs of decidualization in 2.

Conclusion.—Transdermal estradiol and twice-weekly administration of Crinone vaginal progesterone gel is a new and viable HRT regimen. It is a practical option for a no-bleed treatment that assures both high endometrial protection and the inherent safety associated with administering physiologic hormones nonorally.

▶ Many postmenopausal women wish to take natural, not synthetic, hormones to relieve vasomotor symptoms and vaginal dryness. Oral progesterone is given once daily and is associated with drowsiness. In this study vaginal progesterone and a transdermal estradiol patch were each given twice weekly and there was no evidence of proliferative endometrium. Bleeding control was good, but information about side effects was not stated. Randomized studies comparing this therapeutic regimen with others should be undertaken, as this pilot study indicates that vaginal progesterone may have advantages compared with oral progesterone or synthetic progestins.

D. R. Mishell, Jr, MD

Transdermal Progesterone and Its Effect on Vasomotor Symptoms, Blood Lipid Levels, Bone Metabolic Markers, Moods, and Quality of Life for Postmenopausal Women

Wren BG, Champion SM, Willetts K, et al (Royal Hosp for Women, Randwick, Australia)
Menopause 10:13-18, 2003   12–16

Introduction.—There is debate concerning how transdermal progesterone is metabolized and its effect on postmenopausal symptoms. Transdermal cream containing either progesterone or placebo was compared in a parallel, double-blind, randomized, placebo-controlled investigation to determine whether transdermal progesterone has any influence on mood, sexual feelings, vasomotor function, or bone and lipid metabolism.

Methods.—Eighty postmenopausal women were randomly assigned to treatment with transdermal cream containing either progesterone 32 mg daily or placebo. Participants were evaluated with the Greene Climacteric Scale and the Menopause Quality of Life Questionnaire, along with blood analysis for lipids and bone markers during a 12-week evaluation period.

Results.—There were no reported changes in vasomotor symptoms, mood characteristics, or sexual feelings. No changes in blood lipid levels or bone metabolism markers were observed, despite a small elevation in blood progesterone levels.

Conclusion.—Use of the transdermal route to administer progesterone 32 mg daily does not appear to provide adequate hormone to enter the body to achieve a biologic effect on lipid levels, bone mineral markers, vasomotor symptoms, or moods.

▶ Transdermal administration of progesterone cream has been widely advocated by many clinicians to alleviate postmenopausal hot flushes and prevent osteoporosis. Many women utilize this therapy despite a paucity of evidence regarding a beneficial effect of transdermal progesterone. The results of this placebo-controlled, randomized trial found that progesterone cream did not result in significantly better short-term effects on mood, vasomotor symptoms, or markers of bone resorption than did placebo. Women should be advised that despite widespread publicity there is a lack of proven benefit of transdermal progesterone cream upon menopausal symptoms or bone loss.

D. R. Mishell Jr, MD

A Randomized Controlled Trial of Estrogen Replacement Therapy in Long-term Users of Depot Medroxyprogesterone Acetate

Cundy T, Ames R, Horne A, et al (Univ of Auckland, New Zealand)
J Clin Endocrinol Metab 88:78-81, 2003   12–17

Background.—The long-term use of the injectable contraceptive depot medroxyprogesterone acetate (DMPA) has been associated with decreased bone mineral density (BMD), especially in the lumbar spine. The cause of this bone loss is unknown. However, the relative estrogen deficiency induced by DMPA use may be responsible.

Methods.—Thirty-eight premenopausal women with a mean age of 37 years were enrolled in a randomized, double-blind, controlled trial of oral estrogen replacement therapy. All participants had a minimum 2-year duration of DMPA use and below-average baseline lumbar spine BMD. Nineteen women were assigned to conjugated estrogens, 0.625 mg/d orally, and 19 to placebo. In all women, regular DMPA injections were continued during the study period. Twenty-six patients completed the 2 years of the study.

Findings.—During the 2-year study, mean lumbar spine BMD increased by 1% in the estrogen-treated group and declined by 2.6% in the placebo group. Between-group differences at 12, 18, and 24 months were 2%, 3.2%, and 3.5%, respectively. Less significant differences occurred in the femoral neck, Ward's triangle, greater trochanter, total body, legs, and trunk. No major adverse events occurred.

Conclusions.—Estrogen deficiency is probably the cause of DMPA-related bone loss. The current data suggest that such bone loss can be arrested by estrogen replacement treatment.

▶ Many studies have shown that women receiving DMPA injections for long periods of time have decreased BMD. However, after stopping DMPA there appears to be a reversal of bone loss. Furthermore, there are no reports of an increased incidence of fracture in former DMPA users compared with nonusers. If women taking DMPA are concerned about having decreased bone density, estrogen therapy can be given together with DMPA.

D. R. Mishell, Jr, MD

Phytoestrogen Supplements for the Treatment of Hot Flashes: The Isoflavone Clover Extract (ICE) Study: A Randomized Controlled Trial
Tice JA, Ettinger B, Ensrud K, et al (Univ of California, San Francisco; Univ of Minnesota, Minneapolis; Kaiser Permanente Med Care Program, Oakland, Calif; et al)
JAMA 290:207-214, 2003   12–18

Background.—Isoflavone-containing dietary supplements are among the new options being tried for the treatment of menopausal symptoms. Few data on this treatment are available. The efficacy and safety of 2 different isoflavone-containing supplements derived from red clover were compared with placebo for the treatment of menopausal hot flashes.

Methods.—The trial included 252 recently postmenopausal women experiencing hot flashes, at least 35 per week. Vegetarians, those who frequently consumed soy products, and those who took medications affecting isoflavone absorption were excluded. After 2 weeks on placebo, the women were randomly assigned to receive 1 of 2 supplements—Promensil or Rimostil, providing 82 and 57 mg/d of total isoflavones, respectively—or placebo. At the end of 12 weeks of treatment, patient diary data were used to compare the change in frequency of hot flashes between the groups. Quality-of-life effects of adverse outcomes were monitored as well.

Results.—Ninety-eight percent of women enrolled completed the trial. The 3 groups all had similar reductions in mean daily hot flash count: about 5 per day. Quality-of-life outcomes and adverse effects were also similar among groups. Promensil was associated with a more rapid reduction in hot flashes compared with placebo; this effect was not significant for Rimostil.

Conclusions.—The isoflavone-containing supplements Promensil and Rimostil do not significantly reduce menopausal hot flashes compared with placebo. The effect of Promensil on the rate of reduction in hot flashes supports the existence of some biologic effect. However, neither supplement shows a clinically significant effect.

▶ Dietary supplements containing isoflavone in both soy products and red clover are used by many postmenopausal women for the treatment of menopausal symptoms, particularly hot flashes. This large, well-done randomized trial compared the effects of 2 widely used dietary supplements containing either 41 or 29 mg of isoflavones per tablet with a placebo tablet. Although there was a sizable reduction in hot flashes with the soy products, the magnitude of reduction was not significantly different from placebo. Clinicians should strongly advise patients not to take soy or red clover to reduce menopausal symptoms, as these costly agents are no better than placebo.

D. R. Mishell, Jr, MD

Effect of Soy-Derived Isoflavones on Hot Flushes, Endometrial Thickness, and the Pulsatility Index of the Uterine and Cerebral Arteries
Penotti M, Fabio E, Modena AB, et al (Istituti Clinici di Perfezionamento, Milan, Italy; Istituto Auxologico Italiano, Milan, Italy; Univ of Parma, Italy; et al)
Fertil Steril 79:1112-1117, 2003   12–19

Background.—Soy and its derivatives are major components of Asian diets. These dietary components are the prevalent source of isoflavones, a category of phytoestrogens. The soy isoflavones include genistine and daidzine. The effects of soy-derived isoflavones on hot flushes, endometrial thickness, and the vascular reactivity of uterine and cerebral arteries were investigated.

Methods and Findings.—Sixty-two healthy postmenopausal women, aged 45 to 60 years, volunteered for the double-blind, randomized, placebo-controlled study. Participants received soy-derived isoflavones, 72 mg, or placebo. Both groups had a 40% decline in the number of hot flushes (Fig 1). The isoflavones did not affect endometrial thickness or the arterial pulsatility index of the uterine or cerebral arteries.

Conclusions.—In this series, daily administration of 72 mg of soy-derived isoflavones was no more effective than placebo in decreasing hot flushes. The isoflavones also had no effect on endometrial thickness or on the pulsatility index of the uterine or cerebral arteries.

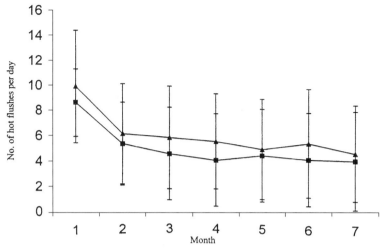

FIGURE 1.—Number of hot flushes per month. *Closed triangles*, Treated group; *closed box*, placebo group. (Courtesy of Penotti M, Fabio E, Modena AB, et al: Effect of soy-derived isoflavones on hot flushes, endometrial thickness, and the pulsatility index of the uterine and cerebral arteries. *Fertil Steril* 9:1112-1117, 2003. Copyright American Society for Reproductive Medicine. With permission from the American College of Surgeons.)

▶ Many women are now using alternative medical compounds instead of estrogen for relief of hot flushes and other symptoms of estrogen deficiency. The results of this well-done randomized trial indicate that ingestion of high doses of soy isoflavones did not diminish the incidence of hot flushes more than placebo therapy. The majority of randomized trials of soy and other alternative medical compounds agree with the results of this study, which indicate that these agents are no more effective than placebo for improvement of vasomotor symptoms.

D. R. Mishell, Jr, MD

A Randomized Placebo-Controlled Crossover Trial With Phytoestrogens in Treatment of Menopause in Breast Cancer Patients
Nikander E, Kilkkinen A, Metsä-Heikkilä M, et al (Helsinki Univ; Natl Public Health Inst, Helsinki; Univ of Helsinki)
Obstet Gynecol 101:1213-1220, 2003   12–20

Background.—Phytoestrogens are popular with the public as a treatment for the symptoms of menopause. A placebo-controlled, double-blind, crossover study was performed to compare phytoestrogens with placebo for treatment of the symptoms of menopause in breast cancer survivors.

Study Design.—The study group consisted of 56 breast cancer survivors who complained of incapacitating hot flashes after the onset of spontaneous menopause. These women were randomly assigned to either 114 mg of phytoestrogens daily for 3 months or a placebo, followed by a 2-month washout period and then 3 months of crossover to the other regimen. The results of general and pelvic examinations, blood samples, the Kupperman index for menopausal symptoms, visual analogue scale for symptoms, and a rating of physical and mental working capacity were recorded before and after each treatment period. Study participants also kept weekly diaries of health, side effects, bleeding, and medication use. The women indicated their treatment preference at the end of the study.

Findings.—Phytoestrogens were well tolerated. The Kupperman index; quality of life parameters; and levels of follicle-stimulating hormone, luteinizing hormone, estradiol, and sex hormone–binding globulin were not significantly different between the 2 treatment arms. Among the 56 women, 44.6% preferred the phytoestrogen regimen, 26.8% preferred the placebo, and 28.6% had no preference.

Conclusion.—Phytoestrogens did not relieve hot flashes or other symptoms of menopause in breast cancer survivors.

▶ Phytoestrogens are present in soybeans and red clover and are widely used as a so-called natural alternative to estrogen to treat hot flashes and other menopausal symptoms. This well-designed, randomized, crossover study demonstrates that daily ingestion of high doses of phytoestrogens was no more effective than placebo for relief of hot flashes or improvement of mood and quality of life. Women should be informed that the beneficial effect of phytoestrogens upon menopausal symptoms is no greater than placebo. Other studies have demonstrated that estrogen prevents hot flashes significantly more than placebo. Therefore, estrogen is superior to phytoestrogens for the relief of hot flashes.

D. R. Mishell, Jr, MD

13 Abortion

Circulating Levels of Inhibin A, Activin A and Follistatin in Missed and Recurrent Miscarriages
Muttukrishna S, Jauniaux E, Greenwold N, et al (Royal Free-UCL Med School, London; Imperial College Med School, London; Oxford Brookes Univ, England)
Hum Reprod 17:3072-3078, 2002   13–1

Introduction.—Normal pregnancy is associated with high circulating levels of serum inhibin A, activin A, and follistatin. However, little is known about the biologic roles of these proteins in pregnancy. Inhibin A, activin A, and follistatin were evaluated as possible serum markers of early pregnancy loss.

Methods.—The study used blood samples from 10 women with sporadic missed miscarriage, 15 control women undergoing pregnancy termination at 8 to 12 weeks' gestation, and 12 women with a history of unexplained recurrent miscarriages at 6 to 12 weeks' gestation. In each sample, levels of inhibin A, activin A, and follistatin were measured along with human chorionic gonadotropin (hCG), estradiol, and progesterone.

Results.—Levels of inhibin A, hCG, estradiol, and progesterone were approximately 2- to 3-fold lower in women with sporadic miscarriages compared with control subjects (Fig 1). Among the women with recurrent miscarriages, patterns of change in inhibin A and hCG were significantly different for women with subsequent miscarriage compared with those with subsequent live birth. Levels of inhibin A and hCG at 6 to 7 weeks were approximately 4-fold lower in the women with subsequent miscarriages, whereas estradiol levels were approximately 2-fold lower (Fig 3). Inhibin A levels were near the limit of detection. Normal control subjects showed a positive correlation between serum inhibin A and hCG and between progesterone and estradiol, whereas sporadic miscarriages showed a positive correlation between inhibin A and progesterone.

Conclusions.—Serum inhibin A is a potentially useful and specific biochemical marker of early pregnancy loss. The inhibin A level drops significantly before the first symptoms of recurrent miscarriage appear. Levels of inhibin A and hCG are strongly correlated in women with miscarriage, suggesting their possible use in predicting the outcomes of future pregnancies.

▶ Trophoblastic tissues synthesize the proteins inhibin A, activin A, and follistatin. In normal pregnancies levels of inhibin A increase until 12 weeks of

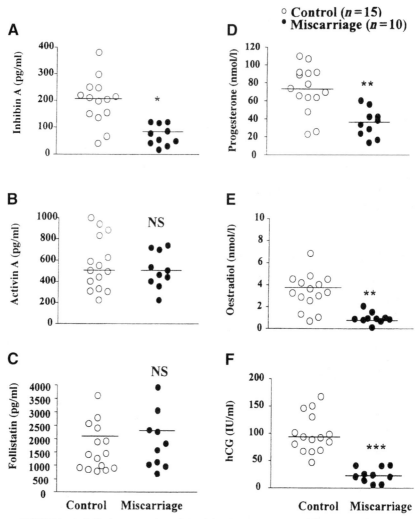

FIGURE 1.—Individual concentrations of (A) inhibin A, (B) activin A, (C) follistatin, (D) progesterone, (E) estradiol, and (F) hCG in the maternal serum of control pregnant women undergoing pregnancy termination (n = 15) and patients with missed abortions (n = 10) at 8 to 12 weeks' gestation. *Straight lines* across are the medians. Student *t* test results: *P < .05; **P < .01; ***P < .001. *Abbreviation:* NS, Not significant. (Courtesy of Muttukrishna S, Jauniaux E, Greenwold N, et al: Circulating levels of inhibin A, activin A and follistatin in missed and recurrent miscarriages. *Hum Reprod* 17:3072-3078, 2002. Copyright European Society for Human Reproduction and Embryology, by permission of Oxford University Press.)

gestation, after which they decline to a nadir and remain low in the second trimester. The results of this study indicate that there is a good correlation between levels of inhibin A (but not activin A or follistatin) and progesterone and hCG. In women with recurrent pregnancy loss, levels of both hCG and inhibin A were lower at 6 to 7 weeks' gestation in women who subsequently had a miscarriage than in those who had a viable birth. Perhaps inhibin A levels as

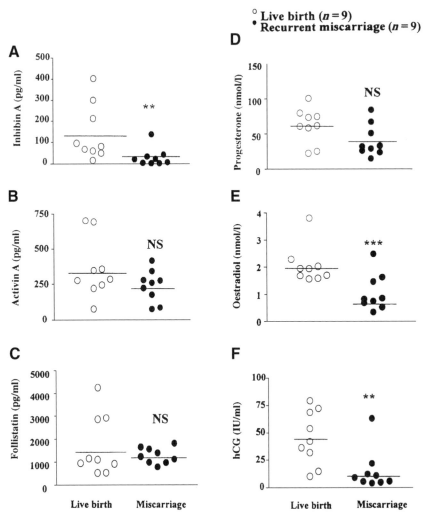

FIGURE 3.—Individual concentrations of (A) inhibin A, (B) activin A, (C) follistatin, (D) progesterone, (E) estradiol, and (F) hCG in the maternal plasma of recurrent miscarriage patients who subsequently had live births (n = 9) or recurrent miscarriages (n = 9). Samples were taken at 6 to 7 weeks' gestation. *Straight lines* across are the medians. Paired student *t* test results: * * * *P* < .001; * * *P* < .01. *Abbreviation:* NS, Not significant. (Courtesy of Muttukrishna S, Jauniaux E, Greenwold N, et al: Circulating levels of inhibin A, activin A and follistatin in missed and recurrent miscarriages. *Hum Reprod* 17:3072-3078, 2002. Copyright European Society for Human Reproduction and Embryology, by permission of Oxford University Press.)

well as hCG levels should be measured at 6 to 7 weeks' gestation in women with recurrent early pregnancy loss to provide a better prognosis for the pregnancy than measuring hCG alone.

D. R. Mishell, Jr, MD

Plasma Folate Levels and Risk of Spontaneous Abortion

George L, Mills JL, Johansson ALV, et al (Karolinska Institutet, Stockholm; NIH, Bethesda, Md; Danderyds Hosp, Stockholm)
JAMA 288:1867-1873, 2002   13–2

Background.—Some studies have suggested that folate deficiency is a risk factor for spontaneous abortions; however, some have suggested that folate supplementation is a risk factor for spontaneous abortions. Sweden has not introduced folic acid fortification. This large, population-based, case-control study examined the association between plasma folate levels and the risk of early spontaneous abortions in Sweden.

Study Design.—The study group consisted of 468 women who had spontaneous abortions at 6 to 12 weeks of pregnancy from 1996 through 1998 in Uppsala County, Sweden. The control group consisted of 921 pregnant women from the same county, matched to case subjects by gestational week. Interviews were conducted to obtain information on potential risk factors for spontaneous abortions. Blood was collected for plasma folic acid and cotinine assay. Maternal plasma folate levels were compared with the risk of a spontaneous abortion.

Findings.—Women with low folate levels were at an increased risk of having spontaneous abortions, whereas women with normal or high folate levels had no increased risk of spontaneous abortions. Low maternal folate levels were associated with a significantly increased risk of a spontaneous abortion when a fetal karyotype abnormality existed but not when the fetal karyotype was normal.

Conclusions.—Low maternal serum folate levels are associated with an increased risk of a spontaneous abortion when the fetal karyotype is abnormal. Higher levels of folate are not associated with an increased risk of a spontaneous abortion. Folic acid fortification will not increase the rate of spontaneous abortions.

▶ Some previous studies have reported that folic acid deficiency is associated with an increased risk of a spontaneous abortion, but others have not found an association. This well-done case-control study found that low plasma folate levels were associated with an increased risk of spontaneous abortions when the fetal karyotype was abnormal but not when it was normal. Women wishing to conceive have been advised to ingest folic acid supplements to reduce the incidence of neural tube defects. Folic acid supplementation may also reduce the risk of a spontaneous abortion.

D. R. Mishell, Jr, MD

Increased Prevalence of Insulin Resistance in Women With a History of Recurrent Pregnancy Loss

Craig LB, Ke RW, Kutteh WH (Univ of Tennessee, Memphis)
Fertil Steril 78:487-490, 2002   13–3

Background.—From 2% to 4% of couples of reproductive age experience recurrent pregnancy loss (RPL), and many factors have been suggested as etiologic contributors. Even with recent advances in investigative tools, 30% to 40% of the cases are not explained. Women who have polycystic ovary syndrome have a higher incidence of pregnancy loss. These women also generally have increased rates of anovulation, androgen excess, insulin resistance (IR), and infertility. The rate of IR among women with polycystic ovary syndrome is about 40%. Whether IR is independently related to RPL was assessed.

Methods.—The participants were consecutive patients referred for RPL between April 2000 and January 2001. Evaluations were carried out for genetic, endocrinologic, anatomic, immunologic, microbiologic, and lifestyle factors influencing pregnancy. Both partners underwent karyotype assessment. Additional tests included hysterosalpingogram or hysteroscopy; midluteal serum progesterone determinations; serum levels of prolactin, thyrotropin, and lupus anticoagulant; IgG, IgM, and IgA anticardiolipin and antiphosphatidyl serine antibodies; and cervical cultures for mycoplasma, ureaplasma, and chlamydia. The definition of pregnancy loss used was any natural abortion that occurred before 20 weeks' gestation or before achievement of a fetal weight of 500 g. None of the participants had multiple losses with intermixed viable pregnancies, ectopic pregnancies, or molar pregnancies. A fasting insulin and serum glucose sample was drawn from each of the 74 participants. A control group consisted of 74 age-, weight-, and race-matched women who had at least one previous live born infant and no more than one previous miscarriage. The diagnosis of IR was applied to all women whose fasting insulin levels were at least 20 µU/mL or whose fasting glucose-to-fasting insulin ratio was less than 4.5.

Results.—Twenty women (27.0%) in the study group and 7 (9.5%) in the control group had IR. Sixteen of the 20 study group women and all 7 of the controls with IR had a fasting glucose–to–fasting insulin ratio of less than 4.5. Forty-five percent of the patients with IR and 53% of the women without IR had other causes of RPL. No correlation was apparent between the presence of IR and other identifiable causes of RPL.

Conclusions.—IR was found in 27.0% of the women with RPL but only 9.5% of the control group. Thus, the incidence of IR among women referred for evaluation of RPL was increased over that found in comparable women without RPL. Women who are to be evaluated for RPL should undergo assessment for IR, including a fasting insulin and glucose level determination.

▶ Women with polycystic ovary syndrome (PCOS) who become pregnant have a high rate of miscarriage. About 40% of women with PCOS also have IR. Whether the presence of IR in women with PCOS is associated with an increased incidence of miscarriage has not been investigated. In this study, the presence of IR was found to be 3 times more likely in women with RPL than an age- and weight-related control group. If the findings of this study are confirmed, women with unexplained RPL should have a fasting insulin and glucose level measured. If the glucose-to-insulin ratio is less than 4.5, it may be beneficial to treat these women with metformin in an attempt to increase the incidence of viable birth.

D. R. Mishell, Jr, MD

Management of Miscarriage: A Randomized Controlled Trial of Expectant Management versus Surgical Evacuation
Wieringa-de Waard M, Vos J, Bonsel GJ, et al (Univ of Amsterdam)
Hum Reprod 17:2445-2450, 2002   13–4

Background.—Surgical uterine evacuation is, in many countries, the standard treatment for women with a miscarriage. Several observational studies have advocated expectant management as an alternative to surgical uterine evacuation in these patients. Only 1 randomized clinical trial has been reported that compared both of these options in a hospital setting, and the results suggested similar outcomes for both management options. However, in this study, the duration of expectant management was restricted to 3 days. A longer period of expectant management and more information concerning patient preference are needed, particularly if it is confirmed that no significant differences exist in effectiveness, costs, and availability. These 3 variables of expectant management were compared with those of surgical evacuation in the management of miscarriage in a randomized, controlled study.

Methods.—The study included patients with an established diagnosis of early fetal demise or incomplete miscarriage at a gestational age of less than 16 completed weeks. A total of 122 women were selected randomly to either surgical evacuation or expectant management, and 305 women who refused to be selected in this manner were managed according to their preference.

Results.—No differences were noted in the number of emergency curettages and complications between the 2 treatment options. At 6 weeks, the efficacy of expectant management was 47%, compared with 95% for surgical evacuation. After 7 days of expectant management, 37% of women had a spontaneous complete miscarriage. Intention-to-treat analysis after 6 weeks showed similar effectiveness for the 2 modalities (92% vs 100%). Results in the group who were treated according to their preference were comparable with results in the randomized groups.

Conclusions.—In the management of miscarriage, an expectant management period of 7 days after diagnosis may prevent 37% of surgical procedures.

▶ A large group of women with first trimester uterine bleeding with either an incomplete abortion (n = 126) or early fetal demise (n = 64) were managed expectantly for 1 week. During this week, 37% had a spontaneous complete miscarriage. Some women may wish to delay having a rapid curettage to treat this problem if informed that by waiting 1 week, they have a 37% chance of not requiring the procedure.

D. R. Mishell, Jr, MD

Early Intrauterine Pregnancy Failure: A Randomized Trial of Medical Versus Surgical Treatment
Muffley PE, Stitely ML, Gherman RB (Naval Med Ctr, Portsmouth, Va; Bethesda Naval Hosp, Md)
Am J Obstet Gynecol 187:321-326, 2002   13–5

Background.—Curettage is the traditional treatment for early pregnancy failure. Medical treatment, with the synthetic prostaglandin E-1 analogue, misoprostol, could provide an alternative. This randomized clinical study compared medical and surgical treatment of patients with early pregnancy failure.

Study Design.—The study group consisted of 50 adult women with failed early intrauterine pregnancies who were randomly assigned to receive either surgical treatment with suction curettage or medical treatment with 1 to 2 doses of intravaginal misoprostol. Data were analyzed on an intention-to-treat basis.

Findings.—In the medical treatment group, 60% of the pregnancy terminations were successful, without requiring surgery. Over 60% of patients in the medical group required 2 doses. All surgical treatments were successful. There were no significant differences between the hematocrits of the 2 groups or the time needed to achieve negative human chorionic gonadotropin test results.

Conclusion.—Medical treatment of early intrauterine pregnancy failure with intravaginal misoprostol is noninvasive, effective, and well tolerated. Patients seemed to prefer it to surgical methods. The authors believe that medical treatment is a reasonable alternative and will eventually replace surgical treatment as the initial treatment for early pregnancy failure.

▶ Several studies have reported the management of early pregnancy failure with vaginal administration of 800 μg of misoprostol every 24 hours for 2 doses. Successful evacuation of the gestational tissue occurs in about 60% to 85% of women so treated. Clinicians may wish to offer this therapy to women with early pregnancy failure if they do not wish to have a curettage.

D. R. Mishell, Jr, MD

Management of Missed Abortion: Comparison of Medical Treatment With Either Mifepristone + Misoprostol or Misoprostol Alone With Surgical Evacuation: A Multi-Center Trial in Copenhagen County, Denmark
Grønlund A, Grønlund L, Clevin L, et al (Gentofte Univ Hosp, Denmark; Herlev Univ Hosp, Denmark; Glostrup Univ Hosp, Denmark)
Acta Obstet Gynecol Scand 81:1060-1065, 2002   13–6

Background.—Standard treatment for missed abortion has long been surgical evacuation (SE). The efficacy of 2 medical regimens was compared with that of SE in women with missed abortion.

Methods.—Between October 1999 and October 2000, 3 Danish centers enrolled 176 women in the prospective study. Regimens were alternated every 4 months. The women received mifepristone, 600 mg orally, plus misoprostol, 0.4 mg vaginally (Mf + Ms); misoprostol 0.4 mg vaginally (Ms); or conventional SE.

Findings.—Complete expulsion occurred within 1 week in 74% of women receiving Mf + Ms, 71% of those receiving Ms, and 96% receiving SE. Bleeding duration was 6.9, 7.1, and 2.5 days, respectively. A significantly better response to medical treatment was documented in women with an initial plasma chorionic gonadotrophin level between 2000 and 20,000 IU/L and a gestational age of less than 75 days than in women not meeting these criteria. Initial p-progesterone was unrelated to the success of medical therapy.

Conclusions.—In most women with missed abortion, vaginal misoprostol, 0.4 to 0.6 mg, is an effective treatment. Pretreatment with the anti-progesterone mifepristone does not appear to improve treatment success rates. Patient selection based on gestational age and initial plasma chorionic gonadotrophin levels may significantly increase the success rate of medical treatment.

▶ This prospective crossover study compared 2 methods of medical therapy with surgical evaluation of the uterus among a group of women with early pregnancy failure, either an anembryonic gestation or embryonic demise. Administration of 0.4 mg misoprostol vaginally resulted in 72% successful evaluation of the uterine contents. Use of 600 mg mifepristone 2 days prior to the same dose of misoprostol did not significantly improve the incidence of success but did result in a longer duration of bleeding. Additional doses of misoprostol also did not increase success. Several studies, including this one, have shown that in women with early pregnancy failure administration of a single dose of 0.4 to 0.8 mg of misoprostol results in about a 70% to 80% successful rate of evacuation of the uterine contents.

D. R. Mishell, Jr, MD

A Prospective Randomized Study to Compare the Use of Repeated Doses of Vaginal With Sublingual Misoprostol in the Management of First Trimester Silent Miscarriages

Tang OS, Lau WNT, Ng EHY, et al (Univ of Hong Kong)
Hum Reprod 18:176-181, 2003   13–7

Introduction.—Fifteen percent of first-trimester pregnancies end in spontaneous miscarriage. Surgical evacuation of the uterus is standard practice for managing miscarriage in many parts of the world and is successful in up to 98% of patients. This approach is associated with some serious adverse events, including postabortion pelvic infection, perforation of the uterus, and Asherman's syndrome. These complications may be irreversible and can seriously compromise future fertility. Repeated doses of sublingual misoprostol were compared with vaginal misoprostol for medical management of first-trimester miscarriages in a randomized, controlled trial.

Methods.—Eighty women who had silent miscarriages (at <13 weeks) were randomly assigned to treatment with either sublingual or vaginal doses of 600 µg misoprostol every 3 hours for a maximum of 3 doses. Treatment outcome was initially evaluated on day 7 after misoprostol with transvaginal US of the pelvis. Surgical evacuation was performed if a gestational sac was still present or if there was a significant amount of the products of conception in the uterus, along with clinical evidence of heavy vaginal bleeding.

Results.—The success rates of medical management were identical in both groups (87.5%; 95% confidence interval, 74%-95%) and there were no serious complications. The rate of diarrhea was higher in the sublingual versus vaginal route group (70% vs 27.5%; $P < .005$). More women in the sublingual group had fatigue than in the vaginal route group (65% vs 40%; $P = .043$). Other side effects were similar for both groups. Overall patient acceptability of medical management was good. Most women indicated they would select medical management if they were allowed to choose again and would recommend this approach to other women.

Conclusion.—The misoprostol regimen is useful in the management of silent miscarriage. It was associated with high success and patient acceptability rates. Sublingual misoprostol administration may be a good alternative for women who do not want repeated vaginal administration of the drug.

▶ Pelvic sonography is being performed with increased frequency in early pregnancy. As a result the diagnosis of early pregnancy failure is also being made more frequently. Early pregnancy failure occurs from anembryonic gestation, when a gestational sac more than 18 mm is present without an embryo visualized and embryonic or fetal death, when an embryo more than 4 mm in length withoout cardiac activity is present. The management of early pregnancy failure can be performed by surgical evacuation of the intrauterine contents or by observation, also called expectant management. Several studies have reported that the use of misoprostol alone or after mifepristone has about a 60% to 80% success rate for treatment of early pregnancy failure. Different therapeutic doses and regimens of misoprostol have been used. The 2 regimens reported in this study had a 87.5% success rate, which is very good. The mean duration of bleeding was 12 days, but some women bled for more than a month. Side effects such as nausea, diarrhea, headache, and abdominal pain were common. Women with early pregnancy failure may be offered treatment with misoprostol, but they also need to know about the high frequency of side effects and prolonged duration of bleeding.

D. R. Mishell, Jr, MD

Abortion Incidence and Services in the United States in 2000
Finer LB, Henshaw SK (Alan Guttmacher Inst, New York)
Perspect Sex Reprod Health 35:6-15, 2003   13–8

Introduction.—About half of unintended pregnancies and in excess of one fifth of all pregnancies in the United States end in abortion. No nationally representative statistics on abortion incidence or the number, types, and locations of abortion service providers have been reported since 1996. Reported was national data from the Alan Guttmacher Institute (AGI) concerning the number of abortions performed and abortion rates for 1999 through the first half of 2001.

Methods.—Versions of the AGI questionnaire for 3 major categories of providers of abortion services were created: clinics, physicians, and hospitals. Data were collected for 1999, 2000, and the first half of 2001. Trends were determined by comparing the survey results with data from previous AGI surveys.

Results.—Between 1996 and 2000, the number of abortions dropped by 3% to 1.31 million and the abortion rate decreased 5% to 21.3/1000 females aged 15 to 44 years (by comparison, the rate dropped 12% between 1992 and 1996). The abortion ratio in 2000 was 24.5 per 100 pregnancies ending in abortions or live births. In 2000, 34% of females aged 15 to 44 years lived in 87% of counties with no provider; 86 of the nation's 276 metropolitan areas had no provider. Approximately 600 providers performed an estimated 37,000 early medical abortions during the initial 6 months of 2001; these procedures represented about 6% of all abortions performed during that period. Abortions performed by dilation and extraction were estimated at 0.17% of all abortions performed in 2000.

Conclusion.—The incidence and number of abortion providers continued to fall during the late 1990s, yet at a slower rate than earlier in the decade. Medical abortions began to have a small yet significant role in abortion provision.

▶ Data from this comprehensive nationwide survey provide useful information regarding many aspects of elective pregnancy termination in the United States. Between 1996 and 2000, there has been a steady decrease in the number of elective abortions performed in the United States, as well as a decrease in the number of abortion providers. There are no abortion providers in nearly

90% of the counties in the United States, and one third of reproductive age women live in these counties.

The most disturbing statistic in this report is the fact that about one fourth of all pregnancies in the United States since 1995 continue to be electively terminated by abortion. Women who do not wish to become pregnant and are sexually active should be strongly encouraged to use one of the several effective methods of contraception available in this country so they do not have an unintended pregnancy.

D. R. Mishell, Jr, MD

Contraceptive Use Among U S Women Having Abortions in 2000-2001
Jones RK, Darroch JE, Henshaw SK (Alan Guttmacher Inst, New York)
Perspect Sex Reprod Health 34:294-303, 2002   13–9

Introduction.—Approximately half of unintended pregnancies end in abortion. Forty-nine percent and 42% of women, respectively, who underwent abortion in 1987 and from 1994 to 1995 reported they and their partners were not using a contraceptive method. It is not known what percentage of pregnancies among method users were the result of inconsistent or incorrect contraceptive use and what proportion is from method failure. Described is the extent to which contraceptive nonuse, problems with contraceptive use, and failure of contraceptive methods result in unintended pregnancies that end in abortion in the United States.

Methods.—A self-administered questionnaire was used to assess contraceptive use patterns among a nationally representative sample of 10,683 women receiving abortion services in 2000 to 2001. Data were also collected concerning social and demographic characteristics, reasons for nonuse, problems with the most commonly used methods, and the impact emergency contraceptive pills had on abortion rates. Eight hospitals and 92 nonhospital facilities successfully administered surveys to all women who had an abortion during a specified period that ranged from 2 to 12 weeks between July 2000 and June 2001.

Results.—More than half of the respondents (56%) were women in their 20s; women in their 30s accounted for 22% of abortions and adolescents for 19%. Seventeen percent were married, 67% had never married, and 16% had been previously married; 31% were cohabiting and most (61%) had 1 or more child. Forty-six percent had not used contraception in the month they conceived, primarily because of perceived low risk of pregnancy and concerns about contraception (33% and 32% of nonusers, respectively). Use of the male condom was the most frequently reported method among all women (28%), followed by the birth control pill (14%) (Table 1). Inconsistent method use was the major cause of pregnancy in 49% of condom users and 76% of pill users; 42% of condom users reported condom breakage or slippage as a reason for pregnancy. Notable proportions of pill and condom users reported perfect method use (13% and 14%, respectively). Up to

TABLE 1.—Percentage Distribution of Women Obtaining Abortions in 2000, by Contraceptive Method Used in the Month of Conception, and of Women at Risk of Unintended Pregnancy in 1995, by Contraceptive Method Used

Method	Women Having Abortions, 2000	Women at Risk of Unintended Pregnancy, 1995*
Any method	53.7	92.5
Long-acting	1.1	40.5
Sterilization	0.1	35.8
IUD	0.1	0.7
Implant/injectable	0.9	4.0
Pill	13.6	24.9
Male condom	27.6	18.9
Withdrawal	7.3	2.8
Periodic abstinence	2.2	2.1
Other†	1.9	3.3
No method	46.3	7.5
Never used	8.1	0.1
Previously used	38.2‡	7.4
Total	100.0	100.0
Unweighted N	10,683	7,725
Weighted N (in 000s)	1,313	41,796

*Based on special tabulations from the 1995 National Survey of Family Growth. Includes women using a contraceptive method in the survey month and fertile women using no method who had intercourse in the previous 3 months and were not pregnant, seeking pregnancy, or postpartum and whose partner was not sterile.
†Female condom, diaphragm, foam, sponge, suppository or any other method.
‡Includes women who used only emergency contraceptive pills to prevent the current pregnancy.
(Courtesy of Jones RK, Darroch JE, Henshaw SK: Contraceptive use among U.S. women having abortions in 2000-2001. *Perspect Sex Reprod Health* 34:294-303, 2002.)

51,000 abortions were averted by use of emergency contraceptive pills in 2000.

Conclusion.—Women and men need accurate information concerning fertility cycles and about the risk of pregnancy when a contraceptive is not used or used imperfectly. The increased use of emergency contraceptive pills could further decrease levels of unintended pregnancy and abortion.

▶ Unintended pregnancy is a major problem in the United States. About half of all pregnancies are unintended and half of these pregnancies, one fourth of all pregnancies, are terminated by elective abortion. The abortion rate in the United States is higher than all Western European countries as well as Japan. The data from this survey indicate that half of all women having an elective abortion were using no method of contraception in the month they conceived and the other half were using methods of contraception, mainly the condom and oral contraceptives, but usually inconsistently. Women at risk of unintended pregnancy should be advised to use effective methods of contraception consistently and correctly.

D. R. Mishell, Jr, MD

Factors Affecting the Outcome of Early Medical Abortion: A Review of 4132 Consecutive Cases

Ashok PW, Templeton A, Wagaarachchi PT, et al (Univ of Aberdeen, Scotland; Grampian Univ Hosps NHS Trust, UK)

Br J Obstet Gynaecol 109:1281-1289, 2002   13–10

Background.—In a previous study of medical abortion with mifepristone 200 mg followed by vaginally administered misoprostol 800 µg, the authors found an increased failure rate at gestations of 50 days or longer. They report their results in a large series of patients treated with mifepristone followed by up to 2 doses of vaginal misoprostol.

Methods.—The experience included 4132 consecutive women undergoing early medical abortion over an 8-year period. Mean gestation was 51 days of amenorrhea, up to 63 days; 47% of the women were primigravidas. Each patient took a single 200-mg dose of mifepristone; 36 to 48 hours later, they were admitted for administration of vaginal misoprostol, 800 µg. In the latter half of the experience, a second 400-µg dose of misoprostol was given if abortion was not imminent within 4 hours. The second dose was given either orally or vaginally, depending on the amount of bleeding present. The women were discharged home after 8 hours, or after abortion had occurred. The study definition of success was complete evacuation of the uterus, with no need for surgical intervention.

Results.—Approximately 2% of women aborted with mifepristone only. Of the 4036 who proceeded to receive misoprostol, 98% had complete abortion with no surgical intervention. Thus 2.3% of women required surgical intervention, with a 1.6% rate of surgical evacuation for incomplete abortion, 0.3% for missed abortion, 0.3% for continued pregnancy, and 0.1% as an adjunct to laparoscopy performed to exclude ectopic pregnancy. Ninety-five percent of women receiving the complete regimen passed products of conception while still on the ward. Overall efficacy was similar for women with more or less than 50 days' gestation. Women with less than 50 days' gestation were more likely to abort with mifepristone only, whereas those with 50 or more days were more likely to have continuing pregnancy. Women with previous pregnancies were more likely to require surgical intervention. The overall failure rate and the continuing pregnancy rate were higher in women with previous abortions. Adding the second dose of misoprostol eliminated the gestation-related difference observed when just 1 dose was used.

Conclusions.—The described regimen, including a second dose of misoprostol if indicated, is effective for early medical abortion. This modified regimen reduces the continuing pregnancy rate while eliminating the lower success rate in women over 50 days' gestation. The failure rate is highest in women with previous abortions and, in those with no previous abortions, multiparous women.

▶ The use of 600 mg of mifepristone followed by a single 400-µg dose of oral misoprostol is more effective for terminating pregnancies of 49 days gestation or less then pregnancies of a greater gestational age. In this study, after 200 mg of mifepristone was ingested, 800 µg of misoprostol was placed in the vagina. If abortion was not imminent 4 hours later, a second 400 µg of misoprostol was placed in the vagina or ingested. With use of 2 doses of misoprostol the success rate of termination of pregnancies from 50 to 63 days' gestation and 49 days or less was similar, 98% in each group. The use of the second dose of misoprostol removed the effect of gestational age upon failure of the method. This treatment protocol can be used to successfully perform medical abortions in pregnancies up to 63 days' gestation.

D. R. Mishell, Jr, MD

A Prospective Randomized, Double-Blinded, Placebo-Controlled Trial Comparing Mifepristone and Vaginal Misoprostol to Vaginal Misoprostol Alone for Elective Termination of Early Pregnancy
Jain JK, Dutton C, Harwood B, et al (Univ of Southern California, Los Angeles; Univ of Pittsburgh, Pa; Univ of California, San Francisco)
Hum Reprod 17:1477-1482, 2002   13–11

Introduction.—Vaginal misoprostol is effective as a single agent for medical abortion. A regimen of mifepristone and misoprostol was compared with misoprostol alone for termination of early pregnancy in a randomized, double-blind, placebo-controlled investigation.

Methods.—Two hundred fifty women with gestations of 56 days or more were randomly assigned to receive either 200 mg mifepristone orally or placebo followed 48 hours later by 800 µg vaginal misoprostol. The administration of misoprostol was repeated every 24 hours to 3 doses if abortion did not occur. Abortion success was considered complete abortion without the use of surgical aspiration.

Results.—Medical abortions were successful in 114 (95.7%) of 119 participants after mifepristone followed by vaginal misoprostol. A total of 110 (88.0%) of 125 women successfully aborted after placebo and vaginal misoprostol. The higher success rate of complete abortion with mifepristone and misoprostol regimens was statistically significant compared with the placebo and misoprostol regimen ($P < .05$).

Conclusion.—A regimen of mifepristone and misoprostol was significantly more effective for terminating pregnancies of 56 or more days compared with misoprostol alone. The 88% efficacy observed with vaginal misoprostol alone may be clinically acceptable when mifepristone is not available.

▶ Mifepristone followed by misoprostol is an effective means to electively terminate pregnancies up to at least 8 weeks' gestational age. In many countries mifepristone is unavailable or expensive to purchase. Misoprostol is widely available and inexpensive. This study is the first randomized trial comparing the use of mifepristone followed by vaginal misoprostol with placebo followed by 1, 2, or 3 doses of 800 µg of misoprostol administered vaginally for termination of pregnancies less than 8 weeks' gestational age. The use of the latter regimen resulted in an 88% rate of successful medical abortion compared with the 96% success rate with use of mifepristone followed by misoprostol. Side effects were similar with the 2 treatment regimens. In places where mifepristone is unavailable or too costly to use, vaginal misoprostol can be offered to women wishing to terminate pregnancies less than 8 weeks' gestational age by medical therapy with an estimated effectiveness rate of nearly 90%.

D. R. Mishell, Jr, MD

Early Pregnancy Termination With Vaginal Misoprostol Before and After 42 Days Gestation
Zikopoulos KA, Papanikolaou EG, Kalantaridou SN, et al (Med School of Ioannina, Greece)
Hum Reprod 17:3079-3083, 2002   13–12

Background.—Some women prefer medical abortion to avoid the risks of surgery and anesthesia. Misoprostol is a prostaglandin E_1 analogue that has been used for medical abortions. The efficacy of vaginal misoprostol for medical abortions of less than 42 days' gestation was compared with use for those of 42 to 56 days' gestation.

Study Design.—The study group consisted of 160 women, aged 18 to 30 years, who requested medical pregnancy termination at a gestational age of no more than 56 days. At the first clinic visit, 800 µg misoprostol were administered vaginally. On the second and third day, participants returned for assessment of pregnancy. If intrauterine pregnancy was detected, treatment was repeated (up to 3 times). Medication for possible side effects was administered prophylactically. Treatment outcome was evaluated on day 4. All women who had a successful medical abortion received a further dose of both oral and vaginal misoprostol. A symptom log was maintained by all participants. Patient satisfaction was assessed at end of treatment.

Findings.—The overall complete medical abortion rate was 91.3%. When the gestational age was less than 42 days, the complete abortion rate was 96.3%; it was 86.3% in those with gestational age of 42 to 56 days. The 2 groups did not differ significantly regarding side effects. Women who had a successful medical abortion were significantly more satisfied than those who did not.

Conclusions.—Vaginal misoprostol is safe and effective for women seeking a medical abortion up to 56 days of gestation, but it appears to be more effective before 42 days of gestation.

▶ In a randomized study, summarized in the preceeding abstract, we have shown that mifepristone followed by misoprostol is significantly more effective than misoprostol alone for elective termination of first-trimester pregnancy. However, in many countries mifepristone is not available for clinical use. As shown in this and other studies, use of vaginal misoprostol alone results in a more than 85% successful pregnancy termination rate. It is concerning that in this study, 2 of the 80 women with gestations after 42 days required a blood transfusion and 2 others emergency curettage. Other studies performed with misoprostol did not report this high rate of complications. It is also unclear why 2 additional doses of misoprostol were given after the pregnancies were evacuated. Other studies limit the use of misoprostol to 3 doses with similar rates of success.

D. R. Mishell, Jr, MD

A Comparison of Oral Misoprostol With Vaginal Misoprostol Administration in Second-Trimester Pregnancy Termination for Fetal Abnormality
Dickinson JE, Evans SF (Univ of Western Australia, Perth; Women and Infants Research Found, Perth, Australia; King Edward Mem Hosp for Women, Perth, Australia)
Obstet Gynecol 101:1294-1299, 2003   13–13

Background.—When severe fetal anomalies are detected, there can be a need for second-trimester pregnancy termination. Misoprostol is frequently used for medical termination of pregnancy. Oral and vaginal misoprostol for the termination of second trimester pregnancy were compared in a randomized clinical trial.

Study Design.—The study group consisted of 84 women who were admitted to King Edward Memorial Hospital for Women in Perth, Australia, for second-trimester pregnancy termination between March 2001 and July 2002. There was no restriction on the number of fetuses or a history of previous uterine surgery. Women were randomly assigned to receive 400 μg of misoprostol intravaginally every 6 hours for up to 48 hours, 400 μg of misoprostol orally every 3 hours for up to 48 hours, or 600 μg of misoprostol intravaginally followed by 200 μg of misoprostol orally every 3 hours for up to 48 hours.

All women who had not delivered within 48 hours were considered protocol failures. The women completed a questionnaire regarding pain, control, and their overall opinion of the treatment. At the time the study was halted, 28 women had been randomly assigned to vaginal, 27 to oral, and 27 to vaginal plus oral misoprostol. Analysis was based on intention to treat.

Findings.—At the time of interim safety analysis, a significant difference was noted between the groups and the trial was halted. There was a significant difference in median time to achieving delivery among the treatment arms. Within 24 hours, 85.7% of women in the vaginal group, 44.8% in the oral group, and 74.1% in the oral/vaginal group had delivered. At 48 hours, 0% in the vaginal, 20.7% in the oral, and 3.7% in the oral/vaginal misoprostol groups had not delivered (Fig 1). Women had no preferences among the treatment regimens.

Conclusion.—Intravaginal misoprostol is superior to oral misoprostol in achieving second trimester pregnancy termination.

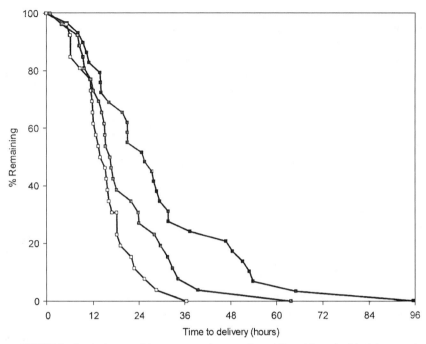

FIGURE 1.—Survival curves of the percentage of pregnancies undelivered for each of the 3 dosage regimens. Group 1 (*lightly shaded squares*) versus group 2 (*solid squares*) versus group 3 (*heavily shaded squares*) (*P* = .042). (Reprinted with permission from The American College of Obstetricians and Gynecologists courtesy of Dickinson JE, Evans SF: A comparison of oral misoprostol with vaginal misoprostol administration in second-trimester pregnancy termination for fetal abnormality. *Obstet Gynecol* 101:1294-1299, 2003.)

▶ Administration of misoprostol vaginally is more effective than oral administration and a vaginal dose of 400 µg every 6 hours terminated 86% of second trimester pregnancies in 24 hours and 100% in 48 hours. Although some prior studies excluded the use of misoprostol in women with a prior cesarean delivery, nearly 20% of the women in this study had a prior cesarean delivery and there were no women who had a uterine rupture. At present, vaginal placement of 400 µg of misoprostol every 6 hours appears to be the best regimen for administration of this agent for terminating second trimester pregnancies in women with and without a history of prior cesarean delivery.

D. R. Mishell, Jr, MD

A Randomized Controlled Trial Comparing Two Protocols for the Use of Misoprostol in Midtrimester Pregnancy Termination
Bebbington MW, Kent N, Lim K, et al (Univ of British Columbia, Vancouver, Canada)
Am J Obstet Gynecol 187:853-857, 2002   13–14

Introduction.—Misoprostol (Cytotec) is a synthetic prostaglandin E_1 analogue that is useful in the induction of labor at term and is effective in producing medical abortion in both the first and second trimesters. The efficacy of misoprostol administered orally was compared with vaginal application for induction of midtrimester termination of pregnancy.

Methods.—Between September 1, 1998, and November 1, 2001, women seen for midtrimester termination of pregnancy were randomly assigned to receive either misoprostol orally in a dose of 200 μg every hour for 3 hours followed by 400 μg every 4 hours or vaginally in a dose of 400 μg every 4 hours. This protocol was followed for 24 hours; thereafter, management was at the discretion of the attending physician. The major outcome measure was the induction-to-delivery interval.

Results.—Of 114 randomly assigned women, 49 received vaginal misoprostol and 65 received oral dosing. The 2 groups were similar in maternal age, parity, indication for pregnancy termination, gestational age, and maternal weight. The mean induction-to-delivery interval was significantly shorter for the vaginal than for the oral group (19.6 hours vs 34.5 hours; *P* < .01). Significantly more women in the vaginal group were delivered within 24 hours (85.1% vs 39.5%; *P* < .01) (Figure), and more women in the oral group needed changes in the method of induction when undelivered after 24 hours (38.2% vs 7%; *P* < .01).

Mean blood loss was similar for the 2 groups. Length of stay was significantly shorter in the vaginal group (32.3 hours vs 50.9 hours; *P* < .01). The one complication was an increase in febrile morbidity in the vaginal group (25% vs 6.7%; *P* = .046). This did not necessitate an increased use of antibiotics; all fevers resolved postpartum without further complications.

Conclusion.—Vaginal administration of misoprostol produced a shorter induction-to-delivery interval than oral administration of misoprostol in patients undergoing midtrimester termination of pregnancy.

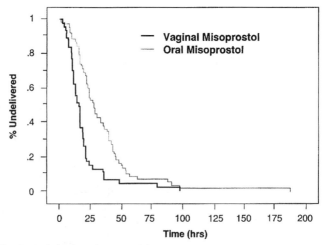

FIGURE.—Survival plot for induction-to-delivery interval. (Reprinted by permission of the publisher courtesy of Bebbington MW, Kent N, Lim K, et al: A randomized controlled trial comparing two protocols for the use of misoprostol in midtrimester pregnancy termination. *Am J Obstet Gynecol* 187:853-857. Copyright 2002 by Elsevier.)

▶ The results of this study are in agreement with the study of Dickenson et al (see Abstract 13–13) indicating that vaginal administration of 400 µg of misoprostol every 4 hours is more effective than oral administration of misoprostol for second trimester pregnancy termination. In both studies, 86% of patients had successful pregnancy termination by 24 hours with vaginal misoprostol, and no uterine rupture occurred when women with prior cesarean delivery were treated.

D. R. Mishell, Jr, MD

Medical Abortion at 64 to 91 Days of Gestation: A Review of 483 Consecutive Cases
Hamoda H, Ashok PW, Flett GMM, et al (Univ of Aberdeen, Scotland)
Am J Obstet Gynecol 188:1315-1319, 2003   13–15

Background.—In 2000, 45% of abortions in England and Wales were performed between 9 and 12 weeks of gestation. In Scotland, 27.7% of abortions in 2001 were performed between 10 and 13 weeks of gestation. The antiprogestogen mifepristone in combination with a prostaglandin analog was licensed in 1991 for the termination of pregnancies of 63 days or fewer amenorrhea. Four years later, this drug was also approved for the termination of pregnancies of more than 13 weeks' gestation. Between 10 and 13 weeks of gestation, surgical methods are used almost exclusively, and few reports in the literature are available regarding medical methods. A randomized trial comparing medical and surgical abortion at 10 to 13 weeks of gestation showed no statistically significant difference in the number of women who experienced complete abortion without the need for surgical intervention (94% vs 98%). A study of medical abortion at 64 to 91 days of gestation with mifepristone and repeated doses of misoprostol, using an inpatient approach is discussed.

Methods.—The study intended 891 women who underwent an abortion between 64 and 91 days of gestation from October 2000 to April 2002. Of these, 483 women underwent medical abortion and were included in this study. Misoprostol was administered vaginally into the posterior fornix. When products of conception were not passed, further doses of misoprostol were given orally or vaginally at 3-hour intervals to a maximum of 5 doses. When products of conception were not passed after the final dose of misoprostol, a US was performed to exclude ongoing pregnancy, missed abortion, or incomplete abortion. A surgical abortion was performed when any of these conditions was diagnosed.

Results.—Complete abortion occurred in 458 (94.8%) of 483 cases, with decreasing efficacy with increasing gestational age. Surgical evacuation was performed in 1 woman at 9 to 10 weeks of gestation, in 8 women at 10 to 11 weeks of gestation, in 7 women at 11 to 12 weeks of gestation, and in 9 women at 12 to 13 weeks of gestation. Indications for surgery included ongoing pregnancy in 8 patients, missed abortion in 3 patients, incomplete abortion in 13 patients, and emergency curettage for bleeding in 1 patient. The

**Cumulative
Percentage**

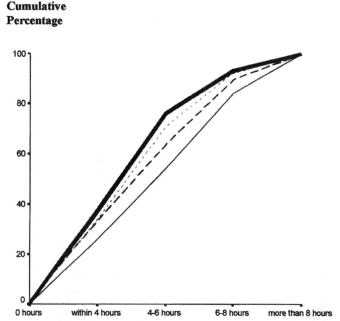

FIGURE 2.—Cumulative percentage of complete abortion in relation to gestational weeks and of induction-to-abortion interval in hours. *Thick solid line*, 9 to 10 weeks of gestation; *small dashed line*, 10 to 11 weeks of gestation; *long dashed line*, 11 to 12 weeks of gestation; *thin solid line*, 12 to 13 weeks of gestation. (Reprinted by permission of the publisher courtesy of Hamoda H, Ashok PW, Flett GMM, et al: Medical abortion at 64 to 91 days of gestation: A review of 483 consecutive cases. *Am J Obstet Gynecol* 188:1315-1319. Copyright 2003 by Elsevier.)

mean number of misoprostol doses was 2.3. Of the women who had a complete abortion, 152 (32.6%) aborted within 4 hours of receiving misoprostol (Fig 2). The mean induction-to-abortion interval was 5.5 hours, and most patients (93.6%) were treated as day cases.

Conclusions.—Medical abortion between 64 and 91 days of gestation is effective and has a high uptake. It is suggested that the choice of medical abortion be extended to women in this gestational group.

▶ Currently, mifepristone followed by misoprostol is approved for medical termination of pregnancies less than 7 weeks' gestational age. Previous studies have shown that use of these agents up to 9 weeks' gestational age is an effective means of medical abortion. The results of this study indicate that ingestion of 200 µg of mifepristone followed by 1 or more doses of misoprostol in women with a gestational age of 64 to 91 days resulted in a 95% successful abortion rate. Women wishing to have medical abortion should not be restricted to those with a gestational age less than 7 weeks but should be offered this choice for pregnancy termination up to a gestational age of 13 weeks (91 days).

D. R. Mishell, Jr, MD

Abortions and Breast Cancer: Record-Based Case-Control Study
Erlandsson G, Montgomery SM, Cnattingius S, et al (Karolinska Institutet, Stockholm)
Int J Cancer 103:676-679, 2003   13–16

Background.—Some authorities suggest that after abortion, breast epithelium is left in a proliferative state with an increased susceptibility to carcinogenesis. The possible association between abortion and subsequent breast cancer risk was investigated in a case-control study.

Methods.—Data were obtained from 2 population-based Swedish registers and medical records. Information on induced and spontaneous abortions and a number of potential confounding variables was prospectively gathered. The case group consisted of 1988 women diagnosed as having breast cancer between 1973 and 1991, at a mean age of 40 years. Each case subject was matched to 2 control subjects.

Findings.—Compared with women who had no abortions, women who had had at least 1 abortion had a reduced risk of breast cancer, with an odds ratio (OR) of 0.84. The adjusted OR declined in a stepwise fashion with number of abortions, being 0.59 for 3 or more abortions compared with no abortions. Patterns for induced and spontaneous abortions were comparable.

Conclusions.—In this large case-control study, a history of induced or spontaneous abortions did not correlate with an increased breast cancer risk. The current data suggest that pregnancy, regardless of outcome, has a protective effect against breast cancer.

▶ The occurrence of spontaneous abortion has been previously reported not to alter the risk of developing breast cancer. Several studies have reported that induced abortion may increase the risk of breast cancer, but other studies have not shown a change in risk of breast cancer after having an induced abortion. The results of this large case-control study found that a history of either spontaneous or induced abortion was not associated with an increased risk of developing premenopausal breast cancer. Studies suggesting that an induced abortion increases the risk of breast cancer may have been subject to recall bias. In this study the information of pregnancy history was obtained prospectively from antenatal care records. The results of this study suggest that pregnancies terminating in spontaneous or induced abortion are actually associated with a reduced risk of developing breast cancer with an odds ration of 0.84 for a history of 1 or more abortions compared with no abortions.

D. R. Mishell, Jr, MD

14 Infection

Prevalence of Vulvovaginal Candidiasis and Susceptibility to Fluconazole in Women
Bauters TGM, Dhont MA, Temmerman MIL, et al (Ghent Univ, Belgium)
Am J Obstet Gynecol 187:569-574, 2002   14–1

Background.—Epidemiologic research has demonstrated a continuous increase in the prevalence of vulvovaginal candidiasis. An increasing number of these cases is being caused by non-*Candida albicans* species. Identifying the non-*C albicans* species is thus increasingly important before antifungal treatment is initiated. A membrane filtration technique was developed for the rapid presumptive differentiation of 4 major *Candida* species. The prevalence of vaginal colonization by *Candida* was determined with the rapid detection method; the determinants of vaginal candidiasis were examined and susceptibility for fluconazole was evaluated.

Methods and Findings.—Vaginal swabs were collected from 612 unselected women at 1 outpatient clinic. Thirty-nine of these women (6.3%) had clinical candidiasis. Overall, the yeast colonization rate was 20.1%. C *albicans* was isolated most commonly, in 68.3% of the patients, followed by C *glabrata* in 16.3% and C *parapsilosis* in 8.9%. Clinical candidiasis positively correlated with estrogen impregnation status. In vitro susceptibility for fluconazole, by the National Committee for Clinical Laboratory Standards method, identified resistance in 21.2% of the isolates.

Conclusions.—In this series of women, more than one fifth were colonized with *Candida* species. Hyperestrogenemia correlated with an increased vulvovaginal colonization by *Candida*. Unexpectedly, 21% of the isolates were resistant to fluconazole.

▶ There is a continuing increase in the prevalence of vulvovaginal candidiasis. The results of this study in an unselected series of women visiting a gynecologic clinic found that 20% had some type of candidiasis isolated in the vagina. C *albicans* was present in nearly 70% of the isolates, and 21% of the isolates were resistant to fluconazole. Patients with symptomatic vulvovaginal yeast infections who do not respond to fluconazole treatment should have tests for susceptibility of the organisms. It is of interest that candidiasis was most frequently present when estrogen levels were high, such as during pregnancy, oral contraceptives use, or postmenopausal estrogen use.

D. R. Mishell, Jr, MD

A Multiplex Polymerase Chain Reaction–Based Diagnostic Method for Bacterial Vaginosis

Obata-Yasuoka M, Ba-Thein W, Hamada H, et al (Univ of Tsukuba, Japan)
Obstet Gynecol 100:759-764, 2002   14–2

Background.—The most common lower genital tract infection in young women is bacterial vaginosis. A polymerase chain reaction (PCR)–based diagnostic technique for bacterial vaginosis was developed with bacterial vaginosis–related anaerobes.

Methods.—The multiple PCR assay was based on primers specific to 16S ribosomal DNA, *nanH*, and an internal spacer region of ribosomal DNA. Vaginal swabs were obtained from nonpregnant and pregnant women and evaluated by using the Gram stain–based Nugent scoring system. Of 853 Gram stain–interpretable samples, 172 were selected randomly and analyzed by multiplex PCR assay.

Findings.—The PCR assay sensitivity ranged from 10^3 to 10^4 colony-forming units per vaginal swab. According to the Nugent scoring system, the prevalence of bacterial vaginosis was 21.6%; of the intermediate category, 26%; and of the normal category, 52.4%. With the multiplex PCR-based diagnostic technique, 20.3% of the samples were classified as bacterial vaginosis. Compared with Gram stain analysis, multiplex PCR had a diagnostic sensitivity of 78.4%, a specificity of 95.6%, and positive and negative predictive values of 82.9% and 94.2%, respectively.

Conclusions.—A multiple PCR-based diagnostic test for bacterial vaginosis with detection of multiple anaerobes in vaginal swab samples has been developed. This method is useful for diagnosing or screening for bacterial vaginosis.

▶ Development of a PCR assay for the diagnosis of bacterial vaginosis will be of use to clinicians. The test could be used to screen pregnant women and those undergoing elective gynecologic surgical procedures as well as in vitro fertilization procedures. The presence of bacterial vaginosis has been reported to increase the complication rate of pregnancy, the miscarriage rate after in vitro fertilization, and the infection rate after gynecologic surgery. If the PCR detects bacterial vaginosis, therapy can be instituted to lower the adverse action of these events.

D. R. Mishell, Jr, MD

BVBlue Test for Diagnosis of Bacterial Vaginosis

Myziuk L, Romanowski B, Johnson SC (Univ of Alberta, Edmonton, Canada; Gryphus Diagnostic LLC, Birmingham, Ala)
J Clin Microbiol 41:1925-1928, 2003   14–3

Objective.—The standard method of diagnosing bacterial vaginosis is the Amstel criteria: abnormal vaginal discharge, vaginal pH greater than 4.5, positive amine odor test, and clue cells on vaginal Gram smear, usually based on a Nugent system score of 7 or higher. The diagnostic process would be simplified by the availability of a point-of-care test. The BVBlue system, a chromogenic test based on the detection of high sialadase enzyme in vaginal fluid, was evaluated for the diagnosis of BV.

Methods.—The analysis included 57 women, mean age 31 years, evaluated for possible BV. All were assessed with the Amstel criteria and Gram stain. At the same time, a sample of vaginal fluid was collected for the BVBlue test. The swab was placed in the testing vessel and incubated for 10 minutes, after which 2 drops of developer solution were added. An immediate blue or green color change indicated elevated sialadase level and a positive result. The BVBlue findings were compared with the other diagnostic assessments, including the Amstel criteria.

Results.—The BVBlue test was positive in 12 women, a rate of 21%. A decrease in *Lactobacillus* spp. was noted in 92% of women with sialadase activity compared with just 2% of those without sialadase activity. In addition, clue cells were noted in 92% of sialadase-positive specimens compared with none of the sialadase-negative specimens. The kappa coefficient for agreement between BVBlue and the Nugent score was 0.894, indicating excellent agreement. Compared with the Nugent score, BVBlue offered a sensitivity of 91.7% compared with 50.0% for the Amstel criteria. Specificities were comparable: 97.8% and 100.0%, respectively. A history of sexual contact within the past week was noted for 72% with sialadase activity versus 45% for those without. Positive results on the BVBlue test were approximately 3 times more frequent among women with a previous history of BV.

Conclusions.—The BVBlue system appears to offer a useful point-of-care diagnostic test for BV. A positive BVBlue result is associated with elevated vaginal fluid pH, amines, and clue cells. Diagnostic sensitivity and specificity values agree closely with those of the Nugent score.

▶ The development of a quick and easy test to assist in the diagnosis of bacterial vaginosis would not need to use a microscope to identify clue cells. The test described detects sialidase activity. Women with bacterial vaginosis have vaginal bacteria that secrete sialidase in the vaginal fluid. Sialidase is secreted from anaerobic gram-negative bacterial rods such as *Bacteroides* and *Gardnerella*. The test utilized in this study correlated very well with the Amstel criteria, and the test is available 10 minutes after incubation of the swab of vaginal secretions. This rapid, easily performed, accurate test should help busy clinicians diagnose bacterial vaginosis.

D. R. Mishell, Jr, MD

Does Pre- and Postoperative Metronidazole Treatment Lower Vaginal Cuff Infection Rate After Abdominal Hysterectomy Among Women With Bacterial Vaginosis?
Larsson P-G, Carlsson B (Central Hosp, Skövde (Kärnsjukhuset), Sweden; Linköpings Universitet, Sweden)
Infect Dis Obstet Gynecol 10:133-140, 2002   14-4

Introduction.—Bacterial vaginosis (BV) is a well-described risk factor for postoperative infection after abdominal hysterectomy and is characterized by a 1000 to 10,000-fold increase in the concentration of various bacteria, including anaerobic bacteria. Vaginal bacterial flora scored as intermediate (no or few lactobacilli and no diagnosis of BV; a flora between normal and BV) appear to be of similar clinical significance as BV. It has been suggested that intermediate flora and BV be merged into a single group called "abnormal vaginal flora." The effect of preoperative and postoperative metronidazole treatment regarding the postoperative infection rate among women with abnormal vaginal flora were compared with women with lactobacilli flora in an open randomized trial.

Methods.—Participants were women undergoing elective total abdominal hysterectomy for benign reasons between 1992 and 1996 and were younger than 50 years or were still menstruating if older than 50 years. Two hundred thirteen patients were randomly assigned to either treatment with metronidazole rectally for a minimum of 4 days or no treatment. On preoperative gynecologic examination, a vaginal smear was obtained and Gram stained. Women with BV or intermediate flora were merged to 1 group called abnormal vaginal flora.

Results.—Seventy-one women were excluded, leaving 142 eligible for analysis. Of 59 diagnosed with abnormal vaginal flora, there were no vaginal cuff infections in the treated arm compared with a rate of 27% in the no treatment arm ($P < .01$). Treatment decreased the vaginal cuff infection rate from 9.5% to 2% in the 83 women with lactobacilli flora (P = not significant). Treatment had no effect on the incidence of wound infections. Intention-to-treat analysis revealed a significant decrease in vaginal cuff infections among women randomized to treatment.

Conclusion.—Preoperative and postoperative treatment for a minimum of 4 days with metronidazole rectally significantly decreases the rate of vaginal cuff infections in women with abnormal vaginal flora undergoing elective total abdominal hysterectomy for benign reasons.

▶ The results of this study suggest that the presence of BV increases the risk of developing vaginal cuff infection after a total abdominal hysterectomy. Women scheduled for an elective abdominal hysterectomy should have the vaginal secretions analyzed to determine if BV is present. If BV is present, treatment with metronidazole should be given for at least 4 days to reduce the incidence of postoperative vaginal cuff infection.

D. R. Mishell, Jr, MD

Bacterial Vaginosis Is a Strong Predictor of *Neisseria gonorrhoeae* and *Chlamydia trachomatis* Infection

Wiesenfeld HC, Hillier SL, Krohn MA, et al (Univ of Pittsburgh, Pa)
Clin Infect Dis 36:663-668, 2003   14–5

Background.—Bacterial vaginosis is associated with an alteration of the Lactobacillus-predominant normal vaginal flora to an environment dominated by anaerobes, *Gardnerella vaginalis*, and *Mycoplasma hominis*. In studies of women in 2 African countries, bacterial vaginosis has recently been associated with an increased susceptibility to sexually transmitted diseases (STDs), including HIV-1. However, data that link abnormal vaginal flora to non-HIV STDs are limited. The relationship between bacterial vaginosis and STDs among women recently exposed to men with urethritis was investigated.

Methods.—The study included 255 nonpregnant women, 15 to 30 years old, who were treated at the STD clinic of a Pittsburgh hospital and a reproductive health care provider from 1998 to 2001. All of the study participants reported recent sexual contact with a male partner in whom either gonococcal or chlamydial urethritis or nongonococcal urethritis had been diagnosed. The women underwent a comprehensive gynecologic examination. Samples of vaginal fluid were obtained for pH measurement, Whiff amine testing, and microscopy with an additional swab for Gram stain interpretation. Samples from the posterior vaginal fornix were cultured for *G. vaginalis*, and endocervical samples were tested for the presence of *Neisseria gonorrhoeae* and *Chlamydia trachomatis*.

Results.—Compared to study participants with normal vaginal flora, those with bacterial vaginosis were 4.1 times more likely to test positive for *N gonorrhoeae*. Study participants with bacterial vaginosis were also significantly more likely to test positive for *C trachomatis* compared with participants without bacterial vaginosis. Study participants colonized vaginally by hydrogen peroxide–producing lactobacilli were less likely to be diagnosed with chlamydial infection or gonorrhea than those without these lactobacilli.

Conclusions.—Bacterial vaginosis is a strong predictor of gonorrhea and chlamydial infection in women who reported recent exposure to a male partner with urethritis. These findings are supportive of the importance of vaginal flora in preventing the acquisition of STD.

▶ Changes in the bacterial flora of the vagina associated with bacterial vaginosis are a risk marker for acquisition of *C trachomatis* and *N gonorrhoeae*. The presence of normal bacterial flora in the vagina helped prevent the acquisition of these organisms among a group of women having intercourse with men who recently had urethritis.

D. R. Mishell, Jr, MD

Genital Human Papillomavirus Infection: Incidence and Risk Factors in a Cohort of Female University Students

Winer RL, Lee S-K, Hughes JP, et al (Univ of Washington, Seattle)
Am J Epidemiol 157:218-226, 2003   14–6

Background.—Genital human papillomavirus (HPV) infections are the cause of genital warts and squamous intraepithelial lesions. In addition, some types of HPV infections are causally related to the development of anogenital cancers. These infections have a high prevalence, and current evidence suggests that at least 50% of sexually active women have been infected with one or more types of HPV infection. The primary route of transmission is sexual contact, but rates of acquisition and risk factors for infection are largely unknown. Also unknown is the potential risk of infection from nonpenetrating sexual contact, including the possible association between oral-penile contact and oral HPV, which is associated with oral cancer. The cumulative incidence of HPV infection was estimated in a cohort of female university students, and the characteristics of women and their sex partners that have the potential to increase the risk of HPV infection in women were investigated.

Methods.—The study group comprised 603 women aged 18 to 20 years who were enrolled at a university in the state of Washington. The women were examined every 4 months, and at each visit, a sexual and health questionnaire was completed, and cervical and vulvovaginal samples were collected to detect HPV DNA.

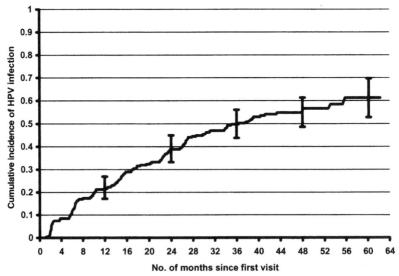

FIGURE 1.—Cumulative incidence of human papillomavirus (*HPV*) infection among women sexually active and HPV negative at enrollment (n = 296) in Washington State, 1990-2000. *Vertical bars,* 95% confidence intervals at 12, 24, 36, 48, and 60 months. (Courtesy of Winer RL, Lee S-K, Hughes JP, et al: Genital human papillomavirus infection: Incidence and risk factors in a cohort of female university students. *Am J Epidemiol* 157(3):218-226, 2003. By permission of Oxford University.)

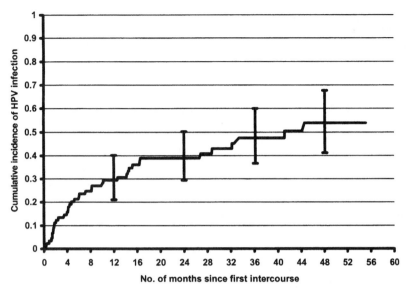

FIGURE 2.—Cumulative incidence of human papillomavirus (*HPV*) infection from time of first sexual intercourse (n = 94) among women in Washington State, 1990-2000. *Vertical bars*, 95% confidence intervals at 12, 24, 36, 48, and 60 months. (Courtesy of Winer RL, Lee S-K, Hughes JP, et al: Genital human papillomavirus infection: Incidence and risk factors in a cohort of female university students. *Am J Epidemiol* 157(3):218-226, 2003. By permission of Oxford University.)

Results.—At 24 months, the cumulative incidence of first-time infection was 32.3% (Fig 1). Virgins and nonvirgins had comparable incidences calculated from time of new-partner acquisition (Fig 2). Factors predictive of incident infection were smoking, oral contraceptive use, and report of a new male sex partner, particularly a new partner known for less than 8 months before sex occurred. Always using a male condom with every new partner did not provide any protection against infection. Infection was rare in virgins, but any type of nonpenetrative sexual contact was associated with an increased risk of infection. Only 5 of 2619 oral specimens (0.2%) were positive for oral HPV. Detection of oral HPV was not associated with oral-penile contact.

Conclusions.—The incidence of HPV infection associated with the acquisition of a new sex partner is high, and nonpenetrative sexual contact is a plausible route of transmission in virgins.

▶ Genital HPV infection is extremely common among young women in the United States. Among virginal and sexually active HPV-negative women, nearly 40% were infected with HPV within 2 years after initiating or continuing sexual activity. It is disturbing that use of condoms did not reduce the incidence of HPV transmission, and that the most common HPV type detected was HPV-16, which is a precursor of cervical dysplasia and cancer. It is very important for sexually active women to have annual Pap smears to detect and treat cervical dysplasia before it progresses to cervical cancer.

D. R. Mishell, Jr, MD

Effect of a Clinical Practice Improvement Intervention on Chlamydial Screening Among Adolescent Girls
Shafer M-AB, Tebb KP, Pantell RH, et al (Univ of California, San Francisco; Kaiser Permanente, San Francisco; Kaiser Permanente, Oakland, Calif; et al)
JAMA 288:2846-2852, 2002   14–7

Introduction.—*Chlamydia trachomatis* infection is a serious health problem that disproportionately affects adolescent girls. Annual *C trachomatis* screening of sexually active adolescent girls is recommended by health professional organizations and is a Health Employer Data and Information Set performance measure; this goal is not being met. The effectiveness of a system-level, clinical practice improvement intervention designed to increase *C trachomatis* screening by using urine-based tests for sexually active girls during their routine checkups at a pediatric clinic was examined.

Methods.—Participating organizations were a randomized cluster of 10 pediatric clinics in the Kaiser Permanente of Northern California HMO, where adolescent girls aged 14 to 18 years had a total of 7920 routine checkup visits between April 2000 and March 2002. Five clinics were randomly assigned to provide usual care and 5 to provide the intervention. The intervention required that the HMO leadership be engaged by presenting evidence of a gap between current and best practice for *C trachomatis* screening; a team be created to champion the project; barriers be identified and solutions developed through monthly meetings; and progress be monitored by site-specific screening proportions. The primary outcome measure was the *C trachomatis* screening rate for sexually active 14- to 18-year-old girls during routine checkups at each participating clinic.

Results.—The population of adolescent girls was ethnically diverse. The average age was 15.4 years. Twenty-four percent of girls in the intervention group and 23% of controls were sexually active. Of 1017 patients eligible for screening in the intervention group, 478 (47%) were screened; of 1194 eligible for screening in the control group, 203 (17%) were screened. At baseline, the proportion screened was 0.05 (95% confidence interval [CI], 0.00-0.17) for the intervention group and 0.14 (95% CI, 0.01-0.26) for controls. At months 16 to 18, screening rates were 0.65 (95% CI, 0.53-0.77) for the intervention group and 0.21 (95% CI, 0.09-0.33) for controls (time period by study group interaction, $F_{6,60} = 5.33$; $P < .001$). The average infection rate for the intervention clinics was 5.8% (23 positive results out of 393 total urine tests and 3986 clinic visits) compared with 7.6% in controls (12 positive test results out of 157 tests and 3934 clinic visits).

Conclusion.—Implementation of the intervention was feasible in the setting of a large HMO, and significantly increased the *C trachomatis* screening rates for sexually active adolescent girls during routine checkups.

▶ There is a very high rate of *C trachomatis* (CT) infection of adolescent females in the United States. In this study, 6% to 8% of the adolescents screened were infected with CT. It is now recommended by several professional organizations that sexually active adolescent girls and women up to the age of 25 be screened for the presence of CT annually. It is important to detect CT in women because about 75% of the infections are asymptomatic and, if untreated, can cause salpingitis that results in infertility and ectopic pregnancy. The techniques described in this article markedly enhanced the percentage of adolescent girls screened for CT in a large HMO.

D. R. Mishell, Jr, MD

15 Infertility

Prolonged Use of Oral Contraception Before a Planned Pregnancy Is Associated With a Decreased Risk of Delayed Conception
Farrow A, Hull MGR, Northstone K, et al (Brunel Univ, Isleworth, England; Univ of Bristol, England)
Hum Reprod 17:2754-2761, 2002   15–1

Background.—Fecundity can be measured epidemiologically by the time needed to conceive. About 90% of fertile couples conceive within 12 months of trying, and a delay of more than 12 months is usually assumed to fit a clinical definition of infertility or subfertility. There has been increasing concern in the last 2 decades that prolonged oral contraceptive use may be associated with impaired fertility. The association between the total duration of oral contraceptive use and the time needed to conceive was investigated.

Methods.—This prospective study included 8497 planned pregnancies among a population that recruited 85% of eligible couples in Southwest England who were expecting the birth of a child over a 21-month period. The couples completed questionnaires at 18 weeks' gestation to determine parity, paternity, cohabitation, use of the contraceptive pill, smoking and alcohol status, educational achievement, height, weight, and time taken to conceive. Factors independently related to conception in 12 months or less were identified through logistic regression analysis.

Results.—Nearly three quarters of the participants (74%) conceived in 6 months or less; 14% conceived in 6 to 12 months, and 12% conceived after 1 year. Previous prolonged use of oral contraceptives was statistically significantly associated with a decreased risk of delayed conception (Table 4). The prolonged use of oral contraception was also associated with improved fecundity, independent of other factors. The possibility of selection bias in this study is unlikely because similar odds ratios were calculated for nulligravid women.

Conclusion.—These findings should provide reassurance to women with prolonged use of oral contraceptives, as it appears that these women experience no adverse effects in terms of the time needed to conceive.

▶ Many women believe that prolonged use of oral contraceptives (OCs) will result in a decreased ability to conceive or delay the time until conception occurs, compared with non–OC users. The results of this large study indicate that prolonged use of oral contraceptives actually decreased the duration of

TABLE 4.—The Effect of the Duration of Oral Contraceptive Use on the Odds Ratios for Achieving Conception Within 12 Months for All Women in the Study

	≥5 Years (Ref.)	3-4 Years	1-2 Years	<1 Year	Never	χ^2 (P-Value)
Years of oral contraceptive use	3849 (59.1%)	1311 (20.1%)	678 (10.3%)	407 (6.2%)	279 (4.3%)	
Conception within 12 months (n = 5754; 88.2%)	1.00	0.71 (0.56-0.91)	0.52 (0.39-0.70)	0.46 (0.33-0.65)	0.67 (0.43-1.06)	33.24 (< 0.0001)

Note: 95% confidence intervals. Adjustment was made for woman's and man's age at starting to try to conceive (+ quadratic term for woman's age), woman's body mass index (+ quadratic term), education, exposure to smoking, parity, housing type, and years of cohabitation.

(Courtesy of Farrow A, Hull MGR, Northstone K, et al: Prolonged use of oral contraception before a planned pregnancy is associated with a decreased risk of delayed conception. *Hum Reprod* 17:2754-2761, 2002. Copyright European Society for Human Reproduction and Embryology, by permission of Oxford University Press.)

time to conception among both nulliparous and parous women attempting to become pregnant, compared with OC nonusers of similar age. Women who had not used OCs were about one third less likely to conceive in 1 year, compared with an age-matched group of women who had used OCs for more than 5 years before stopping these agents in order to become pregnant.

An earlier report found that long-term OC users who became pregnant after stopping their use were less likely to have a miscarriage than women who became pregnant without prior use of OCs. Women should be reassured that long-term OC use does not adversely delay the time to conception or having a miscarriage in these pregnancies and may actually reduce the risk of each of these problems.

D. R. Mishell, Jr, MD

Infertility Drugs and the Risk of Breast Cancer: Findings From the National Institute of Child Health and Human Development Women's Contraceptive and Reproductive Experiences Study
Burkman RT, Tang M-TC, Malone KE, et al (Henry Ford Health System, Detroit; Fred Hutchinson Cancer Research Ctr, Seattle; Ctrs for Disease Control and Prevention, Atlanta, Ga)
Fertil Steril 79:844-851, 2003   15–2

Background.—The relationship between exogenous reproductive hormones and breast cancer has been widely studied as part of the continuing effort to identify risk factors for breast cancer. Other factors, such as menstrual cycle characteristics and infertility, including a variety of treatment approaches, have been studied. Results from some of these studies have indicated that increased numbers of ovulatory menstrual cycles may increase the risk of breast cancer. Women with infertility caused at least partly by ovulatory dysfunction may be treated with drugs that stimulate ovulation and alter levels of endogenous reproductive hormones. Some studies, but not all, have shown an association between pharmacologic therapy for infertility and breast cancer risk. Whether such an association exists was determined in a multicenter study in 5 large US cities.

Methods.—This population-based case-control study included 4575 women, 35 to 64 years old, with histologically confirmed primary invasive breast cancer and 4682 control subjects (women without breast cancer) identified in the same geographic locations using random-digit telephone dialing. Patients and control subjects were asked to complete a standardized questionnaire that focused on reproductive health, family history, and the use of oral contraceptives and other hormones and infertility drugs. Data on the type of breast cancer were obtained from the case patients. The main outcome measures were the odds ratios indicating the association between the use of various infertility drugs and invasive breast cancer.

Results.—Overall, no association was noted between a history of drug use and the risk of breast cancer. However, compared with women who never used any fertility medications, women who used human menopausal gonadotropin (hMG) for 6 months or more for at least 6 cycles had a relative risk of breast cancer ranging between 2.7 and 3.8.

Conclusions.—A history of infertility drug use was generally not associated with an increased risk of breast cancer, but the long-term use of certain infertility drugs, particularly hMG, may increase the risk of breast cancer. More studies are needed to confirm this potential association.

▶ The relation of drugs used to induce ovulation and the subsequent development of breast cancer remains uncertain with some studies showing an increased risk and others no increase. The results of this case-control study found no overall relation between use of these drugs and the development of breast cancer, but use of hMG for more than 6 cycles may be associated with a 3-fold increased risk of breast cancer. Additional studies are needed before a relation between use of some or all ovulation-inducing agents in infertile women and an increased risk of breast cancer is either confirmed or refuted.

D. R. Mishell, Jr, MD

A Randomized Clinical Trial of Treatment of Clomiphene Citrate–Resistant Anovulation With the Use of Oral Contraceptive Pill Suppression and Repeat Clomiphene Citrate Treatment

Branigan EF, Estes MA (Bellingham In Vitro Fertilization and Infertility Ctr, Wash)
Am J Obstet Gynecol 188:1424-1430, 2003   15–3

Background.—One of the more common causes of infertility in women is chronic anovulation. In most cases, women with chronic anovulation are treated initially with clomiphene citrate (CC), 50 to 250 mg. One large study reported that 50% of patients ovulate at the 50-mg dose and that 74% of patients ovulate at the 100-mg dose. However, less than 50% of these women will become pregnant despite successful ovulation.

It has been reported that more than 25% of women with chronic anovulation will fail to ovulate on any dose of CC. For these CC-resistant women, adjunctive therapy includes weight loss, insulin-sensitizing agents, bromocriptine, glucocorticoids, extended doses or continued doses of CC, and surgery. All of these options are accompanied by some risk and are not useful in all CC-resistant patients. The effectiveness and endocrine response of oral contraceptive ovarian suppression followed by clomiphene citrate in CC-resistant patients was investigated.

Methods.—The study enrolled 48 patients from a private tertiary infertility clinic. The patients were randomly assigned to either oral contraceptive/CC or to CC only. On day 3, 17β-estradiol, follicle-stimulating hormone, luteinizing hormone, and androgens were assayed before and after treatment. The main outcome measures were follicle growth, ovulation, and pregnancy. The statistical significance of the findings was determined by the Student *t* test and analysis of variance.

Results.—The group treated with oral contraceptive/CC had a significantly higher percentage of patients who ovulated and a significantly higher percentage of ovulatory cycles and pregnancies compared with patients who received CC only. The oral contraceptive/CC group also had significantly lower levels of 17β-estradiol, luteinizing hormone, and androgen. There were no significant changes in these hormone levels in the group that received CC only.

Conclusion.—In patients with chronic anovulation who were previously resistant to CC, suppression of the ovary with oral contraceptives provided excellent rates of ovulation and pregnancy. The mechanism of this improved response may be the declines in ovarian androgens, luteinizing hormones, and 17β-estradiol.

▶ Various modalities have been used to induce ovulation in anovulatory women with adequate amounts of circulatory estrogen who fail to ovulate following use of CC. Methods utilized include metaformin, dexamethasone, human menopausal gonadotropin, and partial ovarian destruction. The results of this randomized trial indicate that administration of oral contraceptives for 6 to 7 weeks followed by CC resulted in a 71% ovulation rate among a group of women who previously had not ovulated with high doses of CC.

It is much easier and less costly to administer oral contraceptives than human menopausal gonadotropin to anovulatory women who do not ovulate with CC. Clinicians may wish to utilize this form of therapy as a way to initially manage anovulatory women who do not respond to CC therapy. However, additional studies in other settings are needed to confirm the good results of this study.

D. R. Mishell, Jr, MD

Pregnancy Outcomes Among Women With Polycystic Ovary Syndrome Treated With Metformin
Glueck CJ, Wang P, Goldenberg N, et al (Jewish Hosp, Cincinnati, Ohio)
Hum Reprod 17:2858-2864, 2002   15–4

Background.—Metformin has been shown to facilitate conception in oligoamenorrheic women with polycystic ovary syndrome (PCOS). Whether metformin would safely decrease the rate of first-trimester spontaneous abortion (SAB) and increase the number of live births without teratogenicity was determined.

Methods and Findings.—Seventy-two oligoamenorrheic women with PCOS who conceived with metformin, 2.55 g/d, were evaluated prospectively in an outpatient clinic. Of the 84 fetuses conceived, 63 normal live births (75%) have occurred to date. Fourteen (17%) ended in SAB. The remaining 7 pregnancies (8%) are ongoing at 13 weeks or more, with no evidence of congenital defects or other abnormalities on sonography. Before metformin treatment, 40 of the 72 women had had a total of 100 pregnancies, which resulted in 34 live births and 62 first-trimester SAB. With metfor-

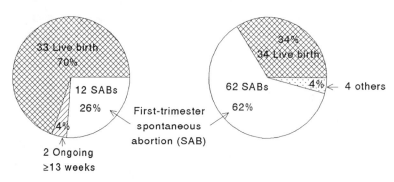

Current (receiving metformin)
46 pregnancies, 47 fetuses

Previous (not receiving metformin)
100 pregnancies

FIGURE 2.—Current (on metformin) and previous (no metformin) pregnancy outcomes in 40 women with polycystic ovarian syndrome. Without metformin the 40 women had 100 pregnancies with 34 (34%) live births and 62 (62%) first trimester spontaneous abortions (SAB). On metformin, the 40 women had 46 pregnancies, 47 fetuses (1 twin pregnancy, 6 women with 2 singleton pregnancies, 33 women with 1 singleton pregnancy). Metformin reduced first trimester SAB from 62% to 26% (McNemar's $S = 32$, df $= 1$; $P <$ .0001). (Courtesy of Glueck CJ, Wang P, Goldenberg N, et al: Pregnancy outcomes among women with polycystic ovary syndrome treated with metformin. *Hum Reprod* 17:2858-2864, 2002. Copyright European Society for Human Reproduction and Embryology, by permission of Oxford University Press.)

min, these 40 women have had a total of 46 pregnancies with 47 fetuses, resulting in 33 live births (70%), 2 ongoing pregnancies (4%), and 12 SAB (26%) (Fig 2). No maternal lactic acidosis occurred. There were no cases of maternal or neonatal hypoglycemia. Fasting entry serum insulin was a significant factor in total first-trimester SAB, with an odds ratio of 1.32. Gestational diabetes developed in 4% of pregnancies with metformin, compared with 26% in previous pregnancies without metformin. No major congenital defects have been identified in the 63 live births or in the 7 continuing fetuses. The weight and length of the 63 babies born did not differ significantly from those of a normal neonatal population. At 6 months, their height was greater than and their weight comparable to that in a normal pediatric population. Motor and social development were also normal.

Conclusions.—Metformin given during pregnancy to women with PCOS is associated with a decrease in SAB and gestational diabetes. This treatment was not teratogenic, with no adverse effects on birth weight or height, or weight, height, and motor and social development at 3 and 6 months' follow-up.

▶ Use of the insulin-sensitizing drug metformin has been shown to induce ovulation in women with PCOS. Women with PCOS who conceive have a high rate of SAB. In this cohort of women with PCOS, the SAB rate of pregnancies conceived without metformin was 62%. In this study, metformin was continued throughout pregnancy or through the first trimester, and the SAB rate was 17% (26% in the 40 women with prior pregnancies). The data from this observational study suggest that continuing metformin throughout pregnancy in women with PCOS who conceive reduces the incidence of first-trimester SAB as well as the development of gestational diabetes. These results need to be confirmed by performing a randomized controlled trial comparing the use of metformin with placebo.

D. R. Mishell, Jr, MD

Sequential Treatment of Metformin and Clomiphene Citrate in Clomiphene-Resistant Women With Polycystic Ovary Syndrome: A Randomized, Controlled Trial

George SS, George K, Irwin C, et al (Christian Med College, Vellore, Tamil Nadu, India)

Hum Reprod 18:299-304, 2003   15–5

Background.—The importance of insulin resistance in clomiphene-resistant women with polycystic ovary syndrome (PCOS) has been recognized, resulting in the use of insulin sensitizers. The efficacy of sequential treatment with metformin and clomiphene citrate was compared with that of conventional gonadotropins in a randomized, controlled study.

Methods.—Sixty clomiphene-resistant women with PCOS were assigned to receive either metformin for 6 months, followed by ovulation induction with clomiphene citrate (group 1), or human menopausal gonadotropin for ovulation induction (group 2). Hormonal profiles were assessed at treatment initiation and after treatment completion.

Findings.—Pregnancy rates did not differ significantly between groups 1 and 2, being 16.7% and 23.3%, respectively. Group 1 had significant improvement in menstrual function and ovulation after treatment (40% and 46.7%, respectively). This group also had a significant reduction in fasting insulin concentrations. No changes occurred in other biochemical parameters. In group 2, the ovulation rate was 43.3%, with a high rate of dropout. Cost analysis for medications per pregnancy indicated a cost of $71 in group 1 and $277 in group 2.

Conclusions.—Sequential treatment with metformin and clomiphene citrate is effective and safe in clomiphene-resistant women with PCOS. Such sequential therapy significantly improves ovarian function in this population. A significant decline in fasting insulin levels was also associated with this treatment.

▶ Infertile anovulating women with PCOS who fail to ovulate after treatment witih clomiphene citrate have been treated with human menopausal gonadotropin (hMG) with limited success. The results of this randomized trial indicate that similar pregnancy rates occur in women with PCOS who fail to ovulate with clomiphene citrate when they are treated with hMG or metformin followed by clomiphene citrate. Since metformin is less expensive and easier to administer than hMG, metformin therapy should be given initially to anovulatory women with PCOS who fail to ovulate with clomiphene citrate.

D. R. Mishell, Jr, MD

Use of Dexamethasone and Clomiphene Citrate in the Treatment of Clomiphene Citrate–Resistant Patients With Polycystic Ovary Syndrome and Normal Dehydroepiandrosterone Sulfate Levels: A Prospective, Double-Blind, Placebo-Controlled Trial
Parsanezhad ME, Alborzi S, Motazedian S, et al (Shiraz Univ of Med Sciences, Iran)
Fertil Steril 78:1001-1004, 2002   15–6

Purpose.—Twenty to thirty percent of women with polycystic ovary syndrome (PCOS) do not respond to front-line therapy with clomiphene citrate (CC). The efficacy of adding dexamethasone to CC was evaluated for the treatment of PCOS in women with normal levels of dehydroepiandrosterone sulfate (DHEAS) who are resistant to initial CC therapy.

Methods.—This double-blind, randomized trial included 230 infertile women with PCOS who were resistant to CC but had normal serum DHEAS levels. The definition of CC resistance included failure to achieve ovulation and a normal luteal phase after at least 5 cycles with an increasing dose of CC; all patients did not ovulate despite a 250-mg dose of CC for 5 days combined with 10,000 IU of human chorionic gonadotropin. Women assigned to the treatment group received 200 mg CC from cycle day 5 to 9, plus 2 mg dexamethasone from day 5 to 14; those in the control group received the same dose of CC plus placebo from days 5 to 14. The 2 groups were compared for follicular development, hormonal status, ovulation rate, and pregnancy rate.

Results.—Mean dominant follicle diameter was 18.4124 mm in the treatment group versus 13.8585 in the control group. Evidence of ovulation occurred in 88% of women receiving CC plus dexamethasone compared with 20% of those receiving CC plus placebo. Women in the treatment group also had significant reductions in DHEAS and hormone levels. The pregnancy rate was 40.5% in the treatment group compared with 4.2% in the control group.

Conclusions.—For women with PCOS and normal DHEAS levels who do not respond to CC, adding dexamethasone to subsequent CC treatment has beneficial effects. The combination of dexamethasone and CC brings improvement in follicular development, hormone levels, and pregnancy rate. This treatment should be tried before proceeding to gonadotropin administration or surgery.

▶ Daily administration of 0.5 mg dexamethasone has been used to induce ovulation in women with PCOS who have elevated levels of DHEAS and fail to ovulate with high doses of CC alone. The results of this randomized trial indicate that women with PCOS and normal levels of DHEAS who fail to ovulate with CC alone also have a high incidence of ovulatory cycles and subsequent pregnancy when they receive very high doses of dexamethasone for 10 days in the follicular phase of the cycle. If other studies confirm these findings, the therapy described in this trial may be used to treat anovulatory women with

PCOS who fail to ovulate with CC instead of using human menopausal gonadotropins with their associated high incidence of complications.

D. R. Mishell, Jr, MD

Effect of Diagnosis, Age, Sperm Quality, and Number of Preovulatory Follicles on the Outcome of Multiple Cycles of Clomiphene Citrate–Intrauterine Insemination
Dickey RP, Taylor SN, Lu PY, et al (Fertility Inst of New Orleans, La; Louisiana State Univ, New Orleans)
Fertil Steril 78:1088-1095, 2002   15–7

Background.—With infertility treatments such as clomiphene citrate (CC) and intrauterine insemination (IUI), an upper limit is set as to the number of successful treatment cycles; beyond that limit, pregnancies are less likely. However, other than a possible increased likelihood of ovarian cancer with long-term use of ovulation-inducing agents, no scientific reason supports these usually 3-cycle limits. Factors influencing likelihood of pregnancy when IUI is used include endometriosis, tubal factor, age, poor initial sperm quality, and single preovulatory follicle. Whether the low pregnancy rates with these factors are overcome by repetitive cycles of combined CC-IUI therapy was assessed along with how many cycles should be tried.

Methods.—During a 15-year period, 4000 women (8051 IUI cycles) were treated; 3381 CC-IUI cycles were analyzed. Ovulation induction used CC alone or with human chorionic gonadotropin (hCG). Patients with a history of pelvic inflammatory disease, pelvic surgery, symptoms of dyspareunia or severe dysmenorrhea, or evidence of endometriosis had laparoscopy before CC-IUI initiation; others had diagnostic laparoscopy after 3 CC-IUI cycles without pregnancy. IUI was done when husband semen quality failed to meet World Health Organization (WHO) criteria ($\geq$ 20 million/mL, total $\geq$40 million, progressive motility $\geq$50%, and $\geq$30% normal forms) or when fewer than 5 progressively motile sperm were found on repeated overnight postcoital testing. Ovulation induction began on the cycle's third day; based on initial cycle body weight, 50 or 100 mg of CC was used. Progesterone level was measured 5 to 7 days after ovulation. With fresh sperm, a single IUI was done within 24 hours of a luteinizing hormone surge or 24 to 36 hours after hCG injection; with cryopreserved donor sperm, IUI was done 36 hours after hCG injection. Per-cycle pregnancy rate (PR) and cumulative PR were determined.

Results.—In 313 of the 3381 CC-IUI cycles, clinical pregnancies occurred (9.2%); 72 spontaneous abortions (23.0%) and 13 ectopic pregnancies (4.2%) were included. The average per-cycle PR was 9.7% during the first 4 CC-IUI cycles, falling to 2.8% in cycles 5 and 6. No pregnancies in 57 attempts occurred beyond the sixth cycle. For all diagnoses, PRs were constant for at least 4 cycles when women aged 43 years or older and cycles with sperm below IUI quality were excluded (Fig 1). Patients with ovulation dysfunction had a cumulative PR of 46% after 4 cycles and 65% after 6 cycles.

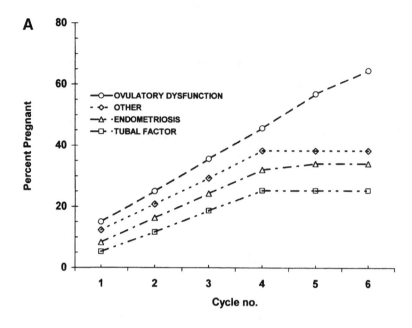

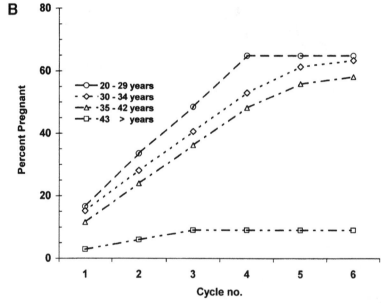

FIGURE 1.—Cumulative pregnancy rate. A, By diagnosis. Diagnoses were as follows: (1) ovulatory dysfunction: anovulatory, polycystic ovaries, or luteal insufficiency; (2) endometriosis: with or without tubal involvement; (3) tubal factor: unilateral tubal obstruction or tubal adhesions without endometriosis; (4) other: cervical factor, male factor, or unexplained infertility and normal cycles without endometriosis or tubal factor. Patients aged ≥43 years and cycles with total initial motile sperm count of <5 million or motility of <30% excluded. B, By age. Patients with endometriosis, tubal impairment, and cycles with total initial motile sperm count of <5 million or motility of <30% were excluded. (Courtesy of Dickey RP, Taylor SN, Lu PY, et al: Effect of diagnosis, age, sperm quality, and number of preovulatory follicles on the outcome of multiple cycles of clomiphene citrate–intrauterine insemination. *Fertil Steril* 78:1088-1095, 2002. Copyright American Society for Reproductive Medicine. Copyright 2002, with permission from the American College of Surgeons.)

For women younger than 30, when endometriosis, tubal factor, and sub–IUI-quality sperm were omitted, the cumulative PR was 65% and plateaued after 4 cycles. When donor sperm were used, cumulative PRs were 61% after 4 cycles and 76% after 6 cycles (excluding endometriosis, tubal factor, and age ≥43). A 73% plateaued PR after 4 cycles was found with at least 3 preovulatory follicles of at least 15 mm on the day hCG was injected or when LH surge occurred (omitting endometriosis, tubal factor, age ≥43, and sub–IUI-quality sperm). Eliminating women aged 43 or older and patients with endometriosis and tubal factor, no significant difference in PR was found during the first 4 cycles regardless of whether husband sperm met WHO criteria, did not meet WHO criteria but was sufficient for IUI, or donor sperm was used. A link was found between PR and the number of follicles of at least 15 mm when hCG was injected; the PR increased from 9.8% per cycle with 1 follicle to 17.7% with 3 or more follicles.

Conclusions.—Pregnancies occurred at a constant rate over at least 4 CC-IUI cycles in the 3381 cycles evaluated. Patients with ovulatory dysfunction had cumulative PRs of 65% after 6 cycles. Continuing CC-IUI for 5 and 6 cycles compensated for conditions linked to reduced per-cycle PRs, specifically, age greater than 30, lower quality sperm, and fewer than 3 preovulatory follicles present, if the women do not have endometriosis or tubal factor. Thus, CC-IUI can be recommended for at least 4 cycles before more aggressive interventions are undertaken.

▶ The use of CC, 100 mg/d, for 5 days beginning on cycle day 2 in ovulating women with unexplained infertility, results in pregnancy rates of about 10% to 15% per cycle when IUI is also used. In this study, the cumulative PR after 4 cycles of CC plus IUI in women without tubal disease or endometriosis was nearly 40%. The PR did not increase with 2 more cycles of CC plus IUI. Women with unexplained infertility should be offered the opportunity of treatment with 4 cycles of CC plus IUI before in vitro fertilization.

D. R. Mishell, Jr, MD

Assisted Reproductive Technology in the United States: 1999 Results Generated From the American Society for Reproductive Medicine/ Society for Assisted Reproductive Technology Registry
Society for Assisted Reproductive Technology and the American Society for Reproductive Medicine (Birmingham, Ala)
Fertil Steril 78:918-931, 2002   15–8

Background.—The Society for Assisted Reproductive Technology and the American Society for Reproductive Medicine collect yearly data on the assisted reproductive technology (ART) procedures and outcomes performed in the United States each year. The 1999 results are presented.

Methods.—The report includes mandatory information reports by 370 ART programs. The medical director of the reporting clinic verified the accuracy of all data; on-site validation visits were made to a random sample of 29 clinics.

Findings.—During 1999, the 370 programs initiated approximately 88,000 cycles of ART treatment. Nearly 67,000 of these consisted of in vitro fertilization (IVF) and fresh transfer of embryos from the patient's own oocytes; intracytoplasmic sperm injection (ICSI) was performed in approximately 27,000 cycles. Approximately 800 cycles of fresh nondonor gamete intrafallopian transfer and 950 of zygote intrafallopian transfer were performed, with ICSI used in approximately 700. Donor oocytes and fresh embryo transfer were used in approximately 6500 cycles, including 2500 with ICSI and 800 with embryo transfer to a host uterus. There were 12,000 nondonor cryopreserved embryo thaw procedures, along with 2500 donor oocyte or embryo-derived cryopreserved embryo thaw procedures. All these activities led to approximately 22,000 deliveries and 31,000 newborns; more than one third of deliveries were multiple gestations.

The retrieval rate of all initiated IVF cycles was 86%, with 93% of retrievals leading to transfer. The clinical pregnancy rate was 30.5% per cycle and 38% per transfer. Delivery rates were 25% and 32%, respectively. The clinical pregnancy loss rate was 17%, with an ectopic pregnancy rate of approximately 2%. Success rates in 1999 were 32% for women younger than 35 years, 26% for those aged 35 to 37 years, 18% for those aged 38 to 40 years, and 8% for those older than 40 years. Women younger than 35 accounted for 45% of all IVF cycles; the report includes detailed information on outcomes of IVF, by age, for couples with and without male factor infertility. Outcomes data are also presented in terms of ART clinic volume.

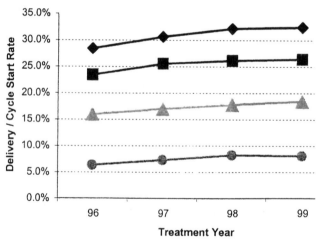

FIGURE 1.—Annual comparison of IVF delivery rates. *Diamonds* represent women less than 35 years, *squares* represent women 35 to 37 years, *triangles* represent women 38 to 40 years, and *circles* represent women more than 40 years. (Courtesy of Society for Assisted Reproductive Technology and the American Society for Reproductive Medicine: Assisted reproductive technology in the United States: 1999 results generated from the American Society for Reproductive Medicine/Society for Assisted Reproductive Technology Registry. *Fertil Steril* 78:918-931, 2002. Copyright American Society for Reproductive Medicine. Copyright 2002, with permission from the American College of Surgeons.)

Conclusions.—The 1999 data suggest significant increases in the number of programs performing ART, along with a 7.5% increase in the number of reported cycles compared with the previous year. Success rate increased by 0.4% overall, or by 1.2% compared with the previous year. The report highlights include the dramatic effect of patient age on success rate (Fig 1) and the declining impact of male factor infertility, presumably related to the effective use of ICSI.

▶ The results of this annual analysis of ART in the United States provides useful information for infertile couples considering use of these techniques in order to have a viable birth. It is of interest that large-volume clinics had higher viable birth rates (32% per initiated cycle) than low-volume clinics (24%). Age of the woman also strongly affected viable birth rates, 33% per initiated cycle for women younger than 35 years compared with 8% for women older than 40 years. It is of interest that 43% of all IVF cycles in the United States in 1999 used ICSI. The use of this technique allowed couples with male factor infertility to have the same delivery rate as couples with other diagnoses of infertility.

D. R. Mishell, Jr, MD

Intracytoplasmic Sperm Injection Versus In Vitro Fertilization: A Randomized Controlled Trial and a Meta-analysis of the Literature
Tournaye H, Verheyen G, Albano C, et al (Dutch-Speaking Brussels Free Univ, Belgium)
Fertil Steril 78:1030-1037, 2002   15–9

Background.—In cases of male infertility caused by poor sperm quality, intracytoplasmic sperm injection (ICSI) has been used to successfully increase the fertilization rate. However, concerns have been raised about its safety. Whether increasing the sperm concentration during standard in vitro fertilization (IVF) procedures could reduce the need for ICSI procedures in cases of male infertility was investigated.

Study Design.—The study group consisted of 73 couples who were using artificial reproductive technology because of moderate male infertility. The first cumulus-oocyte complex aspirated was randomly assigned to either ICSI or IVF, and subsequent oocytes were assigned to alternating procedures. For conventional IVF, each oocyte was inseminated with 5000 (standard) or 20,000 (high insemination concentration, HIC) motile spermatozoa. All resulting embryos were evaluated on the basis of morphologic characteristics and 2 or 3 were transferred.

Findings.—The overall fertilization rate was significantly lower after standard IVF than after ICSI or HIC IVF. The rates for ICSI and HIC IVF were comparable. Once fertilization occurred, the mean cleavage rate was the same for all procedures. No differences in embryo morphologic characteristics were observed between procedures.

Conclusions.—ICSI is a more efficient technique than standard IVF, but not more efficient than HIC IVF. HIC IVF may provide an alternative to the use of ICSI in cases of moderate male infertility.

▶ Currently a high proportion of IVF procedures, with and without abnormalities in the semen analysis cycle, are being performed with ICSI. There are concerns about the long-term effects of ICSI on malformation risks and child development. As shown in this study, oocytes used in IVF that are inseminated with a concentration of 200,000 motile spermatozoa from men with moderate abnormalities in the semen analysis had a much lower fertilization rate than when ICSI was used. However, when a concentration of 800,000 motile spermatozoa were used in the IVF procedure, the fertilization rates were the same as ICSI. When the male partner has abnormalities in the semen analysis, with the use of HIC of sperm, it appears that pregnancy rates after IVF are similar to the use of ICSI. Therefore the use of ICSI with its theoretical concerns about safety may be unnecessary.

D. R. Mishell, Jr, MD

Outcome of First and Repeated Testicular Sperm Extraction and ICSI in Patients With Non-obstructive Azoospermia
Friedler S, Raziel A, Schachter M, et al (Assaf Harofeh Med Ctr, Zerifin, Israel)
Hum Reprod 17:2356-2361, 2002   15–10

Background.—The value of repeating testicular sperm extraction (TESE) for patients in whom no sperm are found during the first attempt is not clear. The outcome of 2 to 5 repetitive TESE procedures as opposed to the first trial in patients with nonobstructive azoospermia was evaluated.

Methods.—Eighty-three patients with nonobstructive azoospermia underwent open testicular biopsy for TESE between 1995 and 1999. Testicular sperm extraction was done twice in 22 patients, 3 times in 8 patients, 4 times in 6 patients, and 5 times in 3 patients. The distribution of main testicular histology was germ cell aplasia in 55%, maturation arrest in 29%, and germ cell hypoplasia in 16%.

Findings.—The first TESE yielded mature sperm for intracytoplasmic sperm injection in 39% of the patients (sp+) and failed in 61% (sp−). A second TESE yielded mature sperm in 1 of 4 patients in the sp− group as well as in 16 of 18 patients in the sp+ group. In the original sp+ group, 8 of 8 patients were sp+ again on the third trial, 5 of 6 on the fourth trial, and 3 of 3 on the fifth trial. When compared with the first trial outcome, all further trials did not differ significantly in rate of fertilization, implantation, or clinical pregnancy per cycle. No pregnancies were achieved after the fifth TESE (Table 3, B). With the exception of maturation arrest, pregnancies occurred in all histologic groups.

Conclusions.—Repeating TESE appears to have clinical value, as pregnancies can be achieved in each repetitive trial. Repeated trials also do not appear to result in increased complications.

TABLE 3, B.—Outcome of First and Repetitive Testicular Sperm Extraction (*TESE*)–ICSI Cycles

TESE Trial	1st TESE	Repetitive TESE
No. of ICSI cycles	32	33
No. of ova injected/cycle	9.2 ± 4.6	9.0 ± 4.9
No. of ova fertilized/cycle	5.0 ± 3.4	5.4 ± 2.8
Fertilization rate (%)	54	49
No. of embryos cleaved/cycle	4.7 ± 3.4	4.8 ± 3.0
No. of embryos replaced/embryo transfer	3.0 ± 1.5	4.0 ± 1.8
Implantation rate (%)	10/105 (9.5)	6/112 (5.4)
Clinical pregnancy rate/embryo transfer (%)	6/31 (19)	5/31 (16)
Clinical pregnancy rate/ICSI cycle (%)	6/32 (19)	5/33 (15)
Pregnancy outcome	4 (delivered) 2 (early miscarriages) 3 (delivered)	1 (missed twin, singleton delivered) 1 (IUFD at 34th week of gestation)

Abbreviations: ICSI, Intracytoplasmic sperm injection; *IUFD,* intrauterine fetal death.

(Courtesy of Friedler S, Raziel A, Schachter M, et al: Outcome of first and repeated testicular sperm extraction and ICSI in patients with non-obstructive azoospermia. *Hum Reprod* 17:2356-2361, 2002. Copyright European Society for Human Reproduction and Embryology, by permission of Oxford University Press.)

▶ The use of TESE followed by intracytoplasmic sperm injection (ICSI) in men with nonobstructive azoospermia has resulted in viable births. In this study, about 40% of men with nonobstructive azoospermia had testicular sperm retrieved that allowed ICSI to be performed. Of the pregnancies that occurred in these treatment cycles, two thirds resulted in viable births. In this study, repetitive TESE was repeated in about half of these men, and about 10% to 20% of the subsequent ICSI cycles resulted in pregnancies in the second to fourth, but not the fifth cycle of TESE. Men with nonobstructive azoospermia who have sperm present after TESE, but ICSI does not result in a viable birth, may be offered several additional cycles of TESE followed by ICSI because pregnancy may occur.

D. R. Mishell, Jr, MD

Pregnancy Course and Health of Children Born After ICSI Depending on Parameters of Male Factor Infertility
Ludwig M, for the German ICSI Follow-up Study Group (Univ Hosp, Lübeck, Germany; et al)
Hum Reprod 18:351-357, 2003   15–11

Background.—Intracytoplasmic sperm injection (ICSI) may use sperm obtained by ejaculation or those of testicular or epididymal origin. No increased risk of major malformations has been detected among the children conceived with the ICSI method, but some concern has arisen concerning risks that may be associated with the source of the sperm. A prospectively collected database was evaluated regarding the pregnancies that occurred after ICSI and whether there were differences between pregnancies established after the use of sperm from ejaculates, testicular biopsies, or epididymal aspirates.

Methods.—Data were obtained from 3198 couples in Germany who were pregnant after an ICSI procedure and the transfer of fresh embryos. All were enrolled before the 16th week of gestation (a point when the further course of pregnancy cannot be foreseen) and were included only if the pregnancy was continuing at the 16th week. Analysis was carried out for differences in the course of the pregnancy and in the outcome between those using ejaculated, epididymal, or testicular sperm. A total of 2809 pregnancies were included; 2687 pregnant patients (95.7%) consented to a second contact and examination of their offspring after birth, a total of 3372 fetuses/children. Data concerning sperm count and origin were available for 2545 pregnancies that produced 3199 fetuses/children.

Results.—Comparing the pregnancies/children with the sperm data, no statistically significant differences were noted between the groups with respect to live births, stillbirths, pregnancy terminations, or spontaneous abortions; complication rates; rate of singleton, twin, or triplet births; birth data; rate of major malformations; major malformations linked to their indication; or major malformation rates and number of sperm found in the ejaculate.

Conclusions.—There is no increased risk for established pregnancies and live infants when epididymal or testicular sperm rather than ejaculated sperm are used for an ICSI procedure. The risk of a major malformation was similar in the 3 groups, and the data for children who were born were similar, with no significant differences. These findings confirm those of previous studies showing that the use of epididymal or testicular sperm rather than ejaculated sperm does not influence the course of the pregnancy, the outcome, or the birth data of the children born. It should be noted that enrollment before the 16th week of gestation does not allow estimations of early abortion rates or the rate of ectopic pregnancies.

▶ ICSI is the optimal method to treat severe male factor infertility. ICSI is used with both ejaculated sperm and sperm recovered from the testis or epididymis in men with both obstructive and nonobstructive azoospermia. An earlier study from this group reported that children born after ICSI had a significantly increased risk of major malformations (relative risk, 1.25) compared with children who were conceived spontaneously. In this study, among pregnancies of more than 16 weeks' gestation, there were no differences in malformation or pregnancy outcomes among children conceived with ICSI from ejaculated sperm (n = 2887), testicular sperm (n = 227), or epididymal sperm (n = 25). There was also no relation between the number of sperm in the ejaculate and the malformation rate. These data should be presented to couples considering the use of ICSI with sperm obtained from testicular and epididymal origin.

D. R. Mishell, Jr, MD

Developmental Outcome at 2 Years of Age for Children Born After ICSI Compared With Children Born After IVF
Bonduelle M, Ponjaert I, van Steirteghem A, et al (Dutch-speaking Brussels Free Univ, Belgium)
Hum Reprod 18:342-350, 2003   15–12

Background.—Medical outcome studies on children born after intracytoplasmic sperm injection (ICSI) have been done, but few have addressed developmental outcomes. The results of a standard developmental test in 2-year-old children born after ICSI were compared with the results in children born after in vitro fertilization (IVF).

Methods and Findings.—Four hundred thirty-nine children born after ICSI and 207 born after IVF were studied at 24 to 28 months. The 2 groups did not differ in maternal educational level, maternal age, gestational age, parity, birth weight, neonatal complications rate, or malformation rate at 2 years of age. Developmental outcomes assessed by the Bayley scale also did not differ between the groups. A multivariate regression analysis for singletons indicated that parity, sex, and age significantly affected the test result, with boys having lower scores than girls. However, the fertility procedure did not influence test results. Children born after ICSI to fathers with low sperm concentration, low sperm motility, or poor morphology had developmental outcomes comparable to those in children with fathers with normal sperm parameters.

Conclusions.—Children born after ICSI do not appear to have a lower psychomotor development than children born after IVF. Paternal risk factors associated with male-factor infertility had no effect on developmental outcome.

► Infertile couples considering ICSI may be concerned that this procedure would have an adverse effect on the development of children born after ICSI was used to achieve fertilization. The results of this study indicate that children born after ICSI do not have lower psychomotor development at 2 years of age than children born after standard IVF. The sperm quality of the father also does not influence the psychomotor development of children born after ICSI. Couples considering ICSI should be informed about the results of this study.

D. R. Mishell, Jr, MD

16 Ectopic Pregnancy

Sites of Ectopic Pregnancy: A 10 Year Population-Based Study of 1800 Cases
Bouyer J, Coste J, Fernandez H, et al (INSERM U569-IFR69, Le Kremlin Bicêtre, France; Hôpital Antoine Béclère, Clamart, France; CHU Hôtel-Dieu, Clermont-Ferrand, France)
Hum Reprod 17:3224-3230, 2002   16–1

Background.—The incidence of ectopic pregnancy (EP) among women in developed countries rose by a factor of 3 to 4 in the 1980s and 1990s, but some countries have noted a decline more recently. The site of implantation of the EP influences how severe the problem becomes as well as immediate and delayed adverse effects. With the use of a population-based sample, the distribution of EP sites was assessed, as was variance over time. The immediate complications and factors that determine the site of EP were investigated, along with rates of subsequent fertility and EP recurrence.

Methods.—Three departments of the Auvergne region of central France were included in a registry consisting of all women aged 15 to 44 years who live permanently in this area and who had either surgical or medical interventions for EP. Follow-up was continued until age 45 years, with recording of all reproductive outcomes. The study focused on 1933 EPs registered from January 1992 to December 2001. A total of 133 women with medical treatment only were excluded because implantation site data were lacking, but for 1679 subjects the site was known. Any relationship between EP site and known risk factors for EP was assessed. Fertility was determined by recurrence of EP and intrauterine pregnancy. "Natural" fertility was evaluated, with women having in vitro fertilization or not trying to become pregnant excluded from follow-up.

Results.—Of the EPs that occurred, 4.5% were extratubal and 75% of the tubal pregnancies were ampullary. The frequency of cervical EPs was less than 1 in 455 EPs. Over time, the site of implantation varied. A significant increase from interstitial to abdominal sites was found in the proportion of EPs diagnosed before 6 weeks' gestation. Human chorionic gonadotropin levels, which indicate pregnancy activity, fell progressively from interstitial to abdominal sites of EP, even after adjustment for pregnancy term at diagnosis. The proportion of EPs initially managed conservatively showed a progressive increase from interstitial to abdominal sites.

The high proportion of failure in interstitial (14.6%) and fimbrial (11.3%) EPs explained the difference in rates of failure of the first treatment attempt. The proportion of women using intrauterine devices (IUDs) increased as one moved from interstitial to ovarian EP sites. Damaged tubes were more likely among women with proximal implantation sites than among those with distal sites. The only factor that remained significantly associated with EP site on multivariate analysis was current use of an IUD.

Of the 1228 women who were followed up for a mean of 3.2 years, 693 attempted to become pregnant again; only 9 who desired a repeat pregnancy had experienced an abdominal pregnancy, so subsequent fertility among women with an abdominal EP could not be evaluated. Of the other 684 women, 78 had another EP, for a 2-year cumulative rate of recurrent EP of 0.22 that did not differ by site of implantation. The 2-year cumulative rate for intrauterine pregnancy was 0.76, with a progressive increase from interstitial to ovarian sites. Of all the women studied, 113 had a second EP.

Conclusion.—The complications that develop with EP vary greatly depending on site of implantation. Use of an IUD was significantly correlated with a lower incidence of interstitial pregnancy. Women who had distal and extratubal EPs tended to have a higher rate of subsequent fertility than those with other sites of implantation. There was some degree of correlation between the sites of 2 successive EPs if they were homolateral.

▶ The results of this large study indicate that about 70% of EPs occur in the ampullary portion of the oviduct and that cervical EPs are extremely rare. It is estimated that only about 0.1% to 0.2% of EPs are cervical pregnancies. It is of interest that of 684 women with an EP trying to become pregnant, 489, or 70%, became pregnant within 2 years. About 22% of these pregnancies were ectopic and 76% intrauterine. Thus, about 53% of women with an EP wishing to conceive had an intrauterine pregnancy in the subsequent 2 years.

Other studies have shown that nulliparous women with an EP are less likely to have a subsequent intrauterine pregnancy than parous women with an EP. With these data, women with an EP who wish to have a child can be counseled to determine if they wish to utilize in vitro fertilization or attempt to conceive spontaneously.

D. R. Mishell, Jr, MD

Cervical Ectopic Pregnancy: A Case Report and Literature Review
Gun M, Mavrogiorgis M (Queen Elizabeth Hosp, Woodville South, Australia)
Ultrasound Obstet Gynecol 19:297-301, 2002   16–2

Background.—Cervical ectopic pregnancy has been associated in the past with high morbidity and adverse consequences for the fertility of affected patients. Early diagnosis with the use of US has led to a significant decline in complications. A case of cervical pregnancy and its diagnosis and management were discussed.

Case Report.—Woman, 39, with a 2-week history of painless vaginal bleeding, was admitted to the emergency department. Quantitative human chorionic gonadotropin was 23,060 IU/L at presentation. This exceeded what was expected for a 5- to 6-week gestation. A transabdominal US was performed on day 1 that showed a well-formed gestational sac containing a live fetal pole just above the vaginal vault, and a diagnosis of cervical pregnancy was made. Conservative management to preserve fertility was started with a single systemic dose of methotrexate at 50 mg/m² body surface area. On day 3, both transabdominal and transvaginal US were repeated, with no fetal heart beat being identified. The only change was that the sac was less rounded. A second dose of systemic methotrexate was given on day 7. On day 11, there was heavy bleeding and a drop in hemoglobin to 8.2 g/dL. A bilateral uterine artery embolization was performed. After a right femoral artery puncture, a 4F guide wire was used to select the left uterine artery. Embolization with Gelfoam was performed until the blood flow ceased. The procedure was repeated on the right internal iliac and right uterine arteries. Bleeding ceased and the human chorionic gonadotropin dropped to 3375 IU/L. A US examination on day 15 showed a reduction in the volume of the sac (1.7 mL), which had become echogenic, with a hypoechoic endometrium and thinning of the echogenic rim of the sac.

Conclusion.—The early diagnosis of cervical pregnancy with the use of US and conservative treatment regimes has decreased the morbidity and improved the ongoing fertility of affected patients.

▶ The presence of a cervical ectopic pregnancy is uncommon but can result in severe hemorrhage and may be fatal. If uterine preservation is desired, treatment with methotrexate may be attempted. Unlike the high success rate following treatment of small unruptured tubal ectopic pregnancies with methotrexate, the failure rate of methotrexate alone for the treatment of cervical pregnancy is high. The additional use of uterine artery embolization, as reported in this case report, appears to increase the success rate following methotrexate therapy of cervical ectopic pregnancy. Thus, if methotrexate alone is unsuccessful, it is advisable to perform uterine artery embolization, provided facilities and personnel with sufficient training in this procedure are available.

D. R. Mishell, Jr, MD

Interstitial Ectopic Pregnancy: A Contemporary Case Series

Verity L, Ludlow J, Dickinson JE (King Edward Mem Hosp for Women, Subiaco, Australia; Univ of Western Australia, Perth)

Aust N Z J Obstet Gynaecol 43:232-235, 2003   16–3

Background.—The term "interstitial ectopic pregnancy" (EP) refers to a rare (2% to 4% of all EPs) ectopic gestation lateral to the uterotubal junction. Six cases were described and conclusions drawn regarding clinical presentation, diagnosis, and management.

Case 1.—Woman, 36, nulliparous, had amenorrhea lasting 6 weeks and heavy vaginal bleeding of 4 days' duration plus abdominal discomfort. Laparoscopy revealed a left interstitial EP. The mass was directly injected under laparoscopic control with 50 mg methotrexate; 2 more IM methotrexate doses were given 2 and 4 days later. The mass resolved in 6 months.

Case 2.—Woman, 45, nulliparous, was seen 6 weeks after embryo transfer with 4 days of vaginal bleeding and right iliac fossa pain. On transvaginal US, a well-defined mass measuring 2 × 2 cm with a 6-mm central echo-free area was noted in the right isthmus, with blood flow in adjacent tissues. A right interstitial pregnancy was suspected and confirmed laparoscopically. A direct 50-mg injection of methotrexate was administered. Serial measurements of β human chorionic gonadotropin (βHCG) showed a progressive fall to undetectable levels 31 days after surgery.

Case 3.—Woman, 22, nulliparous, had 6 weeks of amenorrhea and intermittent pelvic pain lasting 3 weeks. An eccentrically located 4-week–size gestation sac was found on transvaginal US. Laparoscopy was not performed. A 75-mg IM dose of methotrexate was given; then, after βHCG levels rose to 1890 IU/L 4 days later, a second dose was administered. βHCG levels were undetectable 49 days after the last injection.

Case 4.—Woman, 20, in her first pregnancy, had 8 weeks of amenorrhea and experienced 7 days of suprapubic pain and 1 day of vaginal bleeding; the quantitative βHCG level was 5560 IU/L. A right interstitial area with increased vascularity measuring 3 × 3 cm was revealed by transvaginal US, suggesting right interstitial pregnancy. She was given 2 doses of IM methotrexate, 50 mg each 48 hours apart, and had a steady decline in βHCG levels over 60 days.

Case 5.—Woman, 24, multiparous, had experienced painless vaginal bleeding 8 weeks after her last period. An eccentrically located gestation sac measuring 3.5 × 3 cm was noted in the left cornu. It contained a 13-mm fetal pole that lacked cardiac pulsation. Systemic methotrexate was given in two 95-mg doses (1 mg/kg). Serial quantitative βHCG monitoring showed steady declines until 30 days after treatment, when the patient stopped coming for follow-up.

Case 6.—Woman, 38, in her first pregnancy had vaginal bleeding at about 6 weeks gestation and serum βHCG levels of 7900 IU/L. A right-sided eccentrically placed gestation sac with a fetal pole and cardiac activity was found on transvaginal US. Repeat US 6 days later suggested right interstitial pregnancy, and the patient was given a single 80-mg IM dose of methotrexate (1 mg/kg) on an outpatient basis. Normal transvaginal US findings were noted within 2 months.

Conclusion.—Early nonsurgical interventions were successful for non-ruptured small interstitial pregnancies. Transvaginal US suggested the diagnosis; high-resolution US performed by an expert, experienced gynecologic sonographer is recommended. In this study, sensitive quantitative serum βHCG assays supported the diagnosis and monitored treatment. Conservative methods were successful, although route of administration varied. Systemic methotrexate was sufficient in 3 cases; none required open surgery nor were there serious complications or major side effects.

▶ Pregnancies located in the interstitial portion of the oviduct lateral to the uterotubal junction are called interstitial pregnancies. EPs located in this area of the oviduct are uncommon and difficult to diagnose sonographically because of their proximity to the uterine cavity. For this reason, the diagnosis is often delayed until the second trimester when rupture of the EP and interperitoneal hemorrhage occur.

In this series of 6 consecutive cases of interstitial pregnancy, the diagnosis was made in the first trimester by transvaginal sonography. Despite the initial βHCG level being between 5000 and 10,000 mIu/mL in 4 of the 6 cases, all were successfully treated with either local or systemic methotrexate. All patients with a possible EP should have transvaginal sonography performed early in gestation by an experienced sonographer. If an interstitial pregnancy is diagnosed and the βHCG level is less than 10,000 mIU/mL, methotrexate can be used as therapy.

D. R. Mishell, Jr, MD

Presumed Diagnosis of Ectopic Pregnancy
Barnhart KT, Katz I, Hummel A, et al (Univ of Pennsylvania, Philadelphia; Univ of San Francisco)
Obstet Gynecol 100:505-510, 2002   16–4

Background.—Ectopic pregnancy (EP) is a common cause of morbidity and mortality among women in their reproductive years. Because there is no noninivasive method to detect ectopic pregnancy definitively, diagnosis requires exclusion of intrauterine pregnancy, usually by dilation and curettage (D&C). In an attempt to simplify the management of women with presumed EP, some physicians treat these women with methotrexate, without D&C for definitive diagnosis, to save time, reduce costs, and avoid surgery with its potential complications. This retrospective study evaluated the accuracy of diagnosis of presumed EP to determine whether this strategy was effective.

TABLE 1.—Ultimate Diagnosis of Women With Presumed
Ectopic Pregnancy

Final Diagnosis	SAB (%)	Ectopic Pregnancy (%)
All patients	69 (61.6)	43 (38.4)
hCG > 2000 mIU/mL	19 (45.7)	16 (54.3)
hCG < 2000 mIU/mL	24 (31.2)	53 (68.8)

Three groups are demonstrated: all patients, those with hCG of >2000, and those with hCG of <2000.
Abbreviation: SAB, Spontaneous abortion.
(Courtesy of Barnhart KT, Katz I, Hummel A, et al: Presumed diagnosis of ectopic pregnancy. *Obstet Gynecol* 100:505-510, 2002. Reprinted with permission from The American College of Obstetricians and Gynecologists.)

Study Design.—The study group consisted of 112 women with presumed ectopic pregnancies treated at the University of Pennsylvania from 1998 through 1999. During this time, all women with presumed EP underwent D&C before treatment. Women were included if their human chorionic gonadotropin (hCG) level was above the discriminatory zone without visible intrauterine pregnancy or their hCG level plateaued below the discriminatory zone. The primary outcome was the final diagnosis, EP or miscarriage. The diagnosis of miscarriage was based on the presence of chorionic villi at D&C or decline and resolution of serum hCG levels after D&C. Patient characteristics were compared between those with a final diagnosis of EP and those with a final diagnosis of miscarriage.

Findings.—Overall, 38.4% of the women were diagnosed with miscarriage and 61.6% with EP (Table 1). There were no significant differences in race, age, gravity, parity, hCG trends, or time to diagnosis between these 2 groups. Women were more likely to have a final diagnosis of EP if their initial hCG level was below 2000 mIU/mL. US was significantly correlated with the diagnosis, but it was not definitive.

Conclusions.—The presumed diagnosis of EP, without definitive D&C, is inaccurate almost 40% of the time. Therefore D&C remains necessary to distinguish EP from intrauterine miscarriage before treatment. Inclusion of this procedure will avoid unnecessary treatment delay while establishing a definitive diagnosis to aid in patient management.

Usefulness of Pipelle Endometrial Biopsy in the Diagnosis of Women at Risk for Ectopic Pregnancy

Barnhart KT, Gracia CR, Reindl B, et al (Univ of Pennsylvania, Philadelphia; Providence Health System, Portland, Ore)
Am J Obstet Gynecol 188:906-909, 2003   16–5

Background.—Dilation and curettage (D&C) is the standard for the diagnosis of ectopic pregnancy (EP), but it is expensive, inconvenient, and associated with a small risk of complications. Pipelle endometrial biopsy is a simpler, less expensive technique that is used to accurately diagnose endometrial cancer. Use of the Pipelle biopsy was compared with D&C for the diagnosis of EP.

Study Design.—The study group consisted of 32 hemodynamically stable women who presented to the emergency department of the University of Pennsylvania for a diagnosis of potential EP. A standard Pipelle biopsy was performed in the operating room just before a standard D&C. Both samples were sent for pathologic analysis, and results of pathology were compared to final diagnosis. Sensitivity, specificity, and positive and negative predictive values were calculated.

Findings.—According to the results of D&C, 31% of these patients had samples that were consistent with a miscarriage. Pipelle biopsy had a sensitivity of 30%, a specificity of 100%, a positive predicitive value of 100%, and a negative predictive value of 76%. D&C frozen section had a sensitivity of 87.5%, a specificity of 100%, a positive predictive value of 100%, and a negative predictive value of 95.3%.

Conclusions.—When a patient has suspected EP, endometrial sampling is necessary to distinguish an EP from miscarriage. Pipelle sampling has poor sensitivity and is not sufficient for the diagnosis of EP. Until a more sensitive noninvasive technique is developed, D&C remains the gold standard to distinguish EP from miscarriage.

▶ Before initiating medical or surgical therapy of a presumed EP it is important to establish its diagnosis. Measurement of human chorionic gonadotropin in serum and pelvic sonography cannot differentiate the diagnosis of EP from early pregnancy failure (also called impending miscarriage). As shown in the first of these 2 articles (Abstract 16–4), it is necessary to determine whether or not chorionic villi are present in the uterine cavity. Use of an endometrial biopsy instrument does not yield sufficient tissue to determine whether chorionic villi are present. These 2 articles provide important information for clinicians taking care of patients with pelvic pain and/or bleeding in early pregnancy. All patients with these symptoms need a diagnostic evaluation to determine whether or not an EP is present.

D. R. Mishell, Jr, MD

The Ultrasonographic Appearance of Tubal Pregnancy in Patients Treated With Methotrexate

Gamzu R, Almog B, Levin Y, et al (Tel Aviv Univ, Israel)
Hum Reprod 17:2585-2587, 2002   16–6

Background.—There has been an increase in the incidence of extrauterine pregnancy (EUP) to a rate of about 2% of all pregnancies. Accompanying this increase has been a significant decline in mortality rate, which is in part caused by an increased awareness and early, accurate diagnosis. The medical treatment of tubal pregnancy with methotrexate has gained popularity and is considered highly effective. The US appearance of a tubal EUP mass treated with methotrexate was reported only once in a small cohort. The effects of methotrexate treatment on the US appearance of EUP were evaluated, and the hypothesis that the US appearance is not predictive of treatment success was tested.

Methods.—This prospective cohort study included 56 women with tubal EUP who received a single-dose protocol of methotrexate. EUP was diagnosed when an intrauterine gestational sac was not identified by transvaginal US, accompanied by an abnormal rise or plateau in human chorionic gonadotropin concentration. Serial transvaginal US evaluations were performed weekly until human chorionic gonadotropin normalization occurred or the size of the ectopic mass declined to 1 cm².

Results.—An ectopic tubal mass was identified on transvaginal US in 45 (80%) of 56 women, with a mean size of 4 ± 0.5 cm². After the first week of methotrexate injection, the mean size of the ectopic mass increased significantly to 6 ± 0.8 cm². The initial size of the ectopic mass was not related to the success of the treatment or to serum human chorionic gonadotropin levels. US resolution of the ectopic mass occurred in 27 women after a mean of 42 ± 2.4 days.

Conclusions.—There is no relation between the initial size of a tubal pregnancy and the success of methotrexate treatment. In patients with a tubal pregnancy, methotrexate treatment is followed by an initial increase in the size of the ectopic mass. Thus, such an enlargement of the ectopic mass should not be considered as a higher risk for failure of methotrexate treatment.

▶ It appears that the initial serum level of human chorionic gonadotropin (hCG) is a better predictor of successful use of methrotrexate for treatment of unruptured tubal pregnancy than the size of the adnexal mass. In this study, the mean diameter of the tubal mass was 4 cm, yet there was a high rate of successful use of methotrexate. Of the 45 women with a tubal mass, 39 were successfully treated with methrotrexate. Women with an ectopic pregnancy and evidence of cardiac activity in the mass or an hCG level of 10,000 mIU/mL or greater were not treated with methotrexate. If the adnexal mass is larger than 4 cm, but the hCG level is less than 10,000 mIU/ml and there is no cardiac activity, methotrexate therapy can be used to treat the ectopic pregnancy.

D. R. Mishell, Jr, MD

Predictors of Success With Methotrexate Treatment of Tubal Ectopic Pregnancy at Grady Memorial Hospital
Potter MB, Lepine LA, Jamieson DJ (Emory Univ, Atlanta, Ga)
Am J Obstet Gynecol 188:1192-1194, 2003   16–7

Background.—Methotrexate is the widely accepted medical treatment for tubal ectopic pregnancy, with the most commonly used protocol employing a single dose. The experience of patients at a single institution (Grady Memorial Hospital, an inner-city teaching hospital serving a population that is largely indigent) with single-dose methotrexate was reviewed retrospectively.

Methods.—Over 15 months, patients coming for care who were diagnosed with tubal ectopic pregnancy received a single IM dose of 50 mg/m² of methotrexate. According to the protocol, patients had β human chorionic gonadotropin (β-hCG) measurements during workup, on the first, fourth, and seventh days after methotrexate injection and during follow-up as needed. A repeat dose was given to patients whose levels did not fall at least 15% between the fourth and seventh days or fall a minimum of 15% each week thereafter. The resolution of the β-hCG level to less than 50 mIU/mL was interpreted as a successful response to methotrexate therapy.

Results.—Eighty-one women were eligible and 69 (85%) had successful responses to methotrexate treatment. Resolution of the ectopic pregnancies required a median of 26 days overall. When the patient required a second dose, the median time to resolution was 48 days, while those requiring a single dose had a median time to resolution of 20 days. The appropriate fall in the β-hCG level between days 4 and 7 was not present in 15 women (19%), but only 9 received a second methotrexate dose. Before treatment, the median β-hCG level was 971 mIU/mL. Patients for whom methotrexate was efficacious had a significantly lower median β-hCG level (793 mIU/mL) than those who did not respond (3804 mIU/mL). The success rate fell as the pretreatment β-hCG level rose. When the level was under 1000 mIU/mL, the success rate was 98%; when it was between 1000 and 4999 mIU/mL, the success rate was 80%; and when it was over 5000 mIU/mL, the success rate was only 38%.

On univariate analysis, the median peak β-hCG, the median rise of β-hCG from the first through the fourth day, the presence of an adnexal mass, and the presence of an adnexal yolk sac were significantly predictive of failure for methotrexate treatment. On multivariate logistic regression, only the presence of an adnexal yolk sac remained independently predictive of treatment failure. Treatment failed in 5 of the 7 patients who had an adnexal yolk sac.

Conclusion.—The 85% success rate with methotrexate is comparable to other published findings regarding the treatment of tubal ectopic pregnancy. An additional finding was that the presence of a yolk sac proved to be a risk factor for treatment failure.

► A single dose of methotrexate is being used by many clinicians to treat unruptured ectopic pregnancy with a small or absent adnexal mass and βHCG levels below 10,000 mIUl/mL. In this large series, 85% of patients with small, unruptured ectopic pregnancies were treated successfully with 1 or 2 doses of methotrexate. The presence of a yolk sac was an independent risk factor for failure of methotrexate therapy. If a yolk sac is seen in the adnexa sonographically, it may be best to treat the ectopic pregnancy surgically instead of medically.

D. R. Mishell, Jr, MD

Predictors of Success in Methotrexate Treatment of Women With Unruptured Tubal Pregnancies

Nazac A, Gervaise A, Bouyer J, et al (Université Paris-Sud, Clamart, France; INSERM U292, Le Kremlin Bicêtre, France)
Ultrasound Obstet Gynecol 21:181-185, 2003   16–8

Background.—Early diagnosis of ectopic pregnancy (EP) permits the use of a nonsurgical approach. Administration of methotrexate is a common medical treatment for tubal pregnancy, but factors that determine success have not been clarified. The predictors of successful methotrexate treatment of unruptured tubal pregnancy were examined.

Study Design.—The study group consisted of 137 women with unruptured EP, a hematosalpinx visualized by US, a pretherapeutic score of less than 13, and human chorionic gonadotropin (hCG) levels either stable or increasing. These patients received methotrexate, either 50 mg/m² IM or 1 mg/kg directly into the sac under US guidance with a technique similar to that used for in vitro fertilization. Study participants had hCG assays on days 2 and 7 and then weekly. An additional IM dose of methotrexate was administered if hCG levels did not decline as expected. Failure was defined as a need for surgical treatment. A logistic regression model was used to determine patient and treatment characteristics associated with successful medical treatment.

Findings.—The overall success rate for methotrexate treatment of EP was 79.6%. The 2 factors independently associated with successful medical treatment of EP were initial hCG level no more than 1000 mIU/mL and local administration of methotrexate.

Conclusions.—When EP is discovered early, medical management with administration of methotrexate can be used successfully. The 2 factors that influence successful medical management are route of administration and hCG levels.

▶ Women with unruptured EP and serum hCG levels above 5000 mIU/mL are less likely to be successfully treated with systemic methotrexate than women with lower hCG levels. In this nonrandomized study, injection of methotrexate into the gestational sac of the EP resulted in a 92.5% incidence of success compared with IM systemic injection, which yielded a 67% incidence of success. These data need to be confirmed by a prospective randomized trial. If they are confirmed clinicians should consider injecting methotrexate directly into the EP under sonographic guidance. The technique is similar to that used for follicle aspiration when performing in vitro fertilization.

D. R. Mishell, Jr, MD

Failed Methotrexate Treatment of Cervical Pregnancy: Predictive Factors
Bai SW, Lee JS, Park JH, et al (Yonsei Univ, Seoul, Korea)
J Reprod Med 47:483-488, 2002   16–9

Background.—In the past, the resultant massive intraperitoneal bleeding associated with an ectopic pregnancy required emergency procedures to save the patient's life rather than to preserve her fertility. Today, early detection and follow-up after treatment made possible with transvaginal US and the measurement of human chorionic gonadotropin (hCG) levels make it possible to preserve fertility without the need for surgery. The effects of pretreatment serum hCG concentrations, size of the gestational sac, and presence of peritoneal fluid and fetal cardiac activity on treatment results when systemic methotrexate was used to treat cervical pregnancies were investigated.

Methods.—Thirty-two women with cervical pregnancies who were treated with systemic methotrexate injections were enrolled in the study. The diagnosis of a cervical pregnancy was made when the urinary hCG concentration was positive, a gestational sac was not visualized in the uterine cavity, a perceptible gestational sac was present in the cervix, and an increase in the serum hCG concentration was less than 50% of the initial level for a period of 48 hours. When the serum hCG concentration decreased to less than 15% or continued to increase, treatment was repeated. The efficacy of the therapy was determined by evaluation of pretreatment serum concentrations of hCG, the size of the gestational mass, fetal cardiac activity, and the presence of hemoperitoneum in the peritoneal cavity.

Results.—Of the 32 women enrolled in the study, 24 (75%) were treated successfully with systemic methotrexate therapy (success group) and 8 (25%) had surgery because of the failed systemic methotrexate therapy (failure group). Seven women had hysterectomies when an increase in serum hCG concentration or intractable vaginal bleeding occurred. No significant differences were present in age, gravidity, parity, or history of cesarean section or dilation and evacuation. Between the 2 groups, the failure group had significantly increased serum hCG levels ($P = .025$), significantly higher rates of pretreatment serum hCG ($P = .02$), and significantly higher rates of the presence of fetal cardiac activity ($P = .027$) than did the success group. No difference was found in the size of the gestational sac, presence of peritoneal fluid, or gestational age between the 2 groups; however, serum hCG concentrations were found to be related to fetal cardiac activity ($P = .001$). Of 13 women with initial serum hCG concentrations of 10,000 mIU/mL or more, 11 had fetal cardiac activity and 4 of these 11 were treated successfully with methotrexate. The level of serum hCG had an independent correlation with the outcome of treatment, irrespective of the relationship between fetal cardiac activity and serum hCG level.

Conclusions.—The failure of methotrexate treatment was high when the pretreatment hCG level was greater than 10,000 mIU/mL or fetal cardiac activity was detected by transvaginal US; surgery was then required. No relationship between gestational sac diameter and the outcome of methotrexate treatment was shown. However, a high pretreatment serum hCG level and the presence of fetal cardiac activity are the most important predictive factors in the failure of methotrexate treatment of a cervical pregnancy.

▶ In this large series of women with cervical ectopic pregnancies, it was found that a serum hCG level more than 10,000 mIU/mL or the presence of cardiac activity in the embryo or fetus were indicators of poor success with methotrexate therapy alone. If a cervical ectopic pregnancy is present with these risk factors, it seems advisable to follow methotrexate by uterine artery embolization if the woman does not wish to have a hysterectomy.

D. R. Mishell, Jr, MD

Cervical Pregnancy Successfully Treated With a Sequential Combination of Methotrexate and Mifepristone

Sexton C, Sharp N (Royal United Hosp Bath, England)
Aust N Z J Obstet Gynaecol 42:211-213, 2002   16–10

Background.—Cervical pregnancy is a rare but life-threatening complication of pregnancy. Until recently, total abdominal hysterectomy has been the treatment used to reduce the risk of severe hemorrhage. Methotrexate has become the medical treatment most often used for ectopic pregnancy. A case of cervical pregnancy successfully treated with methotrexate and mifepristone was reported.

> *Case Report.*—Girl, 16 years, with lower abdominal pain and vaginal bleeding was referred to an early pregnancy assessment clinic. Transvaginal US showed a slightly enlarged uterus with thickened endometrial interface and a fluid-filled sac, 15×20 mm, situated within the upper cervix. A decidual reaction with vascularity consistent with a cervical ectopic pregnancy was shown surrounding the sac. The patient's serum quantitative β–human chorionic gonadotropin (β-hCG) was 6269 IU. The patient was admitted to the hospital to begin methotrexate therapy. The first day, the dose of methotrexate was 85 mg. After 3 days, when the patient did not show a strong response to the methotrexate, a single dose of oral mifepristone, 400 mg, was administered. On day 5, the patient experienced more vaginal bleeding with cramping pelvic pain. The following 3 days showed the β-hCG measurement to be considerably lower and the bleeding settled; the cervical ectopic pregnancy was reduced in size to a sac 13×20 mm and was less vascular. The serum hCG measurement was repeated until a negative result was achieved 2 weeks after the initial diagnosis. There were no side effects with the administration of either methotrexate or mifepristone

Conclusion.—Methotrexate and mifepristone in combination are seen to be a safe and effective treatment for cervical ectopic pregnancy. Their use may be important to avoid the risk of precipitating hemorrhage, a major concern in cervical ectopic pregnancy.

▶ Cervical pregnancy is a rare event, and it is unlikely that a randomized trial could be performed to determine whether the addition of mifepristone following methotrexate results in increased efficacy to that of methotrexate alone. Nevertheless, if a single dose of methotrexate given to women with cervical pregnancy results in no decrease in hCG levels, clinicians may wish to consider giving 400 mg mifepristone instead of additional methotrexate, as was done successfully in this case. There are some data suggesting that the treatment of an unruptured tubal pregnancy with methotrexate plus mifepristone may be more effective than methotrexate alone.

D. R. Mishell, Jr, MD

17 PMS

Female Sexual Dysfunction in Postmenopausal Women: Systematic Review of Placebo-Controlled Trials
Modelska K, Cummings S (Univ of California, San Francisco)
Am J Obstet Gynecol 188:286-293, 2003   17–1

Background.—Female sexual dysfunction (FSD) is common after menopause but has not been well studied. A systematic literature review of randomized, double-blind, placebo-controlled clinical trials was performed to examine the efficacy of medical treatment for FSD in postmenopausal women.

Study Design.—A computerized search was performed of literature published from January 1990 to February 2002 on medical treatment of FSD in postmenopausal women. Conference proceedings and published article bibliographies were hand searched.

Findings.—Only 6 randomized, placebo-controlled trials that assessed the effects of medical therapy on sexual function in postmenopausal women were found. A single trial of sildenafil, a selective inhibitor of phosphodiesterase 5, found that it did not improve sexual function. A single trial of hormone replacement therapy found that it did improve sexual desire and arousal. Treatment with transdermal testosterone or estrogen-androgen replacement also significantly increased sexual desire and frequency of intercourse, but not vaginal lubrication or pain during intercourse. Transdermal testosterone was associated with adverse effects, such as hirsutism. Treatment with tibolone, a synthetic steroid, was associated with significantly improved vaginal blood flow and lubrication, but not with increased frequency of intercourse or orgasm.

Conclusions.—Research into the treatment of sexual dysfunction in postmenopausal women is not yet sufficient to determine optimal treatment. Additional controlled clinical trials with larger samples sizes and longer follow-up periods will be necessary to answer this question.

▶ FSD is a common problem, estimated to occur in as many as 50% of women in the United States. FSD is very common in postmenopausal women and several therapies have been utilized to treat this problem, particularly the use of exogenous androgens. This extensive review found there is a parity of randomized, placebo-controlled trials of agents used to treat FSD. Only 6 randomized controlled trials have been conducted to assess the effects of various therapies to treat FSD in postmenopausal women. Two of these studies reported improvement in sexual function when androgens were given to postmenopausal women, particularly with use of transdermal testosterone. Sildenafil citrate was of no benefit in treating FSD in postmenopausal women and there are no studies that investigated the effect of selective estrogen receptor modalities on FSD. Because FSD is such a common problem it is important that additional studies be undertaken to determine the effect of a variety of agents used to treat postmenopausal women with FSD.

D. R. Mishell, Jr, MD

Comparative Effects of Oral Esterified Estrogens With and Without Methyltestosterone on Endocrine Profiles and Dimensions of Sexual Function in Postmenopausal Women With Hypoactive Sexual Desire

Lobo RA, Rosen RC, Yang H-M, et al (Columbia Univ, New York; UMDNJ-Robert Wood Johnson Med School, New Brunswick, NJ; Solvay Pharmaceutical Inc, Marietta, Ga)
Fertil Steril 79:1341-1352, 2003   17–2

Background.—It has been proposed that androgens influence female libido. The effects of estrogen alone were compared to that of estrogen plus testosterone in postmenopausal women with hypoactive sexual desire.

Study Design.—The study group consisted of 221 healthy postmenopausal women who were receiving estrogen and who had hypoactive sexual desire associated with menopause onset. Participants were randomly assigned to daily treatment with esterified estrogen alone or in combination with methyltestosterone for 16 weeks (Fig 1). Response to treatment was investigated with the Sexual Interest Questionnaire and the Brief Index of Sexual Functioning for Women at baseline, and 4, 8, 12, and 16 weeks of treatment. Testosterone, sex hormone–binding globulin, and estrone levels were assessed. Safety and tolerability were evaluated.

Findings.—Treatment with the estrogen-testosterone combination significantly increased bioavailable testosterone and suppressed sex hormone–binding globulin. Sexual desire and frequency increased from baseline and were significantly greater in the women treated with the combination therapy. Treatment with combination therapy was well tolerated, although hirsutism and acne were increased in the combination treatment group. By week 18, the combination therapy group had a significant decrease and the estrogen alone group had a significant increase in HDL cholesterol.

Conclusions.—In this double-blind, randomized study, treatment with a combination of esterified estrogen and methyltestosterone increased bioavailable testosterone, suppressed sex hormone–binding globulin, and increased both sexual desire and frequency compared with postmenopausal women receiving estrogen alone. These findings support the influence of testosterone on sexual desire in postmenopausal women.

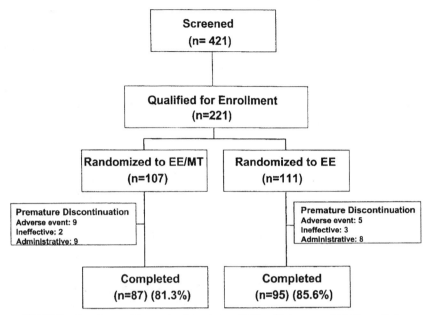

FIGURE 1.—Recruitment of the sample. *Abbreviations: EE*, Esterified estrogen; *EE/MT*, esterified estrogen and methyltestosterone. (Reprinted from Lobo RA, Rosen RC, Yang H-M, et al: Comparative effects of oral esterified estrogens with and without methyltestosterone on endocrine profiles and dimensions of sexual function in postmenopausal women with hypoactive sexual desire *Fertil Steril* 79:1341-1352. Copyright 2003, with permission from the American College of Surgeons. Copyright American Society for Reproductive Medicine.)

▶ Tablets containing a combination of esterfied estrogen and methyl testosterone have been marketed in the United States for several years to treat postmenopausal women with decreased libido. In this randomized study comparing the effects of esterfied estrogen with and without methyltestosterone, it appears that the formulation with testosterone enhanced sexual interest and desire significantly more than estrogen alone among a group of mainly white, college-educated postmenopausal women. The results of this study were obtained by analyzing a self-administered questionnaire. An earlier, more sophisticated study by Meyers et al[1] reported that conjugated estrogen plus methyltestosterone did not increase sexual behavior or sexual arousal. It is concerning that the formulation with methyltestosterone caused a 12% decrease in HDL cholesterol levels. Studies should be performed comparing oral methyltestosterone with transdermal testosterone to compare their effect on libido and lipid changes.

D. R. Mishell, Jr, MD

Reference

1. Myers LS, Dixen J, Morrissette D, et al: Effects of estrogen, androgen, and progestin on sexual psychophysiology and behavior in postmenopausal women. *J Clin Endocrinol Metab* 70:1124-1131, 1990.

Efficacy of Intermittent, Luteal Phase Sertraline Treatment of Premenstrual Dysphoric Disorder

Halbreich U, Bergeron R, Yonkers KA, et al (State Univ of New York, Buffalo; Ottawa Hosp Research Inst, Ont, Canada; Yale Univ, New Haven, Conn; et al)
Obstet Gynecol 100:1219-1229, 2002   17–3

Background.—Premenstrual dysphoric disorder, which appears in the week before menstrual bleeding and ends after menses onset, can cause disabling emotional, behavioral, and physical symptoms. The efficacy and tolerability of sertraline taken in the luteal phase for this disorder were reported.

Methods.—Two hundred eighty-one women meeting criteria for premenstrual dysphoric disorder were studied. All completed 2 prospective screening cycles and 1 single-blind placebo cycle. They were then randomly assigned to 3 cycles of placebo or to sertraline in a flexible daily dose of 50 to 100 mg. The Daily Record of Severity of Problems and the Clinical Global Impression Severity and Improvement scales were used to determine outcomes.

Findings.—Women given sertraline had significantly better Clinical Global Impression Improvement scale scores and cycle 3 Daily Record of Severity of Problems change scores. By cycle 1, 50% of the sertraline group had responded to treatment compared with 26% given placebo. Sertraline also significantly improved quality of life and functioning outcomes. The patients tolerated intermittent luteal administration of sertraline well. Only approximately 8% of sertraline recipients and less than 1% of placebo recipients quit the study because of adverse effects.

Conclusions.—Sertraline administered intermittently during the luteal phase appears to be significantly more effective than placebo in relieving the symptoms of premenstrual dysphoric disorder. This agent also appeared to be tolerated well.

▶ This well-done placebo-controlled trial found that administration of the selective serotonin reuptake inhibitor (SSRI) sertraline, in doses of 50 or 100 mg/d in the luteal phase of the cycle, significantly improved the behavioral but not the physical symptoms of women with premenstrual dysphoric disorder (PMDD). The main side effects of sertraline were nausea and dry mouth, each reported by about 10% of subjects. Luteal phase sertraline appears to be an effective, safe way to diminish the behavioral symptoms of PMDD and improve the quality of life of women with PMDD.

D. R. Mishell, Jr, MD

Premenstrual Daily Fluoxetine for Premenstrual Dysphoric Disorder: A Placebo-Controlled, Clinical Trial Using Computerized Diaries

Cohen LS, Miner C, Brown E, et al (Harvard Med School, Boston; Eli Lilly and Company, Indianapolis, Ind; Univ of Pennsylvania, Philadelphia; et al)

Obstet Gynecol 100:435-444, 2002   17–4

Background.—Premenstrual dysphoric disorder is a significant mood disturbance affecting 3% to 8% of women in their reproductive years. The efficacy of premenstrual daily fluoxetine was evaluated in women with premenstrual dysphoric disorder.

Methods.—Two hundred sixty women were enrolled in the study. After a 2-cycle screening and 1-cycle single-blind placebo period, the women were randomly assigned to placebo or to 10 or 20 mg fluoxetine for 3 cycles. Doses were taken daily from 14 days before the next expected menses through the first full day of bleeding. The women recorded their symptoms in a computerized version of the Daily Record of Severity of Problems.

Findings.—Women receiving 20 mg of fluoxetine daily had significantly improved mean Daily Record of Severity of Problems luteal scores than did women receiving placebo (Fig 3). The 10-mg dose did not appear to be significantly superior to placebo in mean scores. Total scores on the daily Record of Severity of Problems showed significant improvement by the first treatment cycle in both active treatment groups. However, only the 20-mg

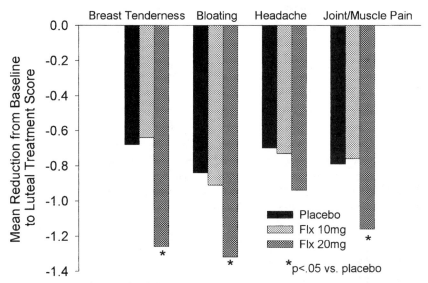

FIGURE 3.—Reduction in luteal physical symptom scores baseline to treatment. Reduction from mean luteal baseline score to mean luteal treatment score (across 3 treatment cycles). Pairwise comparisons between treatment groups were based on the least-square means from an analysis of variance model with treatment and investigator in the model (treatment by investigator interaction was not significant and was dropped from final model). *Abbreviation: Flx,* Fluoxetine. (Courtesy of Cohen LS, Miner C, Brown E, et al: Premenstrual daily fluoxetine for premenstrual dysphoric disorder: A placebo-controlled, clinical trial using computerized diaries. *Obstet Gynecol* 100:435-444, 2002. Reprinted with permission of the American College of Obstetricians and Gynecologists.)

dose continued to be significantly better than placebo throughout the active treatment phase. Both doses of fluoxetine were significantly superior to placebo in relieving mood-related symptoms, though only the larger dose was superior in relieving the physical symptoms of breast tenderness, bloating, and joint and muscle pain. The women tolerated fluoxetine well. The 3 groups did not differ in number of discontinuations because of adverse events.

Conclusions.—Premenstrual daily dosing with fluoxetine can alleviate the mood, physical, and social functioning symptoms of premenstrual dysphoric disorder. A 20-mg dose appears to be much more effective than 10 mg with comparable tolerability.

▶ Daily dosing of fluoxetine has been previously shown to be effective therapy for premenstrual dysphoric disorder (PMDD) and is approved by the Food and Drug Administration for treatment of PMDD. The results of this study indicate that ingestion of 20 mg/d of fluoxetine for 14 days in the luteal phase of the cycle also provides safe, effective therapy for PMDD. Women with PMDD can take fluoxetine daily or only in the luteal phase to reduce the symptoms of PMDD.

D. R. Mishell, Jr, MD

Recurrence of Symptoms of Premenstrual Dysphoric Disorder After the Cessation of Luteal-Phase Fluoxetine Treatment

Pearlstein T, Joliat MJ, Brown EB, et al (Butler Hosp, Providence, RI; Lilly Corporate Ctr, Indianapolis, Ind)
Am J Obstet Gynecol 188:887-895, 2003   17–5

Background.—Recently, intermittent doses of 20 mg fluoxetine daily have been approved for the treatment of premenstrual dysphoric disorder (PMDD). Data from 2 clinical trials were analyzed to determine PMDD symptom severity after fluoxetine treatment was discontinued.

Methods.—Data were obtained from 2 separate multicenter, randomized, double-blind, placebo-controlled studies. Symptom recurrence after the discontinuation of daily and weekly luteal-phase fluoxetine treatment was analyzed. Relapses were assessed with the daily record of severity of problems, the Sheehan disability scale, the premenstrual tension scale-clinician rates, and the clinical global impression-severity.

Findings.—Analysis indicated that PMDD symptoms increased significantly after discontinuation of fluoxetine treatment. Although scores did not return to baseline, the benefits of fluoxetine were no longer significantly superior to those of placebo.

Conclusions.—After 3 cycles of fluoxetine therapy for PMDD, discontinuation is associated with symptom recurrence during the next cycle. This rapid recurrence of symptoms supports the hypothesis that PMDD is a clinical entity distinct from depression.

▶ Several studies have reported that daily or luteal phase administration of fluoxetine significantly reduces the symptoms of PMDD. On the basis of these studies the Food and Drug Administration has approved the use of daily or luteal-phase intermittent doses of fluoxetine for treatment of PMDD. This study indicates that after 3 cycles of fluoxetine treatment of PMDD, the symptoms recur rapidly if the drug is discontinued in the fourth cycle. Thus women with PMDD should be encouraged to continue long-term therapy with luteal-phase intermittent use of fluoxetine for treatment of PMDD.

D. R. Mishell, Jr, MD

18 Contraception

Evaluation of the Efficacy of a Nonlatex Condom: Results From a Randomized, Controlled Clinical Trial
Walsh TL, Frezieres RG, Peacock K, et al (California Family Health Council, Los Angeles; Harbor-Univ of California, Torrance; Univ of California, Los Angeles; et al)
Perspect Sex Reprod Health 35:79-86, 2003   18–1

Introduction.—Natural rubber latex causes an allergic reaction, especially after sustained exposure, in approximately 3% of the United States population. Styrene ethylene butylene styrene (SEBS), a synthetic material, shares many of the characteristics of natural latex, but it does not initiate an allergic response in persons with known allergies to natural latex. The SEBS condom was compared with 2 commercial latex condoms in a prospective contraceptive efficacy investigation that included a nested breakage, slippage, and acceptability trial to ascertain the rate of condom failure, product acceptability, and adverse events.

Methods.—Between 1998 and 2000, 830 monogamous couples were randomly assigned to either a nonlatex condom or a commercial natural latex condom for 6 months as their only birth control method. Couples completed detailed condom use reports for the first 5 condoms used. The reports included data concerning product performance (breakage, slippage), frequency and timing of problems, and adverse events. Couples used diary forms to document coital acts, condom use, onset of menses, and any problems with the use of condoms. Pregnancy rates linked with typical and consistent condom use were determined. Rates of clinical failure (condom breakage or slippage) were ascertained for the initial 5 condom uses.

Results.—During the initial 5 uses, the nonlatex condom had a higher rate of breakage or slippage during intercourse or withdrawal compared with the latex condom (4.0% vs 1.3%); the breakage rate for the nonlatex condom was approximately 8-fold that of the latex condom. The 6-cycle typical-use pregnancy rate did not vary significantly between users of nonlatex and latex condoms (10.8% vs 6.4%). The 6-cycle consistent-use pregnancy rate was higher for the nonlatex versus latex condom users group (4.9% vs 1.0%).

Conclusion.—It appears that condom breaks exert an upward influence on the consistent-use and perfect-use pregnancy rates of the SEBS condom. Clinical failure rates for latex and nonlatex condoms were 1.3% and 4.0%, respectively. Nonlatex condoms remained intact during 96% of uses, markedly decreasing the female partner's exposure to semen compared with unprotected intercourse.

▶ About 3% of individuals may develop an allergic reaction to the use of latex condoms. This study showed that a nonlatex condom was associated with slightly higher slippage, breakage, and perfect-use pregnancy rates than the latex condom. *If* the latex condom is used perfectly each time, the 1-year pregnancy rate was only 1.5%, with a low incidence of breakage and slippage of the condom. Condoms, when used perfectly, are effective contraceptives as well as barriers for transmission of sexually transmitted infection.

D. R. Mishell, Jr, MD

Quick Start: A Novel Oral Contraceptive Initiation Method
Westhoff C, Kerns J, Morroni C, et al (Columbia Univ, New York)
Contraception 66:141-145, 2002   18–2

Introduction.—Conventional approaches to the initiation of oral contraceptives (OCs) necessitate waiting for the next menstrual period to take the first pill. This approach delays the onset of contraceptive protection, particularly in women who do not have a regular menstrual cycle. Pregnancy can result while waiting. Also, delaying the start of pill taking to the correct time may be confusing, and motivation can wane. This clinic encourages patients to take the pill at the clinic when it is first prescribed and to continue daily pill taking regardless of the menstrual cycle day. Called Quick Start, the method was compared with continuation after other approaches to initiation in a prospective, observational cohort investigation.

Methods.—All patients starting or restarting combined OCs were eligible for participation. Patients were interviewed concerning past contraceptive use, motivation to prevent pregnancy, relationship characteristics, and basic demographic information. They were offered several approaches to OC initiation. The primary outcome measure was short-term continuation to the second pack of pills, described as having begun the second pack.

Results.—Telephone follow-up of 91% of the cohort showed that women who swallowed the first OC in the clinic were more likely to continue the OC until the second package compared with women who planned to start the OC later (adjusted odds ratio, 2.8; 95% confidence interval, 1.1-7.3). Other factors correlated with short-term continuation were partner's knowledge of planned OC use, older age, and participant's agreement that she would be "very unhappy about becoming pregnant in the next 6 months."

Conclusion.—Directly observed OC initiation during the clinic visit, regardless of menstrual cycle day, has the potential for increasing OC continuation and reducing unintended pregnancy without any new health care costs.

▶ Although this study was not a randomized trial, it appears that initiating OC use on the day of the initial clinic visit enhances continuation of OC use, compared with initiating use at a later date. Other studies have shown that up to 25% of women given an OC prescription fail to initiate OC use. Initiating OC use at the time of the clinic visit did not adversely affect bleeding patterns or enhance the incidence of adverse events. There appears to be no medical reason to delay start of OCs until menses begins. Starting OCs at the time of the first clinic visit may decrease the risk of an unplanned pregnancy and deserves further study.

D. R. Mishell, Jr, MD

Acceptance of Altering the Standard 21-Day/7-Day Oral Contraceptive Regimen to Delay Menses and Reduce Hormone Withdrawal Symptoms
Sulak PJ, Kuehl TJ, Ortiz M, et al (Texas A&M Univ, Temple)
Am J Obstet Gynecol 186:1142-1149, 2002   18–3

Introduction.—In women who continue to use oral contraceptives (OCs) for more than 1 year, side effects are common and usually occur during the 7-day hormone-free interval. The format 21 days of active pills of estrogen and progestin followed by 7 days of inactive pills was arbitrarily created to allow monthly withdrawal bleeding and mimic spontaneous menstrual cycles. The acceptance and long-term follow-up of a large series of women taking OCs with hormone withdrawal symptoms who were permitted to extend the number of days of active pills to the length they desired were pro-

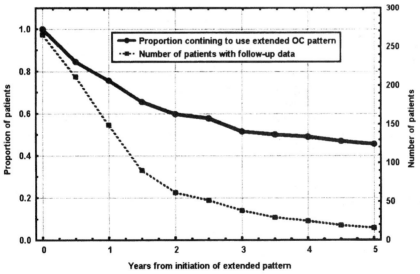

FIGURE 1.—Graph constructed by using survival methods for 267 patients initiating extended OC patterns. Proportion of patients continuing extended patterns and number of patients with available follow-up data are shown. (Reprinted by permission of the publisher courtesy of Sulak PJ, Kuehl TJ, Ortiz M, et al: Acceptance of altering the standard 21-day/7-day oral contraceptive regimen to delay menses and reduce hormone withdrawal symptoms. *Am J Obstet Gynecol* 186:1142-1149. Copyright 2002 by Elsevier.)

spectively examined, along with the option to decrease the number of hormone-free days to less than 7.

Methods.—Patients taking OCs with hormone withdrawal symptoms during the hormone-free interval who were counseled by a single obstetrician-gynecologist concerning changing their standard 21/7 regimen were assessed. All women used a monophasic 30 to 35 μg pill and underwent an initial counseling visit between December 1993 and October 2000.

Results.—Of 318 patients who were counseled about extending the number of active pills, 292 (92%) had documented follow-up after initial counseling (Fig 1). The main reason for extending the number of active pills was to reduce symptoms of headache (35%), dysmenorrhea (21%), hypermenorrhea (19%), and premenstrual symptoms (13%). The other 12% of patients made changes for purposes of convenience, endometriosis, and other reasons, including menstrual-related acne. Twenty-five (9%) participants chose not to extend, with a preference for monthly menses as the most frequent reason (40%), followed by the belief that symptoms were not severe enough to warrant extension (32%). Of 267 participants who initiated an extended regimen, 57 discontinued OCs, 38 returned to a standard regimen, and 172 were continuing the extended regimen at last follow-up. A survival analysis performed at 5 years showed that 46% of the cohort continued as extended OC pattern. The regimen of extended OC use was 12 weeks of active pills (median, 9 weeks; range to 104 weeks) with a pill-free interval of 6 days (median, 5 days; range 0-7 days).

Conclusion.—Most patients with hormone withdrawal symptoms on OCs will initiate a regimen of extending active pills, frequently with a shortened hormone-free interval to decrease the frequency and severity of related symptoms.

▶ The results of this case series indicate that among a large group of OC users who developed headaches, dysmenorrhea, and other symptoms during the 7-day hormone-free interval about 90% initiated an extended pattern of OC use after counseling. The women were given a monophasic OC and took the pills continuously for a medium of 9 weeks. Nearly half the women also shortened the pill-free interval to 4 or 5 days instead of 7 days. Unfortunately this study was not randomized, but about half the women initiating the extended pattern were still taking OCs 5 years later. Clinicians may wish to suggest the option of extended use for women using OCs who develop adverse symptoms during the pill-free interval.

D. R. Mishell, Jr, MD

Oral Contraceptive Use by Teenage Women Does Not Affect Body Composition

Lloyd T, Lin HM, Matthews AE, et al (Penn State College of Medicine, Hershey, Pa)

Obstet Gynecol 100:235-239, 2002   18–4

Background.—Perceived weight gain is the most common reason for discontinuing oral contraceptives (OC). The effects of recent OC formulations on body composition among teenage girls was investigated in a longitudinal study.

Study Design.—The study group consisted of 39 OC users, who had used OCs continuously for at least 6 months and who were still using OCs at age 21 years. There were 27 girls who had never used OCs. The groups were well-matched at baseline. Follow-up visits occurred every 6 months for the

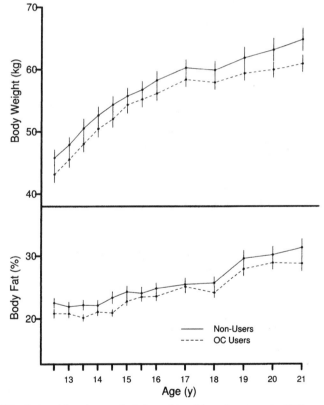

FIGURE 2.—Body weight and percent body fat tracking of the oral contraceptive (OC) users and nonusers. The number of nonusers was 27. The values at all time points for the OC users group (n = 36) include all those individuals who would eventually become OC users (n = 39), regardless of when they started. (Reprinted with permission from The American College of Obstetricians and Gynecologists, from Lloyd T, Lin HM, Matthews AE, et al: Oral contraceptive use by teenage women does not affect body composition. *Obstet Gynecol* 100:235-239, 2002.)

first 4 years of study participation and then annually. Cardiolipin profiles were obtained from fasting blood samples. Systolic and diastolic blood pressure measurements were obtained. Dual energy x-ray absorptiometry was used to assess percent body fat and lean body mass.

Findings.—Between the ages of 12.5 and 21 years, gains in height, weight, body mass index and percent body fat were not significantly different between users and nonusers of OCs (Fig 2). During this same period, OC users had significantly greater increases in total serum cholesterol, serum low-density cholesterol, and serum triglyceride levels than did OC nonusers.

Conclusions.—The use of OCs by teenage girls is associated unfavorably with blood lipid pattern changes but is not associated with weight gain or increased percent body fat. Teenage girls should be counseled that use of OCs will not result in unfavorable body composition changes.

▶ Even though the major reason why teenage girls discontinue using OCs is weight gain, the results of this longitudinal study indicate that OC use by teenagers does not alter their body weight, body mass index, percent body fat, or lean body mass compared with teenagers not using OCs. Teenagers who gain weight have an increase in percentage body fat between ages 12 and 21 years. The magnitude of the increase is not affected by OC use, and teenagers should be counseled more strongly about this effect so that they will be less likely to discontinue OC use.

D. R. Mishell, Jr, MD

Venous Thromboembolism in Young Women: Role of Thrombophilic Mutations and Oral Contraceptive Use
Legnani C, Palareti G, Guazzaloca G, et al (Azienda Ospedaliera di Bologna, Italy; Università di Ferrara, Italy)
Eur Heart J 23:984-990, 2002   18–5

Background.—The mutations, R506Q factor V and G20210A prothrombin, are the most common causes of familial thrombophilia. Oral contraceptive use is also associated with an increased risk of venous thromboembolism. The interaction between oral contraceptive use and these 2 mutations was investigated in a case-control study of women of reproductive age who had deep vein thrombosis of the lower limbs.

Study Design.—The study group consisted of 301 women of reproductive age with deep vein thrombosis of the lower limbs. The control group consisted of 650 healthy women of reproductive age from the same community. Of the 301 women with deep vein thrombosis, 55.8% had been using oral contraceptives when thrombosis developed. In the control group, 26.6% used oral contraceptives. Blood was collected to identify prothrombin and factor V mutations in these women. The relative risk for deep vein thrombosis was calculated as a function of oral contraceptive use and mutation prevalence.

TABLE 3.—Risk of Deep Vein Thrombosis According to the Presence of G20210A Prothrombin Mutation, R506Q Factor V Mutation, and Use of Oral Contraception

	Women With DVT (n = 297)*	Healthy Women (n = 650)	OR† (95% CI)
No defect, no OC	118	444	1 (Reference)
No defect, OC	86	166	2·4 (1·7-3·5)
G20210A prothrombin mutation, no OC	11	18	2·0 (0·8-4·8)
R506Q factor V mutation, no OC	30	15	8·9 (4·4-18·2)
G20210A prothrombin mutation + R506Q factor V mutation, no OC	1	0	—
G20210A prothrombin mutation, OC	18	2	58·6 (12·8-267)
R506Q factor V mutation, OC	26	4	41·0 (13·5-125)
G20210A prothrombin mutation + R506Q factor V mutation, OC	7	1	86·5 (10·0-747)

*Patients with homozygous R506Q (n = 2) and with combined homozygous R506Q + G20210A prothrombin mutation (n = 2) were excluded.
†Adjusted for age and presence of other thrombophilic defects.
Abbreviations: OC, Oral contraceptives; *DVT*, deep vein thrombosis; *OR*, odds ratio.
(Reprinted from Legnani C, Palareti G, Guazzaloca G, et al: Venous thromboembolism in young women: Role of thrombophilic mutations and oral contraceptive use. *Eur Heart J* 23:984-990, copyright 2002, with permission from the RCOG, copyright The European Society of Cardiology.)

Findings.—Of the women with deep vein thrombosis, 19.3% were carriers of R506Q, 9.6% were carriers of G20210A, and 2.7% were carriers of both mutations. Among control subjects, 2.9% were carriers of R506Q, 3.1% were carriers of G20210A, and 1 woman was a carrier of both mutations. The relative risk of deep vein thrombosis associated with being a carrier of R506Q was 10.3, the relative risk associated with being a carrier of G20210A was 4.7, and the relative risk associated with being a carrier of both was 45.6. The relative risk associated with oral contraceptive use was 2.4. The relative risk associated with contraceptive use plus R506Q was 41.0, with contraceptive use plus G20210A was 58.6, and with contraceptive use plus both mutations was 86.5 (Table 3). In women who did not use oral contraceptives, the risk of deep vein thrombosis was significantly increased in carriers of R506Q but not in carriers of G20210A.

Conclusions.—Oral contraceptive use is a risk factor for deep vein thrombosis among women of reproductive age. Oral contraceptive use strongly interacts with both R506Q and G20210A mutations to further increase the risk of deep vein thrombosis in these women. Women should be informed of this increased thrombotic risk so they can decide for themselves whether they wish to be screened for these 2 common mutations before initiating oral contraceptives.

▶ The factor V mutation causes activated protein C resistance and occurs in about 20% of individuals with venous thromboembolism (VTE). This mutation occurs in 3% to 5% and increases the risk of developing VTE about 10- fold in women of reproductive age not using oral contraceptives (OCs) and about 30- to 40-fold in women using OCs. Another thrombophilic mutation, G20210A, is also common and is present in 2% to 3% of the population. This mutation is found in about 6% of individuals with VTE and increases the risk 2- to 4-fold.

The results of this study found that the risk of VTE in women of reproductive age not using OCs with the G20210A mutation was insignificantly increased about 2-fold but was increased 58-fold in women using OCs.

Universal screening for these mutations before OC use is currently not recommended because of the high cost of screening and the low absolute risk of VTE. Screening is now recommended only for women with a family history of VTE; however, the sensitivity of a positive family history is low for predicting the presence of either mutation. Women may wish to be informed about the increased risk of VTE with the presence of either mutation and OC use so that they can decide whether they wish to be screened before initiation of OC use or before becoming pregnant.

D. R. Mishell, Jr, MD

Pregnancies Diagnosed During Depo-Provera Use
Borgatta L, Murthy A, Chuang C, et al (Boston Univ; Planned Parenthood Federation of America Inc)
Contraception 66:169-172, 2002   18–6

Introduction.—Until 1998, affiliated Planned Parenthood clinics were compelled to report contraceptive failures to the Insurance Division of Planned Parenthood Federation of America, Inc. This provides an opportunity to examine the rate of contraceptive failure for Depo-Provera (depot medroxyprogesterone acetate), the most widely used long-term reversible contraceptive in the United States. Contraceptive failures among women using Depo-Provera were evaluated by reviewing reports to the Insurance Division of the Planned Parenthood Federation of America, Inc. Cases were included if the Depo-Provera had been administered at a Planned Parenthood center and pregnancy had either been diagnosed or reported to a Planned Parenthood center.

Results.—Between 1994 and 1998, 402 pregnancies were reported. The crude rate of reported pregnancies was 0.42 pregnancies/1000 women using Depo-Provera per year. Pregnancy was diagnosed after the first trimester in 46% of women. Seventy-seven women (19.1%) received additional Depo-Provera injections during pregnancy. Of women whose date of conception could be calculated, 113 (45%) of 258 became pregnant after injection. There was no increase in either the ectopic pregnancy rate or fetal anomalies.

Conclusion.—Pregnancy during Depo-Provera use is unusual, yet does occur. These pregnancies are commonly unrecognized (45%) until beyond the first trimester.

▶ Pregnancy occurring among users of Depo-Provera is uncommon. There is an increased rate of ectopic pregnancies among women conceiving with other progestin-only methods of contraception, such as subdermal implants. It is reassuring to know that only 4 ectopic pregnancies and 260 known intrauterine pregnancies were reported in this study, for an ectopic pregnancy rate of 1.5%, similar to the rate of noncontraceptive users who become pregnant. It is also reassuring that no fetal anomalies were reported in these pregnancies. Women who use Depo-Provera and develop symptoms of pregnancy should have a pregnancy test performed as Depo-Provera is not completely effective.

D. R. Mishell, Jr, MD

IUD Use and the Risk of Endometrial Cancer
Benshushan A, Paltiel O, Rojansky N, et al (Hebrew Univ, Jerusalem)
Eur J Obstet Gynecol Reprod Biol 105:166-169, 2002   18–7

Background.—The intrauterine device (IUD) is one of the most common forms of birth control used worldwide. However, the long-term effects of IUDs on the uterus have not been extensively studied. The effects of IUD use on the incidence of endometrial cancer were reported.

Methods.—One hundred twenty-eight women, aged 35 to 64 years, with a histologically verified diagnosis of endometrial cancer were compared with 255 healthy women randomly selected from the same geographic area. Factors independently associated with endometrial cancer in a univariate analysis were assessed in a multivariate logistic model after adjusting for age.

Findings.—Endometrial cancer was significantly and independently associated with nulliparity, with an odds ratio (OR) of 2.7; a history of infertility, with an OR of 1.8; and a body mass index of 27 or greater, with an OR of 2.3. The use of oral contraceptives and IUDs had a protective effect against endometrial cancer, with ORs of 0.29 and 0.37, respectively.

Conclusions.—The use of an IUD appears to protect against endometrial cancer risk. The mechanism underlying this protective effect may be the intense inflammatory response that results in other lysosomal and inflammatory actions, which may include cells responsible for early elimination of hyperplastic endometrial epithelial cells. Alternatively, the more complete shedding of the endometrium associated with IUD use may reduce hyperplasia of the endometrium, a known risk factor for endometrial carcinoma.

▶ There are now several case-control studies, including this one, that indicate that use of an IUD reduces the risk of subsequently developing endometrial cancer by about 50%. Women should be informed about this noncontraceptive benefit of the IUD when deciding which method of contraception they wish to use.

D. R. Mishell, Jr, MD

The Levonorgestrel Two-Rod Implant for Long-Acting Contraception: 10 Years of Clinical Experience
Wan LS, Stiber A, Lam L-y (New York Univ)
Obstet Gynecol 102:24-26, 2003   18–8

Background.—The levonorgestrel subdermal implant has been used by millions of women throughout the world, and its efficacy and convenience for long-acting contraception have been widely reported. While Norplant was marketed in the United States in 1991, it never attained wide use because of the need for a minor surgical incision for insertion and removal. The use of Norplant in the United States plummeted when problems with its removal were reported, and the implant was recalled in the United States in 2001 due to manufacturing problems. It remains unavailable in the United States. A 2-rod version of the implant is currently marketed in Europe and has recently been approved for 5 years of use by the US Food and Drug Administration. Experience with this new 2-rod implant from 1990 to 2000 was described.

Methods.—Volunteers aged 18 to 40 years who desired long-acting contraception were recruited from the Bellevue Hospital Women's Health Clinic in New York. The study was originally designed for 5 years but was later extended to 6 years.

Results.—A total of 249 women received the 2-rod implant and were observed for a total of 823 women-years. Two pregnancies were reported during the study, for a pregnancy rate of 0.24 per 100 woman-years. One pregnancy occurred in the first month of use and the other after 6 years. Menstrual irregularity was the most significant side-effect; no serious side effects were observed during the study. Insertion of the device was easy and took less than 2 minutes. The average removal time was 4.5 minutes.

Conclusion.—The levonorgestrel 2-rod implant is a safe, effective, and convenient long-acting contraceptive method. The 2-rod system is easier to insert and remove than the Norplant system and is equally effective.

▶ The levonorgestrel 2-rod implant is a very effective, long-term, rapidly reversible progestin-only contraceptive method. Insertion and removal of the 2 rods is much more rapid than insertion and removal of the 6 capsules containing levonorgestrel. Although the 2-rod system is marketed in several countries outside the United States, it is not marketed in this country despite being approved by the US Food and Drug Administration. It is unfortunate that women in the United States do not have the opportunity to use this very effective, long-acting method of steroid contraception.

D. R. Mishell, Jr, MD

Microinsert Nonincisional Hysteroscopic Sterilization
Cooper JM, for the Selective Tubal Occlusion Procedure 2000 Investigators Group (Women's Health Research, Phoenix, Ariz; et al)
Obstet Gynecol 102:59-67, 2003   18–9

Background.—Most interval sterilization procedures in the United States and other developed countries involve laparoscopy under general anesthesia in an outpatient setting. It is estimated that 89% of interval tubal sterilizations in the United States are performed laparoscopically. The conventional incisional approaches to interval sterilization, including laparoscopy and minilaparoscopy, carry risks associated with general anesthesia. In addition, these incisional approaches can, in rare cases, cause vascular damage; injury to the bowel, bladder, or uterus; or unintended laparotomy. Laparoscopic tubal sterilization may also be associated with significant postoperative pain.

A transcervical approach is an attractive alternative to the transabdominal approach as it eliminates the need for general anesthesia and incisional surgery. The safety, effectiveness, and reliability of a tubal occlusion microinsert for permanent contraception were assessed. Included in this assessment were patient recovery and overall satisfaction with the procedure.

Methods.—This prospective phase III trial enrolled 518 previously fertile women seeking sterilization. Microinsert placement was attempted in 507 women. Microinserts were placed bilaterally in the proximal fallopian tube lumens under hysteroscopic visualization. All procedures were performed as outpatient procedures.

Results.—The bilateral placement was accomplished in 464 of 507 (92%) patients. The most common reasons for failure to accomplish satisfactory placement were tubal obstruction and stenosis or difficult access to the proximal tubal lumen. Over half of the women rated the average pain during the procedure as either mild or none. Tolerance of device placement was rated as good to excellent by 88% of patients. The average time to discharge was 60 minutes. The majority of women (60%) returned to normal functioning within 1 day, and 92% missed 1 day or less of work. After 3 months, correct microinsert placement and tubal occlusion were confirmed in 96% and 92% of patients, respectively. Comfort was rated as good to excellent in 99% of women at follow-up. Ultimately, 87% of women could rely on the microinsert for permanent contraception. No pregnancies have been recorded in 9629 woman-months of exposure to intercourse.

Conclusion.—Hysteroscopic interval tubal sterilization with microinserts is well tolerated and provides rapid recovery, a high level of patient satisfaction, and effective permanent contraception.

▶ Sterilization of the woman by tubal occlusion except shortly after delivery is called "interval sterilization." Methods to perform tubal occlusion by transcervical techniques have been tried for many years with a varying incidence of effectiveness. Hysteroscopic placement into the tubal ostia of the devices described in this report is effective, with a minimal amount of patient discomfort, avoidance of general anesthesia, and a high rate of successful insertion of the devices. Complications were uncommon in this series. Clinicians with training in hysteroscopic procedures should consider offering this method of tubal sterilization to women requesting interval sterilization.

D. R. Mishell, Jr, MD

Low Dose Mifepristone and Two Regimens of Levonorgestrel for Emergency Contraception: A WHO Multicentre Randomised Trial

von Hertzen H, for the WHO Research Group on Post-Ovulatory Methods of Fertility Regulation (WHO, Geneva; et al)

Lancet 360:1803-1810, 2002   18–10

Introduction.—A single dose of mifepristone, 10 mg, and 2 doses of levonorgestrel, 0.75 mg, administered within 72 hours of unprotected intercourse are effective as emergency contraception. No trials have compared the efficacies of the 2 compounds or assessed a single dose of levonorgestrel, 1.5 mg. Thus, a randomized, double-blind, 3-arm trial was performed in 15 family-planning clinics in 10 countries to assess these efficacies.

Methods.—All participants were seen for emergency contraception within 120 hours of a single act of unprotected intercourse, were healthy, had regular menstrual cycles, and had to be willing to abstain from unprotected intercourse during the treatment cycle. Women were randomly assigned to 1 of 3 regimens as follows: 10 mg of single-dose mifepristone, 1.5 mg of single-dose levonorgestrel, or 2 doses of 0.75 mg of levonorgestrel administered 12 hours apart. The main outcome measure was unintended pregnancy; other outcome measures were side effects and timing of the subsequent menstrual period. Analysis was by intention to treat; some patients were excluded from the final analyses.

Results.—Of 4071 women with known outcomes, the pregnancy rates were 1.5% (21/1359) for those in the mifepristone group, 1.5% (20/1356) for those in the single-dose levonorgestrel group, and 1.8% (24/1356) for those in the 2-dose levonorgestrel group. The relative risk of pregnancy for single-dose versus double-dose levonorgestrel was 0.83 (95% confidence interval, 0.46-1.50). The relative risk for the 2 regimens combined compared with mifepristone was 1.05 (95% confidence interval, 0.63-1.76). Side effects were mild and did not vary significantly between groups. Most women menstruated within 1 day of the expected date. Women who received levonorgestrel had earlier menses compared with those who received mifepristone.

Conclusion.—The 3 regimens evaluated are efficacious as emergency contraception and prevent a large proportion of pregnancies if administered within 5 days of unprotected intercourse. Mifepristone and levonorgestrel are similar in efficacy. A 1.5-mg single levonorgestrel dose may be used instead of two 0.75-mg doses 12 hours apart.

▶ A single dose of 10 mg of mifepristone is an effective means of emergency contraception. However, mifepristone is not marketed in this dosage and is difficult to obtain in the United States. Two doses of 750 µg of levonorgestrel taken 12 hours apart is an effective means of emergency contraception and is widely available. The results of this study indicate that taking the two 750-µg tablets of levonorgestrel on 1 occasion is as effective as the 2-dose regimen. The results of this study also indicate that this emergency contraceptive regimen is nearly as effective when taken between 72 and 120 hours after coitus as when taken prior to 72 hours. This important information should be provided to women who need emergency contraception 4 to 5 days after unprotected intercourse.

D. R. Mishell, Jr, MD

Modifying the Yuzpe Regimen of Emergency Contraception: A Multicenter Randomized Controlled Trial
Ellertson C, Webb A, Blanchard K, et al (Ibis Reproductive Health, Cambridge, Mass; Abacus Centre for Contraception and Reproductive Health, Liverpool, England; Population Council, Johannesburg, South Africa; et al)
Obstet Gynecol 101:1160-1167, 2003   18–11

Introduction.—The Yuzpe regimen is the best-evaluated emergency contraceptive approach for prevention of unintended pregnancy after unprotected intercourse. This regimen consists of ordinary combined oral contraceptives containing levonorgestrel and ethinyl estradiol. Women usually take 1 dose within 72 hours after unprotected intercourse and a second dose 12 hours later. Since the rules for the Yuzpe regimen did not originate from a rigorous evidence base, it may be that modifications could make the therapy more accessible, comfortable, and convenient without compromising efficacy. The Yuzpe regimen was evaluated to determine whether (1) women could use combined oral contraceptives other than those that contain levonorgestrel, and (2) eliminating the second dose improves comfort and convenience.

Methods.—Women seen within 72 hours after unprotected intercourse were randomly assigned to receive either the standard 2-dose Yuzpe, a variant of Yuzpe substituting norethindrone for levonorgestrel, or only the first dose of Yuzpe, followed 12 hours later with a placebo.

Results.—Perfect-use failure rates were low for all 3 groups and did not vary in a statistically significant fashion (standard Yuzpe 2.0%, norethindrone-ethinyl estradiol 2.7%, and single dose of Yuzpe 2.9% in 589, 547, and 546 patients, respectively). The typical-use failure rates were significantly higher yet similar across groups (Table 2). Women taking the single dose reported half the rate of vomiting, compared with the other 2 groups. Taking pills with food did not appear to decrease nausea or vomiting. Taking the pills sooner after unprotected intercourse did not make them more effective.

Conclusion.—Oral contraceptives containing norethindrone-ethinyl estradiol work about as well for emergency contraception as the levonorgestrel-ethinyl estradiol formulations. They may be offered when first-line therapies are not available.

▶ The emergency contraceptive regimen originally described by A. Yuzpe consists of 2 tablets of an oral contraceptive containing 50 µg of ethinyl estradiol and 0.5 mg of norgestrel taken on 2 occasions 12 hours apart. Other types of oral contraceptives and use of a single dose instead of 2 doses with a 12

TABLE 2.—Perfect- and Typical-Use Failure Rates (Pregnancy Rates) and Effectiveness Rates (Proportional Reductions in Pregnancy), by Study Regimen

| | Pregnant | n | % Pregnant | 95% CI* | Failure Rate | | | Effectiveness Rate | | |
					P*	Odds Ratio	95% CI†	% Reduction in Pregnancy	95% CI‡	P‡
Perfect use§										
Standard two-dose Yuzpe	12	589	2.0	1.1, 3.5	Ref.	Ref.	Ref.	72.8	51.2, 84.9	Ref.
Norethindrone–ethinyl estradiol	15	547	2.7	1.5, 4.5	.44	1.36	0.59, 3.20	61.3	34.3, 77.2	.38
Single dose of Yuzpe	16	546	2.9	1.7, 4.7	.35	1.45	0.64, 3.39	60.1	33.5, 76.1	.34
Typical use‖										
Standard two-dose Yuzpe	17	675	2.5	1.5, 4.0	Ref.	Ref.	Ref.	66.5	44.8, 79.7	Ref.
Norethindrone–ethinyl estradiol	18	650	2.8	1.6, 4.3	.86	1.10	0.53, 2.30	60.0	34.7, 75.4	.62
Single dose of Yuzpe	23	648	3.5	2.3, 5.3	.34	1.42	0.72, 2.87	52.4	26.1, 69.3	.30

Note: All comparisons are to the standard 2-dose Yuzpe control group (reference category).
*95% exact binomial confidence intervals (CIs); P values are based on Fisher exact tests comparing the rates from each experimental group with those from the standard 2-dose Yuzpe control group.
†95% exact.
‡95% CIs based on normal approximation; z tests compare the effectiveness rates from each experimental study group with those from the standard 2-dose Yuzpe control group.
§Includes only women who started therapy in the assigned time period, who took both doses, and who had no further acts of unprotected intercourse after treatment.
‖Includes all women with known pregnancy outcomes.
(Reprinted with permission from The American College of Obstetricians and Gynecologists courtesy of Ellertson C, Webb A, Blanchard K, et al: Modifying the Yuzpe regimen of emergency contraception: A multicenter randomized controlled trial. *Obstet Gynecol* 101:1160-1167, 2003.)

hour dosing interval were not studied. The results of this trial suggest that other oral contraceptive formulations, specifically one containing norethindrone, may have similar effectiveness to the original regimen designed by Yuzpe.

A single dose of an oral contraceptive with ethinyl estradiol and norgestrel had similar effectiveness as 2 doses with less side effects. The most effective steroidal emergency contraceptive appears to be 1500 µg of levonorgestrel administered as 2 doses of 750 µg taken 12 hours apart. If this formulation is unavailable, combination formulations containing ethinyl estradiol and levonorgestrel should be used. If this formulation is unavailable, a formulation with norethindrone plus ethinyl estradiol is also effective.

D. R. Mishell, Jr, MD

A Randomised Study Comparing a Low Dose of Mifepristone and the Yuzpe Regimen for Emergency Contraception
Ashok PW, Stalder C, Wagaarachchi PT, et al (Univ of Aberdeen, Scotland; Grampian Univ Hosps NHS Trust, Scotland)
Br J Obstet Gynaecol 109:553-560, 2002   18–12

Background.—Mifepristone is an orally active synthetic norsteroid. When given in the early luteal phase of the menstrual cycle, it is believed to inhibit implantation. This randomized trial compared mifepristone to the Yuzpe regimen for emergency contraception up to 72 hours after intercourse.

TABLE 2.—Pregnancy Rates by Groups and Time Interval From Coitus to Treatment

Coitus to Treatment Interval	Pregnancies n (%)	RR (95% CI)
All women		
Mifepristone ($n = 487$)	3 (0.6)	6.04 (1.75 to 20.75)
Yuzpe regimen ($n = 471$)	17 (3.6)	
<24 hours		
Mifepristone ($n = 135$)	0 (0)	2.03 (1.79 to 2.29)
Yuzpe regimen ($n = 134$)	3 (2.2)	
25-48 hours		
Mifepristone ($n = 212$)	1 (0.5)	7.03 (0.85 to 57.66)
Yuzpe regimen ($n = 217$)	7 (3.2)	
49-72 hours		
Mifepristone ($n = 140$)	2 (1.4)*	4.27 (0.87 to 20.98)
Yuzpe regimen ($n = 120$)	7 (5.2)	

*User failures.
Abbreviation: RR, Relative risk.
(Reprinted from Ashok PW, Stalder C, Wagaarachchi PT, et al: A randomised study comparing a low dose of mifepristone and the Yuzpe regimen for emergency contraception. *Br J Obstet Gynaecol* 109:553-560. Copyright 2002, with permission from Elsevier Science.)

Study Design.—The study group consisted of 1000 women, aged 16 to 45 years, who were randomly assigned to receive either the Yuzpe regimen or mifepristone for emergency contraception. The primary outcome measure was pregnancy. Secondary outcome measures included side effects and patient satisfaction. Crude, expected, and prevented pregnancy rates were calculated.

Findings.—The crude pregnancy rate was 3.6% with the Yuzpe regimen and 0.6% with mifepristone. Mifepristone prevented 92% of pregnancies, and the Yuzpe regimen prevented 56% of pregnancies. Increased time between intercourse and treatment was associated with contraceptive failure in the Yuzpe regimen but not with mifepristone treatment. The menstrual period was delayed in 24.5% of those treated with mifepristone and in 13.1% of those treated with the Yuzpe regimen (Table 2). The mifepristone regimen was better tolerated and had fewer side effects. More women were satisfied with mifepristone as emergency contraception than with the Yuzpe regimen and would recommend it to a friend.

Conclusions.—Mifepristone is an effective emergency contraceptive when taken within 72 hours of unprotected intercourse. It is well tolerated and has few side effects and high patient acceptability.

▶ This well-done, large, randomized controlled trial of 2 agents for emergency contraception found that a single 100-mg dose of mifepristone was significantly more effective than 2 tablets of a combination oral contraceptive given at a 12-hour interval, the Yuzpe regimen. Pregnancy rates were 0.6% with the former regimen, and 3.6% with the latter. The failure rate was higher when the Yuzpe regimen was given more than 24 hours after intercourse but the same was not true for the use of mifepristone. In addition, side effects were greater with the Yuzpe regimen than with mifepristone. Although mifepristone is not approved for emergency contraception in the United States, its high rate of efficacy and low incidence of side effects warrant use of this agent to prevent unintended pregnancy after a single act of unprotected midcycle intercourse.

D. R. Mishell, Jr, MD

Extending the Time Limit for Starting the Yuzpe Regimen of Emergency Contraception to 120 Hours
Ellertson C, Evans M, Ferden S, et al (Ibis Reproductive Health, Cambridge, Mass; Abacus Centre for Contraception and Reproductive Health, Liverpool, England; Planned Parenthood of Greater Iowa, Des Moines; et al)
Obstet Gynecol 101:1168-1171, 2003   18–13

Introduction.—Current protocols state that the Yuzpe regimen of emergency contraception can be initiated up to 72 hours after unprotected intercourse. In parallel to a double-masked, randomized, controlled trial of 2 modifications to the Yuzpe regimen, a prospective, observational trial was performed to determine whether the window for emergency hormonal contraception can be extended to 120 hours.

Methods.—A total of 111 women were evaluated who requested emergency contraception between 72 and 120 hours after unprotected intercourse and refused postcoital copper intrauterine devices, preferring the Yuzpe regimen. Failure rates were compared for this cohort with the rates of 675 otherwise similar women who initiated the same therapy within 72 hours.

Results.—Both perfect use (1.9%) and typical use (3.6%) failure rates were low in women for whom the Yuzpe regimen was initiated between 72 and 120 hours after unprotected intercourse. These rates were similar to those for the standard Yuzpe regimen (2.0% during perfect use and 2.5% during typical use). The small sample size of 111 participants provided just 25% power to identify a doubling in the failure rates (2% to 4%) and 59% power to identify a tripling in the failure rates (2% to 6%).

Conclusion.—The 72-hour cutoff for the Yuzpe regimen of emergency contraception may be needlessly restrictive. Women who request this therapy more than 72 hours after unprotected intercourse should be allowed to receive therapy, especially if they decline postcoital insertion of a copper intrauterine device and would otherwise have no other choices for decreasing the risk of pregnancy.

▶ There are now several studies which suggest that the use of emergency contraception, either levonorgestrel alone or a combination of norgestrel and ethinyl estradiol, remain at least partially effective for prevention of pregnancy when administered between 72 and 120 hours after a single act of midcycle unprotected sexual intercourse. Women who delay requesting emergency contraception beyond 72 hours but less than 120 hours should be offered such therapy, even though it may be less effective than when it is administered prior to 72 hours after coitus. The most effective type of emergency contraception administered between 72 and 120 hours after unprotected coitus is insertion of a copper intrauterine device. However, many women do not wish to have an intrauterine device inserted and would prefer levonorgestrel or oral contraceptives.

D. R. Mishell, Jr, MD

Advance Supply of Emergency Contraception: Effect on Use and Usual Contraception—A Randomized Trial
Jackson RA, Schwarz EB, Freedman L, et al (Univ of California, San Francisco; San Francisco Gen Hosp)
Obstet Gynecol 102:8-16, 2003   18–14

Background.—The abortion rate in the United States is one of the highest of any developed nation. Emergency contraception has proved safe and effective and could decrease the abortion rate by up to 50%. However, the use of emergency contraception remains limited. There is insufficient knowledge among both patients and providers regarding emergency contraception, and access is limited by difficulties in obtaining prescriptions or unavailability of emergency contraception pills at local pharmacies. The majority of women in the United States are unfamiliar with emergency contraception, which significantly limits its potential effectiveness.

Among the strategies for increasing access are pharmacist dispensation, over-the-counter availability, and advance provision by health care providers. The effectiveness of advance provision of emergency contraception for increasing its use and whether it adversely affects usual contraceptive practices were evaluated.

Methods.—This randomized, controlled trial compared advance provision of emergency contraception with usual care in 370 postpartum women from an inner-city public hospital. The study participants were followed up for 1 year, and 85% attended at least 1 follow-up session. All of the participants received routine contraceptive education. The intervention group received a supply of emergency contraception and a 5-minute educational session. The control group received only the routine contraceptive counseling provided to all women before discharge (usual care). The use of emergency contraception and changes in contraceptive behavior were compared between groups.

Results.—Women in the intervention group were 4 times as likely to have used emergency contraception as women in the control group (17% vs 4%). However, women in the intervention group were no more likely to have switched to a less effective method of birth control (30% and 33%, respectively) or to be using contraception less consistently (18% and 25%, respectively). Roughly half of the women in each group reported at least 1 episode of unprotected sex during follow-up, but women in the intervention group were 6 times as likely to have used emergency contraception after unprotected intercourse (25% vs 4%).

Conclusion.—The advance provision of emergency contraception significantly increased its use and did not adversely affect the use of routine contraception in this population. Advance provision of emergency contraception is safe and appropriate for all postpartum women before discharge from the hospital.

▶ Numerous studies have shown that use of emergency contraceptive steroids by women within 3 days of unprotected midcycle sexual intercourse effectively reduces the risk of pregnancy by 75% to 85%. Unfortunately, there are many barriers that limit the accessibility of emergency contraception (EC). This study shows that routine provision of 1 dose of EC at the time of postpartum discharge significantly increased the subsequent use of EC during the first year post partum, compared with a control group not given EC. Unfortunately, only one fourth of the women given EC who had unprotected intercourse used EC, but this rate was 6 times higher than the 4% of control women who used EC after unprotected intercourse.

Provision of EC did not decrease use of effective methods of contraception. Clinicians should offer to provide EC to all sexually active women, even if using an effective reversible method of contraception, so if EC is needed, it will be readily available.

D. R. Mishell, Jr, MD

19 Endocrinology

Long-term Follow-up of Functional Hypothalamic Amenorrhea and Prognostic Factors
Falsetti L, Gambera A, Barbetti L, et al (Univ of Brescia, Italy)
J Clin Endocrinol Metab 87:500-505, 2002   19–1

Objective.—Women with functional hypothalamic amenorrhea (FHA) have abnormally low pulsatile GnRH secretion, with clinical manifestations ranging from inadequate luteal phase to hypothalamic amenorrhea. Clinically, FHA may be associated with various types of stress or with weight loss related to decreased energy intake or intense exercise. However, the neuroendocrine abnormalities involved remain unclear. The long-term outcomes of women with FHA were analyzed, along with prognostic factors for recovery.

Patients.—The analysis included 93 patients with FHA seen at a department of gynecologic endocrinology from 1990 to 1992. At admission, the patients' mean age was 23 years, mean body mass index was 20 kg/m², and mean duration of secondary amenorrhea was 15 months. After diagnostic investigation, the patients were given advice on nutrition and exercise to maintain proper energy balance; depending on their contraceptive desires, treatment consisted of hormone replacement therapy or oral contraceptives. Outcomes and prognostic factors were analyzed after an average follow-up of 8 years.

Outcomes.—Seventy-one percent of the women recovered. The chances of recovery were unrelated to anamnestic causes of FHA and the echocardiographic findings of the ovary. However, recovery was more likely for women with a higher baseline body mass index and androstenedione level and with a lower baseline cortisol level. Body mass index either increased or remained stable in all women whose FHA resolved but decreased or remained stable in those whose FHA persisted. Recovery rates were 74% for women receiving hormone replacement therapy and 80% for those receiving no therapy compared with 42% for those receiving oral contraceptives (Fig 1).

Conclusions.—This long-term follow-up study suggests that FHA is reversible in most cases. The chances of recovery are affected by the initial body mass index, androstenedione level, and cortisol level. Elimination of psychological stressors and correction of energy balance may be important factors in promoting recovery from FHA.

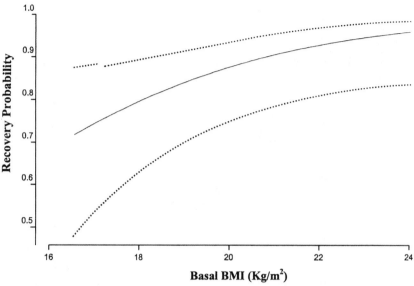

Adjusted to: Cortisol=19; A=1.6; Therapy=Therapy

FIGURE 1.—Relationship between basal body mass index and recovery probability. (Courtesy of Falsetti L, Gambera A, Barbetti L, et al: Long-term follow-up of functional hypothalamic amenorrhea and prognostic factors. *J Clin Endocrinol Metab* 87(2):500-505, 2002. Copyright The Endocrine Society.)

▶ FHA is a common cause of secondary amenorrhea. The results of this prospective study of a large group of women with FHA followed up for a mean of 8 years showed that 70% developed normal ovulatory cycles. Factors positively associated with recovery included an increase in body mass index and the use of hormone replacement therapy instead of oral contraceptives. Women with FHA should be encouraged to gain weight. Whether use of hormone replacement therapy instead of oral contraceptives increases the likelihood of recovery of normal cycles is not proven in this nonrandomized study, but it may be advisable to use the former therapy instead of oral contraceptives, as there may be a causal relation.

D. R. Mishell, Jr, MD

A Retrospective Cohort Study Comparing Microwave Endometrial Ablation With Levonorgestrel-Releasing Intrauterine Device in the Management of Heavy Menstrual Bleeding
Henshaw R, Coyle C, Low S, et al (South East Regional Health Service, Adelaide, South Australia; Univ of Adelaide, South Australia)
Aust N Z J Obstet Gynaecol 42:205-209, 2002   19–2

Background.—Heavy menstrual bleeding can have significant effects on quality of life. Two new treatment options are the levonorgestrel-releasing intrauterine device (LNG-IUD; Mirena) and microwave endometrial abla-

TABLE 2.—Rate Changes in Menstrual Bleeding and
Dysmenorrhoea Scores

	MEA™	LNG-IUD
Pre-treatment bleeding score		
Mean (SD) (range 0-50)	30.0 (11.1)	30.7 (9.4)
Post-treatment bleeding score		
Mean (SD) (range 0-50)	5.3 (7.1)	8.2 (14.3)
p value	< 0.0001	< 0.0001
95% CI	20.5-28.8	16.2-28.7
Pre-treatment dysmenorrhoea score		
Mean (SD) (range 0-50)	11.7 (11.1)	13.2 (10.8)
Post-treatment dysmenorrhoea score		
Mean (SD) (range 0-50)	1.9 (5.5)	6.2 (10.7)
p value	< 0.0001	0.0025
95% CI	5.4-14.1	2.8-11.1

Abbreviations: MEA, Microwave endometrial ablation; *LNG-IUD,* levonorgestrel-releasing intra-uterine device.

(Courtesy of Henshaw R, Coyle C, Low S, et al: A retrospective cohort study comparing microwave endometrial ablation with levonorgestrel-releasing intrauterine device in the management of heavy menstrual bleeding. *Austr NZ J Obstet Gynaecol* 42:205-209, 2002.)

tion (MEA). The LNG-IUD was compared with MEA for the treatment of heavy menstrual bleeding in a retrospective cohort study.

Study Design.—The study group consisted of 39 women treated with MEA and 23 women treated with the LNG-IUD for heavy menstrual bleeding in Australia from 1998 to 2001. The average follow-up duration was 14.6 months. The primary outcome measures were treatment acceptability, treatment efficacy, and patient satisfaction with the treatment. Secondary outcomes included premenstrual symptoms, health-related quality of life, and complications. Each woman served as her own control with regard to changes in bleeding pattern.

Findings.—Both procedures were acceptable, and patient satisfaction was high with both treatments. Both treatments resulted in a significant reduction in menstrual bleeding and dysmenorrhea scores (Table 2). Premenstrual symptoms and quality of life did not differ for the 2 treatments.

Conclusions.—This retrospective cohort study indicates that MEA and the LNG-IUD are equally effective for the management of heavy menstrual bleeding.

▶ Other studies have shown that insertion of the LNG-IUD for treatment of idiopathic menorrhagia is as effective as the hysteroscopic technique of endometrial ablation. MEA is a recently developed technique that allows the endometrium to be destroyed without the use of hysteroscopy. Although this article was a retrospective, uncontrolled subjective assessment of the treatment of menorrhagia with MEA or the LNG-IUD, the results suggest that these 2 techniques have similar levels of efficacy. Because the LNG-IUD is reversible and preserves fertility, unlike endometrial ablation, the LNG-IUD is preferable to endometrial ablation among women with idiopathic menorrhagia who wish to retain fertility.

D. R. Mishell, Jr, MD

Use of a Levonorgestrel-Releasing Intrauterine System to Treat Bleeding Related to Uterine Leiomyomas

Grigorieva V, Chen-Mok M, Tarasova M, et al (Ott Inst of Obstetrics and Gynecology, St Petersburg, Russia; Family Health Internatl, Research, Triangle Park, NC)
Fertil Steril 79:1194-1198, 2003　　　　　　　　　　　　　　　19–3

Background.—Surgical approaches are preferred for the treatment of uterine leiomyomas, including myomectomy and hysterectomy. Leiomyomas are the most common reason for performing a hysterectomy in the United States. The growth of leiomyomas may be inhibited using the levonorgestrel-releasing intrauterine system (LNG IUS; Leiras OY, Turku, Finland). It was postulated that both contraception and long-term treatment of leiomyomas may be possible by using the LNG IUS for women of reproductive age. The efficacy of the LNG IUS was determined by its ability to diminish menstrual blood loss, improve iron deficiency anemia, and reduce the size of the uterus and leiomyomas over the first year of use.

Methods.—Sixty-nine premenopausal women (mean age, 39 years) volunteered for a prospective evaluation of the use of the LNG IUS as their method of contraception. In each case, the uterus was less than 12 weeks' gestational size on pelvic examination and there was at least 1 leiomyoma measuring 2.5 cm or greater in diameter or multiple leiomyomas that included at least 1 measuring a minimum of 1.5 cm in diameter on US evaluation. The pictorial blood loss assessment chart developed by Higham et al was used to estimate menstrual blood loss; in this method, a score over 100 is equivalent to a blood loss of over 80 mL, the defined limit for menorrhagia. Sonographic methods were employed to measure uterine and leiomyoma volumes.

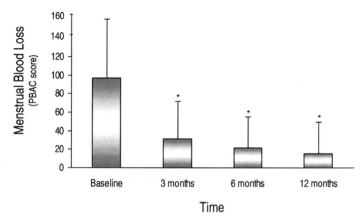

FIGURE 1.—Estimated menstrual blood loss (mean ± standard deviation) before and after insertion of the levonorgestrel-releasing intrauterine system. *Asterisk* indicates *P* < .001 versus baseline. *Abbreviation: PBAC*, Pictorial blood loss assessment chart. (Reprinted by permission from the American Society for Reproductive Medicine courtesy of Grigorieva V, Chen-Mok M, Tarasova M, et al: Use of a levonorgestrel-releasing intrauterine system to treat bleeding related to uterine leiomyomas. *Fertil Steril* 79:1194-1198. Copyright 2003 with permission from the American College of Surgeons.)

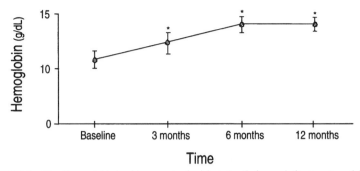

FIGURE 2.—Blood hemoglobin level (mean ± standard deviation) before and after insertion of the levo-norgestrel-releasing intrauterine system. *Asterisk* indicates $P < .001$ versus baseline. (Reprinted by permission from the American Society for Reproductive Medicine courtesy of Grigorieva V, Chen-Mok M, Tarasova M, et al: Use of a levonorgestrel-releasing intrauterine system to treat bleeding related to uterine leiomyomas. *Fertil Steril* 79:1194-1198. Copyright 2003 with permission from the American College of Surgeons.)

Results.—Sixty-seven of the 69 women were eligible for analysis, and 61 women completed the 12 months of observation. Thirty-nine percent of the women had menorrhagia before insertion of the LNG IUS, and 28% had anemia, with a hemoglobin level under 12.0 g/dL, at baseline. Menstrual blood loss fell dramatically, with only 4 patients having excessive menstrual bleeding 3 months after the IUS was inserted. A nearly 6-fold reduction in blood loss was documented after 12 months (Fig 1). Ten percent of the participants had amenorrhea after 3 months, 20% after 6 months, and 40% after 12 months.

Blood hemoglobin (Fig 2) and serum ferritin levels increased significantly, with marked improvement within 3 months and levels significantly higher than baseline at 6 and 12 months. Only 7 women had blood hemoglobin levels under 12.0 g/dL after 3 months, 2 after 6 months, and 1 after 12 months. The average uterine size declined significantly from a mean baseline volume of 138 mL to 122 mL after 12 months. The total leiomyoma volume was statistically significant after 6 months. Side effects of the treatment included spotting and breast tenderness, neither of which required treatment. Two women withdrew from the treatment because of the side effects. No pregnancies occurred.

Conclusion.—By profoundly reducing menstrual blood loss, the LNG IUS was able to effectively address iron deficiency anemia in women with menorrhagia linked to the presence of leiomyomas. It was also able to reduce both uterine and leiomyoma size over the course of 1 year. In addition, effective contraception was provided.

▶ Nearly half of the 600,000 hysterectomies performed in the United States each year are due to the presence of uterine leiomyomas. Increased uterine bleeding is the main reason why hysterectomies are performed in women with uterine leiomyomas. The results of this study indicate that when leiomyomas are present but the uterine size is less than 12 weeks' gestational age and there is no distortion of the uterine cavity, the LNG IUS is an effective treatment of increased menstrual blood loss with resultant increase in hemoglobin levels.

The mean decrease in menstrual blood loss fell from 100 mL before placement of the device to about 30 mL 3 months after insertion of the LNG IUS. In addition, the size of the leiomyomas decreased significantly 6 months after placement of the LNG IUS. Clinicians should consider placement of the LNG IUS as an alternative to hysterectomy in women with uterine leiomyoma and menorrhagia when the uterine size is less than 12 weeks' gestational age.

D. R. Mishell, Jr, MD

Treatment of Nonatypical and Atypical Endometrial Hyperplasia With a Levonorgestrel-Releasing Intrauterine System

Wildemeersch D, Dhont M (Univ Hosp, Knokke, Belgium; Univ Hosp, Ghent, Belgium)
Am J Obstet Gynecol 188:1297-1298, 2003   19–4

Background.—An intrauterine drug delivery system is an alternative route for administering potent progestogens to make uterine tissue incapable of responding to estrogen stimulation. A "frameless" levonorgestrel intrauterine system (IUS) that releases 14 µg of levonorgestrel per day has been found effective in providing strong endometrial suppression. Whether the long-acting levonorgestrel IUS is useful for hyperplasia was investigated.

Methods and Findings.—The IUS consists of a nonresorbable thread with a single knot at its proximal end, which is attached to a 4 cm long, 1.2 mm wide fibrous delivery system that releases approximately 14 µg of levonorgestrel per day. The system was used to treat nonatypical and atypical endometrial hyperplasia in 12 otherwise healthy women aged 46 to 67 years old. All but 1 woman had a thin endometrium of less than 5 mm, as shown on transvaginal US. The remaining woman had a polypoid structure of 20 mm in diameter. The participants were followed up for 3 to 4 years. Repeat endometrial biopsy demonstrated a 100% cure rate. After 12 months of treatment, the polypoid structure in the affected patient decreased in size to 8 mm.

Conclusions.—The levonorgestrel system is an effective technique for suppressing the endometrium in women with nonatypical and atypical hyperplasia. With appropriate follow-up, this treatment may be an alternative to hysterectomy.

▶ The results of this study suggest that insertion of a levonorgestrel-releasing IUS effectively suppresses endometrial hyperplasia with and without atypia. Women with atypical endometrial hyperplasia and medical contraindications for hysterectomy may choose to be treated with a levonorgestrel-releasing IUS. After insertion of the device endometrial sampling should be performed periodically to be certain the hyperplasia regresses. Women with endometrial hyperplasia without atypia may also choose to be treated with this device instead of high doses of oral progestins.

D. R. Mishell, Jr, MD

Prediction of Insulin Sensitivity in Nonobese Women With Polycystic Ovary Syndrome

Cibula D, Škrha J, Hill M, et al (Charles Univ, Praha, Czech Republic; Inst of Endocrinology, Prague, Praha, Czech Republic)
J Clin Endocrinol Metab 87:5821-5825, 2002   19–5

Background.—Women with polycystic ovary syndrome (PCOS) commonly have insulin resistance, which plays a key role in the predisposition to type 2 diabetes. Thus patients with insulin resistance need to be identified. The relation between insulin sensitivity and both endocrine and metabolic indexes was investigated to develop the best model for predicting insulin sensitivity in women with PCOS.

Methods and Findings.—Forty-one nonobese women meeting diagnostic criteria for PCOS were studied. No androgens were associated with the insulin sensitivity index. All euglycemic clamp parameters correlated with sex hormone–binding globulin (SHBG), triglycerides, and body mass index. There was no association with waist-to-hip ratio or waist circumference. The close association between insulin sensitivity and SHBG was demonstrated in a factor analysis and by its presence in all prediction models as the most significant or even the only predictor of the insulin sensitivity index.

Conclusions.—A reduced SHBG level can be used as a single reliable predictor of insulin sensitivity in nonobese women with PCOS. Waist-to-hip ratio, waist circumference, and androgen levels have no such predictive value.

▶ PCOS is relatively common, being estimated to occur in about 4% to 7% of white women. Decreased insulin sensitivity or insulin resistance occurs in both obese and nonobese women with PCOS, although the prevalence of insulin resistance among women with PCOS is not known. The presence of insulin resistance in women with PCOS has been shown to correlate with the subsequent development of type 2 diabetes mellitus. The use of metformin has been advocated to treat women with PCOS and insulin resistance in an attempt to prevent subsequent development of diabetes mellitus. A ratio of fasting glucose/insulin levels less than 4.5 has been used to document the presence of insulin resistance. The results of this study suggest that a low SHBG level is a good predictor of insulin resistance in nonobese women with PCOS. Possibly SHBG measurement can be used as a screening test before performing other studies to determine whether insulin resistance is present. The study also revealed that the waist-to-hip ratio, waist circumference, and androgen levels did not correlate with the presence of insulin resistance.

D. R. Mishell, Jr, MD

Long Term Follow-up of Patients With Polycystic Ovarian Syndrome After Laparoscopic Ovarian Drilling: Clinical Outcome

Amer SAK, Gopalan V, Li TC, et al (Univ of Sheffield, England)
Hum Reprod 17:2035-2042, 2002   19–6

Background.—Laparoscopic ovarian drilling/diathermy (LOD) is used to treat medication-resistant anovulatory infertility associated with polycystic ovarian syndrome (PCOS). A group of women who had PCOS and LOD were compared with women with PCOS who did not receive LOD as a means of examining the long-term effects of LOD treatment in this group of patients.

Study Design.—The study group consisted of 116 women with PCOS who underwent LOD and 34 women with PCOS who did not undergo LOD. The women kept a menstrual cycle record, and serum hormone concentrations were assessed during cycles. Acne, hirsutism, and conception were monitored for up to 9 years of follow-up.

Findings.—The proportion of women with regular menstrual cycles increased significantly after LOD, from 8% to 67%. It then dropped to 37% at 1 to 3 years and then increased to 55% by 4 to 9 years. After LOD, 49% spontaneously conceived during the first year and 42% spontaneously conceived over the next 8 years. Among women with hirsutism, 23% experienced long-term improvement and among those with acne, 40% experienced long-term improvement after LOD. Women who received LOD showed significantly greater improvement at all time periods than women who did not receive this treatment.

Conclusion.—Treatment of women with PCOS with LOD results in long-term improvement in menstrual cycles, conception, hirsutism, and acne.

▶ LOD is a beneficial method to treat anovulating women with PCOS who fail to ovulate when treated with clomiphene citrate. The result of this long-term evaluation of this large series of women with PCOS treated with LOD found that about one third had long-term improvement in menstrual cycle regulation and reproductive performance. About 40% had sustained improvement with acne and 25% had sustained improvement in hirsutism.

D. R. Mishell, Jr, MD

Metformin *versus* Ethinyl Estradiol-Cyproterone Acetate in the Treatment of Nonobese Women With Polycystic Ovary Syndrome: A Randomized Study

Morin-Papunen L, Vauhkonen I, Koivunen R, et al (Univ Hosp of Oulu, Finland; Univ Hosp of Kuopio, Finland)
J Clin Endocrinol Metab 88:148-156, 2003   19–7

Background.—Polycystic ovary syndrome (PCOS) in obese women is characterized by insulin resistance and hyperinsulinemia associated with hyperandrogenism and anovulation. The insulin-sensitizing agent, metformin, can be used to decrease serum androgen levels and improve menstrual cycle and ovulation. Oral contraceptives (OC) are also used to treat menstrual irregularities and hyperandrogenism in women with PCOS. Approximately 20% to 50% of women with PCOS are not obese. The efficacy of treatment of nonobese women with PCOS with either OC or metformin was examined.

Study Design.—The study group consisted of 17 nonobese women with PCOS. The study participants were randomly assigned to either metformin or ethinyl estradiol-cyproterone acetate (EE-CA) for 6 months. All participants were assessed at baseline and after 3 and 6 months of treatment for blood pressure, ovarian status, oral glucose tolerance, serum concentrations of sex steroids, and insulin sensitivity.

Findings.—Metformin treatment had no effect on glucose tolerance or insulin sensitivity, but fasting insulin concentration and waist-to-hip ratio decreased, whereas hepatic insulin clearance increased. Metformin treatment decreased serum testosterone and improved menstrual cycling. EE-CA treatment had no effect on glucose tolerance, serum insulin levels, or insulin sensitivity but increased body mass index and significantly increased serum leptin concentrations. Serum testosterone levels were decreased by EE-CA treatment.

Conclusions.—The OC EE-CA is effective for the treatment of hyperandrogenic symptoms associated with PCOS in nonobese women, but its negative effects on insulin sensitivity and glucose tolerance must be considered before it is prescribed. Metformin treatment improves hyperinsulinemia and hyperandrogenism in nonobese women with PCOS. Metformin appears to be a good treatment alternative for these women. Further study is necessary to understand the role of metformin in the treatment of infertility in nonobese women with PCOS.

▶ Metformin has been used to treat obese women with PCOS because it decreases insulin and serum androgen levels and results in less central obesity and the resumption of ovulatory cycles. From 20% to 50% of women with PCOS are not obese. This study indicates that metformin causes similar metabolic and hormone improvements in nonobese women with PCOS that it does in obese women with PCOS. Nonandrogenic OCs improve the hyperandrogenic symptoms in nonobese women with PCOS. Metformin appears to provide good treatment for nonobese women with PCOS as well as obese women with PCOS.

D. R. Mishell, Jr, MD

Low-Dose Combination of Flutamide, Metformin and an Oral Contraceptive for Non-Obese, Young Women With Polycystic Ovary Syndrome

Ibaáéz L, de Zegher F (Univ of Barcelona; Univ of Leuven, Belgium)

Hum Reprod 18:57-60, 2003   19–8

Background.—Research has shown that combining flutamide and metformin is more effective for normalizing the endocrine-metabolic status of nonobese young women with polycystic ovary syndrome (PCOS) than using either agent alone. Whether the endocrine-metabolic benefits of this combined treatment are maintained in women also taking a low-dose oral contraceptive (OC) was investigated.

Methods.—Twelve young, nonobese women with PCOS being treated with flutamide 125 mg/d and metformin 1275 mg/d elected to take a low-dose OC (20 µg ethinyl estradiol plus 75 µg gestodene). This subgroup was matched to a subgroup continuing on flutamide-metformin treatment alone. The mean age of the total study population was 18.7 years, and the mean body mass index was 21.8 kg/m². Endocrine-metabolic indexes were determined before any treatment, after 12 months on flutamide-metformin, and after another 6 months with or without OC.

Findings.—The beneficial effects of flutamide-metformin on hyperandrogenemia, hyperinsulinemia, and dyslipidemia were maintained in both the groups taking and not taking the OC. Women taking the OC had an additional increase in sex hormone–binding globulin, thereby demonstrating a further decline in the free androgen index.

Conclusions.—In this series, the beneficial effects of combination flutamide and metformin therapy in women with PCOS were maintained in the presence of a low-dose OC. The use of low-dose OC did not adversely influence the combination therapy's positive effects on hyperinsulinemia-dyslipidemia, which are key determinants of long-term complications.

▶ The results of this study found that the use of the insulin-sensitizing agent metformin plus an antiandrogen was beneficial in the management of young nonobese women with PCOS. Many of these women began to ovulate and were at the risk of unwanted pregnancy if they did not wish to conceive. The addition of a low-dose nonandrogen oral contraceptive maintained the benefit of metformin and the antiandrogen and lowered serum androgens levels by raising the levels of sex hormone–binding globulins. The combination of metformin and a low-dose oral contraceptive is useful therapy for women with PCOS and insulin resistance who do not wish to conceive.

D. R. Mishell, Jr, MD

Use of Cyproterone Acetate, Finasteride, and Spironolactone to Treat Idiopathic Hirsutism

Lumachi F, Rondinone R (Univ of Padua, Padova, Italy)
Fertil Steril 79:942-946, 2003   19–9

Background.—Hirsutism affects 5% to 10% of women, with some variation by ethnic group. About 20% of hirsute women may have idiopathic hirsutism, which is defined as hirsutism in a setting of normal ovarian function and normal circulating androgen levels. The clinical determination of the degree of hirsutism is based on the initial study by Ferriman and Gallwey and involves assessment of 11 different body sites, with a score ranging from 0 to 4 assigned to each site. However, some authors believe that hirsutism should be defined by a score of 6 or greater on a modified version of the Ferriman-Gallwey score. The effects of a 12-month administration of cyproterone acetate, finasteride, or spironolactone in patients with idiopathic hirsutism were assessed.

Methods.—This prospective randomized clinical study was conducted in a university hospital and included 41 women with idiopathic hirsutism. The women were 18 to 34 years old (median age, 21 years), and all had requested to use an oral contraceptive. The patients were randomly assigned to receive cyproterone acetate, finasteride, or spironolactone. The main outcome measures were the Ferrimen-Gallwey score before treatment, at 6 and 12 months of treatment, 1 year after the end of treatment, and the androgenic profile before and after treatment.

Results.—The Ferriman-Gallwey score decreased by 38.9%, 38.6%, and 38.5% for patients who used cyproterone acetate, finasteride, and spironolactone, respectively (Fig 1). At 1 year after treatment, the patients who used spironolactone had significantly lower Ferriman-Gallwey scores than pa-

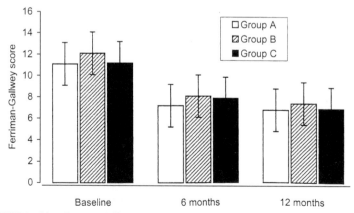

FIGURE 1.—Mean Ferriman-Gallwey scores before and after 6 and 12 months of treatment. Group A = cyproterone acetate recipients; Group B = finasteride recipients; Group C = spironolactone recipients. (Courtesy of Lumachi F, Rondinone R: Use of cyproterone acetate, finasteride, and spironolactone to treat idiopathic hirsutism. *Fertil Steril* 79:942-946. Copyright 2003, with permission from the American College of Surgeons. Reprinted by permission from the American Society for Reproductive Medicine.)

tients who used either cyproterone acetate (6.83) or finasteride (7.42). No significant change was noted in the androgenic profile during treatment.

Conclusions.—Cyproterone acetate, finasteride, and spironolactone have similar short-term results in patients with idiopathic hirsutism, but the beneficial effects of spironolactone and a monophasic oral contraceptive persist for a longer time than the other 2 drugs.

▶ The women with hirsutism and normal circulating androgen levels were previously believed to have idiopathic hirsutism. It is now known that these women have increased rates of conversion of testosterone to dihydrotestosterone in the hair follicle. Spironolactone inhibits this enzymatic activity and decreases the amount of hair present. Because women taking spironolactone frequently have abnormal uterine bleeding, it is best to combine use of this agent with a low-dose estrogen-containing oral contraceptive combined with a progestin with low androgenic activity. The combination of an oral contraceptive and spironolactone in a dose of 100 mg to 200 mg/day is effective therapy for women with hirsutism and normal levels of circulating androgens.

D. R. Mishell, Jr, MD

Long-term Follow-up of Prolactinomas: Normoprolactinemia After Bromocriptine Withdrawal
Passos VQ, Souza JJS, Musolino NRC, et al (Univ of São Paulo, Brazil)
J Clin Endocrinol Metab 87:3578-3582, 2002   19–10

Background.—Medical treatment with dopamine agonist drugs, such as bromocriptine (BRC), is the first choice therapy for both microprolactinomas and macroprolactinomas but usually involves long-term therapy. Whether BRC therapy could be withdrawn from patients with prolactinomas and what factors could be used to predict outcomes were determined retrospectively.

Study Design.—The study group consisted of 280 female and 70 male patients, aged 10 to 70 years, with prolactinomas. All patients were treated with BRC, and 114 also had pituitary surgery. If normoprolactinemia was achieved, the BRC dose was gradually eliminated. Patients who maintained normoprolactinemia after BRC withdrawal were compared with those who did not with regard to age, sex, tumor size, pretreatment serum prolactin levels, initial BRC dose, treatment duration, pregnancy during therapy, and previous surgery and radiotherapy.

Findings.—Of the 350 patients with prolactinomas, 131 achieved normoprolactinemia with BRC treatment. Normoprolactinemia persisted in 27% of these patients, a median of 44 months after BRC withdrawal. No significant differences were found between those with persistent normoprolactinemia and those without with regard to any of the factors examined.

Conclusions.—There is a subset of patients with prolactinomas who achieve normoprolactinemia with BRC treatment and are able to maintain normoprolactinemia after BRC withdrawal. No known factors have been identified that can be used to predict which patients will be able to maintain normoprolactinemia after BRC withdrawal. Therefore, it is suggested that gradual drug withdrawal should be attempted periodically in these patients to avoid unnecessary treatment.

▶ This large study of 350 patients with either prolactin-secreting pituitary microadenomas or macroadenomas found that about one fifth had sustained normalization of prolactin levels after withdrawal of BRC. The patients had received BRC for a median duration of about 4 years. Other studies have reported that prolactin levels remained normal after discontinuation of BRC in 7% to 44% of patients with hyperprolactinemia. Because of the persistently normal prolactin levels in many patients who stop BRC therapy, it is advisable for patients with hyperprolactinemia with either microadenomas or macroadenomas who are taking BRC to discontinue its use at periodic intervals, such as every 2 years, to determine whether their prolactin levels remain normal and would, thus, not need to continue use of this medication.

D. R. Mishell, Jr, MD

20 Sexual Function

The Effect of Interval Tubal Sterilization on Sexual Interest and Pleasure
Costello C, for the US Collaborative Review of Sterilization Working Group
(Ctrs for Disease Control and Prevention, Atlanta, Ga; et al)
Obstet Gynecol 100:511-517, 2002   20–1

Introduction.—Nearly 26% of United States women aged 15 to 44 years who have ever married have undergone interval tubal sterilization. With so many healthy women undergoing this procedure, it is important that they understand the health effects, including the potential physiologic and psychologic effects. Most prior reports concerning the effect of tubal sterilization on sexual functioning have been descriptive in nature. The U.S. Collaborative Review of Sterilization, which represents the largest cohort of women undergoing tubal sterilization, was used to assess whether specific subgroups of women were significantly more likely to have increased or decreased sexual interest or pleasure in the initial 2 years after sterilization.

Methods.—A total of 4576 women were enrolled in this prospective, multicenter cohort investigation between 1978 and 1983. Potential demographic, clinical, and surgical predictors of sexual outcome were examined for significant variation from the overall pattern of unchanged, increased, and reduced sexual interest and pleasure.

Results.—More than 80% of women reported no consistent change in either sexual interest (80%) or pleasure (82%) after undergoing interval tubal sterilization. Among women with consistent change, positive effects were documented 10 and 15 times more often than negative effects for sexual interest and pleasure, respectively. With the exception of women with poststerilization regret, all subgroups were significantly more likely to have increased compared with decreased interest or pleasure. Women with poststerilization regret were most likely to have a negative effect. In multivariate analyses, poststerilization regret was the only factor predictive for reduced interest (odds ratio, 4.0) and diminished pleasure (odds ratio, 5.1). Women reporting regret were significantly less likely to report increased interest or pleasure. It is not known whether regret or reduced sexual interest or pleasure occurred first.

Conclusion.—Interval tubal ligation is not likely to result in changed sexual interest or pleasure. Those who had change were most likely to report positive sexual effects.

▶ We would expect that many women might have improvement in their level of sexual interest and pleasure following permanent sterilization, having been relieved of the fear of unintended pregnancy. This is tempered by the small incidence of patients with post-tubal ovarian dysfunction. Even most patients with poststerilization regret had no change in their interest and pleasure. It will be interesting to see if there is further follow-up of these patients with poststerilization regret to see if their regret is related to their lack of future fertility or if in fact reflects a more global problem with their relationship, as relationship problems are one of the most common causes of sexual dysfunction.

D. S. Miller, MD

▶ The US Collaborative Review of Sterilization provides these prospective analyses on the effect of interval tubal sterilization on women's sexual interest and pleasure. Two-year follow-up was available in this large study population (N = 4576), providing both short- and intermediate-term results. Given the high degree of enthusiasm for sterilization among American women, it was reassuring to discover that 4 of 5 who chose interval sterilization had no change in their sexual pleasure or libido and the majority of those who did report a change, enjoyed a change for the better.

The subset which reported post-sterilization regret comprised 3% of the total. Even in this group, the majority reported no change in sexual pleasure or libido, and of those who did report a change, as many were as likely to report improvement as deterioration.

It is perhaps not surprising that those who had previously used a barrier method were most likely to report improvement in sexual pleasure and interest.

Although data were gathered 15 years ago, sterilization continues to be the most prevalent form of contraception in the US and therefore information on side effects (and benefits) remains relevant.

R. D. Arias, MD

Effect of Raloxifene on Sexual Function in Older Postmenopausal Women With Osteoporosis

Modugno F, Ness RB, Ewing S, et al (Univ of Pittsburgh, Pa; Univ of California, San Francisco)

Obstet Gynecol 101:353-361, 2003   20–2

Introduction.—Raloxifene is a selective estrogen receptor modulator approved for treatment and prevention of postmenopausal osteoporosis. Its mixed estrogen agonists/antagonists effects have raised concerns about an adverse impact on sexual function. The effect of raloxifene versus placebo was examined in older postmenopausal women undergoing treatment for osteoporosis.

Methods.—A subset (12%) of English-speaking women in the United States and Canada participating in the Multiple Outcomes of Raloxifene Evaluation Trial were asked to complete a sexual function questionnaire at baseline and after 36 months of treatment. The Multiple Outcomes of Raloxifene Evaluation Trial was a multicenter, randomized, blinded, placebo-controlled clinical trial in which 7705 postmenopausal women with osteoporosis were randomly assigned to treatment with either raloxifene hydrochloride 60 mg/d or 120 mg/d or placebo. A total of 943 women completed the sexual function questionnaire at both visits. Because preliminary analyses demonstrated no differences by raloxifene dose, both groups were combined and compared with the placebo group. For the sample size, there was 80% power ($\alpha = .05$, 2-sided, ratio of raloxifene to placebo = 2:1) to identify a 10% to 16% difference in the proportion of women who had no change in sexual function between placebo and treatment groups.

Results.—Mean patient ages for the raloxifene and placebo groups were 68.23 years and 68.62 years, respectively. Overall, there were no between-group differences between sexual function and changes in sexual function from baseline to trial end. Particularly, there were no differences in sexual desire or frequency of sexual activity between the placebo and treatment groups. In sexually active women, there were no significant differences in enjoyment, satisfaction, orgasm, or reported sexual problems.

Conclusion.—Sexual function in older postmenopausal women with osteoporosis is not affected by treatment with raloxifene.

▶ Is the glass half full or is the glass half empty? A more important, but not novel, finding in this study is that most elderly women being treated for osteoporosis had no sexual desire or did so less than once a month. What was not defined in this study was whether these patients perceive this as a problem, particularly given the fact that many of them had a partner who was not interested or not able to participate in sexual activity. Nonetheless, it is reassuring to the manufacturers, prescribers, as well as patients taking raloxifene that it does not have a detrimental effect on sexuality.

D. S. Miller, MD

21 HPV

The Interval Between Menarche and Age of First Sexual Intercouse as a Risk Factor for Subsequent HPV Infection in Adolescent and Young Adult Women

Kahn JA, Rosenthal SL, Succop PA, et al (Univ of Cincinnati, Ohio; Univ of Texas at Galveston; Albert Einstein College of Medicine, Bronx, NY)

J Pediatr 141:718-723, 2002   21–1

Background.—The prevalence of sexually transmitted infection with human papilloma virus (HPV) in adolescent and young adult women is 30% to 50%. Among the behavioral risk factors for HPV infection are early age at first sexual intercourse and multiple sexual partners. Cervical immaturity has also been evaluated for its impact on HPV infection and the development of cervical intraepithelial neoplasia, with the suggestion that the time from menarche to age of first sexual intercourse may be a risk factor for HPV infection and cervical intraepithelial neoplasia, with the interval representing a proxy measure for the biological maturity of the cervix.

It was suggested that the interval between menarche and age of first sexual intercourse was significantly shorter for adolescents with HPV infection when compared with noninfected adolescents. Whether there is such an association and whether it is independent of the age of first sexual intercourse were evaluated.

Methods.—A survey was completed of 504 female university students (mean age, 20.4 years), who were then screened for cervicovaginal HPV infection. Samples were tested for HPV types 2, 6, 11, 13, 16, 18, 26, 31 through 35, 39, 40, 42, 45, 51 through 59, 61, 62, 64, 66 through 70, 72, 73, 81, 82, 83, and 85. HPV-positive and HPV-negative subjects were matched.

Results.—The mean age at menarche was 12.3 years, and the mean age at first sexual intercourse was 16.7 years. Women reported a mean lifetime number of sexual partners of 4.2, with a mean number of partners over the preceding 6 months of 1.3. The participants' age at first sexual intercourse and the interval were highly and positively correlated, while age at menarche and age at first sexual intercourse were positively but only slightly correlated. On logistic regression, the interval was significantly related to subsequent HPV infection, with a decrease by 1 year linked to a 12% increase in the odds of subsequent HPV infection. When the age at first sexual intercourse was decreased by 1 year, the odds of subsequent HPV infection increased 20%. On combined analysis, age at first sexual intercourse was still significantly associated with subsequent HPV infection. A short interval is linked with HPV infection, but this relationship is not independent of age at first sexual intercourse.

Conclusion.—A significant association was found between menarche and age at first sexual intercourse and the subsequent development of HPV infection. Other researchers have suggested that sexual activity prolongs the normal maturation process, which increases the risk of infection of immature epithelium. An alternative interpretation of the current findings is that the age at first sexual intercourse is a risk marker for susceptibility to repeated HPV infection as well as first HPV infection. Regardless, age at first sexual intercourse should be considered a risk factor for subsequent HPV infection. This factor is both important and identifiable in research and clinical investigations.

▶ The most logical theory of cervical carcinogenesis involves HPV inoculation at a time when the adolescent cervix is undergoing metaplasia from columnar epithelium to squamous epithelium and thus is presumably more susceptible to incorporation of HPV DNA into cervical epithelial DNA. Most studies have shown that early coitarche and multiple sexual partners, as well as a history of genital warts, are very significant risk factors for cervical cancer.

These authors attempted to use the interval between onset of menarche and age of first sexual intercourse as a proxy measure of cervical epithelial maturation and presumed resistance to HPV inoculation. They found that interval was not consistently significant and very much affected by the early coitarche. Incredibly enough, they did not analyze for number of partners, likely rendering their model not valid. Perhaps this will be the subject of future analysis.

D. S. Miller, MD

Clinical Findings Among Young Women With Genital Human Papillomavirus Infection
Mao C, Hughes JP, Kiviat N, et al (Univ of Washington, Seattle)
Am J Obstet Gynecol 188:677-684, 2003   21–2

Background.—Anogenital warts are most often caused by human papillomavirus (HPV) types 6 or 11, while types 16, 18, 31, and 45 are found in at least 70% of invasive cervical cancer specimens. Such sexually transmitted agents as herpes simplex virus and *Chlamydia trachomatis* that produce cervical inflammation are also related to cervical neoplasia. While HPV infection is linked to considerable morbidity, few data relate genital symptoms to the clinical findings of recent or persistent genital HPV infection. The clinical signs and symptoms indicative of finding HPV DNA in the female genital tract were investigated.

Methods.—The cohort study included 516 university students (aged 18 to 24 years; average age, 19 years). These women were not married, were white, and reported having had a single sex partner. Every 4 months for as long as 4 years, all underwent collection of genital specimens for HPV DNA testing. The symptoms and clinical findings of women with and without HPV DNA were evaluated using multivariate analysis.

Results.—Among women positive for HPV DNA, the percentage of ecto-cervix that had visible columnar epithelium was more often estimated as less than 10% compared with women who were negative for HPV DNA. Cervical erythema was found more often in HPV DNA–positive women than among those who were negative. Bacterial vaginosis (BV) and leukoplakia were more strongly associated with the presence of HPV DNA than any other clinical findings. Generally, HPV DNA was detected before BV was manifest. The cumulative number of sex partners was linked to genital HPV infection; recent (less than 2 days before the visit) intercourse was not.

Strong relationships were noted between finding external genital warts and detecting HPV 6 and 11 DNA; no relationship was found for other HPV types. An association was noted between infection with *Chlamydia* and the detection of HPV 6 or 11 and between the presence of palpable inguinal lymph nodes and the presence of HPV 6 or 11. The median time from the woman's first intercourse to the first detection of HPV DNA was 4 months among the 97 virgins who became sexually active during the study. The median time to the first diagnosis of BV for this group was 12 months.

Conclusion.—Most of the women in whom genital HPV DNA was detected were free of symptoms and clinical findings. There was an increased risk for BV. *Chlamydia* infection, while diagnosed infrequently, was associated with the detection of HPV 6 and 11 DNA.

▶ This is the first study to document that which we have assumed since the significance of HPV infection and cervical carcinogenesis became apparent: that these viral infections of the cervix are usually asymptomatic. The only symptom associated with HPV 6 and 11 is the expected genital warts. The finding that HPV precedes BV accounts for the repeated studies showing failure of treatment of BV to significantly change pap smears. We are reminded again of the significance of multiple sex partners at a young age. A paradoxical finding is that the patients who were HPV negative had more cervical ectopy (correctly described as "cervical eversion") than the HPV-positive patients. One would presume that the cervices of HPV-positive patients were undergoing active metaplasia and thus may have been more susceptible to virus inoculation.

D. S. Miller, MD

22 Pap Smears

Lubrication of the Vaginal Introitus and Speculum Does Not Affect Papanicolaou Smears
Harer WB Jr, Valenzuela G, Lebo D (Arrowhead Regional Med Ctr, Colton, Calif)
Obstet Gynecol 100:887-888, 2002   22–1

Background.—Most gynecology textbooks state that vaginal lubrication should not be used before speculum insertion, but to date, no research on the effects of such lubrication on Papanicolaou smears has been published. The hypothesis that lubrication of the vaginal introitus and external speculum does not adversely affect Papanicolaou interpretation was tested.

Methods and Findings.—One hundred eighty-two patients undergoing Papanicolaou smears were randomly assigned to have warm water only or a water-soluble lubricant to assist speculum insertion. Cytotechnicians and pathologists were unaware of the condition under which the smears were obtained. Two smears from the 93 patients receiving lubricant were unsatisfactory, as were 2 from the 89 receiving warm water only. No significant differences were found in continuous or categoric variables.

Conclusions.—The use of a water-soluble lubricant on the vaginal introitus and external speculum does not adversely affect Papanicolaou smear interpretation. The traditional belief that lubricant cannot be used to improve the patient's comfort during pelvic examination appears to be unfounded.

▶ While not of earthshaking importance, any study where dogma is confronted with evidence should be reviewed. Thus, these authors and those of another article (Abstract 22–2) in the same issue fail to see a difference in unsatisfactory Pap smear rates when a small amount of lubricant was carefully applied to the speculum. It is not stated whether these results apply to liquid-based cytology as only traditional glass smears were evaluated, or whether lubricating actually increased the tolerability of the exam.

D. S. Miller, MD

The Effect of Vaginal Speculum Lubrication on the Rate of Unsatisfactory Cervical Cytology Diagnosis

Amies A-ME, Miller L, Lee S-K, et al (Univ of Washington, Seattle)
Obstet Gynecol 100:889-892, 2002   22–2

Background.—During pelvic examination, nonlubricated plastic specula can adhere to the vaginal introitus, causing discomfort. Whether applying water-soluble gel lubricant to the plastic vaginal speculum would affect the rate of unsatisfactory cervical cytology diagnoses was determined.

Methods.—Five public health family planning clinics were randomly assigned to water-soluble gel or water only as a speculum lubricant. A total of 8534 Papanicolaou smears were collected between July 1998 and December 1999. Cumulative rates of cervical cytology diagnoses were determined for 6 months before, 6 months during, and 6 months after intervention.

Findings.—Rates of unsatisfactory smears were 1.4% with the lubricant and 1.4% without it. The rates of unsatisfactory smears for lubricant use compared with nonlubricant use clinics during the intervention period were 1.4% and 1.3%, respectively. For each 6-month period, no significant differences were noted for the rates of atypical squamous cells of undetermined significance, low-grade squamous intraepithelial lesions, high-grade squamous intraepithelial lesions, or atypical glandular cells of undetermined significance within or between clinics assigned lubricant and nonlubricant.

Conclusions.—The use of a small amount of water-soluble gel lubricant on the outer inferior blade of the plastic vaginal speculum did not impede the interpretation of Papanicolaou smears. Further studies are needed to determine whether lubricant use reduces pain or discomfort associated with speculum examination.

▶ In both of these prospective randomized trials (Abstracts 22–1 and 22–22), cytotechnologists/pathologists were blinded to the use of water-soluble lubricant versus water as an aid to speculum insertion before Pap smear sampling. If lubricant has any effect on the adequacy of Pap smears, or on the difficulty in interpretation, it would appear to be quite small. No difference was found in either of these studies. If the amount of lubricant used in these trials (≤3 cm³) makes it easier for the patient to tolerate the procedure, or for the examiner to conduct the sampling, it would appear that its use should be encouraged.

R. D. Arias, MD

Empiric Treatment of Minimally Abnormal Papanicolaou Smears With 0.75% Metronidazole Vaginal Gel

Ferrante JM, Mayhew DY, Goldberg S, et al (Univ of South Florida, Tampa)
J Am Board Fam Pract 15:347-354, 2002   22–3

Background.—There is no consensus regarding how to treat women with a minimally abnormal Papanicolaou (Pap) smear. Some authors advocate the empirical use of antibiotics to normalize cytologic findings while others advocate a wait-and-see approach. Repeat cytologic findings were compared between women with a minimally abnormal Pap smear who received empiric 0.75% metronidazole vaginal gel and those who received no treatment.

Methods.—The subjects were 114 asymptomatic women with an initial Pap smear showing inflammation, benign cellular changes, reactive cellular changes, or atypical squamous cells of undetermined significance that did not suggest neoplasm. About half the patients were randomly assigned to apply 0.75% metronidazole vaginal gel daily for 5 days, while the other half received no treatment. All patients returned within 3 to 4 months for a repeat Pap smear.

Results.—At the repeat Pap smear, 61 patients (54%) had normal cytologic findings. Reversion to normal cytologic findings was no more frequent in the treatment group (24 of 54 patients, or 44.4%) than in the control group (37 of 60 patients, or 61.7%) ($P = .07$). Only 1 patient had a Pap smear that worsened during follow-up, from reactive cellular changes with inflammation to a low-grade squamous intraepithelial lesion. No subgroup of patients based on demographic variables, sexual history, or Pap smear findings could be identified in which treatment had a significant benefit.

Conclusion.—In asymptomatic women with a minimally abnormal Pap smear, empiric treatment with 0.75% metronidazole vaginal gel does not improve the rate of reversion to normal cytologic findings.

▶ The pressure to "do something" for the woman with a minimally abnormal Pap smear has historically resulted in the use of topical or systemic antibiotics. Though some biologic plausibility for this approach exists, the only controlled trial (prior to this study) of topical antimicrobials failed to show better results than placebo.[1]

In this prospective, randomized trial, metronidazole gel, 0.75%, administered in the absence of apparent infection, did not increase the rate of conversion to a normal Pap. This study, therefore, does not support the empirical use of metronidazole gel in the management of the minimally abnormal Pap. Women with vaginosis at the time of initial evaluation were excluded from study. The treatment of bacterial vaginosis is indicated for control of symptoms and to decrease pregnancy-related morbidity.

R. D. Arias, MD

Reference

1. 2003 YEAR BOOK OF OBSTETRICS, GYNECOLOGY, AND WOMEN'S HEALTH, p 413. (Connor JP, Elam G, Goldberg JM: Empiric vaginal metronidazole in the management of the ASCUS papanicolaou smear: A randomized controlled trial. *Obstet Gynecol* 99:183-187, 2002).

Baseline Cytology, Human Papillomavirus Testing, and Risk for Cervical Neoplasia: A 10-Year Cohort Analysis

Sherman ME, Lorincz AT, Scott DR, et al (NIH, Bethesda, Md; Digene Corp, Gaithersburg, Md; Kaiser Permanente, Portland, Ore)
J Natl Cancer Inst 95:46-52, 2003   22–4

Background.—Cytologic screening programs with Pap smears have dramatically reduced the incidence of cervical cancer and associated mortality in developed nations. However, single Pap tests are limited by suboptimal sensitivity, limited reproducibility, and many equivocal results. The effectiveness of cytologic screening stems from the fact that cervical cancer typically develops slowly, allowing a program of repeated testing and aggressive follow-up to compensate for deficiencies of a single Pap test. Some clinicians have adopted a practice of less frequent screening of women with repeatedly negative Pap tests, but many clinicians favor annual screening to minimize the risk of cervical cancer. Over the past decade, it has been shown that infection with carcinogenic types of human papillomaviruses (HPV) represents a nearly universal event in the development of cervical cancer. Most HPV infections produce only transient minor lesions, but untreated infections may persist and progress to cervical intraepithelial neoplasia (CIN) 3, a cancer precursor. Whether simultaneous screening with a Pap test and HPV testing is useful for the assessment of risk for CIN III or cervical cancer.

Methods.—A total of 23,702 subjects in a study of HPV infection were enrolled. Data were analyzed for 20,810 volunteers who were aged 16 years or older (mean, 35.9 years) with satisfactory baseline Pap tests and suitable samples for HPV testing. The women were followed for up to 122 months to determine the risk for histopathologically confirmed CIN III or cancer.

Results.—A total of 171 women were diagnosed with CIN III or cancer over a 122-month period, of whom 123 (71.9%) had baseline Pap results of atypical squamous cells or worse or a positive HPV test, including 102 of the 118 cases diagnosed within the first 45 months of follow-up. The cumulative incidence of CIN III or cancer was 4.54% in these 45 months among women with a Pap test result indicative of atypical squamous cells or worse, positive HPV tests, or both compared with 0.16% among women with negative Pap and HPV tests. The results were only minimally affected by age, screening behavior, a history of cervical cancer precursors, and a history of treatment of CIN.

Conclusions.—In this 10-year cohort analysis, negative baseline Pap and HPV tests were associated with a low risk for CIN III or cancer in the 45 months after testing, mainly because a negative HPV test was associated with a decreased risk of cervical neoplasia. These findings suggest that negative combined test results should provide further reassurance that the screening interval can be lengthened among low-risk women, whereas positive results will identify a relatively small subgroup of patients that requires more frequent screening.

▶ This large prospective trial confirms what we already knew and adds to our new knowledge. The Pap smear is very good at detecting prevalent disease but does less well at predicting future disease. The HPV test is better at predicting future disease. Patients with a negative HPV test and Pap smear were unlikely to develop CIN III during the subsequent 3 to 4 years. This study provided the pivotal data that allowed Food and Drug Administration recognition of HPV testing as part of a screening test for cervical cancer.

D. S. Miller, MD

23 Intraepithelial Neoplasia

A Prospective Study of High-Grade Cervical Neoplasia Risk Among Human Papillomavirus-Infected Women
Castle PE, Wacholder S, Lorincz AT, et al (Natl Cancer Inst, Bethesda, Md; Digene Corp, Gaithersburg, Md; Kaiser Permanente, Portland, Ore; et al)
J Natl Cancer Inst 94:1406-1414, 2002   23–1

Introduction.—Case-control trials have shown that smoking, parity, and oral contraceptive use are linked with an increased risk of cervical intraepithelial neoplasia grade 3 (CIN3) and cervical cancer in women infected with oncogenic human papillomavirus (HPV). These potential risk factors have not been adequately examined in prospective trials and were thus evaluated in 1812 women enrolled in a 10-year prospective trial of cervical neoplasia.

Methods.—All participants had tested positive for oncogenic HPV DNA and had responded to a questionnaire used to assess smoking, oral contraceptive use, and parity. Absolute risks and crude relative risks with 95% confidence intervals (CIs) for CIN3 or cervical cancer were determined for 3 time intervals as follows: 0 to 8 months; 9 to 68 months; and 69 to 122 months after enrollment. Conditional logistic regression models were used to control for factors that may have impacted risk estimates as follows: the cytologic interpretation of the baseline Papanicolaou (Pap) smear, number of Pap smears during follow-up, age at enrollment, age at the prediagnosis visit, and age at diagnosis.

Results.—Oral contraceptive use and parity were not linked with risk of CIN3 or cervical cancer. Former smokers, women who smoked less than 1 pack of cigarettes per day, and women who smoked 1 or more packs per day had crude relative risks for CIN3 or cervical cancer for the entire follow-up period of 2.1 (95% CI, 1.1-3.9), 2.2 (95% CI, 1.2-4.2), and 2.9 (95% CI, 1.5-5.6), respectively, compared with participants who had never smoked. In the multivariable model, former smokers, women who smoked less than 1 pack per day, and women who smoked 1 or more packs per day had relative risks of 3.3 (95% CI, 1.6-6.7), 2.9 (95% CI, 1.4-6.1), and 4.3 (95% CI, 2.0-9.3), respectively, for CIN3 or cervical cancer compared with never smokers.

Conclusion.—Smoking is linked with an increased risk of invasive cervical cancer in women who are infected with oncogenic HPV. Subsequent trials should assess the role of smoking in the multistage pathogenesis of cervical cancer.

▶ Multiple retrospective epidemiologic studies have found an association between cervical cancer and smoking. This is one of the first prospective studies to confirm that in women who have already been inoculated with HPV. While some putative confounding risk factors were adjusted for such factors as oral contraceptive use, parity, and number of Pap smears, other risk factors likely to be significant, such as age of coitarche and number of past and present partners, were not evaluated. But, importantly, this study reminds us of the devastating consequences of smoking, an effect magnified in developing countries where smoking among women is increasing at a pace far beyond that of their cervical cancer–screening programs.

D. S. Miller, MD

Aberrant Expression of E-Cadherin in Cervical Intraepithelial Neoplasia Correlates With a False-Negative Papanicolaou Smear
Felix JC, Lonky NM, Tamura K, et al (Univ of Southern California, Los Angeles; Southern California Permanente Med Group, Anaheim, Calif; Trylon Corp, Torrance, Calif; et al)
Am J Obstet Gynecol 186:1308-1314, 2002   23–2

Introduction.—E-cadherin is an adhesion molecule that is responsible for cell adhesion in normal cervical epithelium. It is usually absent in the superficial epithelial layers, which allow exfoliation. The association between E-cadherin distribution and Papanicolaou smear was examined in women with cervical dysplasia.

Methods.—Tissue samples from 25 women with cervical dysplasia were examined via immunohistochemistry for E-cadherin, β-catenin and α-catenin expression. The expression pattern of these proteins, whether full thickness or restricted to the basal layers, was correlated with Papanicolaou smear findings.

Results.—Of 12 women with normal Papanicolaou smears, 10 of 11 informative cases revealed E-cadherin expression throughout all epithelial layers. Eight of 10 informative cases associated with an abnormal Papanicolaou smear revealed E-cadherin only at the basal layers; α-catenin was distributed throughout the entire epithelium in samples of all 25 women.

Conclusion.—Expression of E-cadherin throughout all epithelial layers was associated with a false-negative Papanicolaou smear. It is likely that aberrant persistence of E-cadherin in these lesions interrupts the exfoliation of abnormal cells.

▶ Adhesion molecules such as E-cadherin are found in several malignancies, including squamous cell carcinoma of the cervix. The abnormal expression of these molecules is likely a factor in the manifestation of many cancers as a hard mass. As seen in this article, the abnormal expression of these molecules may also prevent shedding of malignant cells from a malignant or premalignant lesion. This may account for some false-negative Pap smears, even when there is a visible lesion.

D. S. Miller, MD

Rate of Human Papillomavirus Clearance After Treatment of Cervical Intraepithelial Neoplasia

Elfgren K, Jacobs M, Walboomers JMM, et al (Karolinska Institutet, Stockholm; Univ Hosp Vrije Universiteit, Amsterdam; Malmö Univ Hosp, Sweden; et al)

Obstet Gynecol 100:965-971, 2002   23–3

Introduction.—Infection with human papillomavirus (HPV) is well known as a prerequisite for the development and maintenance of most cervical cancers and cervical intraepithelial neoplasia (CIN). It has been shown that HPV DNA is usually no longer detected 2 years after effective treatment for CIN, indicating that strategies for follow-up after treatment of CIN based on monitoring the clearance of HPV, the major risk factor for CIN, may be feasible. The rate of clearance of HPV infection after surgical treatment for CIN was examined in 109 women with CIN I to III.

Methods.—All patients were treated with cryosurgery or conization and were observed with cervical HPV DNA testing using general primer polymerase chain reaction and HPV typing at 0, 3, 6, 9, 12, and 24 months after treatment. Penile HPV DNA from current sexual partners was examined.

Results.—Of 104 evaluable women with an adequate sample, 84 (81%) were HPV DNA positive and 20 were HPV DNA negative at the time of treatment or enrollment. Eighteen double infections were identified for a total of 102 cervical infections. At 1-year follow-up, 7 women (9%) remained positive for the same HPV type. Most women had cleared the HPV infection diagnosed at treatment within 3 months. The cryotherapy group had lower CIN grades, were younger, and had a slower HPV clearance rate ($P < .002$), compared with the conization group. The same HPV DNA type was identified in only 4 couples.

Conclusion.—Surgical treatment of CIN typically results in clearance of HPV infection within 3 months. The testing of HPV DNA may be helpful as a rapid intermediate end point for monitoring the efficacy of the therapy.

▶ When HPV testing first came on the market, a few patients had themselves tested even though they had no apparent CIN. Not surprisingly, some of these tests were positive and the patients demanded treatment. I usually deferred, telling them that we did not have a surgical procedure to treat a virus. This study adds to a growing body of literature that contradicts my pronouncement. The authors showed that treatment of CIN did result in clearance of HPV DNA. Presumably, it also cleared the CIN, but that was not clearly stated. Whether excisional treatments of the cervix may successfully treat HPV infection without manifest CIN remains to be determined.

D. S. Miller, MD

Recrudescence of Cervical Dysplasia Among Women Who Are Infected With the Human Immunodeficiency Virus: A Case-Control Analysis

Tate DR, Anderson RJ (John Peter Smith Hosp, Fort Worth, Tex)
Am J Obstet Gynecol 186:880-882, 2002   23–4

Background.—The association between cervical cancer and HIV is well established. In 1988, invasive cervical cancer was added to the list of AIDS-defining illnesses. The prevalence of cervical intraepithelial neoplasia (CIN) has also been shown to be higher among women who are HIV infected (from 20% to 60%) than among women not infected. This is thought to be the result of co-infection with human papillomavirus, which has been reported in approximately 67% of HIV-infected women. The recurrence rate of CIN among HIV-infected women after standard ablative therapy was investigated, and the recurrence rate of CIN after ablative therapy was compared with the rate after hysterectomy.

Methods.—A total of 43 HIV-positive women were compared with 130 patients who were HIV negative after cryotherapy, laser ablation, loop electrosurgical excision procedure, conization, or hysterectomy for cervical dysplasia. All of the patients were followed up for at least 24 months. Patients were excluded if they had preexisting cervical cancer or positive margins after treatment. All of the patients were evaluated by colposcopy, with at least 1 colposcopic-directed biopsy. The severity of cervical dysplasia was similar between the 2 groups, and CIN I was the most common diagnosis at presentation.

Results.—Recurrence was higher in the HIV-positive women for all modalities (73% vs 27%). Higher recurrence rates were seen in patients with CD4 counts of less than 200 cells/mm^3 (55% vs 26%). In addition, the mean viral load was higher for patients with recurrent disease (18,384 vs 3892).

Conclusion.—This study of the recurrence rate of cervical intraepithelial neoplasia in HIV-positive women found that hysterectomy was more effective in preventing recurrence compared with standard ablative therapy (50% vs 86%). However, the recurrence rate in these patients remains high.

▶ As others studies before it have shown, patients with one viral infection, HIV, are much more likely to fail treatments for another virally incited condition, cervical intraepithelial neoplasia, and if the patients' HIV is poorly controlled, as manifested by a low CD4 count or a high viral load, they are even more likely to fail their surgical treatment for CIN. Our nongynecologic HIV physicians have become very good at screening women for human papillomavirus–related diseases in their HIV patients. Yet, many gynecologists continue to use the same management strategies for these patients as they do for HIV-negative patients. It certainly seems that these patients would be better served if, once cervical cancer is ruled out, treatment of a pre-invasive lesion be deferred until the HIV is under control. Then, our surgical treatments may work better for the other virally caused disease, CIN.

D. S. Miller, MD

Treatment of Vulvar Intraepithelial Neoplasia 2/3 With Imiquimod
Jayne CJ, Kaufman RH (Baylor College of Medicine, Houston)
J Reprod Med 47:395-398, 2002   23–5

Background.—The incidence of vulvar intraepithelial neoplasia (VIN) appears to be increasing. Currently, the annual incidence of VIN is 2.1 cases per 100,000 women. Many of these cases appear to be causally related to infection with the human papilloma virus (HPV), particularly high-risk strains such as HPV-16. Complete spontaneous regression of VIN has been documented, but there is evidence that VIN is a precursor to invasive squamous cell carcinoma. There are many treatment options available, including wide local excision, skinning vulvectomy, laser ablation, and topical 5-fluorouracil. However, multiple treatments over a long period are often necessary for individual patients, which is often discouraging to both patient and physician. Imiquimod is an immune response modifier whose primary indication is the topical management of condylomata acuminata. Since many cases of VIN are related to HPV infection, the efficacy of imiquimod in the management of biopsy-confirmed VIN 2/3 was evaluated.

Methods.—The charts of 13 women with a diagnosis of VIN 2/3 and treated with imiquimod were retrospectively reviewed. All of the women were evaluated and treated by 1 gynecologist. The extent of the lesion and the degree of improvement were noted before treatment. Each patient received biopsy confirmation of disease. Response to treatment was categorized as complete regression, at least 75% regression, or not improved.

Results.—The mean duration of therapy was 3.3 months, and the average follow-up after completion of therapy was 5.5 months. Complete regression of the VIN was seen in 8 of 13 patients. Four patients showed 75% regression, and 1 diabetic patient showed no improvement. In 2 women with 75% lesion regression, invasive carcinoma of the vulva was noted in the area of residual disease. One of these women was found to have a superficially invasive squamous cell carcinoma (1 mm of invasion) and the other had an anal tag with invasive squamous cell carcinoma.

Conclusion.—These findings support the consideration of medical management of VIN 2/3 with imiquimod. However, the patient must be carefully evaluated before initiation of imiquimod to exclude the presence of invasive squamous cell carcinoma.

▶ While some patients with VIN may be symptomatic, most patients are not and are not even aware that they have it. They certainly do not incur any mortality as a result of having VIN. The reason that VIN should receive and does receive any attention from health care providers is the fact that a small number of patients may develop invasive cancer. Thus, the prime obligation of those undertaking the care of VIN is to rule out cancer. Accordingly, we should critically evaluate a treatment that invokes an inflammatory response and makes evaluation of the vulva difficult yet does not prevent the development of cancer, or at least obscures an already existent cancer. While imiquimod may have been helpful for some patients with VIN, the overall results are not superior to that of any excisional or destructive treatment and should only be used when cancer has been clearly and convincingly ruled out.

D. S. Miller, MD

24 Surgical Training

Longitudinal Impact of a Female Pelvic Medicine and Reconstructive Pelvic Surgery Fellowship on Resident Education
Cundiff GW, Handa V, Bienstock J (Johns Hopkins Med Insts, Baltimore, Md)
Am J Obstet Gynecol 187:1487-1493, 2002   24–1

Background.—Female pelvic floor dysfunction includes a collection of disorders that have previously been treated by different surgical specialties. The American Board of Obstetrics and Gynecology working with the American Board of Urology has created a new subspecialty of female pelvic medicine and reconstructive pelvic surgery to deal with these disorders. A survey was used to assess residents' perception of the impact of the new fellowships on their education.

Study Design.—A voluntary survey was completed by residents in obstetrics and gynecology at Johns Hopkins at the beginning of the fellowship program and then annually for 3 years. The survey asked the residents to assess the quality of their education and how the fellowships affected their education.

Findings.—The average response rate was 32%. In the initial survey, given within 1 month of the initiation of the fellowship program, the fellowship was perceived as detracting from education. After that, a positive increase was seen in the perceived impact of fellowships, and this impact was sustained over the 3-year period. Residents also reported higher self-assessments of the quality of education over this period.

Conclusions.—The results of this survey suggest that residents in obstetrics and gynecology view fellowships in female pelvic medicine and reconstructive surgery as making a positive contribution to their education.

▶ As with the development of previous subspecialties in obstetrics and gynecology, the development of the fellowship in female pelvic medicine and reconstructive pelvic surgery has generated debate regarding its effects on the quality of resident education. In this study, residents' perceptions were followed up from the inception of the fellowship and then annually for 3 years. Although, initially, the fellows were perceived to detract from the residents' education, the subsequent surveys showed that the fellows' participation was beneficial to their education. This study suggests that, as the residents become accustomed to the presence of a fellow in the role of educator instead of competitor, they are perceived to be beneficial to resident education. The presence of an intermediate level educator with a specific enthusiasm for the challenge at hand can only raise the level of resident education and patient care.

R. D. Arias, MD

Guidelines for the Selection of the Route of Hysterectomy: Application in a Resident Clinic Population

Kovac SR, Barhan S, Lister M, et al (Emory Univ, Atlanta, Ga; Wright State Univ, Dayton, Ohio)
Am J Obstet Gynecol 187:1521-1527, 2002   24–2

Introduction.—Although there is overwhelming evidence in favor of vaginal hysterectomy, no formal guidelines have been adopted to aid physicians in choosing the most clinically appropriate route for hysterectomy. The effectiveness of the Society of Pelvic Reconstructive Surgeons (SPRS) for determining the route of hysterectomy was examined in a resident clinic population.

Methods.—Between October 1, 1994, and December 31, 1999, 407 consecutive women were prospectively assigned to abdominal or vaginal hysterectomy groups according to SPRS guidelines. Age, race, and preoperative and postoperative uterine weights, length of stay, laparoscopic scores, operative times, and complications were compared between groups.

Results.—Vaginal hysterectomy was successfully completed in 91.8% of the cohort. Vaginal hysterectomy had a shorter operative time and length of stay and was associated with fewer complications compared with abdominal hysterectomy ($P < .01$). Laparoscopic assistance was needed in 25.8% of patients to evaluate extrauterine disease.

Conclusion.—Resident physicians who followed the SPRS guidelines decreased the ratio of abdominal-to-vaginal hysterectomy from 3:1 to 1:11. Use of the SPRS practice guidelines in the selection of the route of hysterectomy can increase the ratio of vaginal hysterectomies performed in residency programs and help eliminate existing inconsistencies in health care delivery.

▶ Objective evaluation would indicate that the vaginal route should be the primary method of hysterectomy for benign indications. The implementation of the SPRS guidelines for the route of hysterectomy produced a remarkable reversal in the ratio of abdominal to vaginal hysterectomy in this training program. Residents managed to reduce the rate of abdominal to vaginal cases from 3:1 to 1:11. This reversal is evidence that the use of practice guidelines can dramatically improve patient care as well as resident education.

R. D. Arias, MD

25 Hysterectomy

Abdominal or Vaginal Hysterectomy for Enlarged Uteri: A Randomized Clinical Trial
Benassi L, Rossi T, Kaihura CT, et al (Univ of Parma, Italy)
Am J Obstet Gynecol 187:1561-1565, 2002   25–1

Introduction.—The need to adapt surgical procedures to the demands of modern women has led to the "rediscovery" of the vaginal route for gynecologic procedures. This approach entirely avoids surgical damage to the abdominal wall, thus eliminating pain and dysfunction associated with healing in these tissues. The advantages, disadvantages, and outcomes of vaginal hysterectomy compared with abdominal hysterectomy were compared in patients with an enlarged uterus in a prospective, randomized trial.

Methods.—Sixty patients who underwent vaginal hysterectomies were compared with 59 patients who underwent abdominal hysterectomies from January 1997 through December 2000 for symptomatic uterine fibroids. Excluded were patients with other causes for hysterectomy, including prolapse, bleeding, adenomyosis, and endometrial or cervical carcinoma. In both groups, the range of uterine weights was 200 g to 1300 g. In patients with an enlarged uterus, vaginal hysterectomy was performed with volume reduction techniques, including intramyometrial coring, corporal bisection, and morcellation. Data were recorded concerning patient age, weight, parity, uterine weight, operative time, blood loss, demand for analgesics, eventual surgical complications, length of admission, and hospital charges.

Results.—There were no between-group differences in patient age, weight, parity, or uterine weight. The surgical times were significantly lower in patients who underwent the vaginal versus abdominal route (86 minutes vs 102 minutes; $P< .001$). No intraoperative complications were observed in either group. Surgical bleeding (determined by hemoglobin loss) was not significantly different between groups. There was a higher rate of fever (30.5% vs 16.6%; $P < .05$) and demand for analgesics (86% vs 66%; $P < .05$) in the abdominal compared with vaginal group. Vaginal hysterectomy had a significantly shorter hospital stay (3 days vs 4 days; $P < .001$) and lower cost ($58,581 vs $71,882) than abdominal hysterectomy.

Conclusion.—Vaginal hysterectomy is a valid alternative to abdominal hysterectomy, even in patients with an enlarged uterus.

▶ If further evidence was needed that vaginal hysterectomy provides a safe alternative to the abdominal approach, even for an enlarged uterus, this randomized trial provides it. Standard volume reduction techniques (such as morcellation, bisection, and myomectomy) made the vaginal route feasible for uteri estimated at volumes of 200 to 1300 mL. Patients randomized to vaginal hysterectomy enjoyed increased patient satisfaction, a reduced need for operative analgesia, less febrile morbidity, and a shorter hospital stay. Neither parity nor uterine size (up to 1300 g) precluded the safe conduct of vaginal hysterectomy in this study.

R. D. Arias, MD

Comparative Study of Vaginal, Laparoscopically Assisted Vaginal and Abdominal Hysterectomies for Uterine Myoma Larger Than 6 cm in Diameter or Uterus Weighing at Least 450 g: A Prospective Randomized Study
Hwang J-L, Seow K-M, Tsai Y-L, et al (Shin Kong Wu Ho-Su Mem Med Ctr, Taipei, Taiwan)
Acta Obstet Gynecol Scand 81:1132-1138, 2002   25–2

Introduction.—The success of total vaginal hysterectomy (TVH) in women with an enlarged uterus is affected by vaginal relaxation and uterine mobility, which are important in patients with an enlarged uterus without descensus. Another important factor in the success of this approach is the surgeon's ability to perform uterine morcellation. Perioperative morbidity, preoperative sonographic estimation of uterine weight, and postoperative outcomes of women with uterine fibroids larger than 6 cm in diameter or uteri estimated to weigh a minimum of 450 g were prospectively compared in women undergoing either TVH, laparoscopically assisted vaginal hysterectomy (LAVH), or total abdominal hysterectomies (TAH).

Methods.—Ninety patients who met the criteria of uterine fibroids larger than 6 cm by ultrasonographic examination were included. Patients were randomly assigned to undergo either LAVH, TVH, or TAH (30 patients in each group).

Results.—The LAVH group had significantly longer surgical times compared with the TAH and TVH groups (109, 98, and 74 minutes, respectively; $P < .001$). Blood loss for TVH was significantly lower compared with TAH and LAVH (215, 182, and 343 mL, respectively; $P = .04$). The TVH and LAVH groups had shorter hospital length of stay, lower postoperative pain scores, quicker bowel recovery, and lower postoperative antibiotic use compared with the TAH group. Uterine weight was significantly heavier in the TAH group than the TVH and LAVH groups (1020, 835, and 748 g, respectively; $P = .02$). When a myoma measured between 8 and 10 cm, the uterus weighed about 450 g; sensitivity for this prediction was 57.5%. For a myoma greater than 13 cm, the estimated uterine weight was more than 900 g; sensitivity for this prediction was 71%.

Conclusion.—Both TVH and LAVH can be performed in women with uterine weight of at least 450 g. Preoperative US examination can provide important information concerning the size of the fibroid and the estimated weight of the enlarged uterus before implementing an appropriate surgical method.

▶ The authors conducted a prospective randomized study of 3 methods of hysterectomy in women whose uteri were found to weigh 450 to 1800 g. Both the TVH and LAVH arms had shorter hospital stays, less pain, and quicker return to normal function. The gratuitous addition of laparoscopic interventions in what would have otherwise been an entirely vaginal case only added increased operative time and blood loss.

R. D. Arias, MD

Randomized, Prospective, Double-blind Comparison of Abdominal and Vaginal Hysterectomy in Women Without Uterovaginal Prolapse
Miskry T, Magos A (Royal Free Hosp, London)
Acta Obstet Gynecol Scand 82:351-358, 2003   25–3

Introduction.—There is considerable evidence from observational and uncontrolled trials that demonstrate several advantages of vaginal hysterectomy compared with abdominal hysterectomy, including cosmesis, shorter surgical time, fewer complications, quicker recovery, and lower overall treatment costs. A 2-center, prospective, randomized trial was performed in 36 women with dysfunctional uterine bleeding, uterine fibroids, or pelvic pain to determine, under controlled conditions, whether there are significant differences in the duration of hospitalization and recovery between abdominal and vaginal hysterectomy for indications other than uterovaginal prolapse.

Methods.—The main outcome measure was duration of postoperative hospital stay. Secondary outcome measures were analgesic requirement and return to normal health and function. Patients were advised to resume activities, including work, as soon as they felt well enough. They were asked to complete a daily symptom diary for 2 weeks postoperatively. Visual analog scales were used to evaluate mobility, pain, appetite, energy, and overall well-being. The Short-Form General Health Survey was performed at 6 weeks and 6 months in most patients.

Results.—There were no significant between-group differences in perioperative patient or surgical characteristics. Vaginal hysterectomy was correlated with a decrease in hospital stay compared with abdominal hysterectomy (median stay, 3 days versus 5 days; $P = .01$). Patients in the vaginal hysterectomy group compared with the abdominal hysterectomy group had decreased analgesic requirements (mean 75.4 mg vs 131.4 mg morphine equivalent; $P = .002$), shorter need for IV hydration (mean, 25.3 h vs 32.7 h;

$P = .05$), quicker return of bowel action (median, 3 d vs 4 d; $P = .002$), faster return to normal domestic activities (mean, 4.6 weeks vs 8.5 weeks; $P = .01$) and work activities (mean, 7.0 weeks vs 13.9 weeks; $P = .005$), and completed their recovery more quickly (mean, 7.9 weeks vs 16.9 weeks; $P = .008$).

Conclusion.—Vaginal hysterectomy was correlated with significantly shorter hospital stay and improved patient recovery. Vaginal hysterectomy is recommended for women with and without genital tract prolapse.

▶ These authors randomized women with benign pathology and no pelvic floor defects or prolapse to either an abdominal or vaginal hysterectomy. Preoperative estimate of uterine size varied from normal to 14 weeks. The study design blinded the patient and the operative team to the route of surgery by placing an opaque dressing over the lower abdomen in all cases. Outcomes included duration of hospital stay, analgesic requirements, and time to full recovery.

Sample size excluded statistical evaluation of surgical complications. Not surprisingly, given the relatively small uterine weights, conversion to laparotomy was not required in any of the vaginal procedures, though laparoscopy was used in 1 case to control bleeding.

Women randomly assigned to the vaginal route had less pain and recovered more quickly in both the short and long term. The most striking difference was reduction in time to fitness for work, which was 7 weeks, on average, in the vaginal arm, and 14 weeks in the abdominal arm.

Preoperative randomization and postoperative blinding overcomes 2 biases of the observational literature that have also found the vaginal route superior to the abdominal with regard to recovery time and analgesia requirements.

R. D. Arias, MD

Role of Hysterectomy in Management of Gestational Trophoblastic Disease

Pisal N, North C, Tidy J, et al (Whittington Hosp, London; Weston Park Hosp, Sheffield, England; Central Sheffield Univ Hosps Trust, England)
Gynecol Oncol 87:190-192, 2002   25–4

Background.—Gestational trophoblastic disease is typically treated with chemotherapy, but a role remains for hysterectomy. The incidence, indications, and outcomes of hysterectomy to treat gestational trophoblastic disease at a regional referral center in the United Kingdom were examined.

Methods.—Between January 1986 and December 2000, 5976 new cases of gestational trophoblastic disease were registered at the Weston Park Hospital in Sheffield. This center is 1 of 3 supraregional trophoblastic disease referral centers in the United Kingdom and serves a population of about 22 million. Patients' medical records were reviewed to examine the factors associated with hysterectomy.

Results.—During the study, 301 women (5%) received chemotherapy and 40 (1%) underwent hysterectomy. Compared with patients who received chemotherapy, patients undergoing hysterectomy had a significantly higher pretreatment risk score, as assessed by the Charring Cross Hospital scoring system (7.4 vs 4.6). Patients underwent hysterectomy at a mean of 17 months after the diagnosis of molar disease. The most common indications for hysterectomy were localized chemoresistant disease (12 cases), uncontrolled vaginal or intra-abdominal bleeding (9 cases), and placental site trophoblastic tumor (6 cases). These 40 women were likely to have atypical histologic findings; there were also 3 invasive moles, 13 choriocarcinomas, and 2 dimorphic tumors.

Among 37 patients who underwent hysterectomy for reasons directly related to gestational trophoblastic disease, all but 6 patients (78%) received chemotherapy, including 14 patients (38%) who required more than 1 course of chemotherapy. Of 18 women who underwent hysterectomy before chemotherapy, 10 subsequently needed chemotherapy for persistent trophoblastic disease. In the entire cohort, 10 of 5976 patients died (less than 0.2%), compared with 4 of 40 patients who underwent hysterectomy (10%; $P < .001$).

Conclusion.—At this tertiary referral center, about 1 of 150 women with gestational trophoblastic disease required hysterectomy. These patients represent a high-risk group, as reflected by a high pretreatment risk score, atypical histologic findings, the frequent need for salvage chemotherapy, and higher mortality rates.

▶ Hysterectomy, while not necessary for the treatment of the vast majority of patients with a gestational trophoblastic disease, can be sufficient treatment. Hysterectomy is the most successful treatment for hydatidiform mole. The procedure occasionally may be required in patients who develop multiple chemotherapy–resistant disease within the myometrium. However, the best time to do a hysterectomy is before a resistant trophoblastic tumor develops and thus should be considered early in the course of a patient's disease, if it is compatible with her reproductive goals.

D. S. Miller, MD

The Analgesic Effects of Intraperitoneal and Incisional Bupivacaine With Epinephrine After Total Abdominal Hysterectomy

Ng A, Swami A, Smith G, et al (Leicester Royal Infirmary, England)
Anesth Analg 95:158-162, 2002   25–5

Introduction.—Patient-controlled analgesic (PCA) morphine offers satisfactory analgesia, yet is associated with adverse effects that can limit its use in patients with total abdominal hysterectomy (TAH). The incisional or intraperitoneal administration of local anesthetics during TAH has disappointing results. The administration of local anesthetics into both visceral and cutaneous areas of surgery was evaluated for measurable analgesia in patients who underwent TAH.

Methods.—Forty-six American Society of Anesthesiologists physical status I and II patients undergoing TAH received a standardized anesthetic, PCA morphine, and rectal paracetamol, 1 g every 6 hours. Patients were excluded if they had malignancy, had a history of chronic pain or continuous use of analgesic drugs, or were unable to use the PCA device. Patients were randomly assigned to treatment with either 50 mL bupivacaine, 0.25%, with epinephrine, 5 µg/mL, or 50 mL of normal saline. Thirty milliliters and 20 mL of treatment solution were administered into the peritoneum and incision, respectively, prior to wound closure.

Results.—Seventeen patients in the placebo group and 16 patients in the bupivacaine group completed the trial. Reasons for withdrawal included PCA malfunction, PCA discontinued too early, nausea, chest infection, intra-abdominal drain insertion, and protocol violation. Groups did not differ significantly in age, height, weight, or duration of surgery. Pain on movement on awakening was significantly more intense in the placebo than in the bupivacaine group. Morphine consumption (interquartile range) over 24 hours was 62 mg (53-85 mg) in the placebo group versus 44 mg (33-56 mg) in the bupivacaine group ($P < .01$). This significant difference was due to greater morphine consumption in the placebo group during the initial 4 postoperative hours.

Conclusion.—A combination of intraperitoneal and incisional bupivacaine with epinephrine provides substantial morphine-sparing analgesia for 4 hours after TAH.

▶ In this randomized, blinded study of hysterectomy analgesia, the combination of intraperitoneal installation and incisional injection of bupivacaine and epinephrine significantly decreased the need for morphine in the immediate postoperative period. Both installation and injection were performed following a TAH for benign indications. Previous efforts to reduce pain after laparotomy with intra-operative regional anesthetics have been less successful when a single route of administration was used. This technique may find particular utility in those hospitals where PCA is not available.

R. D. Arias, MD

26 Operative Issues

Randomised Controlled Trial of Glove Perforation in Single and Double-Gloving Methods in Gynaecologic Surgery
Kovavisarach E, Seedadee C (Rajavithi Hosp, Bangkok, Thailand)
Aust N Z J Obstet Gynaecol 42:519-521, 2002   26–1

Background.—Glove perforation during surgery increases the risk of exposure to both the patient and the surgeon. This randomized controlled trial compared perforation rates of single- versus double-gloves for surgeons performing total abdominal hysterectomy (TAH) with or without bilateral salpingo-oophorectomy.

Study Design.—The study group consisted of 170 gynecologic patients undergoing TAH at Rajavithi Hospital from September 1999 through August 2000; patients were randomly assigned to either single or double-glove surgeries. Each glove was evaluated for perforation by filling with air and then immersing in water. The location and number of perforations were recorded.

Findings.—The perforation rate was 22.73% for single gloves and 6.09% for inner gloves. No significant difference was found between the perforation rates of single versus outer gloves. A matched perforation of both outer and inner gloves occurred in 1.22% of pairs.

Conclusions.—The perforation rate was significantly higher with the use of single gloves. The routine use of double gloves is recommended when performing TAH.

▶ Double-gloving significantly reduced the rate of contact between the operator's skin and the patient's blood in this randomized controlled trial of glove perforation. A single operation was included in this trial (TAH), thus reducing the variability associated with different procedures. The rate of perforation in the single-gloving group was similar to the rate found in the outer glove of the double-gloving surgeons. The inner double glove remained intact about 3 times more often than did a single glove, even when the outer glove integrity was breached. Single-gloving surgeons only recognized a breach in glove integrity in 5% of operations. Given the reality of unused glove perforation, a 20% incidence of intraoperative perforation, and a relatively low rate of perforation detection, the authors recommend routine double-gloving while performing TAH.

R. D. Arias, MD

Mechanical Performance of Knots Using Braided and Monofilament Absorbable Sutures

Schubert DC, Unger JB, Mukherjee D, et al (Louisiana State Univ, Shreveport)
Am J Obstet Gynecol 187:1438-1442, 2002   26–2

Introduction.—Most surgeons regard the flat square knot as the gold standard for surgical knots. In gynecologic surgery, sliding knots are frequently used to hold tension on the suture for deep, narrow spaces in the pelvis and vagina. Both braided and monofilament absorbable sutures are commonly used by gynecologic surgeons. The integrity and strength of various flat sliding knots were examined with braided and monofilament absorbable sutures.

Methods.—Four groups were evaluated, each consisting of a single suture type and size, with 5 different knots (square knots, surgeon's knots, modified granny flat knots, and modified identical and nonidentical sliding knots). Each combination was evaluated 10 times (200 total experiments). Suture types were 0-0 and 2-0 Glycomer 631 (Biosyn) and 0-0 and 2-0 coated Lactomer (Polysorb). The knots were tested to failure with a tensiometer. The proportion of knots becoming untied within each group was compared with the ultimate load needed to break tied knots.

Results.—All knots that became untied did so at an average of 49.8 N (range, 14-68 N). In all instances, once a knot began to untie, it continued to completely unravel. Each suture broke at or near the knot. In the 0-0 and 2-0 Lactomer groups, 90% and 60% of modified identical sliding knots, respectively, became untied. This occurred significantly more often than with all other knots.

Conclusion.—Modified identical sliding knots should not be used with 0-0 and 2-0 Lactomer sutures.

▶ These authors used an elegant, scientific approach to an important topic that receives far too little attention. In vaginal surgery, where sliding knots may be preferred due to restricted range of movement, this information is especially important. By choosing suture with smaller gauge or braided surface, one decreases the risk of untied knots. Hopefully, this article will inspire further study in this area. In particular, defining the minimum number of throws necessary by suture type would be instructive.

R. D. Arias, MD

Vaginal Construction With Skin Grafts and Vacuum-Assisted Closure

Hallberg H, Holmström H (Göteborg Univ, Sweden; Sahlgrenska Univ Hosp, Göteborg, Sweden)
Scand J Plast Reconstr Surg Hand Surg 37:97-101, 2003   26–3

Introduction.—The most commonly used method for constructing a vagina in patients with the Mayer-Rokitansky-Kuster syndrome is probably the 1938 approach popularized by McIndoe and Banister. With this method, a cavity is created between the rectum and the urethra-bladder complex and is lined using split-thickness skin grafts. An important disadvantage of this approach is late contraction of the neovagina. To prevent this, full-thickness grafts have been used, but their take is less reliable. Described was the vacuum-assisted closure (VAC) system, a new technique to improve the take of skin grafts, which has been especially valuable in grafting difficult anatomical sites.

Methods.—Three patients aged 16, 17, and 18 with congenital vaginal aplasia underwent vaginal construction with skin grafts and VAC. One patient was treated with split-thickness grafts and the other 2 had full-thickness grafts taken from the groin. All 3 patients fulfilled criteria for the Mayer-Rokitansky-Kuster syndrome.

Results.—For all 3 patients, the grafts took completely. In one patient, the margin of the full-thickness skin graft became detached from the introital mucosa upon removal from the mold. Patients remained on bed rest during the postoperative period. The mold was removed after 6 days in the patient with the split-thickness skin graft. It was recommended that she use the retaining stent after surgery. For psychological reasons, the patient refused this regimen. At 6-month evaluation, there was no contraction of the cavity, which remained 12 to 13 cm deep. She reported having regular vaginal intercourse with full satisfaction from 1 month after surgery.

For the 2 patients with the full-thickness grafts, it was recommended that they test the patency of the vagina daily with a mold. One had vaginal intercourse 28 days postoperatively, and the patient with the introital wound had intercourse after 6 to 7 weeks, with minor problems. Follow-up ranged from 4 to 7 months. The split-thickness grafts appeared more like a normal vaginal cavity with a soft and pliable lining. The full-thickness grafted neovaginas were pale and had few hairs. The vaginal cavity showed no contraction in any patients.

Conclusion.—The VAC system approach, together with skin-lined vaginoplasties, appears to solve the problems of delayed healing and late contracture of the vaginal cavity. It is important to follow these patients up for a few years to determine whether the promising initial results persist.

▶ The VAC device has shown itself to be very useful in gynecology for the closing of poorly healing abdominal wounds. The authors here present a novel, but obvious, extension of this technology to vaginal reconstruction procedures. The biggest problem in achieving good skin take in the vagina is keeping the skin graft in contact with the underlying blood supply. Various molds have been developed to help accomplish this, but they do little to prevent the development of a subgraft fluid collection. The VAC obviates this problem. In gynecologic oncology, this could clearly also be used for vaginal reconstruction with omental pedicle flaps and skin grafts.

D. S. Miller, MD

A Stiff Bristled, Spiral-Shaped Ectocervical Brush: A Device for Transepithelial Tissue Biopsy

Monk BJ, Cogan M, Felix JC, et al (Univ of California, Irvine; Univ of Southern California, Los Angeles; Southern California Permanente Med Group, Anaheim; et al)

Obstet Gynecol 100:1276-1284, 2002   26–4

Introduction.—Brush biopsies have been used in conjunction with other endoscopic procedures for years, particularly for sampling endobronchial lesions in the lung or polypoid lesions in the colon. For cervical tissue examination, endocervical brushing has been shown to be as reliable as endocervical curettage for canal-related disease and has recently been used to obtain colposcopically directed brushings of exocervical lesions before punch biopsy in pregnant women. The efficacy of a new spiral-shaped tissue-sample brush device for cervical transepithelial sampling was assessed.

Methods.—Before large-loop excision of the transformation zone, women with cervical intraepithelial neoplasia underwent a transepithelial brush biopsy of a portion of a colposcopically identified lesion. This was followed by a punch biopsy of the remaining portion. Brush biopsy samples were processed by liquid-based cytology and cell block techniques. Diagnoses were made by consensus of 3 pathologists. Brush biopsy samples without basal cells were not considered adequate. The histologic diagnosis was compared with the brush biopsy and punch biopsy samples. A comparison was made between patient-reported pain and physician-reported bleeding for punch and brush biopsies.

Results.—Fifty-two women were enrolled, 47 of whom successfully completed inclusion protocol. Eight brush biopsy specimens were not adequate. Thirty-nine women had abnormal pathology (human papillomavirus/cervical intraepithelial neoplasia I or worse) on large-loop excision of the transformation zone. Thirty-two women had high-grade or worse lesions. The punch biopsy correlated with high-grade disease in 79.3% of women with a cell block technique and in 76.7% with liquid cytology. Significantly less pain ($P < .001$) and significantly less bleeding ($P < .001$) was reported with the brush biopsy.

Conclusion.—When an adequate sample is obtained, spiral brush biopsy is as good as a standard punch biopsy for identifying cervical pathology, with markedly less pain and bleeding. User education and guidelines for sampling are needed to ensure that an adequate sample is obtained.

▶ The use of a spiral tissue sampling brush in the evaluation of women with cervical intraepithelial neoplasia on Pap smear resulted in correct identification of high-grade squamous intraepithelial lesion in 22 of 29 women with adequate samples. In another 4 women, the specimen was abnormal, though read as low grade, while the definitive specimen (obtained by loop excision of the transformation zone), was high grade.

Cell block and thin-layer cytology were equally effective in evaluating disease in this study.

Seven of 47 cell block preparations were inadequate. The authors suspect that insufficient pressure of the device against the cervix contributed to the lack of basal and parabasal cells in these specimens.

The authors explain the high false-negative rate of diagnosis in the punch biopsies (done on the same women) by bias in favor of the brush, conferred by the study design. The brush sample was taken first, potentially obscuring the lesion for the subsequent punch biopsy. The brush sample was generally less painful and resulted in less blood loss.

The brush sampling technique offers advantages over traditional methods with regard to patient comfort and bleeding. A limitation would seem to be the lack of familiarity with this tissue preparation in the general population of pathologists, at least with regard to cervical tissue.

R. D. Arias, MD

Misoprostol Use in Obstetrics and Gynecology in Brazil, Jamaica, and the United States
Clark S, Blum J, Blanchard K, et al (Population Council, New York; Population Council, Johannesburg, South Africa; Population Council, Sao Paulo, Brazil; et al)
Int J Gynaecol Obstet 76:65-74, 2002   26–5

Introduction.—In most developing countries, access to the latest research results and new drug therapies is limited, particularly when drugs are expensive or necessitate sophisticated delivery systems. Therefore, women in many developing countries do not have access to satisfactory gynecologic and obstetric services. Providers in these settings often modify standard regimens to suit their needs or develop treatments based on available drugs. One example is the widespread off-label use of misoprostol for various reproductive health indications. The current clinical use of misoprostol for the treatment of several reproductive health indications by providers in Brazil, Jamaica, and the United States was examined.

Methods.—The "snowball" method was used to identify potential respondents. Known providers were asked to refer other providers who might be willing to participate. Between February 1999 and May 2000, a telephone survey of 228 obstetricians and gynecologists in Brazil, Jamaica, and the United States (123, 52, and 53 physicians, respectively) was performed to document the use of misoprostol for reproductive health indications and to document some of the variation in regimens used in clinical practice.

Results.—Indications for misoprostol use were sorted into categories: (1) abortion (first trimester induction, second trimester induction, second trimester labor induction, and cervical priming); (2) uterine evaluation (intrauterine fetal death, missed abortion, and incomplete abortion); and (3) labor and delivery (cervical softening, labor induction, and prevention of postpartum hemorrhage). Respondents from all 3 countries used misoprostol for all 10 indications in these categories. Providers in Brazil and Jamaica appeared to be well informed regarding their colleagues' use of misoprostol. In Jamaica, some respondents indicated they were frustrated that misoprostol was not specifically labeled and marketed for reproductive health indications. In Brazil, providers wanted greater access and repeatedly pressured the interviewer regarding information for obtaining new supplies. Providers in all 3 countries mentioned the need for more research and better dissemination of information. Many respondents learned about misoprostol's multiple uses from trusted colleagues. After using the drug for one indication, they realized its potential for other reproductive health indications.

Conclusion.—Providers, and particularly those in developing countries, regard misoprostol as a safe and effective drug that helps fill an important void in their provision of health care.

▶ For many women, misoprostol offers the best hope of safe pregnancy termination—either by completely evacuating the uterus or by initiating an abortion that will then be completed by a skilled provider. The availability of a low-cost, heat-stable prostaglandin analogue has made the possibility of a safe abortion within the reach of women who would otherwise be subjected to the risks associated with illegal surgical abortion.

R. D. Arias, MD

Reduction of Blood Loss During Extensive Pelvic Procedures by Aortic Clamping: A Preliminary Report

Eisenkop SM, Spirtos NM, Lin W-CM, et al (Women's Cancer Ctr, Encino-Tarzana, Calif; Women's Cancer Ctr, Palo Alto, Calif; Huntsville Vascular Specialists PC, Ala)
Gynecol Oncol 88:80-84, 2003   26–6

Background.—The pelvic phase of surgery for gynecologic malignancies is often an extensive undertaking. The effect of intraoperative aortic clamping during extensive pelvic procedures on blood loss, operative time, and morbidity was investigated.

Methods.—Complete aorta occlusion with a vascular clamp was done before the pelvic phase of surgery in 15 women. Thirteen had ovarian cancer; 1, cervical cancer; and 1, extensive pelvic sarcoma. The procedure included heparin and protamine reversal.

Findings.—The median estimated total blood loss was 650 mL in patients requiring en bloc excision of the internal reproductive organs, pelvic peritoneum, and rectosigmoid colon. A median of 2 units of blood was transfused. The median total operative time was 155 minutes. No complications were attributable to aortic clamping.

Conclusions.—Most procedures were completed with a less-than-anticipated blood loss and surgical time. Aortic clamping may reduce blood loss, operative time, and the incidence of transfusion-related morbidity associated with extensive pelvic surgery. Additional study of intraoperative aortic clamping is warranted.

▶ When I heard this paper presented at the Society of Gynecologic Oncologists, the author reported that when he was first discussing with his general surgical colleagues the concept of aortic clamping to facilitate extensive pelvic tumor debulkings, their response was telling, "Why wouldn't you?" The time limit for safest aortic clamping clearly limits its applicability for many radical and ultraradical pelvic procedures that are required in gynecologic oncology. Thus, while it may be lifesaving for a few, it is probably not helpful for most.

This report also illustrates one of the deficits of obstetric and gynecologic as well as gynecologic oncology surgical training, in that virtually all such training programs have very little cross training with other surgical disciplines and thus receive little exposure to other techniques. This is not to our benefit nor to our patients.

D. S. Miller, MD

A Randomized Controlled Trial of a Regular Diet as the First Meal in Gynecologic Oncology Patients Undergoing Intraabdominal Surgery

Pearl ML, Frandina M, Mahler L, et al (State Univ of New York, Stony Brook)
Obstet Gynecol 100:230-234, 2002   26–7

Introduction.—The need to withhold a regular diet has been questioned in patients with gynecologic malignancies who undergo extensive intra-abdominal surgery. The safety and efficacy of a regular diet as the first meal after intra-abdominal surgery were prospectively assessed in a randomized controlled trial of patients undergoing gynecologic oncology procedures.

Methods.—Between February 17, 2000, and October 16, 2001, 254 patients undergoing gynecologic oncology intra-abdominal surgery were ran-

TABLE 3.—Gastrointestinal Information

Category	Clear Liquid (n = 107)	Regular Diet (n = 138)
Morbidity		
Nausea	21 (19.6)	26 (18.8)
Vomiting	10 (9.3)	19 (13.8)
Abdominal distension	10 (9.3)	18 (13.0)
Nasogastric tube use	1 (0.9)	8 (5.8)
Tolerance		
Diet on first attempt	101 (94.4)	121 (87.7)
Regular diet on first attempt	103 (96.3)	
If intolerant, time to tolerance (days)	5.3 ± 1.5	3.6 ± 1.5
Flatus before discharge	55 (51.4)	69 (50.0)
Intervals (days)		
Bowel sounds	1.2 ± 0.5	1.2 ± 0.5
Flatus	2.8 ± 1.4	2.8 ± 1.0
Regular diet*	2.4 ± 2.5	1.1 ± 0.3
Hosptial stay	3.6 ± 3.0	3.4 ± 1.7

Data are mean ± SD or n (%).
*$P < .05$; no other significant differences between groups.
(Courtesy of Pearl ML, Frandina M, Mahler L, et al: A randomized, controlled trial of a regular diet as the first meal in gynecologic oncology patients undergoing intra-abdominal surgery. *Obstet Gynecol* 100:230-234, 2002. Reprinted with permission of the American College of Obstetricians and Gynecologists.)

domly assigned to receive either a clear liquid diet or a regular diet as their first postoperative meal. All patients received their first meal on the first postoperative day if they had no nausea, vomiting, or abdominal distension.

Results.—Both groups were similar in age, disease, surgical procedure distribution, surgery length, and estimated blood loss. The groups were also similar in the incidence of nausea, vomiting, abdominal distension, frequency and duration of nasogastric tube use, passage of flatus before discharge, and the percentage of patients who tolerated their diets on the first attempt. Among patients who did not tolerate the first attempt at either a clear liquid or regular diet, the time to tolerance was similar for both groups. The clear liquid and regular diet groups were similar in time to development of bowel sounds, passage of flatus, hospital stay (Table 3), febrile morbidity, pneumonia, wound complications, and atelectasis. No anastomotic complications or aspirations occurred in either group. The groups were similar in postoperative changes in hematologic indexes and electrolytes.

Conclusion.—A regular diet as the first meal after gynecologic oncology intra-abdominal surgery is both safe and efficacious.

▶ The management of postoperative feeding is one of those areas of surgical practice that has been subject to ritual and dogma. Operative laparoscopy and managed care has required surgeons to reexamine some of their postoperative rituals. Some of us have progressed a long way from previous practices of not allowing clear liquids until bowel sounds or solid food until flatus. The authors of this study have shown that such conservatism is not required for most patients. Most postoperative patients will be able to tolerate a regular diet when it is placed in front of them. However, they did not show that they were able to discharge the patient from the hospital any sooner by this practice. Of note, more patients required nasogastric tubes in the group initially presented a regular diet. The advantage to giving patients a clear liquid diet first is that if they vomit and aspirate clear liquids, they are less likely to have lung injury compared with patients who vomit and aspirate a regular diet.

D. S. Miller, MD

Long-term, Low-Intensity Warfarin Therapy for the Prevention of Recurrent Venous Thromboembolism

Ridker PM, for the PREVENT Investigators (Harvard Med School, Boston; et al)
N Engl J Med 348:1425-1434, 2003   26–8

Background.—The treatment of patients with idiopathic venous thromboembolism usually includes a 5- to 10-day course of heparin followed by 3 to 12 months of oral anticoagulation therapy with full-dose warfarin, with adjustment of the dose to an international normalized ratio between 2.0 and 3.0. However, recurrent venous thromboembolism is a major clinical problem after cessation of anticoagulation therapy, with an estimated incidence of 6% to 9% each year. No therapeutic agent has been shown to provide an acceptable benefit-to-risk ratio for the long-term management of venous thromboembolism. The Prevention of Recurrent Venous Thromboembolism (PREVENT) trial was conducted to test the hypothesis that long-term, low-intensity warfarin therapy could safely and effectively reduce the risk of recurrent venous thromboembolism in patients with a previous idiopathic venous thrombosis.

Methods.—The study enrolled patients with idiopathic venous thromboembolism who had received full-dose anticoagulation therapy for a median of 6.5 months. The patients were randomly assigned to placebo or low-intensity warfarin with a target international normalized ratio of 1.5 to 2.0. Participants were followed up for recurrent venous thromboembolism, major hemorrhage, and death.

Results.—Although the intention was to enroll 750 patients, the study was terminated early after randomization of 508 patients, who were followed up for up to 4.3 years. Of the 253 patients assigned to placebo, 37 had recurrent venous thromboembolism (7.2/100 person-years), as compared with 14 of 255 patients assigned to low-intensity warfarin (2.6/100 person-years). This represented a risk reduction of 64%. The risk reductions were similar for all subgroups, including patients with and without inherited thrombophilia.

Major hemorrhage occurred in 2 patients assigned to placebo and 5 patients assigned to low-intensity warfarin. There were twice as many deaths in the placebo group (8 patients) as in the low-intensity warfarin group (4 patients). Low-intensity warfarin was associated with a 48% reduction in the composite end point of recurrent venous thromboembolism, major hemorrhage, or death and a reduction of 76% to 81% in the risk of recurrent venous thromboembolism on per-protocol and as-treated analyses.

Conclusion.—Long-term, low-intensity warfarin therapy is highly effective for the prevention of recurrent venous thromboembolism.

▶ Patients with "idiopathic" thrombotic events are at high risk for recurrence. Full-dose anticoagulation can decrease that risk of occurrence but with an increased risk of bleeding. Based on the results of this study, low-dose therapy appears to be a safer option. However, this editor reminds the reader that many patients who appear to have idiopathic thrombotic events, in fact, have an identifiable etiology, which is often an occult cancer or more rarely an inherited thrombophilia. Thus, the workup for an "idiopathic" thrombotic event should include an evaluation for occult malignancy.

D. S. Miller MD

SUGGESTED READING

Bern MM, Lokich JJ, Wallach SR, et al: Very low doses of warfarin can prevent thrombosis in central venous catheters: A randomized prospective trial. *Ann Intern Med* 112:423-428, 1990.

27 Cervical Cancers

ThinPrep Detection of Cervical and Endometrial Adenocarcinoma: A Retrospective Cohort Study
Schorge JO, Saboorian MH, Hynan L, et al (Univ of Texas, Dallas)
Cancer 96:338-343, 2002   27-1

Introduction.—The ThinPrep Papanicoloau (Pap) test enhances specimen adequacy, resulting in the cytologic diagnosis of significantly more cervical abnormalities compared with the conventional smear technique. The efficacy of the ThinPrep Pap test for improving identification of glandular lesions has not been well established. Its efficacy in detecting cervical and endometrial adenocarcinomas was compared with that of conventionally prepared Pap smear tests.

Methods.—All ThinPrep-tested cases of atypical glandular cells of undetermined significance (AGCUS) or adenocarcinoma diagnosed between March 1998 and March 2000 were examined. Conventional smears obtained between January 1996 and January 1998, before laboratory conversion to the ThinPrep system, were used for control. Histologic follow-up was documented.

Results.—Of 112,058 ThinPrep Pap tests evaluated, 186 (0.17%) were interpreted as AGCUS/adenocarcinomas versus 77 (0.09%) of 83,464 conventional smears ($P < .001$). The overall sensitivity of a ThinPrep AGCUS/adenocarcinoma smear in identifying either cervical or endometrial adenocarcinoma was 72% versus 41% for controls ($P < .001$). The ThinPrep Pap test was more sensitive in identifying endometrial adenocarcinomas (65% vs 39%; $P = .010$). There was a trend for higher sensitivity in identifying cervical adenocarcinomas (87% vs 55%; $P = .0108$).

Conclusion.—The ThinPrep Pap test is more sensitive than conventional Pap smears in the identification of cervical and endometrial adenocarcinomas.

▶ The widespread availability of conventional Pap smear screening has dramatically reduced the incidence of squamous cervical cancer in the United States. However, endometrial adenocarcinomas are not reliably detected, and the incidence of cervical adenocarcinomas continues to increase. The ThinPrep liquid–based cytology has now captured almost half of the market. These preparations enhance specimen adequacy and have the potential to be a more effective screening method for glandular neoplasia.

The authors performed a large retrospective cohort study to compare the ThinPrep Pap test to conventional smear preparation in detecting cervical and endometrial adenocarcinoma. The overall sensitivity of a ThinPrep to detect AGCUS/adenocarcinoma was superior. Liquid-based cytology preparations may be one way to improve the detection of glandular neoplasia of the cervix and endometrium, but false negative smears remain commonplace.

D. S. Miller, MD

Endocervical Curettage at Conization to Predict Residual Cervical Adeno-carcinoma *in Situ*
Lea JS, Shin CH, Sheets EE, et al (Univ of Texas, Dallas; Brigham and Women's Hosp, Boston; Univ of North Carolina, Chapel Hill; et al)
Gynecol Oncol 87:129-132, 2002   27–2

Introduction.—Cone margin status is the most clinically useful indicator of adenocarcinoma in situ (AIS) of the cervix. Expectant management is not usually recommended unless negative cone margins can be attained. Endocervical curettage (ECC) performed in the operating room at completion of cone biopsy has the potential to ascertain whether residual AIS or "skip" lesions are present in the canal above the endocervical cone margin. A retrospective review was performed to determine whether performing an ECC at the time of conization is useful diagnostically in predicting residual cervical AIS among women who may wish to preserve their fertility.

Methods.—All patients diagnosed with AIS between 1995 and 2000 at 4 institutions were identified. Data were reviewed from medical records of women who were younger than age 40 years, had an ECC performed at the time of the initial cone biopsy, had a clearly demarcated surgical margin pathologically, and underwent a second surgical procedure.

Results.—Twenty-nine (24%) of 123 patients with AIS met inclusion criteria. The median patient age was 33 years (range, 17-39 years). Thirteen participants (46%) were nulliparous. The initial surgery was a cold-knife conization in 17 patients and a loop electrosurgical excision procedure in 12 patients. Twelve (41%) and 15 (52%) ECCs and cone margins, respectively, were histologically positive. Sixteen patients underwent a repeat conization and 13 had a hysterectomy. Residual AIS was identified at the time of the second surgical procedure in 13 (45%) patients. ECC had superior positive predictive value (100% vs 47%; $P < .01$) and negative predictive value (94% vs 57%; $P = 0.01$) compared with cone margin in the prediction of residual AIS. None of the participants undergoing fertility-sparing surgery developed recurrent AIS or adenocarcinoma.

Conclusion.—ECC performed at the time of conization may be helpful in predicting residual AIS in women who wish to preserve their fertility.

▶ ECC performed at the time of conization may be a useful tool for predicting residual AIS in women considering fertility preservation. Few reports have studied the effectiveness of ECC at the time of conization to predict residual

AIS. The experience of this 4-institution study indicates that ECC has a superior predictive value in determining residual AIS compared to cone margin status. Unlike this study, however, the previous reports included postmenopausal women and ECCs performed preoperatively at the time of colposcopy. The positive predictive value of ECC described here is in concordance with that indicated by Goldstein et al.[1]

A prospective, randomized trial will ultimately be necessary to definitely test the hypothesis that ECC performed at the time of conization is predictive of residual AIS. Until then, this study provides some reassurance to patients with retained uteri and their physicians.

D. S. Miller, MD

Reference

1. Goldstein NS, Mani A: The status and distance of cone biopsy margins as a predictor for excision adequacy for endocervical adenocarcinoma in situ. *Am J Clin Pathol* 109:727, 1998.

Radical Vaginal Trachelectomy and Pelvic Lymphadenectomy for Preservation of Fertility in Early Cervical Carcinoma

Burnett AF, Roman LD, O'Meara AT, et al (Univ of Southern California, Los Angeles)
Gynecol Oncol 88:419-423, 2003   27–3

Background.—The standard treatment for cervical cancer results in loss of fertility. Radical vaginal trachelectomy and pelvic lymphadenectomy can be used to treat early cervical cancer while maintaining fertility. An experience with this technique since 1995 is described.

Study Design.—The study group consisted of 21 procedures performed from 1995 to 2001 in young women, aged 23 to 41 years, with early stage cervical cancer (Ib1 and Ia2), who wished to preserve their fertility. All participants were informed that their treatment was not standard treatment. Obstetric and oncologic outcomes were evaluated; the average follow-up was 31.5 months.

Findings.—The average hospital stay was 3 days in this study group. Three patients had postoperative transient neuropathy. Laparotomy was not required. Two patients had radical vaginal hysterectomies, as the cancer could not be cleared by trachelectomy. One patient had postoperative radiotherapy for high-risk features. No tumor recurrence occurred over 31.5 months of follow-up. Three women became pregnant. One woman delivered twins, 1 delivered a singleton, and 1 had rupture of membranes and chorioamnionitis at 20 weeks' gestation.

Conclusions.—Radical vaginal trachelectomy and pelvic lymphadenectomy is an effective treatment for early stage cervical cancer in select young women who wish to preserve fertility.

▶ Radical vaginal trachelectomy and pelvic lymphadenectomy is an innovative surgical technique in the management of early cervical cancer in women who desire preservation of fertility. This article represents the largest series in the United States. The authors report 21 young women with early cervical cancer who underwent this procedure without any recurrence of disease after an average follow-up of 31.5 months. They conclude that radical vaginal trachelectomy and laparoscopic pelvic lymphadenectomy is a feasible and safe procedure for treating early cervical cancer. The long-term viable delivery rate remains to be determined.

R. D. Arias, MD

Radiation Therapy With and Without Extrafascial Hysterectomy for Bulky Stage IB Cervical Carcinoma: A Randomized Trial of the Gynecologic Oncology Group
Keys HM, Bundy BN, Stehman FB, et al (Albany Med College, NY; Roswell Park Cancer Inst, Buffalo, NY; Indiana Univ, Indianapolis; et al)
Gynecol Oncol 89:343-353, 2003   27–4

Background.—Authorities continue to disagree on the role of adjuvant postradiation hysterectomy for patients with large International Federation of Gyngecology and Obstetrics (FIGO) stage IB cervical cancer. The effects of adjuvant hysterectomy after standardized radiation on progression-free survival and survival in this patient population were determined.

Methods.—Two hundred fifty-six eligible patients with exophytic or "barrel"-shaped tumors of 4 cm or larger were randomly assigned to receive either external and intracavitary irradiation or attenuated irradiation followed by extrafascial hysterectomy. In one fourth of the patients, tumors had a maximum diameter of 7 cm or greater.

Findings.—The strongest prognostic factor was tumor size, followed by performance status 2 and age at diagnosis. Hysterectomy did not increase the frequency of grade 3 or adverse effects, which occurred in 10% of each group. Most of these adverse effects resulted from the gastrointestinal or genitourinary tracts only. Patients undergoing radiation plus extrafascial hysterectomy had a lower cumulative incidence of local relapse at 5 years (14% vs 27%). The 2 regimens did not differ significantly in outcomes except for the adjusted comparison of progression-free survival (Fig 4). However, all indicated a lower risk in the adjuvant hysterectomy regimen.

Conclusions.—The use of extrafascial hysterectomy appears to confer no clinically important benefits. However, evidence suggests that patients with tumors of 4 to 6 cm may have benefited from this procedure.

▶ This is a tardy report from the Gynecologic Oncology Group (GOG) on a treatment scheme abandoned by most institutions that once advocated it but

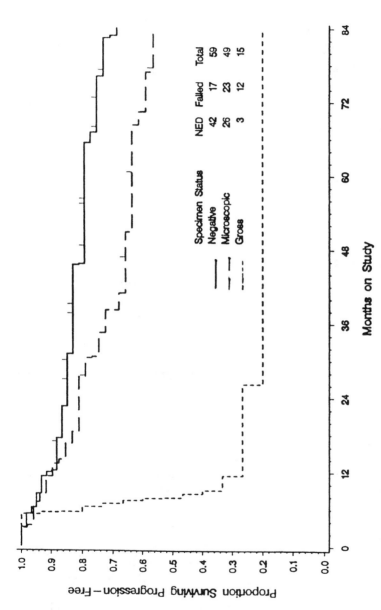

Specimen Status	NED	Failed	Total
Negative	42	17	59
Microscopic	26	23	49
Gross	3	12	15

Months on Study

Proportion Surviving Progression-Free

FIGURE 4.—Progression-free survival by hysterectomy specimen histology. *Abbreviation: NED*, No evidence of disease. (Reprinted by permission of the publisher courtesy of Keys HM, Bundy BN, Stehman FB, et al: Radiation therapy with and without extrafascial hysterectomy for bulky stage IB cervical carcinoma: A randomized trial of the Gynecologic Oncology Group. *Gynecol Oncol* 89:343-353. Copyright 2003 by Elsevier Science Inc.)

still practiced by some gynecologic oncologists. Nonetheless, useful information is contained therein. This is best illustrated in Figure 4. If there really was an advantage for adjuvant hysterectomy, it should be in the patient who had gross residual disease at the end of external beam radiation, where surgery would make up for that which radiation could not accomplish. Unfortunately, that was not the case. The seemingly paradoxic finding of a small advantage for 4- to 6-cm tumors but not in larger tumors is likely due to tumors that are larger than 6 cm, in fact, are not stage IB, but probably have parametrial involvement. Thus, incomplete excision of the parametria would add little to improving the outcome. A subsequent study by the GOG has confirmed these results.[1]

D. S. Miller, MD

Reference

1. Keys HM, Bundy BN, Stehman FB, et al: Weekly cisplatin chemotherapy during irradiation improves survival and reduces relapses for patients with bulky stage IB cervical cancer treated with irradiation and adjuvant hysterectomy: Results of a randomized Gynecologic Oncology Group trial. *N Engl J Med* 340:1154, 1999.

Correlation of Smoking History and Other Patient Characteristics With Major Complications of Pelvic Radiation Therapy for Cervical Cancer

Eifel PJ, Jhingran A, Bodurka DC, et al (Univ of Texas, Houston)
J Clin Oncol 20:3651-3657, 2002   27–5

Introduction.—Various factors that have been evaluated for their possible contribution to the late effects of pelvic radiation include diabetes mellitus, hypertension, pelvic infection, previous abdominal surgery, and age. Patient-related factors that influence the risk of serious late complications of pelvic radiation therapy were examined.

Methods.—The medical records of 3489 patients treated with radiation therapy for International Federation of Gynecology and Obstetrics stage I or II carcinoma of the cervix were reviewed for data concerning patient characteristics, treatment details, and outcomes. Any complication that occurred or persisted in excess of 3 months after treatment that required hospitalization, transfusion, or surgery or caused severe symptoms or patient death was considered a major late complication. Complication rates were determined actuarially. Median follow-up was 85 months; 99% of patients were followed up for a minimum of 3 years or until death.

Results.—Heavy smoking was the strongest independent predictor of overall complications (hazard ratio, 2.30; 95% confidence interval, 1.84-2.87) and had the most striking influence on small bowel complications (hazard ratio for smokers of 1 or more packs per day, 3.25; 95% confidence interval, 2.21-4.78). Hispanics had a significantly lower rate of small bowel complications compared with whites, and African Americans had higher rates of bladder and rectal complications than whites. Thin women were at increased risk of gastrointestinal complications. Obese women were more likely to have serious bladder complications.

Conclusion.—Complications of pelvic radiation therapy are strongly linked with smoking, race, and other patient characteristics. These factors need to be considered before the results of clinical trials are generalized to other cultural or racial groups.

▶ The attitude of some is that once a cancer has occurred there is little reason to discontinue the bad behavior that contributed to its causation. That probably is the case when dealing with the patients for whom only palliation is possible. The authors make a compelling case that smoking increases the complications of treatment and may very likely interfere with the success of radiation therapy. These are all complications that can significantly degrade the patient's quality of life. Thus, for the patient undergoing radiation therapy, it is not too late to stop smoking.

D. S. Miller, MD

28 Uterine Cancers

**Can Ultrasound Replace Dilation and Curettage?: A Longitudinal Evalua-
tion of Postmenopausal Bleeding and Transvaginal Sonographic Measurement of the Endometrium as Predictors of Endometrial Cancer**
Gull B, Karlsson B, Milsom I, et al (Univ of Göteborg, Sweden)
Am J Obstet Gynecol 188:401-408, 2003   28–1

Background.—About 10% of women with postmenopausal bleeding
(PMB) are subsequently diagnosed with endometrial cancer; however, in
60% to 70% of these cases, no organic cause is identified. Both of the traditional methods for diagnosing endometrial cancer (dilation and curettage
and hysteroscopy) carry a small risk of morbidity. Some studies suggest that
transvaginal sonography (TVS) for noninvasive measurement of endometrial thickness (ET) is useful in diagnosing endometrial cancer, but those studies have been limited by relatively short follow-up. This study provides long-
term (10-year or greater) follow-up data from a cohort of women with PMB
who underwent TVS.

Methods.—The subjects were 394 women with PMB examined from November 1987 to October 1990. All patients underwent TVS to measure the
thickness of both endometrial layers; values were grouped as 4 mm or less, 5
to 7 mm, and 8 mm or greater. All patients also underwent dilation and curettage. The medical records of 339 patients (86%) at 10 or more years after
referral were examined to determine the development of endometrial cancer
(with or without atypical hyperplasia), PMB recurrence, and death.

Results.—During follow-up, 39 women (11%) were diagnosed with endometrial cancer, and 44 women (13%) were diagnosed with endometrial
cancer/atypical hyperplasia. Compared with women of the same age from
the general population of the same region, the relative risks for endometrial
cancer alone or with atypical hyperplasia were 63.9 and 72.1, respectively
(Table 1). None of the women with an ET of less than 4 mm was subsequently diagnosed with endometrial cancer. Compared with women with an
ET of 4 mm or less, the relative risk of endometrial cancer in women with an
ET of more than 4 mm was 44.5.

At an ET cutoff value of 4 mm or less, the sensitivity was 100%, specificity
was 60%, the positive predictive value was 25%, and the negative predictive
value was 100%. Among the 257 women who had an intact uterus, 15 patients (5.8%) developed endometrial cancer/atypical hyperplasia. Among
the 66 women with recurrent PMB during follow-up, 15 patients (22.7%)

TABLE 1.—Relative Risk for Endometrial Cancer Alone or Endometrial Cancer/Atypical Hyperplasia in Women With a Referral for Postmenopausal Bleeding, Grouped According to Endometrial Thickness at the Primary Assessment

Endometrial Thickness	No.	Endometrial Cancer			Endometrial Cancer/Atypical Hyperplasia		
		No.	RR (95% CI)	Mean RR (95% CI) for 5-7 and ≥8 mm and Unmeasurable	No.	RR (95% CI)	Mean RR (95% CI) for 5-7 and ≥8 mm and Unmeasurable
≤4 mm	178	0	1.0		2 (1.1%)	1.0	
5-7 mm	51	4 (7.8%)	14.0 (1.6-122.2)	44.5 (6.5-320.1)	4 (7.8%)	7.0 (1.3-37.0)	24.0 (5.9-97.4)
≥8 mm	105	35 (33.3%)	59.3 (8.2-426.8)		38 (36.2%)	32.2 (7.9-130.8)	
Unmeasurable	5	0	0		0	0	
Total	339	39 (11.5%)	63.9 (46.0-88.8)*		44 (13.0%)	72.1 (52.8-98.5)*	

Note: Figures are for 339 women.

Relative risk calculations were performed in comparison with women with an endometrial thickness of 4 mm or less. For the purposes of these calculations, the number of cases of endometrial cancer was increased arbitrarily from 0 to 1.

*Comparison with the risk of endometrial cancer for women of the same age from the general population in the same region of Sweden in which the yearly incidence is 60/100,000 women. The estimated number of cases during the same time period of this study (3 years) therefore would be 180/100,000 women (relative risk, 1.0).

Abbreviations: CI, Confidence interval; *RR,* relative risk.

(Reprinted by permission of the publisher from Gull B, Karlsson B, Milsom I, et al: Can ultrasound replace dilation and curettage? A longitudinal evaluation of postmenopausal bleeding and transvaginal sonographic measurement of the endometrium as predictors of endometrial cancer. *Am J Obstet Gynecol* 188:401-408. Copyright 2003 by Elsevier.)

had endometrial cancer/atypical hyperplasia. However, none of the women whose ET was 4 mm or less at the initial evaluation and who developed recurrent PMB was diagnosed with endometrial cancer/atypical hyperplasia. None of the 191 women without recurrent bleeding developed endometrial cancer/atypical hyperplasia.

Conclusion.—PMB is associated with a 64-fold increased risk of endometrial cancer. In particular, women with recurrent bleeding are at high risk for endometrial cancer/atypical hyperplasia, whereas risk is not increased in women who had no recurrent PMB. None of the women with an ET of 4 mm or less at the initial evaluation subsequently developed endometrial bleeding, even if they did develop recurrent PMB. Thus, TVS is an accurate tool for determining whether women with PMB require further workup to confirm endometrial cancer.

▶ The results of this large study provide additional data to indicate that sonographic measurement of the endometrial echo complex (EEC) should be performed in women with postmenopausal bleeding. In this study, an endometrial curettage was performed concurrently with the US examination. As has been reported in other studies, if the EEC was less than 4 mm thick, no patient had a diagnosis of endometrial cancer. It may not be necessary to perform an endometrial biopsy or curettage in women who experience postmenopausal bleeding and have an EEC ≤4 mm.

D. R. Mishell, Jr, MD

▶ As shown in this article, PMB confers a 60-fold increased risk for the development of endometrial cancer in a patient so afflicted. Tissue sampling of the endometrium in some form is required to rule out cancer. Yet some practitioners are reluctant to do tissue sampling and have turned to TVS measurement of the endometrium in an attempt to predict histology. This is one of the better studies and certainly one of the few that have shown long-term follow-up of patients whose postmenopausal endometrium has been evaluated by sonography. This is not to say that there is no role for sonographic measurement of ET; clearly, sonography can be helpful in patients who have recurrent bleeding after sampling, particularly those who are on hormone replacement therapy.

D. S. Miller, MD

Adequate Staging for Uterine Cancer Can Be Performed Through Pfannenstiel Incisions
Horowitz NS, Powell MA, Drescher CW, et al (Washington Univ, St Louis; Swedish Med Ctr, Seattle)
Gynecol Oncol 88:404-410, 2003   28–2

Background.—The most common approach for exposing the abdominal cavity during surgical staging of gynecologic disease is the vertical midline incision (ML). Recently, the Pfannenstiel incision (PI) has been suggested to provide adequate exposure for staging patients with cervical cancer. Whether the PI provides adequate exposure for patients with uterine cancer was examined.

Methods.—The subjects were 332 women with uterine cancer referred for adjuvant radiotherapy between June 1989 and June 1999. All patients underwent comprehensive surgical staging, 236 (72%) via an ML and 96 (28%) via a PI. Medical records were reviewed to compare operative and histologic findings and outcomes between the 2 groups.

Results.—The 2 groups were similar in terms of age, weight, stage, histologic findings, co-morbidities, and estimated blood loss. The PI was associated with a significantly greater mean number of total lymph nodes retrieved (21 vs 17) and with a comparable mean number of pelvic lymph nodes retrieved (14 vs 12). Para-aortic lymph nodes (PALNs) were slightly, but not significantly, more likely to be dissected in the ML group (72% vs 63%), but when PALNs were obtained, the mean yield was similar in the ML and PI groups (3 vs 4).

Patients in the PI group had significantly fewer intraoperative and postoperative complications (particularly vascular and gastrointestinal problems) than patients in the ML group (7, or 7% vs 32, or 14%). The mean operative time was significantly shorter in the PI group (106 vs 123 minutes), as was the median length of hospital stay (3.0 vs 4.0 days). Estimated 5-year disease-free survival was similar in the PI and ML groups (85% and 83%, respectively), as was estimated 5-year disease-specific survival (85% and 87%, respectively).

Among patients weighing more than 180 lb, the PI approach obtained significantly more total lymph nodes (mean, 23 vs 16) and pelvic lymph nodes (mean, 17 vs 11) than an ML. Although PALNs were sampled significantly more frequently with the ML approach (67% vs 56% of patients), when obtained, the mean PALN yield was similar in the ML and PI groups (4 and 5, respectively). There were also significantly fewer complications in this subgroup associated with the PI approach (1 complication, or 4% vs 7, or 12%).

Conclusion.—The PI can be safely used for comprehensive surgical staging of uterine cancer. Morbidity is lower with the PI, while mortality is the same as with an ML. Furthermore, the PI is associated with shorter operative time and a shorter hospital stay. These benefits suggest that a PI should be considered for surgical staging in appropriately selected patients with uterine cancer.

▶ When confronted with the title of this article, the first response is "Why would you want to?" However, it is always good to confront dogma from time to time and evaluate it critically. As the authors state, it has always been declared but never shown that a PI does not allow for adequate staging of endometrial cancer. This study shows that gynecologic oncologists can perform adequate staging through a PI, with no apparent disadvantage to the patient.

D. S. Miller, MD

Analysis of Survival After Laparoscopy in Women With Endometrial Carcinoma

Eltabbakh GH (Univ of Vermont, Burlington)
Cancer 95:1894-1901, 2002   28–3

Background.—It is unclear whether the laparoscopic surgical approach improves survival in women with endometrial cancer. This question was investigated in women with early-stage endometrial cancer, and the factors that affect survival were examined.

Methods.—The subjects were 186 patients (mean age, 62 years) with stage I endometrial cancer who underwent surgery between January 1996 and June 2001. Their medical records were reviewed to compare clinical, operative, and histologic features and outcomes between the 100 patients who underwent laparoscopy (median follow-up, 27 months) and the 86 patients who underwent laparotomy (median follow-up, 48 months).

Results.—The 2 groups were similar in age, parity, menopausal status, lymphadenectomy, surgical stage, tumor grade, histologic findings, and receipt of postoperative radiation therapy. Tumor recurred in 7 patients (7%) in the laparoscopy group and 9 patients (10%) in the laparotomy group. The site of the recurrence (distant vs local) did not differ significantly between the 2 groups.

The laparoscopy and laparotomy groups had similar estimated recurrence-free survival rates at 2 years (93% vs 94%, respectively) and at 5 years (90% vs 92%); they had similar overall survival rates at 2 years (98% vs 96%) and at 5 years (92% in both groups). Multivariate analyses identified 3 significant and independent predictors of poorer survival. They were advanced surgical stage, poorly differentiated tumors, and unfavorable histologic tumor subtype. However, the surgical approach was not a significant predictor of survival.

Conclusion.—Women with early-stage endometrial cancer who undergo laparoscopy appear to have the same short-term survival as women undergoing laparotomy. Survival appears to depend on surgical stage, tumor histology, and tumor grade.

▶ While we await the results of the Gynecologic Oncology Group randomized trial of laparoscopy versus open surgical staging for endometrial cancer, this study offers some comfort to the laparoscopist that even though the patients who received laparoscopy had a lower BMI than those who underwent laparotomy, the patients who were treated by laparoscopy did not appear to be at a survival disadvantage.

D. S. Miller, MD

Surgical Stage I Endometrial Cancer: Predictors of Distant Failure and Death

Mariani A, Webb MJ, Keeney GL, et al (Mayo Clinic, Rochester, Minn)
Gynecol Oncol 87:274-280, 2002   28–4

Background.—Patients with endometrial adenocarcinoma who are considered at high risk for recurrence or death are often offered adjuvant radiotherapy. Patients whose disease is confined to the uterus, however, may not need radiotherapy because most local recurrences can be treated successfully at the time of failure. In an effort to identify which patients with stage I endometrial cancer would benefit from adjuvant radiation, the predictors of distant failure and death in this population were examined.

Methods.—The subjects were 229 women (mean age, 64 years) with stage I epithelial (all subtypes) endometrial cancer. All patients underwent hysterectomy and lymph node dissection, and in all cases tumor was histologically confined to the uterine corpus. If histologic examination of pelvic lymph nodes showed no disease, para-aortic node dissection was often not performed. Additionally, 67 patients (29%) received adjuvant radiotherapy. For statistical analyses, histologic grade 1 and 2 tumors were combined and compared with histologic grade 3 tumors, and endometrial and adenosquamous tumors were combined and compared with serous, clear cell, mucinous, and undifferentiated tumors. Patients were followed up for a median of 83 months to determine predictors of distant failure and death.

Results.—During follow-up, disease recurred in 22 patients (10%); there were 14 (6%) distant failures, 7 (3%) isolated vaginal recurrences, and 1 (0.4%) simultaneous recurrences at distant and regional sites. Of the 7 patients with isolated vaginal recurrence, only 1 (14%) died of disease; in contrast, 10 of the 15 patients with distant recurrence (67%) died of disease. The 5-year disease-related survival rate was 95%, and 5-year relapse-free survival rate was 91%.

By univariate analysis, significant predictors of a poor prognosis with distant failure included myometrial invasion of 66% or greater, nonendometroid histologic findings, lymphovascular invasion, an absence of associated hyperplasia, and a tumor of 2 cm in diameter or greater. By multivariate analysis, only myometrial invasion of 66% or greater was a significant and independent predictor of an increased risk of poor disease-related survival (relative risk, 12.44), poor relapse-free survival (relative risk, 8.67), and distant failure (relative risk, 24.89). In fact, during 5 years of follow-up, only 2 of 195 patients (1%) with myometrial invasion of less than 66% developed distant failure and died; in contrast, 29 of 33 patients (88%) with myometrial invasion of 66% or greater developed distant failure, and 22 patients (67%) died of disease.

Conclusion.—Myometrial invasion of 66% or greater is the strongest predictor of distant failure and death in patients with stage I (node-negative) endometrial cancer. Deep myometrial invasion (present in 33 patients) was a stronger predictor of poor outcome than a nonendometroid histologic subtype (present in 13 patients). Thus, for patients whose tumor is confined to the uterine corpus, myometrial invasion appears to be the more important predictor of occult distant dissemination. Patients with deep endometrial invasion should have further study to determine the role of adjuvant systemic therapy in preventing distant failure and death.

▶ As have multiple other recent articles,[1-3] this study calls into question the role of adjuvant radiation therapy for surgical stage I endometrial carcinomas. In the authors' experience, myometrial invasion was the most significant predictor of recurrence. The strength of this study was its relatively long-term follow-up. As stated by the authors, if there is a role for adjuvant radiation therapy for surgical stage I endometrial cancer, it is in patients who have deep myometrial invasion, and it is in this group that further radiation trials should be conducted.

D. S. Miller, MD

References

1. 2003 YEAR BOOK OF OBSTETRICS, GYNECOLOGY, AND WOMEN'S HEALTH, pp 468-470. (Straughn JM Jr, Hugh WK, Kelly FJ, et al: Conservative management of stage I endometrial carcinoma after surgical staging. *Gynecol Oncol* 84:194-200, 2002)
2. 2003 YEAR BOOK OF OBSTETRICS, GYNECOLOGY, AND WOMEN'S HEALTH, pp 470-471. (Creutzberg CL, for the PORTEC Study Group: The morbidity of treatment for patients with stage I endometrial cancer: Results from a randomized trial. *Int J Radiat Oncol Biol Phys* 51:1246-1255, 2001)
3. 2001 YEAR BOOK OF OBSTETRICS, GYNECOLOGY, AND WOMEN'S HEALTH, pp 475-476. (Creutzberg CL, for the PORTEC Study Group: Surgery and postoperative radiotherapy versus surgery alone for patients with stage-1 endometrial carcinoma: Multicentre randomised trial. *Lancet* 355:1404-1411, 2000)

Assessment of Prognostic Factors in Stage IIIA Endometrial Cancer
Mariani A, Webb MJ, Keeney GL, et al (Mayo Clinic, Rochester, Minn; Univ of Milano, Milan, Italy)
Gynecol Oncol 86:38-44, 2002   28–5

Introduction.—The prognostic significance of positive results of peritoneal cytology, adnexal spread, and uterine serosal involvement is under debate regarding patients with International Federation of Obstetricians and Gynecologists stage IIIA cancer. The prognostic factors in stage IIIA endometrial cancer were examined.

Methods.—Between 1984 and 1993, 51 patients with stage IIIA endometrial cancer underwent definitive treatment. The authors designated 37 who had positive peritoneal cytologic findings only as stage IIIA1 and 14 who had adnexal or uterine serosal involvement as stage IIIA2. The median patient follow-up was 82.5 months.

Results.—The 5-year disease-related survival (DRS) was 88%. Recurrence-free survival was 73% (79% in patients with stage IIIA1 disease and 57% in patients with stage IIIA2 disease; $P = .04$). The DRS did not significantly vary between stage IIIA1 and IIIA2. In the 37 patients who had stage

IIIA1 tumors, histologic grade 3, nonendometrioid histologic subtype, and lymphovascular invasion (LVI) were significantly predictive of a poor prognosis, with extra-abdominal sites of failure ($P < .05$). There was no recurrent disease in 22 patients with stage IIIA1 disease with endometrial histologic subtype and without LVI (17 patients underwent whole abdominal irradiation or intraperitoneal injection of ^{32}P and 2 had pelvic external radiotherapy).

Of 15 patients with either nonendometrioid histologic subtype or LVI, 9 (60%) had recurrent disease and 7 (47%) died of disease (12 had whole abdominal irradiation or ^{32}P). An extra-abdominal component was observed in 7 of 9 recurrences in this subgroup. Among 14 patients with stage IIIA2 tumors (6 had whole abdominal irradiation, 6 had pelvic external radiotherapy), those who had uterine serosal involvement had a 5-year DRS of 83% and a rate of extra-abdominal failure of 83% versus 100% and 12.5%, respectively, in patients without uterine serosal involvement ($P < .05$).

Conclusion.—The prognosis is excellent for patients with stage IIIA endometrial cancer with endometrioid tumors, no LVI, and positive peritoneal cytologic findings as the only sign of extrauterine disease. Nonendometrioid histologic subtypes, LVI, and uterine serosal involvement are strongly predictive of distant failures and poor prognosis. Patients with either of these histologic factors need to be considered for systemic adjuvant therapy.

▶ International Federation of Gynecology and Obstetrics Stage IIIA carcinoma of the endometrium encompasses disparate pathologic findings including malignant peritoneal cytology, involvement of the uterine serosa, and/or involvement of the adnexa. Previous studies have also shown that positive peritoneal cytology is a significant predictor of bad outcome only in patients who have other signs of extra-uterine disease.[1] This study, too, shows that involvement of lymph vascular spaces portends a worse prognosis. However, not all patients were surgically staged, so this may really be a surrogate marker for patients with undetected metastasis to their pelvic or periaortic lymph nodes. While these patients may be lumped together in stage IIIA, treatment decisions should be determined by the actual pathologic findings. The best treatment for those various findings remains to be determined.[2]

D. S. Miller, MD

References

1. Lurain JR, Rumsey NK, Schink JC, et al: Prognostic significance of positive peritoneal cytology in clinical stage I adenocarcinoma of the endometrium. *Obstet Gynecol* 74:175, 1989.
2. Schorge JO, Molpus KL, Goodman A, et al: The effect of postsurgical therapy on stage III endometrial carcinoma. *Gynecol Oncol* 63:34, 1996.

FIGO Stage III and IV Uterine Papillary Serous Carcinoma: Impact of Residual Disease on Survival

Memarzadeh S, Holschneider CH, Bristow RE, et al (Univ of California, Los Angeles; Cedars-Sinai Med Ctrs, Los Angeles; Northridge Hosp, Calif; et al)
Int J Gynecol Cancer 12:454-458, 2002   28–6

Background.—Uterine papillary serous carcinoma (UPSC) is a type of endometrial carcinoma whose disease course is similar to that of papillary serous adenocarcinoma of the ovary. The extent of residual disease after primary surgical cytoreduction is an important determinant of survival for patients with ovarian cancer. Whether the extent of residual disease after primary surgical cytoreduction influences survival in patients with advanced UPSC was investigated.

Methods.—The subjects were 43 women (median age at diagnosis, 70 years) with International Federation of Gynecology and Obstetrics (FIGO) stage III or IV UPSC who underwent primary surgical cytoreduction between January 1980 and September 2001. Their medical records were reviewed to determine clinical factors, disease status, and overall and disease-free survival over a median follow-up of 20 months (range, 2-156 months).

Results.—The presenting signs and symptoms in these patients with advanced UPSC were similar to those seen in endometrial cancer, but the patterns of metastasis were similar to those seen in primary ovarian papillary serous carcinoma. All patients had extra-uterine disease at staging; disease was microscopic in 18 patients (42%) and macroscopic in 25 patients

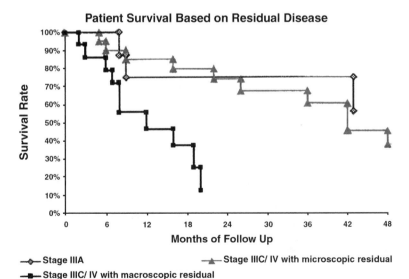

FIGURE 1.—Patient survival based on extent of residual disease following primary cytoreductive surgery. (Courtesy of Memarzadeh S, Holschneider CH, Bristow RE, et al: FIGO stage III and IV uterine papillary serous carcinoma: Impact of residual disease on survival. *Int J Gynecol Cancer* 12: 454-458, 2002. Reprinted by permission of Blackwell Publishing.)

(58%). Survival and recurrence rates were also similar to those seen in papillary serous adenocarcinoma of the ovary.

Median overall survival was significantly worse in the 15 patients with macroscopic residual disease after primary surgical cytoreduction than in the 20 patients with microscopic residual disease (10 vs 40 months) (Fig 1). However, median overall survival in the latter group was similar to that in the 8 patients with stage IIIA disease (ie, preoperative microscopic disease; median survival, 43 months). Disease-free survival was also significantly less in the patients with macroscopic residual disease than in those with microscopic residual disease or microscopic preoperative disease (8 vs 22 and 24 months, respectively).

Conclusion.—Among patients with advanced UPSC, the extent of residual disease after primary surgical cytoreduction is significantly associated with survival. Thus, maximal resection of tumor at the primary surgical staging is recommended for these patients.

▶ Most gynecologic oncologists regard UPSC as a distinct entity of uterine adenocarcinomas, the biology of which more closely resembles that of ovarian cancer than endometrial carcinoma. This retrospective study confirms that impression and a previous work showing that surgical debulking to minimal residual disease improves survival.[1] As no randomized, controlled study has ever shown that tumor debulking in ovarian cancer, much less UPSC, makes a difference, it is incumbent upon the authors to show that their intervention had an impact and that they were not merely illustrating tumor biology. As shown in Figure 1, the survival of patients with gross upper abdominal disease that was resected to minimal residual closely tracked the survival of patients in whom only microscopic disease was found. Thus, a compelling case is made for patients with gross intra-abdominal spread of UPSC to have an attempt at aggressive surgical debulking.

D. S. Miller, MD

Reference

1. Bristow RE, Duska LR, Montz FJ: The role of cytoreductive surgery in the management of stage IV uterine papillary serous carcinoma. *Gynecol Oncol* 81:92, 2001.

Adjuvant Endocrine Treatment With Medroxyprogesterone Acetate or Tamoxifen in Stage I and II Endometrial Cancer—A Multicentre, Open, Controlled, Prospectively Randomised Trial

Kaufmann M, for the South West German Gynecologic Oncology Group (SWGGOG) (Johann Wolfgang Goethe-Universität, Frankfurt/Main, Germany; et al)

Eur J Cancer 38:2265-2271, 2002 28–7

Background.—Previous studies suggest that medroxyprogesterone acetate (MPA) and tamoxifen each improves survival in patients with recurrent endometrial cancer. Whether adjunct MPA or tamoxifen can improve outcomes in patients with early-stage endometrial cancer was examined.

Methods.—The subjects were 388 patients with stage I or II endometrial cancer who underwent abdominal hysterectomy, bilateral salpingo-oophorectomy, and partial colpectomy between April 1983 and October 1989. Patients were randomly assigned to receive 2 years of MPA (133 patients), tamoxifen (121 patients), or observation (134 patients) after surgery. Recurrences, overall survival, and adverse events were compared among the 3 groups.

Results.—During a median follow-up of 56 months, there were 22 local recurrences, 30 distant recurrences, and 32 deaths due to disease. The proportion of patients with recurrence did not differ significantly between the MPA, tamoxifen, and observation groups (10%, 8%, and 11%, respectively). Overall survivals were also similar in the MPA, tamoxifen, and observation groups (66%, 70%, and 66%, respectively). After randomization, 19 patients were diagnosed with second primary tumors. Only 2 second primary tumors were found in the tamoxifen group, compared with 9 tumors in the MPA group and 8 tumors in the observation group.

Adverse events were slightly more common with MPA than with tamoxifen or observation (59%, 49%, and 40%, respectively). Among the 28 patients who dropped out of the study, toxicity was much more common with MPA than with tamoxifen (15 vs 2 withdrawals).

Conclusion.—For patients with early-stage endometrial cancer, adjuvant treatment with MPA or tamoxifen does not prevent recurrence or prolong survival. However, tamoxifen may prevent second primary tumors, and this may have a modest effect on survival.

▶ Even though adenocarcinoma of the endometrium is thought to be caused by unopposed estrogen, we have been very disappointed by the fact that various hormonal therapies have yielded unimpressive results for the treatment of these cancers. Similarly, hormonal agents thought to induce the cancer, like tamoxifen, seem to have little negative or positive impact on recurrence of endometrial cancer. Unfortunately, there appears to be a lack of thorough statistical analysis, as it is implied that there were fewer adverse events, including secondary cancers, in the tamoxifen arm. However, no statistical analysis of those events are provided, so we cannot determine if they are significant.

D. S. Miller, MD

Stage IC Adenocarcinoma of the Endometrium: Survival Comparisons of Surgically Staged Patients With and Without Adjuvant Radiation Therapy

Straughn JM Jr, Huh WK, Orr JW Jr, et al (Univ of Alabama at Birmingham; Florida Gynecologic Oncology, Fort Myers; Univ of Oklahoma, Oklahoma City; et al)

Gynecol Oncol 89:295-300, 2003   28–8

Background.—The role of adjuvant radiation therapy for surgically staged patients with adenocarcinoma of the endometrium is controversial. Outcomes for surgically staged patients with stage IC endometrial cancer who were managed with adjuvant radiation therapy were compared with those of patients who did not receive adjuvant radiation.

Methods.—The subjects were 220 women with stage IC adenocarcinoma of the endometrium who underwent comprehensive surgical staging (including total hysterectomy, bilateral salpingo-oophorectomy, pelvic/para-aortic lymphadenectomy, and peritoneal cytology) between 1988 and 1999. None of the patients had high-risk histologic subtypes, nonepithelial uterine tumors, or previous radiation therapy. Their medical records were examined to identify differences in recurrences, disease-free survival, and overall survival between the patients who did and did not receive adjuvant radiation therapy.

Results.—Of the 220 patients, 121 (55%) did not receive adjuvant radiation, while 56 (25%) received adjuvant brachytherapy, 19 (9%) received whole-pelvis radiation, and 24 (11%) received both types of radiation therapy. The incidence of recurrence did not differ significantly between the patients who received radiation therapy (6 of 99, or 6%; mean follow-up, 53 months) and those who did not (14 of 121, or 12%; mean follow-up, 30 months). Five of the 6 patients in the radiation group who had recurrence had distant recurrence, and all 6 died. Among the 14 patients with recurrence who did not receive radiation therapy, 7 had local recurrence and 7 had distal recurrence.

All 7 patients with local recurrence were salvaged with radiation therapy, and 2 of the patients with distant recurrence were salvaged with surgery and chemotherapy. The overall salvage rate in the patients who did not receive adjuvant radiation was 64%; the mean follow-up after salvage therapy was 30 months. The 5-year disease-free survival rate was significantly better in the patients who received adjuvant radiation (93% vs 75%). However, 5-year overall survival was similar in the patients who did and did not receive adjuvant radiation (92% vs 90%) (Fig 1).

Conclusion.—In patients with stage IC adenocarcinoma of the endometrium who have undergone comprehensive surgical staging, adjuvant radiation therapy improves disease-free survival. However, adjuvant radiation does not improve overall survival, as most local recurrences in the patients who did not receive adjuvant radiation could be salvaged with radiation therapy. Given the low incidence of recurrence and the success rate of salvage therapy, it seems reasonable to avoid the costs and risks of ad-

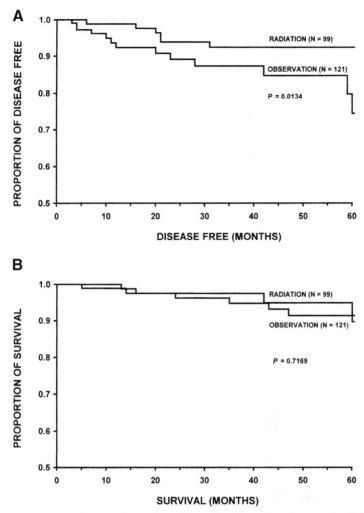

FIGURE 1.—Disease-free survival (**A**) and overall survival (**B**) of stage IC patients treated with observation versus adjuvant radiation. (Reprinted by permission of the publisher from Straughn JM Jr, Huh WK, Orr JW Jr, et al: Stage IC adenocarcinoma of the endometrium: Survival comparisons of surgically staged patients with and without adjuvant radiation therapy. *Gynecol Oncol* 89:295-300. Copyright 2003 by Elsevier.)

juvant radiation therapy for surgically staged patients with stage IC endometrial cancer.

▶ This article is another in a series published over the last several years calling into question routine use of adjuvant radiation therapy in patients with uterine adenocarcinomas confined to the uterus. While the recurrence rate in the patients who did not receive external radiation of some sort was higher, most of those patients could be salvaged, particularly if they were pelvic recurrences, thus allowing for near identical survival in the radiated and unradiated groups (see Fig 1). The reader should note that patients with the so-called high-risk histologies, papillary serous and clear cell, were excluded but hopefully will be the topic for further publication by this group.

D. S. Miller, MD

Survival After Relapse in Patients With Endometrial Cancer: Results From a Randomized Trial

Creutzberg CL, for the PORTEC Study Group (Erasmus MC-Daniel den Hoed Cancer Ctr, Rotterdam, The Netherlands; et al)
Gynecol Oncol 89:201-209, 2003   28–9

Introduction.—The PORTEC trial was a randomized, multicenter trial in which the vaginal, pelvic, and distant relapse rates after postoperative radiotherapy compared with no further treatment for stage I endometrial cancer were examined. Reported are the PORTEC rates of local control and survival after relapse in patients with stage I endometrial cancer.

Methods.—The 715 patients in the PORTEC trial had stage 1 endometrial cancer, either grade 1 or 2 with deep (>50%) myometrial invasion or grade 2 or 3 with <50% invasion. All patients underwent abdominal hysterectomy without lymphadenectomy. Postoperatively, patients were randomly assigned to receive either pelvic radiotherapy at 46 Gy or no further treatment (control subjects).

Results.—A total of 714 patients were evaluated with an intention-to-treat analysis. At a median follow-up of 72 months, the 8-year actuarial locoregional recurrence rates were 4% and 15%, respectively, for the radiotherapy and control groups ($P < .0001$). The 8-year actuarial overall survival rates were 71% for the radiotherapy group and 77% for the control group ($P < .0001$). The 8-year rates for distant metastases were 10% and 6%, respectively ($P = .20$). Most of the locoregional relapses occurred in the vagina, primarily the vaginal vault. Of 39 patients who had isolated vaginal relapse, 35 (87%) were treated with curative intent and 24 (77%) remained in complete remission at further follow-up. Five patients subsequently had distant metastases develop; 2 had a second vaginal recurrence. The 3-year survival rate after the first relapse was 51% for control subjects and 19% for the radiotherapy group ($P = .004$) (Fig 1). The 3-year survival rate after vaginal relapse was 73% compared with 8% for pelvic relapse and 14% after distant relapse ($P < .001$). At 5-year follow-up, the survival after vaginal relapse was 65% for control subjects and 43% for the radiotherapy group.

Conclusion.—Survival after relapse in patients with endometrial cancer was significantly better in patients with no previous radiotherapy compared with those who received radiotherapy. Treatment for vaginal relapse was effective (89%, complete response and 65% 5-year survival in control subjects). There were no significant between-group differences in patients with pelvic relapse compared with those with distant metastases. Pelvic radiotherapy improved locoregional control significantly, yet without a survival

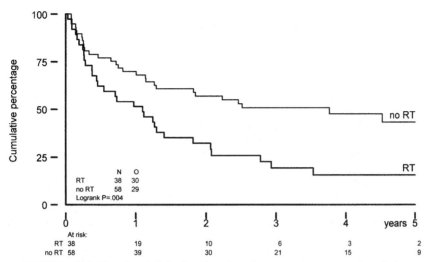

FIGURE 1.—Probability of survival after first relapse for patients assigned to postoperative radiotherapy (*RT*) or no further treatment (*no RT*). (Reprinted by permission of the publisher from Creutzberg CL, for the PORTEC Study Group: Survival after relapse in patients with endometrial cancer: Results from a randomized trial. *Gynecol Oncol* 89:201-209. Copyright 2003 by Elsevier Science.)

benefit. The use of radiotherapy should be restricted to patients at high risk to maximize local control and relapse-free survival.

▶ This is further follow-up of the PORTEC study for which prior publications have been discussed in previous editions of the YEAR BOOK.[1,2] For decades we have been recommending to certain groups of patients with endometrial cancer confined to the uterus that they receive pelvic radiation of some sort even though their risk of recurrence may be less than 10%. This was based on the assumption that a vaginal recurrence of endometrial cancer was untreatable. The authors show that a vaginal recurrence is untreatable in the patient who had been previously radiated. It appears to be quite treatable in the unradiated patient. While the likelihood of recurrence in the patients who were in the control arm and received no adjuvant radiation therapy was higher, very interestingly, their survival was better. I suspect that the survival advantage seen in the control patients was probably due to the late effects of radiation given to the patients who didn't really need it.

D. S. Miller, MD

References

1. 2003 YEAR BOOK OF OBSTETRICS, GYNECOLOGY, AND WOMEN'S HEALTH, p 470. (Creutzberg CL, for the PORTEC Study Group: The morbidity of treatment for patients with stage I endometrial cancer: Results from a randomized trial. *Int J Radiat Oncol Biol Phys* 51:1246-1255, 2001)
2. 2001 YEAR BOOK OF OBSTETRICS, GYNECOLOGY AND WOMEN'S HEALTH, p 475. (Creutzberg CL, for the PORTEC Study Group: Surgery and postoperative radiotherapy versus surgery alone for patients with stage-1 endometrial carcinoma: Multicentre randomized trial. *Lancet* 355:1404-1411, 2000)

Activity of Paclitaxel as Second-Line Chemotherapy in Endometrial Carcinoma: A Gynecologic Oncology Group Study

Lincoln S, Blessing JA, Lee RB, et al (Rush Med College, Chicago; Roswell Park Cancer Inst, Buffalo, NY; Univ of Washington, Seattle; et al)
Gynecol Oncol 88:277-281, 2003   28–10

Background.—The number of chemotherapeutic agents effective in advanced or recurrent adenocarcinoma of the endometrium is limited. A previous phase II trial showed that paclitaxel was effective in patients with advanced or recurrent disease who were naive to chemotherapy. Whether paclitaxel is effective for patients with advanced or recurrent disease who have already been exposed to chemotherapy was examined.

Methods.—The subjects were 50 women with persistent or recurrent adenocarcinoma of the endometrium. All patients had previously received chemotherapy (mainly doxorubicin/platinum–based therapy), and 20 patients had previously received radiotherapy. Paclitaxel was infused over 3 hours at an initial dose of 200 mg/m^2 (or 175 mg/m^2 for patients with prior pelvic radiation) every 21 days. Subsequent courses were not administered until the patient had recovered fully from any nonhematologic toxicity, the granulocyte count was more than 1500 cells/μL, and the platelet count was more than 100,000 cells/μL. Doses were modified based on nadir toxicity (both hematologic and nonhematologic) and adjusted to 200, 175, 135, or 110 mg/m^2.

Results.—Of the 50 patients, 2 were ineligible due to protocol, 3 withdrew from the study (1 developed congestive heart failure, 1 developed bleeding not related to hematologic toxicity, and 1 refused further treatment), and 1 died of toxicity. Of the 44 patients in whom response could be evaluated, 3 (6.8%) had a complete response and 9 (20.5%) had a partial response; thus, the overall response rate was 27.3%. Responders required a median of 2 courses of paclitaxel to respond (range, 1-4 courses), and their response lasted for a median of 4.2 months. Four of the 12 responders had received prior radiation. Median overall survival was 10.3 months.

Of the 48 patients in whom toxicity could be evaluated, 28 (58.3%) had at least 1 episode of grade 3 or 4 neutropenia, and 4 (8.3%) developed grade 3 neurotoxicity. Three patients (6.3%) had grade 3 or 4 gastrointestinal symptoms, but only 1 patient had cardiac toxicity (grade 1). The 1 treatment-related death referred to above occurred in a 73-year-old patient who had undergone extensive surgery for endometrial cancer. About 1 week after her initial paclitaxel treatment, she developed weakness, thrombocytopenia, and febrile neutropenia. Despite resuscitation efforts, she died on day 11.

Conclusion.—Paclitaxel is effective for treating advanced or recurrent endometrial cancer in patients who have had prior chemotherapy. Studies are currently underway to determine the most effective starting dose of paclitaxel and to better define its role in endometrial cancer treatment.

▶ No cytotoxic chemotherapeutic agent is yet approved by the FDA for the treatment of endometrial carcinoma. Previous studies have shown cisplatin, doxorubicin, and ifosfamide to be active agents. Paclitaxel was added to that list on the basis of this study. Paclitaxel has now been combined with the other active agents and evaluated by the Gynecologic Oncology Group in a randomized trial.[1]

D. S. Miller, MD

Reference

1. Fleming GF, Brunetto V, Mundt AJ, et al: Randomized trial of doxorubicin (DOX) plus cisplatin (CIS) versus DOX plus CIS plus paclitaxel (TAX) in patients with advanced or recurrent endometrial carcinoma: A Gynecologic Oncology Group (GOG) study (abstract). Proc ASCO 21:202a, 2002.

29 Mullerian Cancers

Serologic Evidence of Past Infection With *Chlamydia trachomatis*, in Relation to Ovarian Cancer
Ness RB, Goodman MT, Shen C, et al (Univ of Pittsburgh, Pa; Univ of Hawaii, Manoa; Univ of British Columbia, Vancouver, Canada)
J Infect Dis 187:1147-1152, 2003   29–1

Introduction.—Pelvic inflammation may have a role in the development of ovarian cancer. Inflammation involves DNA damage and repair, oxidative stress, and elevation of cytokines and prostaglandins; all of these processes are mutagenic. Pilot data from a population-based case-control trial was used to determine whether immunoglobulin (Ig) G antibodies to *Chlamydia trachomatis*, chlamydial heat shock protein (CHSP) 60, and CHSP10 are linked with an elevated risk of ovarian cancer.

Findings.—Antibodies to *Chlamydia trachomatis*, CHSP60, and CHSP10 were examined in 117 women with ovarian cancer and in 171 age- and ethnicity-matched population-based control subjects. IgG antibodies to serovar D of *Chlamydia* elementary bodies and IgG antibodies to CHSP60-1, CHSP60-2, CHSP60-3, and CHSP10 were identified by an enzyme-linked immunosorbent assay. The probability of having ovarian cancer was 90% higher in women with the highest versus the lowest (optical density, 0.40 or greater vs less than 0.10) levels of *Chlamydia*–elementary bodies antibodies ($P = .05$). There was a monotonic trend ($P = .09$) in ovarian cancer risk linked with CHSP60-1 but not with CHSP60-2, CHSP60-3, or CHSP10.

Conclusion.—Past or chronic persistent infection with *Chlamydia* (the most common cause of pelvic inflammatory disease) and CHSP60-1 (a marker of chronic upper genital tract infection) may be risk factors for ovarian cancer.

▶ It has been more than 30 years since Fathalla articulated our overarching theory of ovarian carcinogenesis: incessant ovulation.[1] However, that theory did not completely explain the ameliorating effect seen with tubal ligations, since that procedure should allow continued ovulation. One can certainly infer from this study and others that have implicated inflammation as a factor in ovarian carcinogenesis that the protective effect from tubal ligation comes not from visualizing the ovaries for a brief period of time but, in fact, comes from obstructing the fallopian tube and presumably preventing ascending infection. Whether *Chlamydia* is necessary or sufficient in this pathophysiology—or whether anything else that causes ovarian inflammation such as endometriosis could also be the culprit—remains to be determined.

D. S. Miller, MD

Reference

1. Fathalla MF: Incessant ovulation—A factor in ovarian neoplasia? *Lancet* 2:163, 1971.

Gynecologic Surgeries and Risk of Ovarian Cancer in Women With BRCA1 and BRCA2 Ashkenazi Founder Mutations: An Israeli Population-Based Case–Control Study

Rutter JL, Wacholder S, Chetrit A, et al (NIH, Bethesda, Md; Chaim Sheba Med Ctr, Tel-Hashomer, Israel; Edith Wolfson Med Ctr, Holon, Israel)

J Natl Cancer Inst 95:1072-1078, 2003   29–2

Background.—There are few preventive or screening options for ovarian cancer, which has the highest case fatality rate of all gynecologic cancers. A family history of ovarian cancer is a strong predictor for development of ovarian cancer and is often indicative of a pathogenic mutation in one breast and ovarian cancer susceptibility genes, *BRCA1* and *BRCA2*. Among the general population, the risk of developing ovarian cancer is reduced in women who have undergone tubal ligation, hysterectomy, or oophorectomy, although peritoneal cancer may develop after bilateral oophorectomy. However, studies performed in genetic screening clinics have reported that women with mutations in the breast and the *BRCA1* and *BRCA2* genes have been found to have a low risk of peritoneal carcinoma after bilateral oophorectomy. This study assessed the level and persistence of reduction of ovarian cancer risk (including the risk of peritoneal cancer) after gynecologic surgery in women who are carriers of the BRCA1/BRCA2 mutations but were not selected from high-risk clinics.

Methods.—A total of 1124 Israeli women with incident ovarian cancer or primary peritoneal cancer were identified, and 847 of these women were tested for the 3 Ashkenazi founder mutations. Gynecologic surgery history was compared among all the case patients, 187 BRCA1 patients and 64 BRCA2 carrier patients, and the 598 noncarrier patients and with the history of 2936 control subjects identified from a population registry. Logistic regression modeling (odds ratio and 95% confidence interval) was used to estimate ovarian cancer risks after gynecologic surgery in mutation carriers and noncarriers.

Results.—A previous bilateral oophorectomy was reported by 8 women with primary peritoneal cancer and 128 control subjects (odds ratio, 0.12; 95% confidence interval, 0.06-0.24). Other gynecologic surgeries were associated with a 30% to 50% reduced risk of ovarian cancer, depending on the type of surgery. Surgery to remove some ovarian tissue was associated with the greatest risk reduction. Reductions in risk were observed in both

BRCA1/BRCA2 carriers and noncarriers. Age of the patient at surgery and the years since surgery did not affect risk reduction.

Conclusions.—The risk of ovarian or peritoneal cancer is reduced in both BRCA1/BRCA2 mutation carriers and noncarriers after gynecologic surgery. The magnitude of the risk reduction depends on the type and extent of surgery.

▶ As discussed in previous editions of the YEAR BOOK, intraoperative observation, partial resection, or complete resection of the ovaries appears to decrease the risk of subsequent ovarian, fallopian tube, or primary peritoneal cancers in patients with or without BRCA mutations.[1,2] This study nicely quantifies the impact of each of these operative maneuvers. The clinical implications of this remain unclear except perhaps to reassure patients who have had previous less-than-complete resection of the ovaries. Nonetheless, these studies need to be viewed carefully as they could be biased in that patients who perceive themselves to be at increased risk may be more willing to submit themselves to such operations and thus the apparent advantage.[3]

D. S. Miller, MD

References

1. Rebbeck TR: Prophylactic oophorectomy in carriers of BRCA1 or BRCA2 mutations. *N Engl J Med* 346:1616, 2002. (2003 YEAR BOOK OF OBSTETRICS, GYNECOLOGY, AND WOMEN'S HEALTH, p 448.)
2. Kauff ND, Satagopan JM, Robson ME, et al: Risk-reducing salpingo-oophorectomy in women with a BRCA1 or BRCA2 mutation. *N Engl J Med* 346:1609, 2002. (2003 YEAR BOOK OF OBSTETRICS, GYNECOLOGY, AND WOMEN'S HEALTH, p 447.)
3. Klaren HM, van'tVeer LJ, Van Leeuwen FE, et al: Potential for bias in studies on efficacy of prophylactic surgery for BRCA1 and BRCA2 mutations. *J Natl Cancer Inst* 95:941, 2003.

Peritoneal Lavage Cytology: An Assessment of Its Value During Prophylactic Oophorectomy

Colgan TJ, Boerner SL, Murphy J, et al (Mount Sinai Hosp, Toronto; Univ of Toronto)
Gynecol Oncol 85:397-403, 2002   29–3

Background.—Prophylactic oophorectomy (PO) is an accepted strategy for the treatment of women with a genetic predisposition to ovarian carcinoma. PO significantly reduces the risk of development of ovarian cancer in these women and also leads to the diagnosis of early-stage carcinomas that may be curable. Peritoneal cytology is an established technique for detection of malignant cells in both endometrial and ovarian carcinoma. The value of peritoneal cytology at the time of PO, if any, has not been established despite recommendations for its use. The primary purpose of lavage at the time of PO is to detect occult primary peritoneal carcinoma. The utility of peritoneal cytology at the time of PO for detection of occult malignancy was assessed for patients who are BRCA-mutation positive.

Methods.—The study group comprised 35 high-risk women not suspected of having any malignancy or ovarian mass. All of these patients underwent peritoneal lavage at the time of PO. BRCA mutation analysis had been performed in 31 of the women. Intensive histopathologic examination was used to identify occult carcinoma in all 35 patients. Lavage specimens were reviewed for the presence of malignant cells and endosalpingiosis. The cytologic review was conducted with no awareness of either the histopathologic or BRCA results.

Results.—No malignancy was detected in 32 of 35 lavage specimens. In the remaining 3 cases, malignant cells were detected. Histopathologic examination confirmed an ovarian/tubal occult carcinoma in 2 of these patients. Two of the 3 women with malignant cells were BRCA1-mutation positive. Endosalpingiosis was detected in the peritoneal lavage specimens of 7 of the 32 women with no evidence of malignancy. All 7 women were BRCA-mutation positive or unknown.

Conclusion.—Peritoneal lavage cytology should be performed at PO to detect occult carcinoma. The significance of occult carcinoma detected by either histopathologic or cytopathologic examination is unclear. Further study is required to determine whether the prevalence of endosalpingiosis detectable by lavage cytology is increased in BRCA mutation–positive patients.

▶ Over the last few years, we have recommended to women at high risk for ovarian cancer that they consider and undergo PO. Thus, we should not be surprised that for a small number of patients we were "just in time" or "a little too late" and an occult carcinoma was found. The interesting thing about this study is not that the peritoneal cytology was positive but that the fallopian tubes seemed to be the frequent source of interesting pathology. Since we often have a difficult time discriminating advanced fallopian tube from ovarian cancer, could the fallopian tube be the source of many of these malignancies, especially those related to BRCA1?

D. S. Miller, MD

Gene Expression Profiles of BRCA1-Linked, BRCA2-Linked, and Sporadic Ovarian Cancers
Jazaeri AA, Yee CJ, Sotiriou C, et al (Natl Cancer Inst, Gaithersburg, Md; Mem Sloan-Kettering Cancer Ctr, New York)
J Natl Cancer Inst 94:990-1000, 2002   29–4

Background.—Germline mutations in BRCA1 and BRCA2 account for 5% to 10% of epithelial cancers. However, the molecular pathways affected by these mutations are unknown. Complementary DNA (cDNA) microarrays were used to compare gene expression patterns in ovarian cancers associated with BRCA1 or BRCA2 mutations with gene expression patterns in sporadic epithelial ovarian cancers and sporadic tumors.

Methods.—Tumor samples were obtained from 61 patients with pathologically confirmed epithelial ovarian adenocarcinoma with matched clinicopathologic features. These samples included 18 with BRCA1 founder mutations, 16 with BRCA2 founder mutations, and 27 samples with neither founder mutation (termed sporadic cancers). The cDNA microarrays contained 7651 sequence-verified features. Gene expression data for these samples were analyzed with a modified 2-sided F test, with $P < .0001$ considered statistically significant. Reverse transcription–polymerase chain reaction was used to study the expression level of 6 genes.

Results.—The greatest contrast in gene expression was between tumors with BRCA1 mutations and tumors with BRCA2 mutations. Overall, 110 genes showed statistically significantly different expression levels. This group of genes was observed to segregate sporadic tumors into 2 subgroups—BRCA1-like and BRCA2-like. This finding suggests that BRCA1-related and BRCA2-related pathways are also involved in sporadic ovarian cancers. In addition, 53 genes were differentially expressed between tumors with BRCA1 mutations and sporadic tumors, and 6 of these genes mapped to Xp11.23 were expressed at higher levels in tumors with BRCA1 mutations than in sporadic tumors. In comparison with the immortalized ovarian surface epithelial cells used as a reference, several interferon-inducible genes were overexpressed in the majority of tumors with a BRCA mutation and in sporadic tumors.

Conclusion.—In epithelial ovarian cancers, mutations in BRCA1 and BRCA2 may result in carcinogenesis through distinct molecular pathways that also appear to be involved in sporadic cancers. These pathways may develop from epigenetic aberrations of BRCA1 and BRCA2 or their downstream effects.

▶ That which is expected is presented as a startling new development in this study. The biological significance of familial or potentially inherited cancer syndromes is that these patients carry in their germlines the mutation, or at least a mutation similar to that which occurs spontaneously in the somatic cells of patients who develop sporadic cancers. We should not be surprised that there are many genetic similarities between BRCA-related ovarian cancers and sporadic ovarian cancers. Thus, the main similarity between BRCA1 and BRCA2 is the name and inheritance and not necessarily function or role in genetic ovarian carcinogenesis.

D. S. Miller, MD

Impact of Adjuvant Chemotherapy and Surgical Staging in Early-Stage Ovarian Carcinoma: European Organisation for Research and Treatment of Cancer–Adjuvant ChemoTherapy in Ovarian Neoplasm Trial

Trimbos JB, for the EORTC-ACTION Collaborators (Leiden Univ Med Ctr, The Netherlands; et al)

J Natl Cancer Inst 95:113-125, 2003   29–5

Background.—None of the previously published randomized trials of adjuvant chemotherapy for early-stage ovarian cancer have had the statistical power to show a difference in the effect on survival between adjuvant and no adjuvant chemotherapy. Also, previous research has not considered the adequacy of surgical staging. In a prospective, unblinded, randomized phase III study, the efficacy of adjuvant chemotherapy in patients with early-stage ovarian cancer was tested, emphasizing the extent of surgical staging.

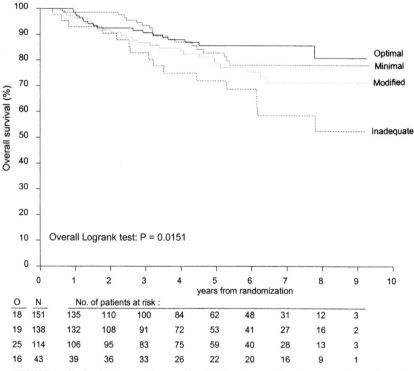

O	N	No. of patients at risk :								
18	151	135	110	100	84	62	48	31	12	3
19	138	132	108	91	72	53	41	27	16	2
25	114	106	95	83	75	59	40	28	13	3
16	43	39	36	33	26	22	20	16	9	1

FIGURE 4.—Kaplan-Meier curves for overall survival in patients with early-stage ovarian carcinoma by staging type. Optimal staging (n = 151) (*solid line*), modified staging (n = 138) (*solid dotted line*), minimal staging (n = 114) (*fine dotted line*), and inadequate staging (n = 43) (*solid/fine dotted line*) are in accordance with the staging guidelines presented in Table 1. The hazard ratio if 2.17 (95% confidence interval [CI] = 1.25 to 3.76; *P* = .005 using the log-rank test) in favor of optimal staging. *Abbreviations:* N, Number of patients; O, number of observations (events). (Courtesy of Trimbos JB, for the EORTC-ACTION collaborators: Impact of adjuvant chemotherapy and surgical staging in early-stage ovarian carcinoma: European Organisation for Research and Treatment of Cancer–Adjuvant Chemotherapy in Ovarian Neoplasm Trial. *J Natl Cancer Inst* 95(2):113-125, 2003. Reprinted by permission of Oxford University Press.)

Methods.—Four hundred forty-eight patients from 40 centers in 9 European countries were enrolled between 1990 and 2000. The patients were randomly assigned to receive adjuvant platinum-based chemotherapy or observation after operation. The median follow-up was 5.5 years

Findings.—The 2 groups did not differ significantly in overall survival. However, recurrence-free survival was significantly better in the adjuvant chemotherapy recipients. Only about one third of patients had had optimal staging. In the observation group, optimal staging correlated with a significant improvement in overall and recurrence-free survival. This correlation was not evident in the adjuvant chemotherapy group. Among patients who had not been staged optimally, adjuvant chemotherapy was associated with significant improvement in overall and recurrence-free survival. Adjuvant chemotherapy appeared to have no benefits among optimally staged patients (Fig 4).

Conclusions.—Adjuvant chemotherapy correlated with significantly improved recurrence-free survival in patients with early-stage ovarian cancer. The benefits of adjuvant chemotherapy appeared to be limited to patients who had not been staged optimally.

▶ Most women with epithelial ovarian cancer confined to the ovary at the time of treatment will be cured by oophorectomy. Depending on how thorough the staging laparotomy, a small to a larger number of those patients will have a recurrence, presumably because of undetected metastasis. Several large clinical trials have yet to identify treatments capable of decreasing this risk of recurrence. The main problem with this study is that most of the patients were not well staged. They did not receive pelvic and periaortic lymphadenectomy, omentectomy, and multiple peritoneal biopsies, including diaphragms and pelvic gutters. While the authors concluded that adjuvant chemotherapy is associated with improved recurrence-free survival, but not overall survival, further scrutiny shows the reasons for this. As is seen in Figure 4, patients in the observation arm who were completely staged did better than those who were not. Fortunately, adjuvant chemotherapy was able to salvage many of those patients with occult metastatic disease not detected by incomplete staging. Thus, the real conclusion of this study is that if a patient has been incompletely staged and appears to have early ovarian cancer, then she may benefit from adjuvant chemotherapy.

D. S. Miller, MD

International Collaborative Ovarian Neoplasm Trial 1: A Randomized Trial of Adjuvant Chemotherapy in Women With Early-Stage Ovarian Cancer

Parmar M, for the International Collaborative Ovarian Neoplasm 1 (ICON1) Collaborators (European Inst of Oncology, Milan, Italy; et al)
J Natl Cancer Inst 95:125-132, 2003   29–6

Background.—Establishing whether platinum-based adjuvant chemotherapy improves outcomes in patients with early-stage epithelial ovarian cancer is important. The effects of adjuvant chemotherapy on overall and recurrence-free survival were determined in women with early-stage epithelial ovarian cancer.

Methods.—In this multicenter, open randomized trial, 84 centers in 5 countries enrolled a total of 477 patients between 1991 and 2000. The patients were randomly assigned to receive either adjuvant chemotherapy immediately after surgery or no adjuvant chemotherapy until indicated clinically.

Findings.—Overall survival was better in women receiving adjuvant chemotherapy than in those who did not, with a hazard ratio of 0.66. The 5-year survival rates were 79% for women receiving adjuvant therapy, compared with 70% for those who did not. In addition, adjuvant chemotherapy increased recurrence-free survival, with 5-year rates of 73% for women receiving adjuvant chemotherapy and 62% for those who did not.

Conclusions.—Platinum-based adjuvant chemotherapy appears to improve survival in patients with early-stagy ovarian cancer. Recurrence-free survival is also prolonged in women receiving such adjuvant therapy.

▶ All the problems with the ACTION trial (Abstract 29–5) appeared to be more at play in this trial. It was stated that this study attempted to replicate "real world conditions." Likely, very few if any of these patients were completely staged but were presumed to have ovarian cancer confined to the ovary. Thus, the findings in this trial magnify those of the ACTION trial in that there was an advantage for chemotherapy in both progression-free and overall survival. Again, this effect is likely caused by the inclusion of many occult stage II and III patients for whom you would expect chemotherapy to make a difference.

D. S. Miller, MD

International Collaborative Ovarian Neoplasm Trial 1 and Adjuvant ChemoTherapy in Ovarian Neoplasm Trial: Two Parallel Randomized Phase III Trials of Adjuvant Chemotherapy in Patients With Early-Stage Ovarian Carcinoma

Trimbos JB, for the International Collaborative Ovarian Neoplasm 1 (ICON1) and European Organisation for Research and Treatment of Cancer Collaborators–Adjuvant ChemoTherapy In Ovarian Neoplasm (EORTC-ACTION) (Leiden Univ, The Netherlands; et al)

J Natl Cancer Inst 95:105-112, 2003   29–7

Background.—Adjuvant chemotherapy may be a strategy for improving survival in women with early-stage ovarian cancer. However, the randomized studies done to date have been too small to adequately address this question. A combined analysis of 2 parallel, randomized clinical trials was presented.

Methods.—The International Collaborative Ovarian Neoplasm 1 (ICON1) and the Adjuvant ChemoTherapy in Ovarian Neoplasm (ACTION) were included in the analysis. Both compared platinum-based adjuvant chemotherapy with observation postoperatively. A total of 925 patients undergoing surgery for early-stage ovarian cancer were enrolled in the studies between 1990 and 2000. The patients were randomly assigned to receive either platinum-based adjuvant chemotherapy or observation until chemotherapy was indicated. The median follow-up was more than 4 years.

Findings.—Two hundred forty-five patients died or had a recurrence during follow-up. At 5 years, overall survival was 82% in the chemotherapy group and 74% in the observation group. Recurrence-free survival at 5 years was 76% and 65%, respectively.

Conclusions.—Platinum-based adjuvant chemotherapy appears to improve 5-year overall survival and recurrence-free survival in women with early-stage ovarian cancer as defined by the inclusion criteria of the ICON1 and ACTION studies. This combined analysis enabled the study of a large number of patients.

▶ Unfortunately, the combining of a study with some of the patients completely staged (ACTION) (Abstract 29–5) and a study with fewer patients staged (ICON1) (Abstract 29–6) does not provide further clarity. There are an unknown number of patients with occult but probably detectable metastatic cancer who were included in this study and who were helped by the adjuvant chemotherapy. At first glance, one would come away satisfied that these patients should receive chemotherapy. Based on the results of this combined analysis, for every 100 patients treated with adjuvant chemotherapy, only 8 actually benefit from it. Ninety-two patients receiving the chemotherapy accrue no benefit either because they didn't need it or they received the chemotherapy and yet still had a recurrence. Since many of these patients with apparent early-stage ovarian cancer are young, the consequences of unnecessary chemotherapy need to be considered. Very clearly, further work must be done in identifying the subgroups of patients who might more substantially benefit from adjuvant chemotherapy, and determining how much chemotherapy they need. Hopefully, the results of GOG #157 will give us further insight into this difficult problem.[1]

D. S. Miller, MD

Reference

1. Bell J, Brady M, Lage J, et al: A randomized phase III trial of three versus six cycles of carboplatin and paclitaxel as adjuvant treatment in early stage ovarian epithelial carcinoma: A Gynecologic Oncology Group Study. *Gynecol Oncol* 88:156, 2003.

Paclitaxel Plus Carboplatin Versus Standard Chemotherapy With Either Single-Agent Carboplatin or Cyclophosphamide, Doxorubicin, and Cisplatin in Women With Ovarian Cancer: The ICON3 Randomised Trial
Parmar MKB, for the International Collaborative Ovarian Neoplasm (ICON) Group (ICON Trials, MRC Clinical Trials Unit, London)
Lancet 360:505-515, 2002   29–8

Background.—Previous research on ovarian cancer has demonstrated that survival and progression-free survival rates are comparable for combined treatment with cyclophosphamide, doxorubicin, and cisplatin (CAP) and single-agent treatment with carboplatin. Paclitaxel plus platinum has since become a widely accepted treatment for ovarian cancer. The safety and efficacy of this combination were compared with that of CAP or carboplatin alone.

Methods.—A total of 130 centers in 8 countries enrolled 2074 women in the randomized trial between February 1995 and October 1998. Women were randomly assigned to receive paclitaxel plus carboplatin or the control treatment—either CAP or single-agent carboplatin, whichever was chosen by the patients and clinician before randomization. The median follow-up was 51 months.

Findings.—During follow-up, 1265 patients died. Survival curves showed no difference in overall survival between paclitaxel plus carboplatin and the control treatment. Patients receiving paclitaxel plus carboplatin had a median overall survival of 36.1 months; those receiving the control treatment had a median survival of 35.4 months. The occurrence of progressive disease or death also did not differ between groups. The median progression-free survival in the paclitaxel plus carboplatin and control groups was 17.3 and 16.1 months, respectively. Treatment with paclitaxel plus carboplatin resulted in more instances of alopecia, fever, and sensory neuropathy than did carboplatin alone and more sensory neuropathy than did CAP. Treatment with CAP resulted in more instances of fever than did paclitaxel plus carboplatin.

Conclusions.—In first-line chemotherapy for ovarian cancer, single-agent carboplatin and CAP are as effective as paclitaxel plus carboplatin. Because treatment with carboplatin alone has a favorable toxicity profile, it is a reasonable choice for the treatment of ovarian cancer.

▶ Similar to the previously published Gynecologic Oncology Group (GOG) study (Abstract 29–7), this report shows no advantage to a platinum and taxane combination over a platinum drug alone for first-line chemotherapy for advanced ovarian cancer.[1] Many of the patients who did not receive first-line paclitaxel received it as salvage therapy. What this study really tells us is that a taxane does not have to be given as part of the initial chemotherapy but could be preceded by other agents. A test of this hypothesis has been incorporated into the current randomized GOG study, protocol #182, which contains several arms of so-called sequential doublets, which consist of 4 cycles of carboplatin and an experimental agent followed by 4 cycles of carboplatin and paclitaxel.

D. S. Miller, MD

Reference

1. Muggia FM, Braly PS, Brady MF, et al: Phase III randomized study of cisplatin versus paclitaxel versus cisplatin and paclitaxel in patients with suboptimal stage III or IV ovarian cancer: A gynecologic Oncology Group study. *J Clin Oncol* 18:106, 2000. (2001 YEAR BOOK OF OBSTETRICS, GYNECOLOGY, AND WOMEN'S HEALTH, p 465.)

Extraovarian Peritoneal Serous Papillary Carcinoma: A Phase II Trial of Cisplatin and Cyclophosphamide With Comparison to a Cohort With Papillary Serous Ovarian Carcinoma—A Gynecologic Oncology Group Study

Bloss JD, Brady MF, Liao SY, et al (Univ of Missouri, Columbia; Roswell Park Cancer Inst, Buffalo, NY; Univ of California at Irvine; et al)
Gynecol Oncol 89:148-154, 2003   29–9

Introduction.—Although the condition was first described in 1959, the etiology, pathogenesis, cell of origin, and clinical characteristics of extraovarian peritoneal serous papillary carcinoma (EPSPC) remains obscure. The probability of response and progression-free and overall survival of a well-defined group of women with EPSPC treated with a combination of cisplatin and cyclophosphamide after cytoreduction surgery was examined in a Gynecologic Oncology Group phase II investigation and compared with those of a group of women with papillary serous ovarian carcinoma (PSOC) who received identical therapy.

Methods.—After primary surgery, patients underwent treatment with cisplatin 75 mg/m² and cyclophosphamide 750 mg/m² every 21 days for 6 cycles. Patient demographics, tumor characteristics, clinical and surgical response to treatment, progression-free survival, and overall survival were assessed. Patients with EPSPC were compared with patients with PSOC who received identical treatment on a separate protocol.

Results.—Women with a diagnosis of EPSPC tended to be older than the PSOC cohort (median age, 65.8 years vs 60.3 years; $P = .04$). The estimated probabilities of complete and partial clinical responses to the treatment regimen were 65% (95% confidence interval [CI], 41%-85%) for EPSPC vs 59% (95% CI, 47%-71%) for women with PSOC. Surgical complete response rates (20% vs 19%) were similar for the 2 groups. Death rates were similar for the 2 groups (hazard ratio, 1.25; 95% CI, 0.834-1.88).

Conclusion.—Women with EPSPC and PSOC have a similar probability of response to treatment with cisplatin and cyclophosphamide and a similar overall survival. It is reasonable to include EPSPC patients in future large-scale treatment trials assessing patients with advanced ovarian cancer.

▶ Since EPSPC was described, there has been a debate as to whether this is a variant of ovarian cancer or a completely separate process. That debate may not be academic, particularly if there are differences in biology that might require different treatment strategies. Our current theories of ovarian carcinogenesis relate to ovarian cancer developing in cysts consequent to incessant ovulation. However, since ovarian cancers are presumed to arise from the epithelium that covers the ovary, is cyst formation really necessary for the development of an ovarian carcinoma from this surface epithelium? It is certainly conceivable that a carcinoma arising on this epithelium could be so small as to escape detection on pathologic exam but could, nonetheless, be the source of metastatic disease. This study shows that the outcomes for patients with EPSPC is similar to that of patients with traditionally defined PSOC and thus supports the rationale of including EPSPC patients in ovarian carcinoma trials as is now done by the Gynecologic Oncology Group.

D. S. Miller, MD

SUGGESTED READING

Eltabbakh GH, Piver MS: Extraovarian primary peritoneal carcinoma. *Oncology* 12:813-819, 1998.

Phase III Randomized Trial of 12 Versus 3 Months of Maintenance Paclitaxel in Patients With Advanced Ovarian Cancer After Complete Response to Platinum and Paclitaxel-Based Chemotherapy: A Southwest Oncology Group and Gynecologic Oncology Group Trial
Markman M, Liu PY, Wilczynski S, et al (Cleveland Clinic Found, Ohio; Ohio State Univ, Columbus, Ohio; Southwest Oncology Group Statistical Ctr, Seattle; et al)
J Clin Oncol 21:2460-2465, 2003   29–10

Background.—Standard initial treatment for ovarian cancer generally includes 5 to 6 courses of a platinum/taxane regimen. Limited randomized study data show no advantage of additional treatment or a consolidation strategy in ovarian cancer or other malignancies. However, findings of non-randomized studies suggest that more protracted treatment with paclitaxel may benefit patients with ovarian cancer. Whether continuing paclitaxel for an extended period prolongs progression-free survival (PFS) and improves survival in women with advanced ovarian cancer who had obtained a clincally defined complete response to a platinum/paclitaxel-based chemotherapy was determined.

Methods and Findings.—By random assignment, 277 patients received 3 or 12 cycles of single-agent paclitaxel every 28 days. Fifty-four PFS events occurred in 222 patients during follow-up. The regimens did not differ significantly in toxicity except for peripheral neuropathy. The median PFS was 21 months in the 3-cycle group and 28 months in the 12-cycle group. The Cox model–adjusted 3-cycle progression hazard ratio compared with the 12-cycle progression was 2.31. These findings resulted in trial discontinuation. As of the date of study termination, overall survival did not differ between groups.

Conclusions.—Twelve cycles of single-agent paclitaxel significantly prolongs PFS in women with advanced ovarian cancer who attain a clinically defined complete response to initial platinum/paclitaxel-based chemotherapy.

▶ This is a much anticipated publication of a study conceived by the Southwest Oncology Group (SWOG) but with most of the patients accrued by the Gynecologic Oncology Group. It has been hailed by some as a milestone and derided by others as a speed bump toward the goal of curing advanced ovarian cancer. As the reader is well aware, most patients will manifest a complete clinical, chemical, and radiologic response to aggressive cytoreductive surgery followed by platinum- and taxane-based chemotherapy. Unfortunately, most of those patients will then have a recurrence, usually within months to a couple of years. Virtually all of those patients will then die of their disease. It is shown that 9 more months of paclitaxel chemotherapy in the experimental arm will prolong the patients' progression-free interval by 7 months but have no significant effect on survival. The reader should note that the hazard for disease progression markedly increased after the paclitaxel was stopped, either after 3 or 12 months. This certainly implies that this is really maintenance therapy that suppresses persistent but clinically undetectable residual cancer. It is also interesting to note that a previous SWOG trial that showed very similar results, in terms of PFS, to the 12-month arm was not cited in this article. But, at least it was acknowledged in the accompanying editorial.[1,2] Needless to say, the various clinical trial groups undertaking prospective studies in front-line ovarian cancer have not changed their trials to incorporate the results of this study. Clearly, further trials are necessary. The reader should also recall that one of the reasons why second-look laparotomy has been abandoned by most centers outside of clinical trials, is that we were unable to show that the detection and prompt treatment of microscopic, persistent ovarian cancer made a difference.[3]

D. S. Miller, MD

References

1. Rothenberg ML, Liu PY, Wilczynski S, et al: Phase II trial of oral altretamine for consolidation of clinical complete remission in women with stage III epithelial ovarian cancer. A Southwest Oncology Group Trial (SWOG-9326). *Gynecol Oncol* 82:317, 2001.
2. Ozols RF: Maintenance therapy in advanced ovarian cancer: Progression-free survival and clinical benefit. *J Clin Oncol* 21:2451, 2003.

3. Miller DS, Spirtos NM, Ballon SC, et al: Critical reassessment of "second-look" exploratory laparotomy in epithelial ovarian cancer: Minimal diagnostic and therapeutic value in patients with persistent cancer. *Cancer* 69:502, 1992.

Consolidation Treatment of Advanced (FIGO Stage III) Ovarian Carcinoma in Complete Surgical Remission After Induction Chemotherapy: A Randomized, Controlled, Clinical Trial Comparing Whole Abdominal Radiotherapy, Chemotherapy, and No Further Treatment

Sorbe B, for the Swedish-Norwegian Ovarian Cancer Study Group (Örebro Univ Hosp, Sweden)
Int J Gynecol Cancer 13:278-286, 2003   29–11

Background.—Primary cytoreductive surgery and induction chemotherapy are standard therapeutic approaches for patients with advanced ovarian carcinomas in FIGO stages III to IV; this regimen produces a clinical tumor response in 60% to 70% of patients and complete surgical remission in 20% to 30% of patients. A pathologic complete response is often recorded in less than 20% of patients; however, potentially curable tumors are mostly found in this group of patients. A major problem in the treatment of ovarian carcinomas is recurrence of tumor within 1 to 3 years after an initially promising tumor response. Consolidation therapy after a complete surgical or pathologic response is a matter of concern. However, the effects of consolidation on the prolongation of life have not been proved. The efficacy and toxicity of whole abdominal radiotherapy were compared with chemotherapy and no further treatment as consolidation treatment in patients with advanced ovarian carcinoma.

Methods.—This prospective randomized trial compared consolidation treatment with radiotherapy or chemotherapy with no treatment in a series of 172 patients with epithelial ovarian carcinoma, FIGO stage III, with complete surgical remission after primary cytoreductive surgery and induction chemotherapy. The primary end point was progression-free survival after the second-look surgery. The secondary end points were overall survival rate and evaluation of acute and late toxicity data.

Results.—In a subgroup of patients with complete surgical and pathologic remission, progression-free survival at 5 years was significantly better in the radiotherapy group (56%) than in the chemotherapy group (36%) and the untreated control group (35%). Overall survival was highest in the radiotherapy group (69% at 5 years), and the radiotherapy group had the lowest number of recurrences. In the subgroup of microscopic residual carcinoma there were no significant differences in survival between the radiotherapy and the chemotherapy-treated patients. Treatment-related side effects occurred most frequently in the radiotherapy group, and severe late intestinal radiation reaction occurred in 10% of patients.

Conclusions.—Although this study found a survival advantage for consolidation therapy in patients with advanced ovarian cancer, there continues to be a need for larger prospective and randomized studies to clearly determine the optimal consolidation therapy for these patients.

▶ This study should have received more attention than it did, being a prospective, randomized, multicenter cooperative group trial that showed a survival advantage for consolidation therapy in patients with advanced ovarian cancer. Unfortunately, it was limited by no power analysis and a now obsolete choice of chemotherapy regimens. Nonetheless, this is another of a series of studies, most retrospective, showing an advantage for whole abdomen radiation therapy for the salvage treatment of minimal residual ovarian cancer.[1]

D. S. Miller, MD

Reference

1. Miller DS, Spirtos NM, Ballon SC, et al: Critical reassessment of "second look" exploratory laparotomy in epithelial ovarian cancer: Minimal diagnostic and therapeutic value in patients with persistent cancer. *Cancer* 69:502, 1992.

A Phase II Study of Docetaxel in Paclitaxel-Resistant Ovarian and Peritoneal Carcinoma: A Gynecologic Oncology Group Study

Rose PG, Blessing JA, Ball HG, et al (Case Western Reserve Univ, Cleveland, Ohio; Roswell Park Cancer Inst, Buffalo, NY; Univ of Massachusetts, Worcester; et al)
Gynecol Oncol 88:130-135, 2003   29–12

Introduction.—Docetaxel is an inhibitor of microtubule depolymerization and has shown activity in paclitaxel-resistant breast cancer and gynecologic cancer. It has also been observed in several human ovarian cancer long-term cell culture lines to be more cytotoxic than paclitaxel on a milliliter to milliliter basis.

This increased toxicity may be due to docetaxel's higher achievable intracellular concentration, its higher affinity for microtubules, and its slower cellular efflux. The Gynecologic Oncology Group performed a large, multi-institutional phase II trial to better determine the antitumor activity, nature, and degrees of toxicity in patients with paclitaxel- and platinum-resistant ovarian cancer deemed as progressive while receiving or within 6 months of therapy.

Methods.—Patients were eligible if they had measurable disease and had not received more than 1 chemotherapy regimen. Docetaxel, 100 mg/m^2, was administered IV over 1 hour every 21 days. A prophylactic regimen of oral dexamethasone, 8 mg twice a day, was initiated 24 hours before docetaxel administration and continued for 48 hours thereafter. Hepatic function was followed closely.

Results.—Sixty patients underwent a total of 256 courses. All 60 patients were evaluable for toxicity and 58 were evaluable for response. Of 22.4% of patients with response, 5.2% were complete responses and 17.2% were partial (95% confidence interval, 12.5%-35.3%). The median response duration was 2.5 months. The likelihood of a response did not seem to be associated with the length of the prior paclitaxel-free interval or the duration of prior paclitaxel infusions. Seventy-five percent of patients experienced grade 4 neutropenia and there was 1 treatment-related death. A decrease in dose was necessary in 36% of patients.

Conclusion.—Docetaxel is active in paclitaxel-resistant ovarian cancer and peritoneal cancer. The significant hematologic toxicity necessitates further investigation to ascertain the optimal dose and schedule.

▶ Docetaxel is a semisynthetic taxane, similar to paclitaxel, extracted from the needles of the European yew. The Gynecologic Oncology Group has established a series of phase II trials evaluating agents for possible activity in patients whose ovarian cancer has progressed or relapsed within 6 months after platinum-based chemotherapy. The 22% response rate in this group of patients is significant as only oral etoposide has approached that response rate in the Gynecologic Oncology Group experience.[1] Unfortunately, the duration of response was short. But the fact that there were responses in patients who had failed previous paclitaxel therapy is important. Further evaluation of docetaxel in combination with other agents should be anticipated.

D. S. Miller, MD

Reference

1. Rose PG, Blessing JA, Mayer AR, et al: Prolonged oral etoposide as second-line therapy for platinum-resistant and platinum-sensitive ovarian carcinoma: A Gynecologic Oncology Group study. *J Clin Oncol* 16:405,1998.

Altretamine (Hexamethylmelamine) in the Treatment of Platinum-Resistant Ovarian Cancer: A Phase II Study
Keldsen N, Havsteen H, Vergote I, et al (Herning Hosp, Denmark; Århus Univ Hosp, Denmark; Univ Hosps, Leuven, Belgium; et al)
Gynecol Oncol 88:118-122, 2003   29–13

Introduction.—Despite an initial good response to chemotherapy, ovarian cancer recurs in most patients and the long-term prognosis is dismal. The response to second-line chemotherapy tends to be poorer, particularly if the disease has progressed during treatment or recurs within a treatment-free interval of 6 to 12 months after initial therapy. A 14% response rate has been reported in 50 patients with platinum-resistant disease treated with altretamine (hexamethylmelamine). The activity of altretamine in women with epithelial ovarian carcinoma who responded (partial response or complete response) to first-line chemotherapy and relapsed within 6 months was evaluated in this multicenter phase II trial. This protocol was later amended to include women with relapse within 12 months.

Methods.—All patients had measurable disease (World Health Organization performance status 2 or below [Karnofsky index >60] and adequate bone marrow function and liver function) and had no more than 1 prior chemotherapy regimen. Altretamine 250 mg/m²/d was administered in 4 divided doses for 2 weeks; this was repeated every 4 weeks. Patient response was assessed after every 2 courses.

Results.—Thirty-one patients received a median of 3 courses of altretamine (range, 1-12 courses). Hematologic toxicity was minimal and gastrointestinal toxicity was common. Twenty-six patients were able to be evaluated for response Three patients (9.7% intent-to-treat) had a partial response, 8 patients had stable disease, and 15 patients had progressive disease after 2 courses of treatment. Median time to progression was 10 weeks (range, 5-51 weeks) and median survival was 34 weeks (range, 7-112+).

Conclusion.—Altretamine should not be used as standard treatment in patients with platinum-resistant recurrent ovarian cancer. This drug may be a useful alternative in patients who prefer oral therapy or when socioeconomic considerations are important.

▶ Altretamine (hexamethylmelamine) was the first cytotoxic drug specifically approved for second-line treatment of ovarian cancer. The outcome in this group of platinum-resistant patients is disappointing but not novel. The response rate and overall survival are comparable to that seen with the most frequently used agents, topotecan and liposomal doxorubicin but inferior to the less commonly used agents docetaxel and oral etoposide.[1-3] While it is a discouraging group of patients to treat, it is only by finding an agent active in platinum-resistant ovarian cancer that we will make progress toward curing more patients with this disease.

D. S. Miller, MD

References

1. Gordon AN, Fleagle JT, Guthrie D, et al: Recurrent epithelial ovarian carcinoma: A randomized phase III study of pegylated liposomal doxorubicin versus topotecan. *J Clin Oncol* 19:3312-3322, 2001.
2. Rose PG, Blessing JA, Ball HG, et al: A phase II study of a docetaxel in paclitaxel-resistant ovarian and peritoneal carcinoma: A Gynecologic Oncology Group study. *Gynecol Oncol* 88:130-135, 2003.
3. Rose PG, Blessing JA, Mayer AR, et al: Prolonged oral etoposide as second-line therapy for platinum-resistant and platinum sensitive ovarian carcinoma: A Gynecologic Oncology Group study. *J Clin Oncol* 16:405, 1998.

Evaluation of Monoclonal Humanized Anti-HER2 Antibody, Trastuzumab, in Patients With Recurrent or Refractory Ovarian or Primary Peritoneal Carcinoma With Overexpression of HER2: A Phase II Trial of the Gynecologic Oncology Group

Bookman MA, Darcy KM, Clarke-Pearson D, et al (Fox Chase Cancer Ctr, Rockledge, Pa; Roswell Park Cancer Inst, Buffalo, NY; Duke Univ, Durham, NC; et al)
J Clin Oncol 21:283-290, 2003   29–14

Introduction.—Growth factors and their receptors have important roles during normal and tumor cell development. Human epidermal growth factor receptor 2 (HER2; also known as HER2/*neu*, p185[HER2], or c-erbB2) is a type I growth factor receptor tyrosine kinase. Abnormal expression of HER2 has been identified in several primary tumors, including breast cancer. The Gynecologic Oncology Group initiated a phase II investigation of single-agent trastuzumab in patients with recurrent or persistent ovarian or primary peritoneal carcinoma to assess the feasibility, toxicity, and efficacy of single-agent monoclonal antibody therapy targeting the HER2/*neu* receptor in these patients.

Methods.—All patients had measurable persistent or recurrent epithelial ovarian or primary peritoneal carcinoma with 2+ or 3+ HER2 overexpression verified by immunohistochemistry. Patients received IV trastuzumab at 4 mg/kg initially, followed by weekly administration of 2 mg/kg. Patients without progressive disease or excessive toxicity were allowed to continue treatment indefinitely. Participants with stable or responding disease at 8 weeks were offered therapy at a higher weekly dose (4 mg/kg) at the time of progression. Sera were examined for the presence of the soluble extracellular domain of HER2, host antibodies against trastuzumab, and transtuzumab pharmacokinetics.

Results.—There were 837 tumor samples screened for HER2 expression. Ninety-five patients (11%) demonstrated the requisite 2+/3+ expression level. Of 45 patients who received prior chemotherapy, 41 were eligible and assessable. Of these, 27 had tumors that exhibited 2+ immmnohistochemical expression of HER2, and 14 had tumors that showed 3+ HER2 expression. All toxicities were mild and there were no treatment-associated deaths. Although an elevated level of the soluble extracellular domain of HER2 was identified in 8 of 24 patients, serum HER2 was not linked with clinical outcome.

There was no indication of host antitrastuzumab antibody formation in any patients. Serum concentrations of trastuzumab gradually rose with ongoing therapy. The overall response rate of 7% included 1 complete response and 2 partial responses. The median duration of treatment was 8 weeks (range, 2-104 weeks). The median progression-free interval was 2.0 months.

Conclusion.—The clinical value of single-agent trastuzumab in recurrent ovarian cancer is restricted by the low rate of HER2 overexpression and the low rate of objective response in patients with HER2 overexpression.

▶ The use of "targeted therapies" has received much attention of late from practitioners as well as stock analysts. The actual data on the use of these therapies are just beginning to emerge. One of the first tested in gynecologic cancers is trastuzumab, which incorporates humanized monoclonal antibodies against HER2 (aka HER2/*neu* or c-erbB2). In breast cancer patients whose tumors overexpress HER2, objective responses were seen in 12% to 15% of cancers. Unfortunately, this activity was not seen against ovarian cancer. Only 11% of patients' tumors were positive for HER2, though 30% had been expected, and even in those, the response rate was a disappointing 7%. It is the expectation of most that targeted therapies will play a significant role in the future of oncology. We await therapies targeted to targets found in ovarian cancer.

D. S. Miller, MD

30 Hormone Replacement Therapy and Cancer

Hormone Replacement Therapy Formulations and Risk of Epithelial Ovarian Carcinoma
Sit ASY, Modugno F, Weissfeld JL, et al (Univ of Pittsburgh, Pa)
Gynecol Oncol 86:118-123, 2002   30–1

Background.—Hormone replacement therapy (HRT) is commonly used for postmenopausal women and has been used increasingly for the prevention of chronic diseases such as osteoporosis and cardiovascular disease. However, adoption of and compliance with HRT has been limited by concerns that HRT may increase the risks of breast and endometrial cancer. There is also concern that HRT may promote ovarian cancer, which is an often-fatal postmenopausal malignancy. Findings in studies of the possible association of HRT with increased rates of ovarian cancer have been inconsistent.

In the only prospective study that directly examined the effect of follicle-stimulating hormone and luteinizing hormone on ovarian cancer, no association was found between gonadotropin levels and the occurrence of ovarian cancer. Estrogen formulations used in HRT vary in their effects on estrogen-sensitive target tissues, such as the ovary. The effects of various HRT formulations and their characteristics of use on the risk of epithelial ovarian carcinoma (EOC) were evaluated.

Methods.—The study group included women participating in a population-based, case-control study set in the Delaware Valley from 1994 to 1998. A total of 484 women aged 45 years or older at diagnosis were compared with 926 community control subjects. Data on HRT formulation, timing, and duration were obtained by interviews. HRT formulations were classified as opposed (estrogen + progestin) or unopposed (estrogen alone). The formulations were then categorized according to the estrogen component as either conjugated equine estrogen (CEE) (the most common formulation) or non-CEE. Multivariate unconditional logistic regression analyses adjusted

TABLE 3.—Odds Ratios of Epithelial Ovarian Carcinoma According to the Types of Hormone Replacement Therapy or Progestins

	All Subjects			Women With Hysterectomy			Women Without Hysterectomy		
	Cases (n = 484)	Controls (n = 926)	Adj OR (95% CI)	Cases (n = 69)	Controls (n = 180)	Adj OR (95% CI)*	Cases (n = 415)	Controls (n = 746)	Adj OR (95% CI)*
Never used HRT	303	541	1.00 (reference)	34	84	1.00 (reference)	269	457	1.00 (reference)
Ever used									
Any HRT	181	385	0.94 (0.74,1.19)	35	96	0.84 (0.47,1.51)	146	289	0.96 (0.74,1.25)
Opp CEE	60	114	1.06 (0.74,1.52)	3	1	7.50 (0.64,88.3)	57	113	0.98 (0.68,1.42)
Unopp CEE	50	104	0.90 (0.61,1.33)	22	62	0.79 (0.40,1.56)	28	42	1.17 (0.69,2.00)
Opp nCEE	20	36	1.08 (0.59,2.00)	0	3		20	33	1.16 (0.63,2.15)
Unopp nCEE	10	35	0.52 (0.25,1.10)	2	22	0.17 (0.04,0.82)	8	13	1.14 (0.44,2.98)
Progestin only	17	50	0.86 (0.47,1.58)	1	5	1.50 (0.12,18.4)	16	45	0.83 (0.45,1.56)

*Adjusted for use of oral contraceptive, number of live births, age at diagnosis, history of tubal ligation, and family history of ovarian cancer.

Abbreviations: Opp CEE, Combination use of conjugated equine estrogen and progestins; *Unopp CEE,* use of CEE alone; *Opp nCEE,* use of an estrogen formulation other than CEE alone; *Opp nCEE,* combination use of non-CEE and progestins; *OR,* odds ratio; *CI,* confidence interval.

(Reprinted by permission of the publisher from Sit ASY, Mondugno F, Weissfeld JL, et al: Hormone replacement therapy formulations and risk of epithelial ovarian carcinoma. *Gynecol Oncol* 86:118-123. Copyright 2002 by Elsevier Science Inc.)

for age at diagnosis, number of live births, use of oral contraceptives, family history of ovarian carcinoma, and history of tubal ligation.

Results.—No association was found between any use of HRT and EOC overall. The use of unopposed non-CEE was associated with a significant decrease in risk among hysterectomized women, but this was not the case for women whose uterus was intact. There were no significant differences in risk of EOC for other HRT formulations (Table 3).

Conclusion.—These findings did not reveal a consistent pattern of increased risk for epithelial ovarian carcinoma and the overall use of hormone replacement therapy by specific formulation.

▶ With the release of the Women's Health Initiative studies, most manufacturers attempted to distance themselves from combined equine estrogen and progestin products. Lacking data to support this, the FDA has lumped all of them together in terms of their product labeling. This is the first study that has attempted to evaluate risk of developing ovarian cancer as it related to categories of hormone replacement therapy products. Unlike a study (Abstract 12–10), it found that unopposed noncontinuous equine estrogen was associated with a significantly decreased risk among hysterectomized women (Table 3) . Unfortunately, this is merely a small comfort to the manufacturers, subscribers, and consumers of hormone replacement therapy products.

D. S. Miller, MD

Estrogen Replacement Therapy for Menopausal Women With a History of Breast Carcinoma: Results of a 5-Year, Prospective Study
Vassilopoulou-Sellin R, Cohen DS, Hortobagyi GN, et al (Univ of Texas, Houston)
Cancer 95:1817-1826, 2002   30–2

Background.—Estrogen replacement therapy (ERT) is an important component of management of some postmenopausal women. There is increasing concern regarding the possible association of ERT with an increased risk of breast carcinoma, and prior breast carcinoma is generally accepted as a contraindication to ERT. However, most women are menopausal at diagnosis for breast carcinoma or develop ovarian failure after chemotherapy. Thus, many women with breast carcinoma may benefit from ERT.

Data on the effect of ERT on breast carcinoma recurrence is encouraging but is limited to a few retrospective studies, prospective single-arm studies, and randomized pilot studies. Outcomes were presented of a randomized, prospective clinical trial to evaluate the efficacy and safety of ERT in select patients with breast carcinoma after a minimum follow-up of 5 years.

Methods.—This prospective clinical trial assessed the safety and efficacy of prolonged ERT in menopausal women with localized (stage I or II) breast carcinoma and a minimum disease-free interval of 2 years if the estrogen receptor status was negative, or 10 years if the estrogen receptor status was unknown. The study included 77 study participants and 222 women with clinical and prognostic characteristics comparable to those of the study participants. Overall, 56 women were taking ERT and 243 women were not. The main outcome measure was the association of ERT with skeletal and lipid changes in the study participants. In addition, the effect of ERT on the development of new or recurrent breast carcinoma and other carcinoma was analyzed in both the study participants and the control subjects.

Results.—Women on ERT and those not on ERT were comparable in terms of tumor size, number of lymph nodes involved, ER status, menopausal status, and disease-free interval; these parameters were similar in the study and control participants. The use of ERT was associated with modest lipid and skeletal benefits, and ERT did not compromise disease-free survival. A contralateral new breast carcinoma developed in 2 of 56 (3.6%) women on ERT. Among the women not on ERT, 33 of 243 (13.5%) developed new or recurrent breast carcinoma. There were no differences between the groups in the development of other carcinomas.

Conclusion.—In this prospective clinical trial with a minimum of 5 years of follow-up, estrogen replacement therapy did not compromise disease-free survival in patients who had previously been treated for localized breast carcinoma.

▶ Not infrequently, the treatment of breast cancer with chemotherapy results in ovarian failure. Some of these patients can be quite young, and in addition to dealing with the consequences of their breast cancer, they must also deal with the climacteric. Some of these patients are so miserable that, in spite of the alarming warnings they receive from their breast surgeons and chemotherapists, they seek out treatment for their estrogen deficiency. A sign of the extent to which patients are intimidated on this issue, is seen by the fact that the authors were not able to complete their prospective study and had to use patients in their collective experience.

It eventually came to the attention of our breast chemotherapy colleagues that most patients treated for estrogen deficiency did not develop immediate and devastating recurrence of their breast cancer. Should we be concerned? Perhaps. If breast cancer, or any other cancer for that matter, recurs after treatment, it is not because of neocarcinogenesis in otherwise normal cells. But, it is due to occult metastases that were not completely treated. Thus, it is unlikely that estrogen replacement therapy in a cancer survivor will make the cancer come back when it wouldn't otherwise. But, it might make the cancer come back sooner.[1]

This has been looked at in several retrospective studies and, interestingly, none have found a worse prognosis for breast cancer survivors who take estrogen replacement therapy.[2] Such is the case in this study, where there appears to be a survival as well as recurrence-free advantage for the women taking estrogen replacement therapy.

D. S. Miller, MD

References

1. Miller DS: Should we offer HRT to ovarian and endometrial cancer survivors? Yes, there is no scientifically valid reason not to do so. *Cont Ob/Gyn* 46:31, 2001.
2. O'Meara ES, Rossing MA, Daling JR, et al: Hormone replacement therapy after a diagnosis of breast cancer in relation to recurrence and mortality. *J Natl Cancer Inst* 93:754, 2001. 2002 YEAR BOOK OF OBSTETRICS, GYNECOLOGY AND WOMEN'S HEALTH, p 519.

31 Breast Disease

Perspectives on the Women's Health Initiative Trial of Hormone Replacement Therapy
Grimes DA, Lobo RA (Family Health Internatl, Research Triangle Park, NC; Columbia Univ, New York)
Obstet Gynecol 100:1344-1353, 2002   31–1

Background.—In July 2002, part of the Women's Health Initiative trial was prematurely halted after the Data Safety and Monitoring Board determined that the use of hormone replacement therapy (HRT) in this trial was associated with increased overall risk (Fig 1). This overview discussed biases inherent in the observational trials that formed the basis for the use of HRT for treatment conditions beyond the symptoms of menopause and assessed

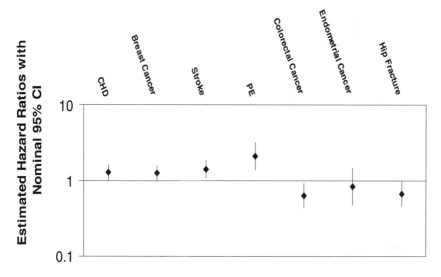

Major Clinical Outcomes

FIGURE 1.—Estimated hazard ratios for major clinical outcomes in the Women's Health Initiative trial of hormone replacement therapy. *Abbreviations: CHD*, Coronary heart disease; *PE*, pulmonary embolism. Source: Writing Group for the Women's Health Initiative Investigators. (Reprinted with permission from The American College of Obstetricians and Gynecologists courtesy of Grimes DA, Lobo RA: Perspectives on the Women's Health Initiative Trial of Hormone Replacement Therapy. *Obstet Gynecol* 100: 1344-1353, 2002.)

the methods and results of the Women's Health Initiative trial to help physicians understand and interpret these surprising findings.

Observational Studies.—Prior to the Women's Health Initiative trial, there was evidence for cardiovascular benefit from HRT, but this primarily came from observational trials rather than controlled clinical trials. Observational trials are subject to several types of inherent biases, which can influence their results. Some of the evidence was based on surrogate markers rather than primary outcome, and use of surrogate markers can frequently be misleading. Selection bias probably accounted for most of the cardiac benefit observed in observational trials, as women who chose to take HRT were healthier, more affluent, better educated, leaner, younger, more likely to drink alcohol moderately, more physically active, and less likely to have a family history of heart disease, to smoke, or to have diabetes.

Another confounding factor is survivor bias. Women who develop illness may stop taking HRT, leaving only the healthy women taking HRT, leading to spurious HRT benefit. Because of these inherent biases, observational research reaches favorable conclusions more frequently than experimental research and is more often incorrect. Controlled, randomized clinical trials are the only way to avoid these biases in research and should be performed whenever possible.

Women's Health Initiative.—Controlled, randomized trials have 2 types of validity: internal and external. Internal validity refers to the trial answering the question it set out to ask. The Women's Health Initiative used excellent methods and can be considered internally valid. External validity refers to generalizability. Women in this trial were asymptomatic and older than the typical HRT user. Whether these findings can be generalized to symptomatic women at the onset of menopause is not known, but the primary focus of this part of the trial was not on treatment for menopause symptoms but on prevention of cardiovascular disease, a common off-label indication for HRT. Conjugated equine estrogen, as used in this trial, is the most commonly prescribed estrogen in the United States.

In the first 2 years of the study, more cardiac events occurred in the HRT group (Fig 1). There was also a doubling in the rate of venous thrombosis and pulmonary embolism in this group. There was a small increase in breast cancer risk. There was a significant reduction in vertebral, hip, and total fractures in the HRT group. The risk of colorectal cancer was also reduced (Fig 1).

Conclusion.—The Women's Health Initiative is the largest controlled, randomized clinical trial of hormone replacement therapy conducted so far. The study group consisted of asymptomatic women, with an average age of 63 years, who had not previously used hormones. The hormone regimen consisted of conjugated equine estrogen (0.625 m) with medroxyprogesterone acetate (2.5 mg). HRT was effective for the treatment of menopause symptoms. In addition, it reduced the risk of osteoporotic fractures and colorectal cancer. Unfortunately, use of HRT was also associated with increased cardiovascular disease, stroke, thomboembolism, and breast cancer. Therefore, HRT should be used sparingly and briefly for the treatment of menopausal symptoms. HRT should not be used for prevention of cardio-vascular disease.

▶ Practicing ob-gyns are in the difficult position of needing to keep up with the most current reports and responding to their patients queries while maintaining a balanced and perspective view of the potential benefits and adverse effects of HRT. This objective response by 2 recognized authorities in this field to the curtailment of the conjugated equine estrogen and medroxyprogesterone acetate arm of the Women's Health Initiative trial is useful background. It is critical to keep in mind that from a pragmatic epidemiologic point of view, there is no consistent hard data to support a clinically meaningful conclusion one way or the other.

Long-term (eg, 20-year) studies with disease-specific survival data, robust numbers, and minimal epidemiologic manipulation of the data are necessary and deserve NIH or similar funding. In the meantime, alendronate, raloxifene, and risedronate can be used for osteoporosis prevention, and exercise, weight control, avoidance of smoking, and blood pressure and lipid control are recommended for heart disease prevention.

In related studies, Sacchini at the Memorial Sloan-Kettering Cancer Center, New York, and the European Institute of Oncology, Milan, Italy, reported on the effects of hormone replacement therapy in a heterogeneous group (*n* = 232) and prognostic factors in breast cancer. Earlier stage breast cancers and more favorable pathologic and biological cancer characteristics were associated with hormone replacement therapy, particularly for durations of more than 5 years.[1] Natrajan in Augusta, Georgia, found that neither risk of recurrence or risk of death were increased by estrogen replacement therapy in patients (*n* = 123) who had been treated for early breast cancer.[2]

W. H. Hindle, MD

References

1. Sacchini V, Zurrida S, Andreoni G, et al: Pathologic and biologic prognostic factors of breast cancers in short- and long-term hormone replacement therapy users. *Ann Surg Oncol* 9:266-271, 2002.
2. Natrajan PK, Gambrell RD Jr: Estrogen replacement therapy in patients with early breast cancer. *Am J Obstet Gynecol* 187:289-295, 2002.

SUGGESTED READING

Nikander E, Kilkkinen A, Metsa-Heikkila M, et al: A randomized placebo-controlled crossover trial with phytoestrogens in treatment of menopause in breast cancer patients. *Obstet Gynecol* 101:1213-1220, 2003.

▶ This well-designed study from the University of Helsinki, Finland, utilized the Kupperman index, visual analogue scales, and validated questionnaires assessing mood changes and working capacity in order to evaluate objectively the use of pure isoflavonoids for the treatment of menopausal symptoms. No therapeutic effect was identified. Furthermore, the levels of follicle-stimulating hormone, luteinizing hormone, estradiol, and sex hormone–binding globulins as well as liver enzymes, creatinine, body mass index, and blood pressure were unaltered by the isoflavonoid treatment. However, 28.6% of the women preferred the placebo therapy. This type of painstaking research will probably be required to scientifically evaluate all the phytoestrogens and other alternative therapies that have been advocated for the treatment of menopausal symptoms. Patients with menopausal concerns should be made aware of this scientific data and similar research as it becomes available.

William H. Hindle, MD

Fugh-Berman A: Bust-enhancing herbal products. *Obstetr Gynecol* 101:1345-1349, 2003.

▶ In the past, estrogen therapy, often at dosages far beyond physiologic levels, was thought by many to be capable of permanently increasing the size of the breasts of physiologically normal women. Extensive clinical experience proved this to be a myth, although some women on the estrogen therapy experienced mastalgia. However, the seemingly endless search for such breast enlarging therapies continues to be led by intense advertising of unregulated formulations, often with testimonials of "astonishing" results.

As with the scientific evaluation of phytoestrogens above, it is important that current commentaries such as this article from the Department of Health Care Sciences, George Washington University School of Medicine, Washington, DC, be published in widely recognized and distributed medical journals. Certainly, women's health care providers should have this information. Hopefully, women with concerns about what they perceive as "undersized" breasts should be made aware of these sound data. The author concludes, "The use of bust-enhancing products should be discouraged because of lack of evidence for efficacy and long-term safety concerns."

William H. Hindle, MD

Twenty-Five-Year Follow-up of a Randomized Trial Comparing Radical Mastectomy, Total Mastectomy, and Total Mastectomy Followed by Irradiation
Fisher B, Jeong J-H, Anderson S, et al (Natl Surgical Adjuvant Breast and Bowel Project, Pittsburgh, Pa)
N Engl J Med 347:567-575, 2002   31–2

Background.—The necessity of radical mastectomy in women with breast cancer has long been a subject of debate. It was the standard surgical treatment for breast cancer through most of the 20th century, but by the mid-1960s, some dissatisfaction with results after radical mastectomy was expressed. In addition, anecdotal information regarding other procedures led some surgeons to advocate more extensive surgery and others to promote more limited surgery. New information regarding tumor metastases also suggested that less radical surgery might be just as effective as the more extensive operations that were being performed. The 25-year findings of a randomized trial initiated in 1971 to determine whether less extensive surgery with or without radiation therapy was as effective as the Halsted radical mastectomy for breast cancer are reported.

Methods.—The study group included 1079 women with clinically negative axillary nodes who underwent either radical mastectomy, total mastec-

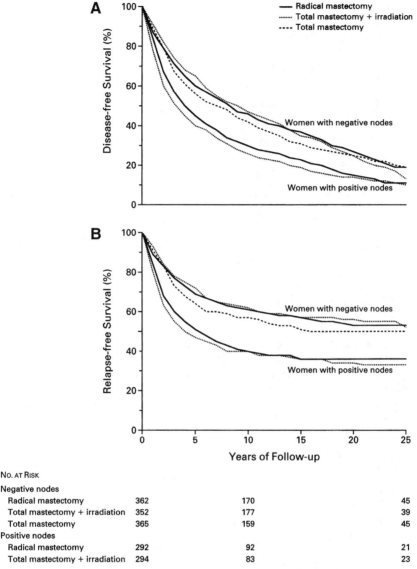

No. at Risk

Negative nodes			
Radical mastectomy	362	170	45
Total mastectomy + irradiation	352	177	39
Total mastectomy	365	159	45
Positive nodes			
Radical mastectomy	292	92	21
Total mastectomy + irradiation	294	83	23

FIGURE 1.—Disease-free survival (**A**) and relapse-free survival (**B**) during 25 years of follow-up after surgery among women with clinically negative axillary nodes and women with clinically positive axillary nodes. There were no significant differences among the groups of women with negative nodes or between the groups of women with positive nodes in either analysis. (Reprinted by permission of *The New England Journal of Medicine* from Fisher B, Jeong J-H, Anderson S, et al: Twenty-five-year follow-up of a randomized trial comparing radical mastectomy, total mastectomy, and total mastectomy followed by irradiation. *N Engl J Med* 347:567-575, 2002. Copyright 2002, Massachusetts Medical Society. All rights reserved.)

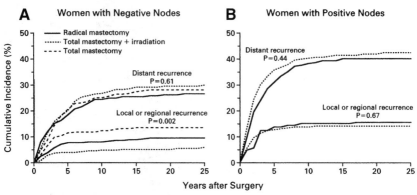

FIGURE 2.—Cumulative incidence of local or regional recurrence and distant recurrence during 25 years of follow-up after surgery among women with clinically negative axillary nodes (**A**) and women with clinically positive axillary nodes (**B**), according to treatment group. In (**A**), the *P* values are for the 3-way comparisons among treatment groups. (Reprinted by permission of *The New England Journal of Medicine* from Fisher B, Jeong J-H, Anderson S, et al: Twenty-five-year follow-up of a randomized trial comparing radical mastectomy, total mastectomy, and total mastectomy followed by irradiation. *N Engl J Med* 347:567-575, 2002. Copyright 2002, Massachusetts Medical Society. All rights reserved.)

tomy without axillary dissection but with postoperative irradiation, or total mastectomy plus axillary dissection only if their nodes became positive. A total of 586 women with clinically positive axillary nodes underwent either radical mastectomy or total mastectomy without axillary dissection but with postoperative irradiation. Kaplan-Meier and cumulative-incidence estimates of outcome were obtained.

Results.—No significant differences were found among the 3 groups of women with negative nodes or between the 2 groups of women with positive nodes in disease-free survival and relapse-free survival (Fig 1). In addition, no significant differences were noted among the 3 groups in the cumulative incidence of distant recurrence as an initial event. Among the women with positive nodes, no significant difference was noted between the 2 groups in the cumulative incidence of local or regional recurrence. The cumulative incidence of local or regional recurrence in the women with negative nodes was lowest for those treated with total mastectomy and radiation (Fig 2). The differences were not significant in the distant disease-free survival rates among the 3 groups with negative nodes. Among the women with positive nodes, no significant difference was noted in distant disease-free survival rates between those who had a radical mastectomy and those who had a total mastectomy plus radiation (Fig 3). Among women with negative nodes, the hazard ratio for death among those who were treated with total mastectomy plus radiation compared with those who underwent radical mastectomy was 1.08 (95% confidence interval [CI], 0.91-1.28; *P* = .38), and the hazard radio among those treated with radical mastectomy compared with those who had total mastectomy was 1.03 (95% CI, 0.87-1.23, *P* = .49). In women with negative nodes, the cumulative incidence of death after a recurrence of breast cancer was 40% and for those with positive nodes, was 67% (Fig 4).

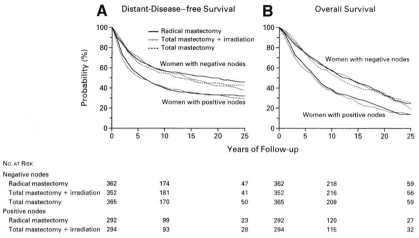

No. at Risk

Negative nodes						
Radical mastectomy	362		174		47	362	218	59
Total mastectomy + irradiation	352		181		41	352	216	56
Total mastectomy	365		170		50	365	209	59
Positive nodes						
Radical mastectomy	292		99		23	292	120	27
Total mastectomy + irradiation	294		93		28	294	115	32

FIGURE 3.—Survival free of distant disease (A) and overall survival (B) during 25 years of follow-up after surgery among women with clinically negative axillary nodes and women with clinically positive axillary nodes. There were no significant differences among the groups of women with negative nodes or between the groups if women with positive nodes in either analysis. (Reprinted by permission of *The New England Journal of Medicine* from Fisher B, Jeong J-H, Anderson S, et al: Twenty-five-year follow-up of a randomized trial comparing radical mastectomy, total mastectomy, and total mastectomy followed by irradiation. *N Engl J Med* 347:567-575, 2002. Copyright 2002, Massachusetts Medical Society. All rights reserved.)

Conclusions.—The study confirms earlier reports that showed no significant benefit from radical mastectomy for the treatment of breast cancer. No significant survival advantage was demonstrated either from the removal of occult positive nodes at the time of surgery or from radiation therapy. Among women with negative nodes, the cumulative incidence of locoregional occurrence was lowest for those who underwent total mastectomy plus radiation. However, among women with positive nodes, ra-

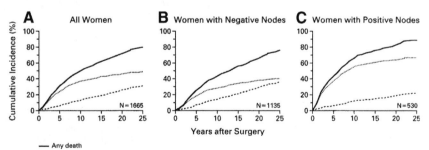

FIGURE 4.—Cumulative incidence of death, of death following recurrence or contralateral of breast cancer, and of death without recurrence or contralateral of breast cancer among women (A), women with clinically negative axillary nodes (B), and women with clinically positive axillary nodes (C). (Reprinted by permission of *The New England Journal of Medicine* from Fisher B, Jeong J-H, Anderson S, et al: Twenty-five-year follow-up of a randomized trial comparing radical mastectomy, total mastectomy, and total mastectomy followed by irradiation. *N Engl J Med* 347:567-575, 2002. Copyright 2002, Massachusetts Medical Society. All rights reserved.)

diation significantly reduced the incidence of only locoregional—not distant recurrence.

▶ The National Surgical Adjuvant Breast and Bowel Projects (NSABP) are exemplary of definitive quality clinical information that can confidently be put to use in clinical practice. This long-term follow-up report of the NSABP B-04 clinical trial (n = 1665) definitively validates "no advantage from radical mastectomy" and no "significant survival advantage from removing occult positive nodes at the time of initial surgery or from radiation therapy." Clinically meaningful contrary evidence is unlikely ever to be presented. Veronesi at the European Institute of Oncology, Milan, Italy, reported (n = 701) confirmatory 25-year follow-up data, supporting the use of breast-conserving surgery for women with 2 cm or smaller breast cancers.[1]

Fisher et al. also published 20-year follow-up data (n = 1851) on the NSABP B-06 clinical trial of total mastectomy and lumpectomy with and without irradiation.[2] The overall 20-year survival rate was 47% for total mastectomy, 46% for lumpectomy alone and 46% for lumpectomy with irradiation. The cumulative local recurrence rate was 13.4% for lumpectomy with irradiation and 39.2% for lumpectomy alone.

W. H. Hindle, MD

References

1. Veronesi U, Cascinelli N, Mariani L, et al: Twenty-year follow up of a randomized study comparing breast-conserving surgery with radical mastectomy for early breast cancer. *N Engl J Med* 347:1227-1232, 2002.
2. Fisher B, Anderson S, Bryant J, et al: Twenty-year follow-up of a randomized trial comparing total mastectomy, lumpectomy, and lumpectomy plus irradiation for the treatment of invasive breast cancer. *N Eng J Med* 347:1233-1241, 2002.

SUGGESTED READING

Khan SA, Stewart MA, Morrow M: Does aggressive local therapy improve survival in metastatic breast cancer? *Surgery* 132:620-627, 2002.
▶ Review of the National Cancer Data Base (1990-1993) revealed 16,023 patients with stage IV breast cancer. About 57% received surgical treatment, of whom 38% had partial mastectomy and 62% had total mastectomy. Free surgical margins improved the 3-year survival of both mastectomy groups, 26% improvement for the partial group and 35% improvement for the total mastectomy group. Surgical resection with free margins showed a superior prognosis with a hazard ratio of 0.61 (95% confidence interval, 0.58-0.65) compared with the nonsurgically treated group.

William H. Hindle MD

Jakub JW, Diaz NM, Ebert MD, et al: Completion axillary lymph node dissection minimizes the likelihood of false negatives for patients with invasive breast carcinoma and cytokeratin positive only sentinel lymph nodes. *Am J Surg* 184:302-306, 2002.
▶ This series of 1380 sentinel node mappings/biopsies revealed that 29.6% had nodal involvement by hematoxylin and eosin (H&E) and that of those that were

negative by H&E, 8.0% were positive by cytokeratin-immunohistochemical (CK-IHC) staining. Of the CK-IHC–positive patients who underwent complete axillary lymph node dissection, 14.5% (9/62) had lymph node involvement by subsequent H&E staining. All 9 cases were associated with cancers larger than 10 mm. With this progressive stepwise surgical approach, the absolute false-negative rate was reduced to 2.6%.

William H. Hindle, MD

Chung MA, Steinhoff MM, Cady B: Clinical axillary recurrence in breast cancer patients after a negative sentinel node biopsy. *Am J Surg* 184:310-314, 2002.
▶ With a median follow-up of 26 months, there were 3 axillary recurrences in the 206 patients studied (1998-2001) for a 1.4% clinical false-negative rate in this series of sentinel lymph node biopsies. A table of 5 published series with a total of 743 patients and a mean 28-month follow-up reveals a mean 0.5% nodal recurrence rate by immunohistochemical evaluation.

William H. Hindle MD

Port ER, Fey J, Gemignani ML: Reoperative sentinel lymph node biopsy: a new option for patients with primary or locally recurrent breast carcinoma. *J Am Coll Surg* 195:167-172, 2002.
▶ This remarkable series of 3490 consecutive sentinel lymph node biopsies (SLNBs) performed at the Memorial Sloan-Kettering Cancer Center, New York, revealed 32 (1%) SLNBs performed after prior axillary surgery. A sentinel lymph node was identified in the 75% (24/32) of the reoperated cases of which 13% (3/24) were positive. The authors state that the reoperative SLNB was more likely to be successful if less than 10 nodes had been removed at the prior surgery. Thus, the indications for SLNB are being extended. Can SLNB as the "standard" be far in the future?

William H. Hindle, MD

Osborne CK, Pippen J, Jones SE, et al: Double-blind, randomized trial comparing the efficacy and tolerability of fulvestrant versus anastrozole in postmenopausal women with advanced breast cancer progressing on prior endocrine therapy: result of a North American trial. *J Clin Oncol* 20:3386-3395, 2002.
▶ The search for more effective and less adverse alternate chemotherapies is ongoing and probably will remain so. Fulvestrant is a seemingly complete estrogen receptor downregulator with no estrogenic activity. In this multicenter trial (n = 400), it was given as a 250-mg monthly injection and compared with anastrozole, 1 mg by mouth daily. Both were well tolerated. Fulvestrant was at least equal in effectiveness compared to anastrozole, and by several end point measures, it appeared to produce superior mean results. Only clinical usage and observations over several years will validate whether this represents a true step forward in the treatment of advanced breast cancer or whether it offers just another option.

William H. Hindle, MD

Partridge SC, Gibbs JE, Lu Y, et al: Accuracy of MR imaging for revealing residual breast cancer in patients who have undergone neoadjuvant chemotherapy. *AJR* 179:1193-1199, 2002.

▶ This pilot study (n = 52) from the University of California, San Francisco, compared preoperative and postoperative MR evaluation with traditional clinical evaluations. Tumor size was estimated by both techniques and then compared with the final pathologic measurements. It was found that MR had a higher correlation with a 100% sensitivity compared to 90% (47/52) for clinical examination. The precise clinical indications and cost effectiveness for MR evaluation in breast cancer patients are still being investigated.

William H. Hindle, MD

A Gene-Expression Signature as a Predictor of Survival in Breast Cancer
van de Vijver MJ, He YD, van 't Veer LJ, et al (Netherlands Cancer Inst, Amsterdam; Ctr for Biomedical Genetics, Amsterdam; Rosetta Inpharmatics, Kirkland, Wash)
N Engl J Med 347:1999-2009, 2002   31–3

Introduction.—Most clinicians agree that patients with poor prognostic characteristics benefit the most from adjuvant therapy. A more accurate method for prognostication in breast cancer that will improve the selection of patients who are appropriate for adjuvant systemic therapy is described.

Methods.—A microarray analysis was used to examine a previously established 70-gene prognostic profile to classify a series of 295 consecutive patients with primary breast cancer as having a gene expression signature that is either linked with a poor or good prognosis. The predictive value of the prognosis profile was assessed by both univariate and multivariate analyses.

Results.—Of 295 patients, 180 had a poor prognosis signature and 115 had a good prognosis signature. The mean overall 10-year survival rates for those with poor and good prognosis signatures were 54.6% and 94.5%, respectively. At 10 years, the probability of remaining free of distant metastases was 50.6% and 80.2% in these 2 groups, respectively. The estimated hazard ratio for distant metastases was 5.1 (95% confidence interval [CI], 2.9-9.0; $P < .001$) for the poor prognosis compared with that of the good prognosis signature group. This ratio continued to be significant when the groups were evaluated according to lymph node status (Fig 2). Multivariate Cox regression analysis demonstrated that the prognosis profile was a strong independent factor in predicting disease outcome.

Conclusion.—The gene expression profile assessed was a more powerful predictor of outcome of distant disease in young patients with breast cancer than standard systems that are based on clinical and histologic criteria.

▶ Because of the heterogeneous nature of breast cancers, there is an urgent ongoing search for accurate prognostic factors that can identify specific cancers that can be targeted with specific favorable treatments. Genetic research appears to be the most logical and fruitful approach to discovering the identity of these specific cancers. This study from The Netherlands Cancer Institute, Amsterdam, used complimentary DNA microassay analysis of 70-gene prognostic profile.[1] The patients (n = 295) had stage I or II breast cancer and were younger than 53 years. Dividing the group into good prognostic profiles and poor prognostic profiles revealed overall 10-year survival rates of 94.5% ver-

FIGURE 2

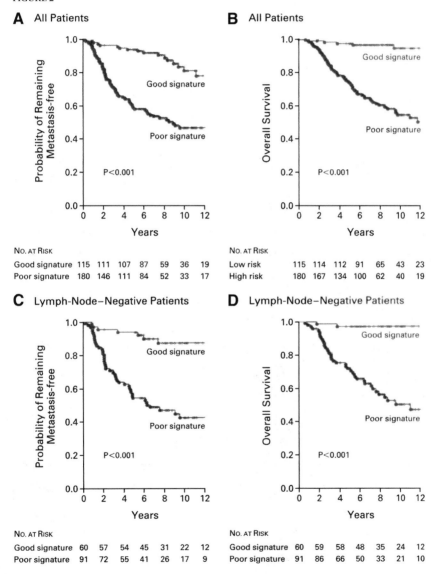

NO. AT RISK

A All Patients							
Good signature	115	111	107	87	59	36	19
Poor signature	180	146	111	84	52	33	17

NO. AT RISK

B All Patients							
Low risk	115	114	112	91	65	43	23
High risk	180	167	134	100	62	40	19

NO. AT RISK

C Lymph-Node–Negative Patients							
Good signature	60	57	54	45	31	22	12
Poor signature	91	72	55	41	26	17	9

NO. AT RISK

D Lymph-Node–Negative Patients							
Good signature	60	59	58	48	35	24	12
Poor signature	91	86	66	50	33	21	10

(Continued)

FIGURE 2 (cont.)

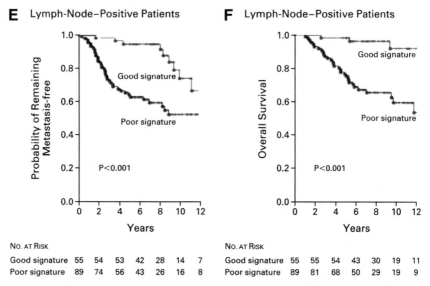

FIGURE 2.—Kaplan-Meier analysis of the probability that patients would remain free of distant metastases and the probability of overall survival among all patients (**A** and **B**), patients with lymph-node–negative disease (**C** and **D**), and patients with lymph-node–positive disease (**E** and **F**), according to whether they had a good-prognosis or poor-prognosis signature. The *P* values were calculated with use of the log-rank test. (Courtesy of *The New England Journal of Medicine* from van de Vijver MJ, He YD, van't Veer LJ, et al: A gene-expression signature as predictor of survival in breast cancer. *N Engl J Med* 347:1999-2009. Copyright 2002, Massachusetts Medical Society. All rights reserved.)

sus 54.6%, and 10-year without distant metastasis rates of 85.2% versus 50.6%. Comparable prognostic profile results were obtained when the patients were stratified into node-negative and node-positive groups; that is, a patient with a good prognosis could be identified regardless of her nodal status. Furthermore, the genetic prognostic profiles were more accurate than the St Gallen[2] or NIH[3] criteria for risk of recurrence. This genetic avenue of approach deserves funding of further exploration and hopefully will become a practical clinical tool.

W. H. Hindle, MD

References

1. van't Veer LJ, Dai H, van de Vijver MJ, et al: Gene expression profiling predicts clinical outcome of breast cancer. *Nature* 415:530-536, 2002.
2. Goldhirsch A, Glick JH, Gelber RD, et al: Meeting highlights: International consensus panel on the treatment of primary breast cancer: Seventh International Conference on Adjuvant Therapy of Primary Breast Cancer. *J Clin Oncol* 19:3817-3827, 2001.
3. Eifel P, Axelson JA, Costa J, et al: National Institutes of Health consensus development conference statement: Adjuvant therapy for breast cancer. *J Natl Cancer Inst* 93:979-989, 2001.

Concordance With Breast Cancer Pathology Reporting Practice Guidelines

Wilkinson NW, Shahryarinejad A, Winston JS, et al (Roswell Park Cancer Inst, Buffalo, NY; State Univ of New York, Buffalo)
J Am Coll Surg 196:38-43, 2003   31–4

Background.—Accurate pathology reporting is an important component of proper medical and surgical treatment of breast cancer. In 1998, the College of American Pathologists (CAP) distributed guidelines for the reporting of cancer specimens (Table 1). Community-wide concordance with CAP breast cancer reporting guidelines was determined.

TABLE 1.—College of American Pathologists Guidelines for Reporting Breast Cancer Specimens: Complete Excision of Tumor Less Than Total Mastectomy With or Without Axillary Contents

Clinical information
    Patient identification
    Responsible physician
    Date of procedure
    Relevant history
        Clinical findings
        Clinical diagnosis
        Operative findings
        Anatomic site of specimen
Macroscopic examination
    Specimen fixation
    Tissue size in three dimensions*
    Location of biopsy site
    Orientation by the surgeon*
    Results of intraoperative consultation
    Tumor size in three dimensions*
    Tumor descriptive features*
    Correlation with imaging studies
    Gross margin designation*
    Margin inking*
    Orientation*
    Status of surgical margins*
    Distance of closet margins*
    Frozen section
Microscopic evaluation
    Tumor size*
    Histologic type*
    Histologic grade*
    Ductal carcinoma in situ pattern and extent*
    Microcalcifications
    Extent of invasion*
    Bloom Scarf Richardson scale*
    Blood/lymphatic vessel invasion*
    Tumor, node, metastasis staging*
    Margins*
    Results of special studies

---

*Reviewed item.
(Reprinted with permission from the American College of Surgeons from Wilkinson NW, Shahryarinejad A, Winston JS, et al: Concordance with breast cancer pathology reporting practice guidelines. *J Am Coll Surg* 196:38-43, 2003.)

TABLE 2.—Margin Evaluation

	Gross Examination (%)	Specimen Inked (%)	Margin Orientation (%)	Micoscopic Margin Status Reported (%)	Distance to Closest Margin Reported (%)
Total (101)	52	77	25	94	69
CH (83)	49	75	16	93	67
RPCI (18)	67	89	72	100	70

Abbreviations: CH, Community hospital; *RPCI*, Roswell Park Cancer Institute.
(Reprinted with permission from the American College of Surgeons from Wilkinson NW, Shahryarinejad A, Winston JS, et al: Concordance with breast cancer pathology reporting practice guidelines. *J Am Coll Surg* 196:38-43, 2003.)

Methods.—The pathology reporting of stage I and II breast cancers was examined for adherence to CAP guidelines. Pathology reports were reviewed from 100 consecutive patients with invasive breast cancer referred to 1 institution from 1998 to 1999 after excisional breast biopsy. Also reviewed were 20 consecutive patients who underwent excisional biopsy at the study institution. Adherence to CAP guidelines for clinically relevant items was determined from the original pathology report for each patient.

Results.—A total of 101 patients met the inclusion criteria. Reports for most of these patients lacked at least 1 of the elements required by the CAP guidelines. Surgical margins were inked in only 77% of patients and the margins oriented in only 25% of patients (Table 2). Many specimens were not oriented by the surgeon. Grade was reported for most patients, but the Bloom Scarf Richardson grade was reported for only 6% of patients (Table 3). The presence or absence of lymphovascular invasion was reported for 57% of patients, and the presence or absence of coexisting in situ disease was reported for 71% of patients (Table 4).

Conclusion.—This study found wide variation in breast cancer pathology reporting. In many cases, key elements affecting treatment were omitted, including gross description and size, orientation and involvement of surgical margins, and description of histologic features. The passive distribution of CAP practice guidelines may be insufficient to accomplish community-wide quality improvement in breast pathology reporting.

TABLE 3.—Microscopic Evaluation of Primary Tumor

	Histologic Type (%)	Tumor Grade BSR (%)	Tumor Grade (%)	Tumor Size (%)	Presence/Absence LVI (%)	Reporting of TNM Staging (%)
Total (101)	100	6	90	90	47	9
CH (83)	100	7	88	88	45	0
RPCI (18)	100	0	100	100	61	50

Abbreviations: BSR, Bloom Scarf Richardson; *CH*, community hospital; *LVI*, lymphovascular invasion; *RPCI*, Roswell Park Cancer Institute.
(Reprinted with permission from the American College of Surgeons from Wilkinson NW, Shahryarinejad A, Winston JS, et al: Concordance with breast cancer pathology reporting practice guidelines. *J Am Coll Surg* 196:38-43, 2003.)

TABLE 4.—Description of In Situ Component (Ductal Carcinoma In Situ/ Lobular Carcinoma In Situ)

	Reported Presence/ Absence of In Situ Component (%)	Reported Extent of In Situ Component (%)	Reported Histologic Type of In Situ Disease (%)
Total (101)	71	47	49
CH (83)	67	37	41
RPCI (18)	94	94	88

Abbreviations: CH, Community hospital; *RPCI*, Roswell Park Cancer Institute.
(Reprinted with permission from the American College of Surgeons from Wilkinson NW, Shahryarinejad A, Winston JS, et al: Concordance with breast cancer pathology reporting practice guidelines. *J Am Coll Surg* 196:38-43, 2003.)

▶ This report documents what has long been suspected, that even when authoritative guidelines have been extensively distributed, many "final reports" in hospital records do not adhere to the guidelines. Thus, material that does not strictly follow published guidelines is not appropriate for definitive evaluation and meaningful clinical research. The heterogeneity and individual biological behavior of breast cancers present enough inherent difficulties without the addition of lumping together and reporting patients with seemingly similar cancers. Subsequently, the literature becomes filled with observational studies on groups of patients with cancers that are not really uniform in their characteristics or presentation. How can meaningful clinical conclusions be drawn from such disparate material?

W. H. Hindle, MD

SUGGESTED READING

Li CI, Anderson BO, Doling JR, et al: Trends in incidence rates of invasive lobular and ductal breast carcinoma. *JAMA* 289:1421-1424, 2003.
▶ Li et al analyzed SEER (Surveillance, Epidemiology, and End Results) data from the National Cancer Institute on 190,458 women aged 30 or older diagnosed with invasive breast cancer (1987-1999). During this study period, the invasive breast cancer incidence rates increased 1.04-fold (95% confidence interval [CI], 1.004-1.07). The lobular carcinoma rates increased 1.52-fold (95% CI, 1.42-1.63) and the mixed ductal-lobular rates increased 1.96-fold (95% CI, 1.80-2.14). However, the ductal carcinoma rates were unchanged.

The authors calculated that the percentage of invasive breast cancers with a lobular component increased from 9.5% to 15.6% (1987-1999). However, this type of epidemiologic study of data from such large numbers of patients should be viewed with caution as to the clinical implications. It would indeed be unfortunate if, in fact, the true incidence of breast lobular carcinoma is increasing in the United States because lobular carcinomas are typically diagnosed at more advanced stages associated with adverse outcomes, compared to ductal carcinomas.

Newcomer et al[1] reported a population-based case-controlled study (n = 2341) of women aged 50 and older with newly diagnosed breast cancer using Wisconsin statewide tumor registry data. Ductal carcinoma, not otherwise specified, accounted for 82% (1920/2341) and lobular carcinoma almost 9% (206/2341). Initial discovery for all the cancers was 48% self-detected, 41% mammographically detected, and 11% detected by clinical breast examination. However, lobular carcinoma was more often detected by clinical breast examination than by the patient. Mammography-detected lobular carcinoma was at about the same frequency as ductal carcinoma (42% vs 40%).

William H. Hindle, MD

Reference

1. Newcomer LM, Newcomb PA, Trentham-Dietz A, et al: Detection method and breast carcinoma histology. *Cancer* 95:470-477, 2002.

African-American Ethnicity, Socioeconomic Status, and Breast Cancer Survival: A Meta-analysis of 14 Studies Involving Over 10,000 African-American and 40,000 White American Patients With Carcinoma of the Breast
Newman LA, Mason J, Cote D, et al (Wayne State Univ, Detroit; Harvard School of Public Health, Boston; Harvard Med School, Boston)
Cancer 94:2844-2854, 2002   31–5

Background.—Compared to white American women, black women have higher breast cancer mortality rates, which have been attributed to socioeconomic factors. Black women with breast cancer also have an increased risk for developing high-grade, estrogen receptor negative disease and an increased risk of being diagnosed with early-onset breast carcinoma, factors which are not explained by socioeconomic considerations. While a crude association is generally supported between black ethnicity and increased breast cancer mortality risk, it diminishes when socioeconomic factors are considered. The independent predictive strength of self-reported black ethnicity regarding survival with breast cancer was assessed through a MEDLINE search and a meta-analysis.

Methods.—The studies sought used a Cox proportional hazards regression model to analyze outcomes for white and black women with breast cancer. A total of 3962 studies were initially identified. The effect of socioeconomic status was controlled.

Results.—Fourteen studies were finally included, covering 10,001 black and 42,473 white American patients who had breast cancer. A statistically significant survival disadvantage was present for black patients in all studies (Figs 1-5). When the various measures of socioeconomic status were considered, a substantial reduction in the relationship between ethnicity and outcome was found. Relatively small sample sizes of affluent black patients with breast cancer were included. On meta-analysis, black ethnicity proved to be a statistically significant independent predictor of outcome for these breast cancer patients, even with adjustments for socioeconomic status. When

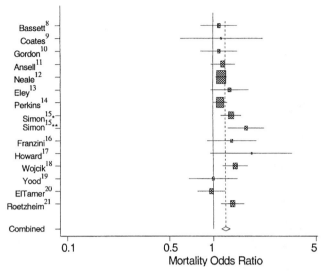

FIGURE 1.—Meta-analysis of all studies. The mortality odds ratios (adjusted for socioeconomic status) are shown for black patients compared with white American patients with breast carcinoma (with all-cause mortality odds ratios entered into the analysis unless only disease specific mortality odds ratios were available): meta-analysis odds ratio, random effects model = 1.215; 95% confidence interval, 1.13-1.30; Q statistic, 21.58 with 14 degrees of freedom. The *size of each box* correlates with the relative sample size of each study population; *horizontal lines* represent 95% confidence intervals. *Names at left* are the lead authors for the referenced studies. *Single asterisk* indicates patients aged less than 50 years; *double asterisk*, patients aged 50 years or older. (Courtesy of Newman LA, Mason J, Cote D, et al: African-American ethnicity, socioeconomic status, and breast cancer survival: A meta-analysis of 14 studies involving over 10,000 African-American and 40,000 white American patients with carcinoma of the breast. *Cancer* 94(11):2844-2854, 2002. ©2002 American Cancer Society. Reprinted by permission of Wiley-Liss, Inc, a subsidiary of John Wiley & Sons, Inc.)

comparisons were made to white American patients, the odds ratio of mortality for black women was 1.22 (range, 1.13 to 1.30). The strongest association between black ethnicity and worse outcome was demonstrated in 3 studies that evaluated patients who were only seen through equal-access systems; this odds ratio was 1.35.

Conclusion.—A number of studies confirm the population-based finding that black American patients who have breast cancer have a worse outcome than their white counterparts. When adjustments were made for socioeconomic factors, the effect of ethnicity was diminished. The flaw appears to be that studies generally include nonsignificant proportions of more affluent black patients, so the studies could not accurately address ethnicity and socioeconomic status. On meta-analysis, ethnicity is shown to be an independent predictor of mortality for black Americans. This indicates that biological and genetic predictors of outcome for breast cancer patients that are related to ethnicity and socioeconomic factors are measured poorly and not completely understood.

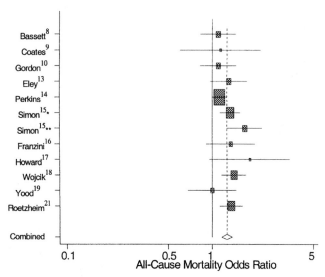

FIGURE 2.—Meta-analysis of studies reporting all-cause mortality showing mortality odds ratios (adjusted for socioeconomic status) for black patients compared with white American patients with breast carcinoma: meta-analysis odds ratio, random effects model = 1.27; 95% confidence interval, 1.17-1.38; Q statistic, 15.16 with 11 degrees of freedom. The *size of each box* correlates with the relative sample size of each study population; *horizontal lines* represent 95% confidence intervals. The *broken vertical line* and *diamond* represent the mortality odds ratio and confidence interval for the pooled analysis, respectively. *Names at left* are the lead authors for the referenced studies. *Single asterisk* indicates patients aged less than 50 years; *double asterisks*, patients aged 59 years or older. (Courtesy of Newman LA, Mason J, Cote D, et al: African-American ethnicity, socioeconomic status, and breast cancer survival: A meta-analysis of 14 studies involving over 10,000 African-American and 40,000 white American patients with carcinoma of the breast. *Cancer* 94(11):2844-2854, 2002. ©2002 American Cancer Society. Reprinted by permission of Wiley-Liss, Inc, a subsidiary of John Wiley & Sons, Inc.)

▶ The effect of African-American ethnicity on the incidence, treatment, outcome, and mortality of breast cancer has attracted intense attention, exemplified by the 3962 published studies in the initial literature search of this report. The multifactorial nature of every aspect of this issue makes analysis of data problematic at best. The authors have attempted to overcome these difficulties with a meta-analysis of 14 studies deemed appropriate for analysis (n = 10,001 study patients and 42,473 control patients). The variability of the studies is apparent in Figures 1 to 5. An odds ratio of 1.22 (95% CI 1.13-1.30) for adverse effects of African-American ethnicity was the summary statistic. Although the methodology of this study is admirable and seems valid, it will probably take definite genetic analysis to finally resolve this controversial issue.

W. H. Hindle, MD

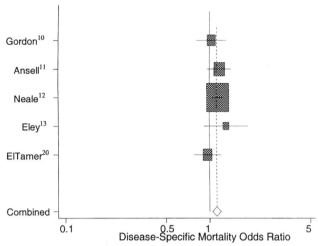

FIGURE 3.—Meta-analysis of studies reporting disease specific mortality. Mortality odds ratios (adjusted for socioeconomic status) are shown for black patients compared with white American patients with breast carcinoma: meta-analysis odds ratio, random effects model = 1.12; 95% confidence interval, 1.05-1.20; Q statistic, 3.20 with 4 degrees of freedom. The *size of each box* correlates with the relative sample size of each study population; *horizontal lines* represent 95% confidence intervals. The *broken vertical line* and *diamond* represent the mortality odds ratio and confidence interval for the pooled analysis, respectively. *Names at left* are the lead authors for the referenced studies. *Single asterisk* indicates patients aged less than 50 years; *double asterisks*, patients aged 59 years or older. (Courtesy of Newman LA, Mason J, Cote D, et al: African-American ethnicity, socioeconomic status, and breast cancer survival: A meta-analysis of 14 studies involving over 10,000 African-American and 40,000 white American patients with carcinoma of the breast. *Cancer* 94(11):2844-2854, 2002. ©2002 American Cancer Society. Reprinted by permission of Wiley-Liss, Inc, a subsidiary of John Wiley & Sons, Inc.)

SUGGESTED READING

Tartter PI, Gajdos C, Smith SR, et al: The prognostic significance of Gail model risk factors for women with breast cancer. *Am J Surg* 184:11-15, 2002.

▶ This report addresses the clinically important issue of eventual outcome related to risk factors, clinical presentations, pathologic finding, cancer characteristic, extent of disease, and treatment. Multivariate analysis revealed a local and distant disease-free survival correlation with lymph node involvement, but with no other factors. When the women were divided into high-risk (n = 106) and low-risk (n = 206) utilizing the Gail model, the unexpected result was that the high-risk group had significantly better disease-free survivals. Thus, in this study, the identified epidemiologic risk factors did not prove to be prognostic factors.

William H. Hindle, MD

Peters F, Kieblich A, Pahnke V: Coincidence of nonpuerperal mastitis and noninflammatory breast cancer. *Eur J Obstet Gynecol Reprod Biol* 105:59-63, 2002.

▶ Although based on only 5 out of 277 women, this report from Germany raises the question of nonpuerperal mastitis as a significant risk factor for the subsequent diagnosis of breast cancer within 12 months of treatment for mastitis. Multivariate analysis and collaboration by other breast centers will be required to confirm this observation and establish the clinical validity of this potential risk factor.

William H. Hindle, MD

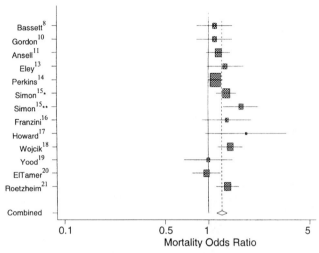

FIGURE 4.—Meta-analysis of studies using income/insurance measures of socioeconomic status. Mortality odds ratios (adjusted for socioeconomic status) are shown for black patients compared with white American patients with breast carcinoma: meta-analysis odds ratio, random effects model = 1.23; 95% confidence interval, 1.14-1.34; Q statistic, 20.0 with 12 degrees of freedom. The *size of each box* correlates with the relative sample size of each study population; *horizontal lines* represent 95% confidence intervals. The *broken vertical line* and *diamond* represent the mortality odds ratio and confidence interval for the pooled analysis, respectively. *Names at left* are the lead authors for the referenced studies. *Single asterisk* indicates patients aged less than 50 years; *double asterisks* patients aged 59 years or older. (Courtesy of Newman LA, Mason J, Cote D, et al: African-American ethnicity, socioeconomic status, and breast cancer survival: A meta-analysis of 14 studies involving over 10,000 African-American and 40,000 white American patients with carcinoma of the breast. *Cancer* 94(11):2844-2854, 2002. ©2002 American Cancer Society. Reprinted by permission of Wiley-Liss, Inc, a subsidiary of John Wiley & Sons, Inc.)

Chen WY, Colditz GA, Rosner B, et al: Use of postmenopausal hormones, alcohol and risk of invasive breast cancer. *Ann Intern Med* 137:798-804, 2002.
▶ Because of the large numbers (n = 44,187) and the length of follow-up, the data from the Nurses' Health Study are always of interest. However, there are known potential pitfalls with the use of pooled data from self-reported questionnaires. Even so, the epidemiologic levels of risk identified were minimal (relative risk, 1.32 and 1.28) and have questionable clinical value.

William H. Hindle, MD

Li R, Gilliland FD, Baumgartner K, et al: Hormone replacement therapy and breast carcinoma risk in Hispanic and non-Hispanic women. *Cancer* 95:960-968, 2002.
▶ This analysis of data from the New Mexico Women's Health Study (n = 366 postmenopausal women with breast cancer and 403 controls) appears to conflict with the report of the Women's Health Initiative in that no breast cancer association was observed with combined estrogen/progestin use in either Hispanic or

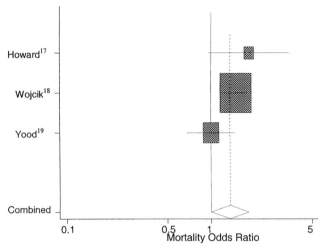

FIGURE 5.—Meta-analysis of studies reporting on breast cancer survival in equal-access health care systems. Mortality odds ratios (adjusted for socioeconomic status) are shown for black patients compared with white American patients with breast carcinoma: meta-analysis odds ratio, random effects model = 1.35; 95% confidence interval, 1.00-1.80; Q statistic, 3.95 with 2 degrees of freedom. The *size of each box* correlates with the relative sample size of each study population; *horizontal lines* represent 95% confidence intervals. The *broken vertical line* and *diamond* represent the mortality odds ratio and confidence interval for the pooled analysis, respectively. *Names at left* are the lead authors for the referenced studies. (Courtesy of Newman LA, Mason J, Cote D, et al: African-American ethnicity, socioeconomic status, and breast cancer survival: A meta-analysis of 14 studies involving over 10,000 African-American and 40,000 white American patients with carcinoma of the breast. *Cancer* 94(11):2844-2854, 2002. ©2002 American Cancer Society. Reprinted by permission of Wiley-Liss, Inc, a subsidiary of John Wiley & Sons, Inc.)

non-Hispanic women. The calculated odds ratios were low but suggested increased risk with "long-term" use of estrogen. Furthermore, this trend was greater for Hispanic women compared to non-Hispanic women. The multifactorial nature of breast cancer and the difficulties of accurate data collection make this and similar epidemiologic studies difficult to interpret and of questionable use in clinical practice.

William H. Hindle, MD

Webb PM, Byrne C, Schnitt SJ, et al: Family history of breast cancer, age and benign breast disease. *Int J Cancer* 100:375-378, 2002.
▶ In this analysis of the questionnaire data from the Nurses' Health Study (n = 80,995), 16,849 (21%) "reported a first diagnosis of benign breast disease." Of the women (n = 1465) who had slides for review from their breast biopsies, the women with a family history of breast cancer were about 3 times more likely to have atypia than women without a family history of breast cancer. The authors took this as support of atypia as a precursor or marker lesion for breast cancer.

William H. Hindle, MD

Oral Contraceptives and the Risk of Breast Cancer in BRCA1 and BRCA2 Mutation Carriers

Narod SA, Dubé M-P, Klijn J, et al (Univ of Toronto; Erasmus Univ, Rotterdam, The Netherlands; Pomeranian Med Univ, Szczecin, Poland; et al)

J Natl Cancer Inst 94:1773-1779, 2002   31–6

Background.—The lifetime risk of developing breast cancer is 50% to 80% in women who inherit a germline mutation in breast cancer susceptibility genes. The cancers typically occur in young women, often before 50 years of age. The use of oral contraceptives has been associated with an increase in the risk of breast cancer in young women. Whether this association is also found in women at high risk for breast cancer because they carry a mutation on either the BRCA1 or BRCA2 breast cancer susceptibility gene was investigated.

Methods.—This matched case-control study enrolled 1311 pairs of women with known deleterious BRCA1 or BRCA2 mutations. They were recruited from 52 centers in 11 countries. Women who had been diagnosed with breast cancer were matched to control subjects by year of birth, country of residence, mutation (BRCA1 or BRCA2), and history of ovarian cancer. Both patients and control subjects completed a questionnaire regarding their

TABLE 3.—Association Between Breast Cancer Risk and Oral Contraceptive Use Stratified by BRCA Mutation

Variable	Odds Ratio (95% CI)	P	P_{Trend}
Oral contraceptive use			
BRCA1 mutation carriers			
Never	1.00 (referent)	.03	
Ever	1.20 (1.02 to 1.40)		
BRCA2 mutation carriers			
Never	1.00 (referent)	.68	
Ever	0.94 (0.72 to 1.24)		
Duration of use, y			
BRCA1 mutation carriers			
Never	1.00 (referent)		
0-4	1.10 (0.92 to 1.31)	.30	
5-9	1.36 (1.11 to 1.67)	.003	
10-14	1.27 (0.99 to 1.64)	.06	
15-30	1.30 (0.91 to 1.87)	.15	
			.006
BRCA2 mutation carriers			
Never	1.00 (referent)		
0-4	0.90 (0.67 to 1.20)	.47	
5-9	0.82 (0.56 to 1.91)	.30	
10-14	1.16 (0.75 to 1.78)	.51	
15-30	1.35 (0.71 to 2.56)	.37	
			.42

Note: All P values were calculated by using a multivariable conditional logistic regression model with adjustment for ethnicity and parity. P_{trend} is based on increments of 5 years of exposure.

Abbreviation: CI, Confidence interval.

(Courtesy of Narod SA, Dubé M-P, Klijn J, et al: Oral contraceptives and the risk of breast cancer in BRCA1 and BRCA2 mutation carriers. *J Natl Cancer Inst* 94:1773-1779, 2002. By permission of Oxford University Press.)

TABLE 4.—Association Between Breast Cancer Risk and Oral
Contraceptive Use in BRCA1 Mutation Carriers

Oral Contraceptives Variable	Odds Ratio (95% CI)	Overall P	P_{Trend}
Contraceptive use			
Never	1.00 (referent)	.03	
Ever	1.20 (1.02 to 1.52)		
Recent use of oral contraceptive			
Never	1.00 (referent)		
Stopped >10 years ago	1.59 (1.30 to 1.94)	<.001	
Stopped within 6-10 years ago	1.10 (0.87 to 1.38)	.44	
Stopped within 1-5 years ago	1.03 (0.81 to 1.32)	.81	
Recent use	0.83 (0.66 to 1.04)	.11	
			.05
Age at first use, y			
Never	1.00 (referent)		
<20	1.36 (1.11 to 1.67)	.003	
20-24	1.35 (1.10 to 1.64)	.004	
25-29	1.03 (0.77 to 1.37)	.85	
30-60	0.75 (0.54 to 1.04)	.08	
			<.001
Age at last use, y			
Never	1.00 (referent)		
15-19	1.14 (0.84 to 1.56)	.41	
20-24	1.35 (1.08 to 1.63)	.006	
25-29	1.20 (0.98 to 1.47)	.08	
30-60	1.11 (0.91 to 1.35)	.30	
			.02

Note: All P values were calculated by means of a multivariable conditional logistic regression model with adjustment made for ethnicity and parity. For duration of use, the overall P value is for a linear trend associated with increments of 5-year exposure. Recent use of oral contraceptives is defined as use within 1 year of the age at diagnosis of the matched case subject.

Abbreviation: CI, Confidence interval.

(Courtesy of Narod SA, Dubé M-P, Klijn J, et al: Oral contraceptives and the risk of breast cancer in BRCA1 and BRCA2 mutation carriers. *J Natl Cancer Inst* 94:1773-1779, 2002. By permission of Oxford University Press.)

use of oral contraceptives. Odds ratios and 95% confidence intervals were derived by conditional logistic regression, and all statistical tests were 2-sided.

Results.—Among women carrying the BRCA2 mutation, any use of oral contraceptives was not associated with an increased risk of breast cancer. For BRCA1 mutation carriers, any use of oral contraceptives was associated with a modest increase in the risk of breast cancer (odds ratio, 1.20; 95% confidence interval, 1.02-1.40) (Tables 3-5). However, compared with BRCA1 mutation carriers who had never used oral contraceptives, those carriers who used oral contraceptives for at least 5 years had an increased risk of breast cancer, as did those who used oral contraceptives before age 30 years, those who were diagnosed with breast cancer before age 40 years, and those who first used oral contraceptives before 1975.

Conclusions.—Women who are carriers of the BRCA1 mutation may have an increased risk for early-onset breast cancer if they first used oral contraceptives before 1975, used them before age 30 years, or used them for 5 or more years. However, oral contraceptives do not appear to be associated

TABLE 5.—Association Between Breast Cancer Risk and Ever Use of Oral Contraceptives Among BRCA1 Mutation Carriers, Stratified by Other Factors

Ever Used Oral Contraceptives	Odds Ratio (95% CI)	P
Year of birth		
1925-1944	1.12 (0.82 to 1.53)	.48
1945-1954	1.20 (0.91 to 1.57)	.20
1955-1980	1.22 (0.94 to 1.59)	.14
Year of diagnosis		
1970-1979	1.98 (1.16 to 3.40)	.01
1980-1989	1.26 (0.94 to 1.70)	.13
1990-2001	1.11 (0.90 to 1.36)	.32
Age at diagnosis, y		
<40	1.38 (1.11 to 1.72)	.003
40-50	0.97 (0.73 to 1.28)	.82
>50	0.91 (0.50 to 1.64)	.76

Note: All P values were calculated by using a multivariable conditional logistic regression model with adjustment for ethnicity and parity. For each subgroup, the referent groups were those who never used oral contraceptives.

Abbreviation: CI, Confidence interval.

(Courtesy of Narod SA, Dubé M-P, Klijn J, et al: Oral contraceptives and the risk of breast cancer in BRCA1 and BRCA2 mutation carriers. *J Natl Cancer Inst* 94:1773-1779, 2002. By permission of Oxford University Press.)

with a risk of breast cancer in BRCA2 carriers, although data for these carriers are limited.

▶ This multicenter report (*n* = 1311 matched pairs) with more than 30 co-authors is probably as "authoritative" as any BRCA1-2 study. However, there are inherent difficulties with recall bias in questionnaire studies compounded by the fact that the exact type, dosage, and duration of oral contraceptive therapy are unknown. The group that "first used oral contraceptives before 1975" had the highest odds ratio in this analysis. The biological activity and dosage of the hormones in oral contraceptives before 1975 was substantially higher than in subsequent formulations. Even so, the odds ratio was less than 2.0, indicating a level of epidemiologic "weak association," that is, results that are probably by chance. With that perspective, these results are actually reassuring (as are all the other studies on oral contraceptive therapy and risk of breast cancer) that if there is any correlation between oral contraceptive therapy and breast cancer risk, the correlation is minimal at most and probably not clinically meaningful.

W. H. Hindle, MD

SUGGESTED READING

Metcalfe KA, Narod SA: Breast cancer risk prevention among women who have undergone prophylactic bilateral mastectomy. *J Natl Cancer Inst* 94:2564-2569, 2002.

▶ This study (n = 75; 1991-2000) from The Centre for Research in Women's Health, Sunnybrook and Women's College Health Sciences Centre, University of Toronto, Canada, interviewed women before and after their bilateral mastectomy as to family history of breast cancer and BRCA1-2 status. Comparisons were made with estimates of risk using the Gail, Claus, and BRCASPRO models. The women estimated their own lifetime risk of breast cancer, on average, as 76% (20%-100%) before surgery and 11.4% (0%-60%) after surgery. "The mean estimated absolute risk reduction the women attributed to prophylactic mastectomy was 64.8%." Except for the known BRCA1-2 carriers, all women significantly overestimated their own breast cancer risk.

Moller et al[1] analyzed patients with familial breast cancer (n = 249) of whom 36 had BRCA1 and 8 had BRCA2 mutations. BRCA1 was associated with estrogen receptor–negative, high grade, and invasive cancer. BRCA1 carriers compared to noncarriers had 5-year survival of 63% versus 91% for invasive cancer and 75% versus 96% for in situ cancer.

The authors describe the observed effects of oophorectomy as "striking." "Twenty-one of the mutation carriers had undergone prophylactic oophorectomy prior to or within 6 months of diagnosis in 13 cases. All but 1 relapse occurred in the 15 who had kept their ovaries ($P = <.01$); no relapse occurred in those whose ovaries had been removed within 6 months ($P = .04$)."[1]

Thompson et al[2] surveyed 11,847 individuals in 699 families and segregated the BRCA1 mutation carriers. Increased risks for other than breast and ovarian cancer were found for pancreatic cancer—relative risk (RR) of 2.26, 95% confidence interval (CI) of 1.26-4.06, $P < .001$; uterine corpus cancer—RR of 2.65, 95% CI of 1.69-4.16, $P = .001$; and cervical cancer—RR of 3.72, 95% CI of 2.26-6.10, $P < .001$.

Bergfeldt et al[3] utilized various Swedish population and health registries to identify 30,552 breast cancer patients matched with 146,117 first-degree relatives. The mean follow-up was 6 years. Ovarian cancer was identified in 122 of the cohort, giving an incidence ratio of 2.0 (95% CI, 1.8-13.1). For women diagnosed with breast cancer before the age of 40 and with a family history of breast cancer, the incidence ratio was 5.6% (95% CI, 1.8-13.1). With a family history of ovarian cancer, the incidence ratio was 17.0 (95% CI, 3.5-50.0). The authors state, "Breast cancer patients with family history of ovarian cancer had nearly a 10% risk of developing ovarian cancer before the age of 70."

William H. Hindle, MD

References

1. Moller P, Borg A, Evans DG, et al: Survival in prospectively ascertained familial breast cancer: Analysis of a series stratified by tumor characteristics, BRCA mutations and oophorectomy. *Int J Cancer* 101:555-559, 2002.
2. Thompson D, Easton DF: The Breast Cancer Linkage Consortium. Cancer incidence in BRCA1 mutation carriers. *J Natl Cancer Inst* 94:1358-1365, 2002.
3. Bergfeldt K, Rydh B, Granath F, et al: Risk of ovarian cancer in breast-cancer patients with a family history of breast or ovarian cancer: A population-based cohort study. *Lancet* 360:891-894, 2002.

A Working Model for the Time Sequence of Genetic Changes in Breast Tumorigenesis

Singletary SE (Univ of Texas, Houston)
J Am Coll Surg 194:202-216, 2002

31–7

Background.—Chemoprevention refers to chemotherapy to inhibit carcinogenesis before the development of invasive cancer. Chemoprevention trials have cancer as the end point and therefore require large sample sizes and long durations. One way to increase the amount of information available from such trials is to use biomarkers as surrogate end points. Appropriate biomarkers should be biologically relevant and characteristic of the specific premalignant lesion. This review used published data to develop a working model of the sequence of genetic changes involved in human breast cancer tumorigenesis. These genetic changes inform the choice of surrogate biomarkers in breast cancer chemoprevention trials.

Cancer Model.—Mutations in several genes are required for onconeogenesis. Progression from normal cell to cancer cell involves the activation of oncogenes and the suppression of tumor suppressor genes. Oncogenes are defined as genes that act to increase cell replication and decrease differentiation. Tumor suppressors are involved in growth inhibition or apoptosis. Certain genes, such as those with angiogenesis activity, are involved in the development of the metastatic phenotype. The accumulation of mutations is often more important that the order in which they occur.

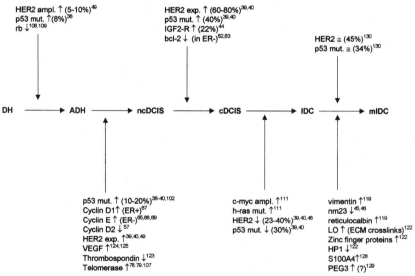

FIGURE 1.—Proposed time course of genetic events related to breast tumorigenesis. *Abbreviations: DH,* Ductal hyperplasia; *ADH,* atypical ductal hyperplasia; *ncDIS,* noncomedo ductal carcinoma in situ; *IDC,* invasive ductal carcinoma; *mICD,* metastatic invasive ductal carcinoma; *ampl,* amplification; *mut,* mutation; *exp,* expression; *ECM,* extracellular matrix; ↑, increase; ↓, decrease. *Note:* See original journal article for references. (Reprinted with permission from the American College of Surgeons courtesy of Singletary SE: A working model for the time sequence of genetic changes in breast tumorigenesis. *J Am Coll Surg* 194:202-216, 2002.)

Conclusion.—The current model for the development of invasive ductal carcinoma involves progression from hyperplasia to ductal carcinoma in situ to invasive carcinoma (Fig 1). The estrogen status of the tumor plays an important role. The early stages of breast cancer appear to be characterized by activation of telomerase and dysregulation of cyclins. High grade ductal carcinoma in situ is often associated with mutation of the tumor suppressor p53. The later stages of breast cancer are associated with the activation of genes associated with the metastatic phenotype. Chemoprevention trials for breast cancer must take into account the estrogen status of the tumor, as well as the biological importance of surrogate biomarkers in breast cancer onconeogenesis.

▶ For the average clinician, this detailed clinical summary requires intense, careful, dedicated reading. The report covers current work in progress on the action and use of surrogate end point biomarkers for breast cancer, with 130 references. It is an understandable background and frame of reference for future therapy to interrupt, and potentially permanently block, the progress of the continuum of the transformation of ductal epithelial hyperplasia to metastatic breast cancer (see Fig 1). How important is the initial genetic status of the epithelial cells? How critical is the sequencing of the changes in malignant transformation? It seems that some invasive cancers "appear de novo" and have not progressed through what we understand of malignant transformation.

What is the tumorigenesis mechanism of these apparently de novo cancers? Once the major cellular pathways of malignant transformation are identified, it will be potentially possible to develop pharmacologic interventions and manipulations that can truly prevent invasive and metastatic breast cancer.

W. H. Hindle, MD

Risk Factors for Fibroadenoma in a Cohort of Female Textile Workers in Shanghai, China

Nelson ZC, Ray RM, Gao DL, et al (Fred Hutchinson Cancer Research Ctr, Seattle; Shanghai Textile Industry Bureau, China)
Am J Epidemiol 156:599-605, 2002   31–8

Background.—Fibroadenomas—benign breast lesions characterized by an overgrowth of fibrous tissue with epithelial elements—are a source of substantial morbidity, anxiety, and cost. Risk factors for fibroadenoma were investigated in a large cohort of female textile workers in Shanghai, China.

Methods.—A total of 265,402 women were enrolled in a randomized study of breast self-examination between October 1989 and October 1991. All the women were interviewed at enrollment and followed up until July 2000. Fibroadenoma developed in 1507 women.

Findings.—Women younger than 35 years had the greatest risk of fibroadenoma. The risk decreased with age after 35 years, declining markedly at

TABLE 1.—Age Distribution of Subjects at the Time of Fibroadenoma Diagnosis in a Cohort of Female Textile Workers in Shanghai, China, 1989-2000

Age Category (Years)	Frequency (No.)	%	Cumulative %
≤34	229	15.2	15.2
35-39	636	42.2	57.4
40-44	464	30.8	88.2
45-49	125	8.3	96.5
50-54	18	1.2	97.7
55-59	14	0.9	98.6
≥60	21	1.4	100.0
Total*	1,507		

*Number of subjects developing fibroadenoma during study.
(Courtesy of Nelson ZC, Ray RM, Gao DL, et al: Risk factors for fibroadenoma in a cohort of female textile workers in Shanghai, China. *Am J Epidemiol* 156:599-605, 2002. By permission of Oxford University Press.)

menopause (Tables 1 and 2). The risk also declined with an increasing number of live births and the duration of oral contraceptive use. The risk increased with the number of previous benign breast lesions and with lower age at first benign lesion. Women receiving instruction in breast self-examination had an increased risk for fibroadenoma diagnosis.

Conclusion.—These data suggest that the development and persistence of fibroadenoma depend on the presence of ovarian hormones. Full-term pregnancies and exposure to exogenous estrogen-progesterone combinations before menopause may decrease the risk of fibroadenomas by enhancing differentiation or decreasing estrogen-induced proliferation in the mammary epithelium. Women who practice breast self-examination will find some fibroadenomas that would otherwise go undetected.

▶ The awesome numbers (*n* = 265,402) in this study by the Shanghai Textile Industry Bureau and Fred Hutchinson Cancer Research Center, Seattle, Wash-

TABLE 2.—Age-Specific Incidence Rates of Fibroadenoma for All Cases and Incident Cases in a Cohort of Female Textile Workers in Shanghai, China, 1989-2000

Age Category (Years)	All Cases*			Incident Cases*,†		
	Instruction Group	Control Group	Total	Instruction Group	Control Group	Total
≤34	369.6	122.0	241.4	198.5	93.4	144.1
35-39	214.9	115.5	164.5	163.4	103.0	132.8
40-44	120.7	74.3	97.3	100.8	70.9	85.7
45-49	44.0	29.8	37.0	41.5	29.1	35.4
50-54	10.6	9.3	10.0	7.4	8.1	7.8
55-59	6.5	3.2	4.9	5.7	2.4	4.1
≥60	3.5	1.8	2.6	3.0	1.8	2.4

*Rates are per 100,000 person-years.
†All fibroadenoma cases occurring at or after 6 months from the subject's entry into the study.
(Courtesy of Nelson ZC, Ray RM, Gao DL, et al: Risk factors for fibroadenoma in a cohort of female textile workers in Shanghai, China. *Am J Epidemiol* 156:599-605, 2002. By permission of Oxford University Press.)

ington, command attention. In this randomized breast self-examination trial, 1507 women (somewhat more than 0.5%) had fibroadenomas (1:176). Instruction in breast self-examination, prior breast lesions, and younger age at diagnosis of a first benign breast lesion increased the incidence. An increasing number of live births; increasing duration of oral contraceptive use; and advancing age, particularly post menopause, decreased the incidence. The authors conclude, "The development and persistence of fibroadenomas are dependent on the presence of ovarian hormones." All these observations are consistent with prior reports on the incidence and biological behavior of fibroadenomas.

W. H. Hindle, MD

Office-Based Ultrasound-Guided Cryoablation of Breast Fibroadenomas
Kaufman CS, Bachman B, Littrup PJ, et al (Univ of Washington, Bellingham; Wayne State Univ, Detroit; Rush Univ, Chicago; et al)
Am J Surg 184:394-400, 2002   31–9

Purpose.—About 1 in 5 surgical biopsies performed for palpable or mammographically detected breast abnormalities yields a diagnosis of fibroadenoma. Approaches using an automated coring device plus a heating or

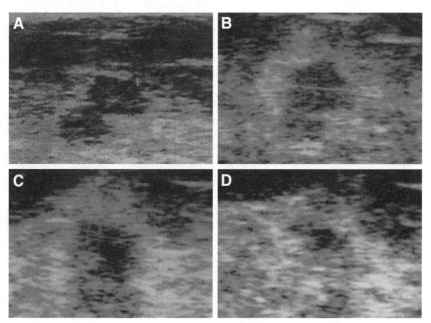

FIGURE 3.—**A**, US finding of bilobed fibroadenoma prior to cryoablation. **B**, US finding of bilobed fibroadenoma 3 weeks post cryoablation. **C**, US finding of bilobed fibroadenoma 3 months post cryoablation. **D**, US finding of bilobed fibroadenoma 6 months post cryoablation. (Reprinted from Kaufman CS, Bachman B, Littrup PJ, et al: Office-based ultrasound-guided cryoablation of breast fibroadenomas. *Am J Surg* 184:394-400, 2002. Copyright 2002 with permission from Excerpta Medica Inc.)

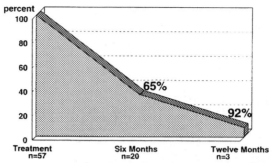

FIGURE 5.—Imaged fibroadenoma volume over time. Volume decreased by 65% at 6 months and 92% at 12 months. (Reprinted from Kaufman CS, Bachman B, Littrup PJ, et al: Office-based ultrasound-guided cryoablation of breast fibroadenomas. *Am J Surg* 184:394-400, 2002. Copyright 2002 with permission from Excerpta Medica Inc.)

cooling element may provide a valuable alternative to open surgery in such cases. An experience with cryoablation of biopsy-confirmed breast fibroadenomas was reported.

Methods.—The study included a total of 57 benign fibroadenomas in 50 patients. In each case, the diagnosis was confirmed at biopsy before cryoablation was performed; the fibroadenomas were no larger than 4 cm in maximum diameter. Treatment was carried out by means of a tabletop cryoablation system with a 2.4-mm cryoprobe, which was placed under sonographic guidance. Each fibroadenoma was treated with 2 cycles of freezing with a period of thawing in between; the treatment algorithm was based on tumor size. Throughout each procedure, skin appearance, skin and probe temperatures, the size of the iceball, and the patient's comfort were closely watched. The results were reevaluated 1 year after the ablation.

Findings.—The first 7 cases were performed in an ambulatory surgical center; the remainder were done in a physician's office, with many patients given only local anesthesia. The mean tumor diameter was 21 mm (range, 7-42 mm). In each case, the iceball completely engulfed the tumor. The procedure was followed by local swelling and ecchymosis, which resolved over time; discomfort was managed by acetaminophen or ibuprofen in most cases. Over 3 to 12 months' follow-up, the lesions gradually shrank and disappeared (Figs 3 and 5). No skin injuries or cosmetic problems were noted; patient satisfaction was high.

Conclusion.—This prospective, nonrandomized experience demonstrates excellent results with sonographically guided cryoablation for biopsy-confirmed fibroadenomas. The procedure was highly effective in shrinking or eliminating the tumors; there were few problems with scarring, and patient satisfaction was high. Cryoablation seems to provide a useful office-based alternative to surgery for these common benign breast tumors.

▶ This multicenter, prospective, nonrandomized pilot study (*n* = 57 fibroadenomas) demonstrates the effectiveness of an office-based, minimally invasive technique for the treatment of fibroadenomas. Most procedures were performed with "only local anesthesia." Apparently, side effects and postoperative discomfort were transient and minimal. Other ablative techniques are currently under investigation elsewhere. In all such procedures, it is essential that a definitive diagnosis be established before the ablative procedure is undertaken, as was done by tissue core-needle biopsy in this study. It is of keen clinical interest that it took 12 months to achieve a mean of 92% reduction in the volume of the treated lesions.

Conservative observational management of biopsy-proven fibroadenomas has been advocated as an alternate nonsurgical treatment of fibroadeomas.[1-3] Again, it is indispensable that a definite diagnosis of fibroadenoma be established prior to conservative management. As with any palpable dominant breast mass, if a definitive diagnosis is not established, the mass should be surgically excised with adequate margins, following the National Surgical Adjuvant Breast and Bowel Project biopsy protocol.[4]

W. H. Hindle, MD

References

1. Hindle WH, Alonzo LJ: Conservative management of breast fibroadenomas. *Am J Obstet Gynecol* 164:1647-1650, 1991.
2. Cant PJ, Madden MV, Coleman MG, et al: Non-operative management of breast masses diagnosed as fibroadenoma. *Br J Surg* 82:792-794, 1995.
3. Dixon JM, Dobbie V, Lamb J, et al: Assessment of the acceptability of conservative management of fibroadenoma of the breast. *Br J Surg* 83:264-265, 1996.
4. Margolese R, Poisson R, Shibata H, et al: The technique of segmental mastectomy (lumpectomy) and axillary dissection: A syllabus from the National Surgical Adjuvant Breast Project workshops. *Surgery* 102:828-834, 1987.

SUGGESTED READING

Franco N, Arnould L, Mege F, et al: Comparative analysis of molecular alterations in fibroadenomas associated or not with breast cancer. *Arch Surg* 138:291-295, 2003.

▶ This retrospective cohort study (n = 32 associated with breast cancer and n = 26 not associated with cancer) from the Centre Georges Francois Leclerc, Dijon, France, did not reveal micro satellite alterations or *p53* gene mutations within the fibroadenomas. Furthermore, histologic evaluation did not reveal any morphological differences between the 2 groups. The authors conclude, ". . .fibroadenomas are not associated with breast carcinogenesis."

In related imaging studies, Chao et al[1] analyzed sonographic features of 2204 fibroadenomas and 110 phyllodes tumors; and Yilmaz et al[2] attempted to differentiate phyllodes tumors (n = 12) and fibroadenomas (n = 19). The phyllodes were larger, more likely lobulated, and occurred in older women than did the fibroadenomas. However, there was substantial overlap in these factors and the sonographic features of the fibroadenomas. Lobulations, heterogeneous hypoechoic internal echoes, and lack of calcifications "suggested" a phyllodes tumor. Furthermore, the authors state, "Sonography cannot distinguish between malignant, borderline or benign phyllodes tumors."

Yilmaz et al reported sonographic findings of round or lobulated shape, marked posterior acoustic enhancement, and intramural cystic areas to correlate with phyllodes tumors compared to fibroadenomas, but, as in the Chao study, there were considerable similarities in both the mammographic and sonographic findings of the 2 tumors. The authors recommend excisional biopsy for definitive histologic diagnosis of "equivocal masses."

William H. Hindle, MD

References

1. Chao TC, Lo YF, Chen SC, et al: Sonographic features of phyllodes tumors of the breast. *Ultrasound Obstet Gynecol* 20:64-71, 2002.
2. Yimaz E, Sal S, Lebe B: Differentiation of phyllodes tumors versus fibroadenomas. *Acta Radiologica* 43:34-39, 2002.

Morris KT, Vetto JT, Petty JK, et al: A new score for the evaluation of palpable breast masses in women under age 40. *Am J Surg* 184:346-347, 2002.

▶ This report (n = 113) from the Department of Surgery, Oregon Health and Science University, Portland, Ore, proposes a modified triple test score of physical examination, fine-needle aspiration, and US imaging in this age group of 40 years and younger. The score is a straightforward summary of 1 for benign, 2 for suspicious, and 3 for malignant for each of the 3 diagnostic modalities. All (n = 108) those scores of 3 or 4 proved to be benign. Two scores of more than 6 were both malignant. Of the 3 scores of 5, 1 was malignant. Thus, only 3% (3/113) required surgical biopsy for definitive diagnosis.

This approach expedites the treatment of malignant masses and allows appropriate follow-up of benign masses. Although the incidence of carcinoma is low in this age group, close follow-up is essential for apparently "benign" lesions that are not excised. Furthermore, if either the patient or her family or her primary care physician continues to be "worried" about the diagnosis, most breast specialists would recommend surgical excision.

William H. Hindle, MD

Severity of Mastalgia in Relation to Milk Duct Dilatation
Peters F, Diemer P, Mecks O, et al (St Hildegardis Hosp, Mainz, Germany; Bioscientía Inst of Lab Chemistry, Ingelheim, Germany)
Obstet Gynecol 101:54-60, 2003   31–10

Background.—The cause of mastalgia is not well understood. The US appearance of milk ducts was investigated in healthy, premenopausal, nonlactating women to examine the association between mastalgia pain and duct size.

Study Design.—The study group consisted of 335 healthy women, aged 17 to 47 years, who were participating in a genital and mammary cancer screening program between 1998 and 1999. Each woman underwent US with color Doppler sonography, and the width of the milk ducts was recorded. The participants then completed a pain chart and linear visual analogue scale for pain for a complete menstrual cycle. Patients with breast pain received another sonogram during the period of worst pain.

Findings.—The width of the milk ducts ranged from less than 0.4 mm (the limit of detection) to 8.0 mm. Breast pain was not reported by 123 study participants, while 212 participants complained of breast pain. The pain was

TABLE 1.—Clinical Data for 335 Premenopausal Women

	Asymptomatic (n = 123)	Cyclical Mastalgia (n = 136)	Noncyclical Mastalgia (n = 76)
Age (y) (mean ± SD)	33.50 ± 6.00	32.85 ± 8.70	34.32 ± 6.69
Parity (mean)	1.35	1.38	1.30
Maximum dilation (mm) (mean ± SD)	1.80 ± 0.84	2.34 ± 1.10	3.89 ± 1.26*
Intensity of pain† (mean ± SD)		34.7 ± 17.2	53.0 ± 19.3*
Dilated ducts = site of pain [n (%)]		24 (17.7)	63 (82.9)*

*P <.001 t test.
†Pain was patient-assessed using a 100-mm analogue scale.
(Reprinted with permission from The American College of Obstetricians and Gynecologists courtesy of Peters F, Diemer P, Mecks O, et al: Severity of mastalgia in relation to milk duct dilatation. *Obstet Gynecol* 101:54-60, 2003.)

cyclical in 64.2% and noncyclical in 35.8% of those who reported pain (Table 1). In women with breast pain, dilated milk ducts were detected in all quadrants of the breast, especially in the retroareolar area (Fig 1). The width of the duct did not appear to vary with the menstrual cycle. The average maximal width of the milk duct was 1.8 mm in asymptomatic women, 2.34 mm in women with cyclical mastalgia, and 3.89 mm in women with noncyclical mastalgia.

Tissue edema was diagnosed in 46.3% of women with cyclical mastalgia. The severity of pain in women with cyclical mastalgia was significantly higher than in those with noncyclical mastalgia. The pain intensity was signifi-

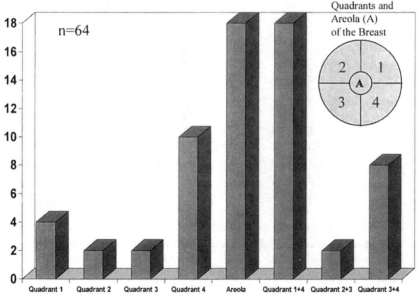

FIGURE 1.—Allocation of milk ducts (more than 0.4mm) to the particular quadrant and the areola of the breast in 64 patients. The *circle* in the top right corner of the figure describes the quadrants of the breast: *1* and *4* = outer quadrants. **A**, indicates the areolar region. (Reprinted with permission from The American College of Obstetricians and Gynecologists courtesy of Peters F, Diemer P, Mecks O, et al: Severity of mastalgia in relation to milk duct dilatation. *Obstet Gynecol* 101:54-60, 2003.)

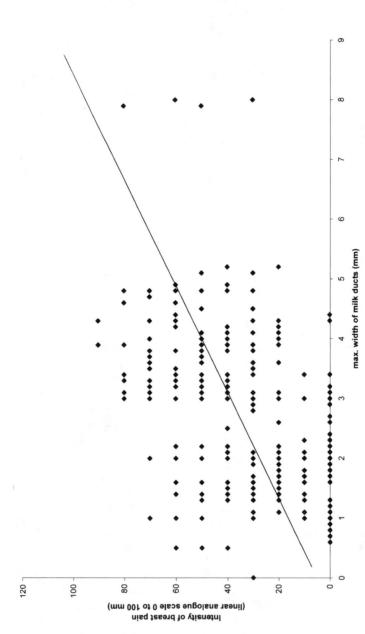

FIGURE 3.—Correlation between the width of the milk ducts and the intensity of breast pain ($n = 168$, $r = 0.5008$, $P < .001$) *Abbreviation: max*, Maximum. (Reprinted with permission from The American College of Obstetricians and Gynecologists courtesy of Peters F, Diemer P, Mecks O, et al: Severity of mastalgia in relation to milk duct dilatation. *Obstet Gynecol* 101:54-60, 2003.)

cantly correlated with milk duct size (Fig 3). Pain was identified at the site of dilated ducts detected by US in 82.9% of women with noncyclical mastalgia.

Conclusion.—Milk duct dilatation is associated with breast pain in healthy, nonlactating women. The reason for the dilatation is not known.

▶ Mastalgia is a common phenomenon in women of reproductive age. However, since it is rarely associated with cancer except in the advanced stages, mastalgia has not received the medical attention, study, and research of cancer-associated symptoms and findings. In fact, many women with mastalgia do not mention their breast symptoms to their primary health care providers. Ob-gyns should inquire about breast pain when taking a woman's history. Physicians will be surprised at the number of women who have or have had "troubling" mastalgia. However, the etiology of cyclic and noncyclic mastalgia remains an enigma, except when the noncyclic pain is associated with specific breast pathology, for example, persistent costochondritis (Tietze's syndrome).

This observational study (n = 335, of which 212 had mastalgia with about two thirds cyclic and one third noncyclic) from Mainz, Germany, used focused US to measure the width of the milk ducts. A positive correlation was found between the intensity of the mastalgia and the width of the milk ducts, and between the site of noncyclic mastalgia and the site of the dilated ducts. These findings are interesting indeed but leave the mechanism of the etiology of the dilated ducts unanswered.

In a related study, Blommers et al reported on a randomized, double-blind, factorial clinical trial evaluating the effectiveness of evening primrose oil and fish oil in the treatment of mastalgia.[1] The study size was (n = 120) divided into 4 subgroups. Mastalgia was decreased by 6 months' treatment, but neither evening primrose nor fish oil demonstrated "clear benefit over control oils." This is surprising as evening primrose oil, particularly due to its minimal side effects, has been a mainstay of mastalgia treatment, especially in the United Kingdom.[2]

W. H. Hindle, MD

References

1. Blommers J, de Lange-de Klerk ESM, Kuik DJ, et al: Evening primrose oil and fish oil for severe chronic mastalgia: A randomized, double-blind, controlled trial. *Am J Obstet Gynecol* 187:1389-1394, 2002.
2. Mansel RE, Hughes LE: Breast pain and nodularity, in Hughes LE, Mansel RE, Webster DJT (eds): *Benign Disorders and Diseases of the Breast.* WB Saunders, London, 2000.

Suggested Reading

Colak T, Ipek T, Kanik A, et al: Efficacy of topical nonsteroidal anti-inflammatory drugs in mastalgia treatment. *J Am Coll Surg* 196:525-530, 2003.

▶ This report (n = 108, 60 cyclic and 48 noncyclic) from the Medical Faculty of Mersin University, Mersin, Turkey, cites references that "More than 70% of women complain of breast pain at some time during their lives."[1,2] In a randomized, placebo-controlled clinical trial, the treatment groups applied 50 mg diclofenac diethylamonium gel topically to the breast 3 times a day for 6 months. The treatment groups had 82% to 88% decrease in pain score compared to 15% to

18% decrease in the placebo groups. The efficacy of this topical nonsteroidal treatment is similar to that reported by Irving.[3] Side effects in both studies were minimal. A double-blinded crossover in the Colak study would have been of keen clinical interest. Furthermore, the study, unfortunately, continues to use the inappropriate "diagnosis" of "fibrocystic disease," which currently is generally accepted to be a "change" or "condition" and not a "disease."

In a related study (n = 110) of focal breast pain without an associated palpable mass, Leung[4] found targeted (focused) US to be useful for patient reassurance. No cancers were identified. Cysts were diagnosed in 13.6% (15/110) and benign solid masses in 2.7% (3/110).

William H. Hindle, MD

References

1. Tavaf-Motamen H, Ader DN, Browns NW, et al: Clinical evaluation of mastalgia. *Arch Surg* 133:211-213, 1998.
2. Gateley CA, Mansel RE: Management of cyclical breast pain. *Br J Hosp Med* 43:330-332, 1990.
3. Irving AD, Morrison SL: Effectiveness of topical non-steroidal anti-inflammatory drugs in the management of breast pain. *J R Coll Surg Edinb* 43:158-159, 1998.
4. Leung JWT, Kornguth PJ, Gotway MB: Utility of targeted sonography in the evaluation of focal breast pain. *J Ultrasound Med* 21:521-526, 2002.

Surgical Decision Making and Factors Determining a Diagnosis of Breast Carcinoma in Women Presenting With Nipple Discharge
Cabioglu N, Hunt KK, Singletary SE, et al (Univ of Texas, Houston)
J Am Coll Surg 196:354-364, 2003   31–11

Background.—Nipple discharge can be benign or pathologic, in the latter case, a sign of breast cancer. There is currently no consensus regarding the utility of diagnostic tests for determining whether breast discharge is benign or pathologic. Nipple discharge characteristics associated with a diagnosis of breast cancer were examined. Also evaluated were the sensitivity, speci-

---

TABLE 2.—Sensitivity, Specificity, and Positive and Negative Predictive Values for Each Diagnostic Procedure in the Detection of Cancer Among Patients With Pathologic Nipple Discharge

Diagnostic Procedure	Sensitivity %	95% CI	Specificity %	95% CI	PPV %	95% CI	NPV %	95% CI
Mammography	68.4	43.5-87.4	75.7	64.3-84.9	41.9	24.6-60.9	90.3	80.1-96.4
Sonography	80	51.9-95.7	61.2	46.2-84.8	38.7	21.9-57.8	90.9	75.7-98.1
Ductography	100.0	75.3-100.0	5.6	1.6-13.8	16.3	8.9-26.2	100	39.8-100.0
Cytology	26.7	7.8-55.1	81.1	68.0-90.6	28.6	8.4-58.1	79.6	66.5-89.4

Abbreviations: CI, Confidence interval; *NPV*, negative predictive value; *PPV*, positive predictive value.
(Reprinted with permission from the American College of Surgeons courtesy of Cabioglu N, Hunt KK, Singletary SE, et al: Surgical decision making and factors determining a diagnosis of breast carcinoma in women presenting with nipple discharge. *J Am Coll Surg* 196:354-364, 2003.)

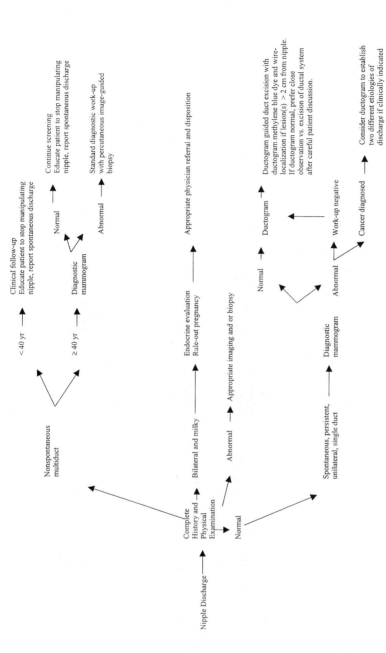

FIGURE 1.—MD Anderson Cancer Center algorithm for evaluation and surgical management of patients presenting with nipple discharge. (Reprinted with permission from the American College of Surgeons courtesy of Cabioglu N, Hunt KK, Singletary SE, et al: Surgical decision making and factors determining a diagnosis of breast carcinoma in women presenting with nipple discharge. *J Am Coll Surg* 196:354-364, 2003.)

ficity, and positive and negative predictive values of the various diagnostic techniques used in determining whether discharge is benign or pathologic.

Study Design.—Medical records were reviewed for all 146 patients who were assessed at The University of Texas MD Anderson Cancer Center for nipple discharge between August 1993 and September 2000. The majority of patients had cytologic analysis of nipple discharge. Of the 146 patients, 52 were classified as having benign discharge and treated conservatively. The remaining 94 patients were classified as having pathologic discharge.

These patients underwent mammographic or sonographic imaging. If this demonstrated any abnormality, the patients had a biopsy or surgical procedure for diagnosis or treatment. Prior to surgery, 42 patients had ductographic localization of the involved duct. The sensitivity, specificity, positive predictive value, and negative predictive value for the detection of cancer were calculated for mammography, sonography, cytology, and ductography.

Findings.—Both mammographic and sonographic abnormalities were independent factors associated with the diagnosis of cancer (Table 2). Ductography was necessary to identify malignant lesions in 33 patients. Patients who had a ductography-guided procedure were more likely to have an underlying lesion specifically identified.

Conclusion.—Discrimination between benign and pathologic nipple discharge should be based on patient history, physical examination, and imaging studies including ductography, if necessary. Ductography combined with surgical excision is useful for the diagnosis and treatment of these lesions (Fig 1).

▶ Nipple discharge is frequently mentioned as a potential sign of breast cancer. In clinical practice, this is rarely the case, unless there is an associated palpable mass. However, many women become acutely concerned when they elicit discharge from their nipples or the discharge occurs spontaneously. Most women of reproductive age can elicit nipple discharge from their breast. Thus, it seems prudent not to recommend that women who wish to perform breast–self examination "squeeze" their nipples to ascertain if they can produce nipple discharge.

At the Breast Diagnostic Center, Women's and Children's Hospital, LAC+USC Medical Center, Los Angeles, approximately 4% of presenting patients complained of nipple discharge.[1] However, only 1% (that is, one fourth of those presenting with nipple discharge) had spontaneous nipple discharge. It is generally agreed that elicited discharge is physiologic and that spontaneous discharge is pathologic and deserves diagnostic evaluation. Galactography (ductography) gives precise identification of the portion of the duct producing the discharge.[2] This precise localization of the lesion allows exact limited surgery and complete excision of the involved portion of the duct. All intraductal lesions should be completely excised, as only histology can definitively diagnose the rare intraductal papillary carcinomas.

An alternate approach based on the experience of the Ochsner Clinic, New Orleans, La—utilizing clinical evaluation, physical examination, and diagnostic breast imaging for women 35 years of age or older—can be useful in areas where galactography is not available.[3] The color of the nipple discharge is important. Non–pregnancy related bloody nipple discharge is most likely to originate from a malignancy. Non–pregnancy related milky discharge is usually bilateral, from multiple ducts, and a manifestation of galactorrhea.[4]

W. H. Hindle, MD

References

1. Hindle WH, Arias RD: Nipple Discharge, in Hindle WH (ed): *Breast Care*. Springer-Verlag, New York, 1999.
2. Tabar L, Dean PB, Pentek Z: Galactography: The diagnostic procedure of choice for nipple discharge. *Radiology* 149:31-38, 1983.
3. King TA, Carter KM, Bolton JS, et al: A simple approach to nipple discharge. *Am Surg* 66:960-965, 2000.
4. Paulson RJ: Galactorrhea, in Hindle WH (ed): *Breast Care*. Springer-Verlag, New York, 1999.

SUGGESTED READING

Dietz JR, Crowe JP, Grundfest S, et al: Directed duct excision by using mammary ductoscopy in patients with pathologic nipple discharge. *Surgery* 132:582-588, 2002.

▶ This observational study (n = 119 patients, 121 procedures) is from the Cleveland Clinic Foundation, Cleveland, Ohio. Ductoscopes with an external diameter of 1.2 mm or 0.9 mm could be passed in 88% (105/119) of patients with "pathologic" nipple discharge. A ductoscopy-directed duct excision was performed in 87% (104/119). Thus, abnormal pathology was diagnosed in 88% (105/119) of the total study patients with 84 papillomas, 16 hyperplasias, and 5 cancers. In 22 of the spinets, the ductal lesions extended beyond 4 cm.

The procedures were performed in an operating room under light IV sedation and local anesthesia. The complications were 1 postoperative hematoma, which resolved spontaneously, and 5 wound infections treated with antibiotics; 1 of the wound infections required incision drainage and packing. Similar studies with comparisons to traditional surgical excisions of intraductal lesions, with cost-effectiveness analysis, will be required before mammary ductoscopy procedures can be recommended for general use.

Wahner-Roedler et al[1] at the Mayo Clinic, Rochester, Minn, reviewed a case of spontaneous unilateral nipple discharge with "negative" physical examination and imaging studies (mammography and US). Subsequently, ductography revealed a 3- to 4-mm intraluminal lesion which needle core biopsy found to be high-grade ductal carcinoma in situ but which mastectomy proved to be multiple foci of invasive mucinous ductal adenocarcinoma. As with reports of others,[2,3] the authors perceive little value for cytologic evaluation of nipple discharge. Ductography is recommended for the evaluation of "pathologic" nipple discharge.[4]

Berna et al[5] at the University General Hospital, Murcia, Spain, reported their experience (n = 11; 1994-1999) with the nonsurgical treatment of mammary duct fistulas. They described "typical" US features and a 20-day regimen of microwave and US. All of the cases responded to the treatment, but 2 required a second treatment cycle. Hopefully, others will duplicate this experience as the treatment of mammary duct fistulas has been frustrating, with a pattern of frequent recurrences. Traditionally, surgical excision has been the final treatment.

William H. Hindle, MD

References

1. Wahner-Roedler DL, Reynolds C, Morton MJ: Spontaneous unilateral nipple discharge: When screening tests are negative—A case report and review of current diagnostic management of pathologic nipple discharge. *The Breast J* 9:49-52, 2003.
2. Danforth DN Jr, Lichter AS, Lippman ME: The diagnosis of breast cancer, in Lipoma ME, Lichter AS, Danforth DN Jr (eds): *Diagnosis and Management of Breast Cancer.* Philadelphia, WB Saunders, 1988, pp 76-77.
3. Di Pietro S, Coopmans de Yoldi G, Bergonzi S, et al: Nipple discharge as a sign of preneoplastic lesions and occult carcinoma of the breast: Clinical and galactographic study in 103 consecutive patients. *Tumori* 65:317-324, 1979.
4. Tabar L, Dean PB, Pentek Z: Galactography: The diagnostic procedures of choice for nipple discharge. *Radiology* 149:31-38, 1983.
5. Berna JD, Sanchez J, Madrigal M, et al: An alternative approach to the treatment of mammary duct fistulas: A combination of microwave and ultrasound. *Am Surgeon* 68:879-899, 2002.

A Prospective Review of the Decline of Excisional Breast Biopsy

Crowe JP Jr, Rim A, Patrick R, et al (Cleveland Clinic Found, Ohio)
Am J Surg 184:353-355, 2002   31–12

Background.—Core biopsies are being performed more often than excisional breast biopsies for the diagnosis of breast cancer. Whether this approach can replace excisional biopsy is not clear. This article investigated the relationship between diagnostic excisional and core biopsies relative to surgical procedures at a single institution over a 5-year period.

Methods and Findings.—Data were collected prospectively on 2631 core biopsies, 2685 excisional biopsies, 2881 surgical procedures for breast cancer, and 51,109 office visits, all of which occurred between 1995 and 2000. The percentage of core biopsies relative to excisional biopsies increased from 31% to 68% (*P* = <0.001) during the study period (Fig 1). However, the percentage of biopsies relative to the number of office visits remained

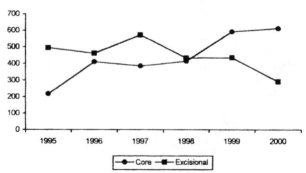

FIGURE 1.—Volume of core biopsies relative to excisional biopsies: Yearly trends (*P* = .001). (Reprinted from Crowe JP Jr, Rim A, Patrick R, et al: A prospective review of the decline of excisional breast biopsy. *Am J Surg* 184:353-355, 2002. Copyright 2002, with permission from Excerpta Medica Inc.)

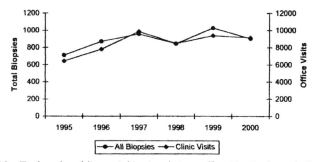

FIGURE 2.—Total number of diagnostic biopsies relative to office visits: Yearly trends (*P* = not significant). (Reprinted from Crowe JP Jr, Rim A, Patrick R, et al: A prospective review of the decline of excisional breast biopsy. *Am J Surg* 184:353-355, 2002. Copyright 2002, with permission from Excerpta Medica Inc.)

stable at 10% to 11% (Fig 2). Also stable was the percentage of breast cancer procedures relative to number of office visits at 5% to 6% (Fig 3).

Conclusion.—At the authors' institution, core biopsies are being done more often than excisional biopsies. However, 1 in 3 biopsies performed over this period at the authors' center was excisional.

▶ This observational study from the Cleveland Clinic Breast Center, Cleveland, Ohio, covers practice and procedure patterns over 5 years (1995-2000). In the last 2 years (see Fig 1), there has been a definitive trend toward an increased number of tissue core-needle biopsies and a commensurate decrease in open surgical excisional biopsies. The authors state that since then, the number of tissue core-needle biopsies "has increased to 68% of all diagnostic breast biopsies in our institution." Similar experiences could probably be found in data from most of the major breast centers in the United States. Since more than 1 million breast biopsies are estimated to be performed every year in the United States,[1] the techniques and total cost per procedure significantly impact the overall cost and allocation of the resources for women's health care. Due to the fractional and diverse delivery system of health care in the United States, trends in major breast centers often do not reflect overall clinical practice.

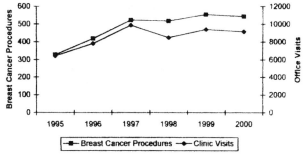

FIGURE 3.—Total number of breast cancer procedures relative to office visits: Yearly trends (*P* = .004). (Reprinted from Crowe JP Jr, Rim A, Patrick R, et al: A prospective review of the decline of excisional breast biopsy. *Am J Surg* 184:353-355, 2002. Copyright 2002, with permission from Excerpta Medica Inc.)

In this Cleveland Clinic study, it is of particular interest that the relationship between the number of biopsies and clinic visits remained constant (Fig 2), as has the relationship between the number of breast cancer procedures and clinic visits (Fig 3). This would suggest that the indications for biopsy and surgical procedures have not changed during the study period.

W. H. Hindle, MD

Reference

1. Edwards MJ, Mahoney D: Image-guided needle breast biopsy. *Breast Dis* 12:13-21, 2001.

SUGGESTED READING

Hansen NM, Grube BJ, Giuliano AE: The time has come to change the algorithm for the surgical management of early breast cancer. *Arch Surg* 137:1131-1135, 2002.

▶ This report from the Joyce Eisenberg Keefer Breast Center, John Wayne Cancer Institute, St. John's Health Center, Santa Monica, Calif, covers 238 sentinel lymph node biopsies (1995-1999) which were negative for cancer both by hematoxylin-eosin and immunohistochemical stains. With a median follow-up of 38.9 (6 to 69) months, there have been no axillary recurrences. However, 4 (4/238) patients have metastatic cancer and 3 (3/238) have died of causes unrelated to their breast cancer. The authors call for a multicenter clinical trial to corroborate these findings and to potentially abandon axillary lymph node dissections for breast cancer patients with negative sentinel node biopsies.

Guenther et al[1] suggested clinical trials evaluating the necessity for axillary lymph node dissection for women with positive sentinel node biopsies based on a prospective cohort study (n = 46; 1996-2001) with a mean cancer size of 1.65 cm (0.4-5.5 cm) and a median 32-month (4-61 months) follow-up of breast cancer patients who did not have axillary dissections due to their refusal or serious co-morbidity. There were no axillary recurrences. However, 1 patient developed distant metastases.

William H. Hindle, MD

Reference

1. Guenther JM, Hansen NM, DiFronzo A, et al: Axillary dissection is not required for all patients with breast cancer and positive sentinel nodes. *Arch Surg* 138:52-56, 2003.

Three- to Six-Year Followup for 379 Benign Image-Guided Large-Core Needle Biopsies of Nonpalpable Breast Abnormalities
Acheson MB, Patton RG, Howisey RL, et al (Northwest Hosp, Seattle)
J Am Coll Surg 195:462-466, 2002   31–13

Background.—How accurately does a benign large-core needle biopsy (LCNB) rule out cancer in nonpalpable breast abnormalities detected at mammography? A group of women with such lesions was followed up for

TABLE 1.—Histology and Location of Tumors Diagnosed in 12 Patients After Benign Core Biopsies on Nonpalpable Mammographically Detected Abnormalities

Benign Core Histology	Tumor Histology	Tumor Location Relative to Original Benign LCNB
Focal fibrocystic disease (4 mm)	Infiltrating ductal	Ipsilateral breast, same site
No abnormality	Infiltrating ductal	Ipsilateral breast, different site
Fibroadenoma	Infiltrating ductal	Ipsilateral breast, different site
Lymph node	Infiltrating ductal	Ipsilateral breast, different site
Florid papillomatosis of nipple	Comedo DCIS	Ipsilateral breast, different site
Focal fibrocystic disease	Infiltrating adenocarcinoma	Ipsilateral breast, different site
Focal fibrocystic disease	Infiltrating lobular	Ipsilateral breast, different site
Papilloma	Infiltrating ductal	Contralateral breast
Fibroadenoma	Infiltrating ductal	Contralateral breast
Fat necrosis	Infiltrating ductal	Contralateral breast
Focal fibrocystic disease	Infiltrating ductal	Contralateral breast
Focal fibrocystic disease	Infiltrating ductal	Contralateral breast

Abbreviations: DCIS, Ductal carcinoma in situ; LCNB, large-core needle biopsy.
(Reprinted with permission from the American College of Surgeons courtesy of Acheson MB, Patton RG, Howisey RL, et al. Three- to six-year followup for 379 benign image-guided large-core needle biopsies of nonpalpable breast abnormalities. *J Am Coll Surg* 195:462-466, 2002.)

up to 6 years to determine the negative predictive value (NPV) of imaging-guided LCNB in these cases.

Methods.—The subjects were 379 women 35 to 94 years of age in whom mammography suggested a breast abnormality but whose lesions were non-

TABLE 2.—BI-RADS–Specific Pathology Diagnoses for 379 Benign Breast Core Biopsies

BI-RADS Diagnosis	All Patients (n = 379)		With FU (n = 312)		No FU (n = 67)	
	n	%	n	%	n	%
Focal fibrocystic disease	191	50.4	159	51.0	32	47.8
Fibroadenoma	87	23.0	64	20.5	23	34.3
Adenosis	21	5.5	19	6.1	2	3.0
Ductal hyperplasia	17	4.5	14	4.5	3	4.5
Fibroadenomatoid hyperplasia	12	3.2	12	3.8	0	0.0
Sclerosing adenosis	12	3.2	11	3.5	1	1.5
No abnormality	11	2.9	8	2.6	3	4.5
Fat necrosis	6	1.6	6	1.9	0	0.0
Lymph node	6	1.6	5	1.6	1	1.5
Foreign body reaction	3	0.8	2	0.6	1	1.5
Atypical ductal hyperplasia	2	0.5	2	0.6	0	0.0
Inflammatory pseudotumor	2	0.5	2	0.6	0	0.0
Scar	2	0.5	2	0.6	0	0.0
Ductal hyperplasia	1	0.3	1	0.3	0	0.0
Florid papillomatosis of nipple	1	0.3	1	0.3	0	0.0
Fibrous tumor	1	0.3	1	0.3	0	0.0
Haematoma	1	0.3	1	0.3	0	0.0
Papilloma	1	0.3	1	0.3	0	0.0
Radial sclerosing lesion	1	0.3	1	0.3	0	0.0
Amyloid tumor	1	0.3	0	0.0	1	1.5

Note: BI-RADS is a trademark of the American College of Radiology, Reston, Va.
Abbreviation: FU, Follow-up.
(Reprinted with permission from the American College of Surgeons courtesy of Acheson MB, Patton RG, Howisey RL, et al. Three- to six-year followup for 379 benign image-guided large-core needle biopsies of nonpalpable breast abnormalities. *J Am Coll Surg* 195:462-466, 2002.)

palpable at clinical examination. All patients underwent imaging-guided LCNB, and results were negative in all cases. Their medical records were reviewed 3 to 6 years after LCNB to determine the incidence of breast cancer.

Results.—Follow-up data were available for 312 patients over a mean of 4.5 years; the other 67 patients were either lost to follow-up or had died of causes other than breast cancer. Of the 312 patients who could be evaluated, only 12 patients were subsequently diagnosed with a malignancy (Table 1). In 6 cases (1.9%), a new lesion developed in the same breast but at a different site; these were considered true-negative findings. In 5 cases (1.6%), a new lesion developed in the contralateral breast. In the remaining patient (0.3%), initial examination missed a 4-mm lesion that had grown to about 11 mm by 8 months later. Re-biopsy indicated an infiltrating ductal carcinoma.

To determine whether the patients with follow-up were similar to those without available follow-up, each of the original 379 benign core biopsy samples was assigned a specific BI-RADS diagnosis. The proportion of patients with a high-risk diagnosis was similar in the groups with and without follow-up (Table 2). The NPV of imaging-guided LCNB of nonpalpable mammographically detected breast abnormalities was 99.7% (311 of 312 cases) (Fig 1).

Conclusion.—Imaging-guided LCNB can accurately rule out breast cancer in nonpalpable mammographically detected breast abnormalities. It cannot rule out the development of new lesions, however, as 3.8% of patients were later diagnosed with malignancy. Given the high NPV of imaging-guided LCNB, mammographic or US screening at 6 and 12 months might be sufficient to rule out malignancy in patients with nonpalpable mammo-

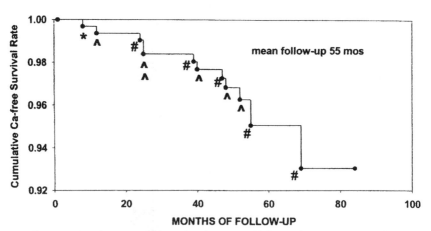

FIGURE 1.—Cumulative cancer-free rate based on censored follow-up for 312 patients with follow-up among 379 with benign large-core needle breast biopsy specimens of nonpalpable mammographically detected abnormalities. *Asterisk* indicates 1 false negative (0.3%) = 4-mm lesion missed on original biopsy, 11 mm at 8 months. *Inverted V* indicates 6 (1.9%) new cancers, ipsilateral breast, different site. *Number sign* indicates 5 (1.6%) new cancers, contralateral breast. *Abbreviation: Ca,* Cancer. (Reprinted with permission from the American College of Surgeons courtesy of Acheson MB, Patton RG, Howisey RL, et al. Three- to six-year followup for 379 benign image-guided large-core needle biopsies of nonpalpable breast abnormalities. *J Am Coll Surg* 195:462-466, 2002.)

graphically detected breast abnormalities before the patient returns to routine mammography screening.

▶ Continuing follow-up of nonpalpable mammographic lesions, which require tissue core-needle biopsy, is critical. Inevitably, though rarely, some lesions diagnosed as benign will prove to be malignant. The NPV of 0.997 (311/312) is reassuring. A ratio of 1 false negative per 312 cases is admirable and sets a high standard for other breast centers.

Why not apply this same diagnostic approach for palpable breast masses utilizing US-guided hand-held tissue core-needle biopsy? The NPV and ratio of false negatives should, theoretically, be even less than with imaged nonpalpable lesions. Performed in the office or outpatient setting, this approach should be meaningfully cost effective and convenient for the patient and the surgeon. Ob-gyns and other primary care physicians for women could certainly be appropriately trained in the performance of this biopsy technique.

In the Seattle Breast Center study above, although "focal fibrocystic disease" may well have been the "BI-RADS diagnosis" given by radiologists, it is unfortunate that authors and editors persist in the use of a term for an entity that is widely accepted not to exist. Fibrocystic changes are not a "disease."[1-3]

W. H. Hindle, MD

References

1. Hindle WH: Fibrocystic changes, in Hindle WH (ed): *Breast Care.* Springer-Verlag, New York, 1999.
2. Love SM, Gelman RS, Silen S: Sounding board: Fibrocystic "disease" of the breast: A non-disease? *N Engl J Med* 307:1010-1014, 1982.
3. Kramer WM, Rush BF: Mammary duct proliferation in the elderly: A histopathologic study. *Cancer* 31:130, 1973.

Randomized Trial of Breast Self-Examination in Shanghai: Final Results
Thomas DB, Gao DL, Ray RM, et al (Fred Hutchinson Cancer Research Ctr, Seattle; Shanghai Textile Industry Bureau, China; Univ of Tromsø, Norway)
J Natl Cancer Inst 94:1445-1457, 2002   31–14

Background.—The ability of breast self-examination (BSE) to reduce breast cancer mortality has not been proven. Whether an intensive program of BSE instruction could reduce the number of women dying from breast cancer was investigated.

Methods.—Between October 1989 and October 1991, 266,064 women working at 519 factories in Shanghai were assigned randomly to BSE instruction or a control group. In the intervention group, initial instruction in BSE was followed by reinforcement sessions 1 and 3 years later. In addition, BSE practice under medical supervision was required at least every 6 months for 5 years. The women in the intervention group also received ongoing reminders to practice BSE monthly. Follow-up extended through December 2000.

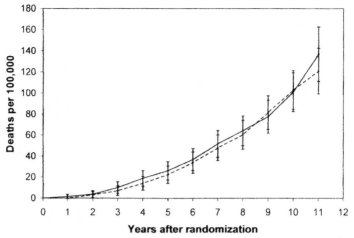

FIGURE 1.—Cumulative breast cancer mortality per 100,000 women in the instruction group (*solid line*) and control group (*broken line*) of the randomized trial of breast self-examination in Shanghai. *Error bars* represent 95% confidence intervals. (Courtesy of Thomas DB, Gao DL, Ray RM, et al: Randomized trial of breast self-examination in Shanghai: Final results. *J Natl Cancer Inst* 94:1445-1457, 2002. By permission of Oxford University Press.)

FIGURE 2

A

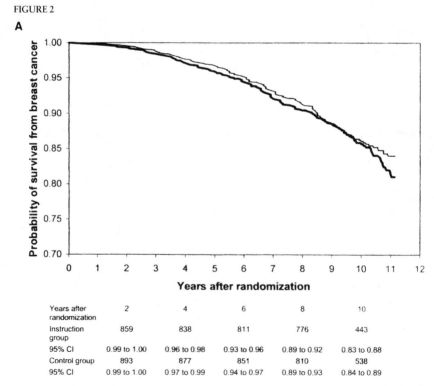

Years after randomization	2	4	6	8	10
Instruction group	859	838	811	776	443
95% CI	0.99 to 1.00	0.96 to 0.98	0.93 to 0.96	0.89 to 0.92	0.83 to 0.88
Control group	893	877	851	810	538
95% CI	0.99 to 1.00	0.97 to 0.99	0.94 to 0.97	0.89 to 0.93	0.84 to 0.89

(*Continued*)

FIGURE 2 (cont.)

B

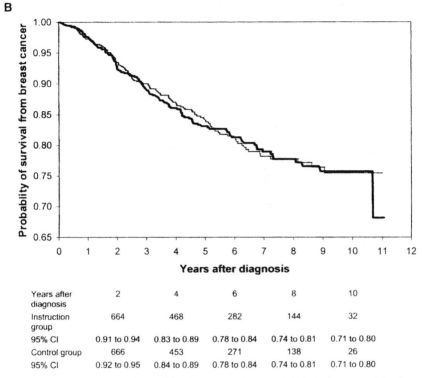

Years after diagnosis	2	4	6	8	10
Instruction group	664	468	282	144	32
95% CI	0.91 to 0.94	0.83 to 0.89	0.78 to 0.84	0.74 to 0.81	0.71 to 0.80
Control group	666	453	271	138	26
95% CI	0.92 to 0.95	0.84 to 0.89	0.78 to 0.84	0.74 to 0.81	0.71 to 0.80

FIGURE 2.—**A,** Probability of survival from breast cancer in case patients by study group and time from entry into the randomized trial of breast self-examination in Shanghai. **B,** Probability of survival from breast cancer in case patients by study group and time from the time of diagnosis. *Thick line* indicates instruction group; *thin line* indicates control group. *Tables* show number of patients at risk and 95% confidence intervals for the probabilities for years 2, 4, 6, 8, and 10 after randomization or diagnosis. *Abbreviation:* CI, Confidence interval. (Courtesy of Thomas DB, Gao DL, Ray RM, et al: Randomized trial of breast self-examination in Shanghai: Final results. *J Natl Cancer Inst* 94:1445-1457, 2002. By permission of Oxford University Press.)

Findings.—Death from breast cancer occurred in 0.1% of both the intervention group (135 of 132,979 women) and the control group (131 of 133,085 women) (Fig 1). Throughout the 10- to 11-year follow-up period, cumulative breast cancer mortality rates were similar for the 2 groups (Fig 2). More benign lesions were diagnosed in the intervention group than in the control group (Table 5).

Conclusion.—Intensive BSE instruction did not decrease mortality from breast cancer. Programs that encourage BSE without mammography probably will not reduce breast cancer mortality. Women who practice BSE need to be told that its efficacy has not been proven and that it may increase their chances of having a benign lesion subjected to biopsy.

TABLE 5.—Numbers of Women With Malignant and Benign Breast Lesions in the Instruction and Control Groups of the Randomized Trial of Breast Self-Examination in Shanghi

Type of Breast Lesion	Instruction Group	Control Group	Total
Carcinoma*			
Invasive	823	862	1685
In situ	33	28	61
Unknown whether invasive†	1	0	1
Total histologically confirmed	857	890	1747
Clinical diagnosis only	7	6	13
Total carcinomas	864	896	1760
Other malignancies of breast	4	3	7
Uncertain whether malignant	5	0	5
Benign breast disease			
Affected No. of women	2387	1296	3683
Total No. of biopsy examinations	2761	1505	4266
Total No. of women with biopsy examinations‡	3253	2189	5442
Total No. of biopsy examinations	3627	2398	6025

*Women with multiple malignancies were counted only once.
†This breast lesion was histologically confirmed as carcinoma, but whether invasive or in situ was not recorded.
‡Excludes clinically diagnosed breast cancers.
(Courtesy of Thomas DB, Gao DL, Ray RM, et al: Randomized trial of breast self-examination in Shanghai: Final results. *J Natl Cancer Inst* 94:1445-1457, 2002. By permission of Oxford University Press.)

▶ With such massive numbers ($n = 266,064$), this Shanghai study cannot be ignored. In fact, with the supervision of the Fred Hutchinson Cancer Research Center, Seattle, the results are probably defining. Although the debate will continue, these data, with 10 to 11 years of follow-up, are as close to definitive and conclusive as will be any future studies on the same issue.

The abstract's conclusions bear repeating: "Intensive instruction in BSE did not reduce mortality from breast cancer. Programs to encourage BSE in the absence of mammography would be unlikely to reduce mortality from breast cancer. Women who choose to practice BSE should be informed that its efficacy is unproven and that it may increase their chances of having a benign breast biopsy." Clinicians are now obligated to give this information to their patients.

W. H. Hindle, MD

Comparison of the Performance of Screening Mammography, Physical Examination, and Breast US and Evaluation of Factors That Influence Them: An Analysis of 27,825 Patient Evaluations
Kolb TM, Lichy J, Newhouse JH (New York; Columbia-Presbyterian Med Ctr, New York)
Radiology 225:165-175, 2002   31–15

Background.—Mammography, US, and physical examination (PE) are each used to screen for breast cancer. Their comparative performance was examined

TABLE 1.—Performance Characteristics of Each Modality

Modality	Sensitivity (%)	Specificity (%)	NPV (%)	PPV (%)	Accuracy (%)
Mammography	77.6 (191/246)	98.8 (27,237/27,579)	99.8 (27,237/27,292)	35.8 (191/533)	98.6 (27,428/27,825)
PE	27.6 (68/246)	99.4 (27,412/27,579)	99.4 (27,412/27,590)	28.9 (68/235)	98.8 (27,480/27,825)
US	75.3 (110/146)	96.8 (12,975/13,401)	99.7 (12,975/13,011)	20.5 (110/536)	96.6 (13,085/13,547)

Note: Screening US was performed and its results reported only in women with dense breasts. Calculations include both invasive and noninvasive cancers. *Data in parentheses* are numbers used to calculate the percentages.

Abbreviations: NPV, Negative predictive value; *PPV,* positive predictive value; *PE,* physical examination.

(Courtesy of Kolb TM, Lichy J, Newhouse JH: Comparison of the performance of screening mammography, physical examination, and breast US and evaluation of factors that influence them: An analysis of 27,825 patient evaluations. *Radiology* 225:165-175, 2002. Radiological Society of North America.)

TABLE 2.—Sensitivity of Each Modality for Cancer Detection in Women With Different Breast Densities

| Modality | BI-RADS Category | | | | |
	1	2	3	4	2-4
Mammography	98.0 (98/100)	82.9 (34/41)	64.4 (38/59)	47.8 (22/46)	64.4 (94/146)
US	NP	65.9 (27/41)	81.4 (48/59)	76.1 (35/46)	75.3 (110/146)
PE	22.0 (22/100)	31.7 (13/41)	28.8 (17/59)	34.8 (16/46)	31.5 (46/146)

Note: Data are percentages. Data in parentheses are numbers used to calculate percentages.
Abbreviations: US, Ultrasonography; PE, physical examination; NP, not performed.
(Courtesy of Kolb TM, Lichy J, Newhouse JH: Comparison of the performance of screening mammography, physical examination, and breast US and evaluation of factors that influence them: An analysis of 27,825 patient evaluations. Radiology 225:165-175, 2002. Radiological Society of North America.)

in a large group of women as a whole and in subgroups based on age, breast density, and hormonal status.

Methods.—The subjects were 11,130 women (mean age, 59.6 years) without signs and symptoms of breast abnormalities. About half the women had fatty breasts and about half had dense breasts. All women underwent screening mammography and PE and women with dense breasts also underwent screening US, for a total of 27,825 screening sessions. A positive abnormality was defined as findings of malignancy on biopsy. A negative abnormality was defined as no finding of malignancy on biopsy or a negative finding on all screening examinations.

Results.—During 1 year of follow-up, 246 cancers were detected in 221 women. Each of the 3 modalities had a high negative predictive value (greater than 99.4%), but their sensitivities differed dramatically (Table 1). PE alone was the least sensitive (27.6%) but the most specific (99.4%). However, PE was significantly less effective than the other 2 modalities in detecting small tumors and early-stage tumors. Screening US alone detected nonpalpable invasive cancer in 42% of women (30 of 71) in whom neither mammography nor PE detected cancer.

For women with dense breasts, the rate of negative biopsy findings increased from 65.9% in women screened with mammography and PE alone to 74.6% after the addition of screening US. Mammography was signifi-

TABLE 3.—Sensitivity of Screening Modalities According to Age

| Modality | Percentage of Women | |
	49 Years or Younger	50 Years or Older
Mammography*	58.0 (29/50)	82.7 (162/196)
PE*	36.0 (18/50)	25.5 (50/196)
US†	78.6 (33/42)	74.0 (77/104)

Note: Data are percentages. Data in parentheses are numbers used to calculate percentages.
*Women with both fatty and dense breasts.
†Only women with dense breasts (BI-RADS category 2-4).
Abbreviations: US, Ultrasonography; PE, physical examination.
(Courtesy of Kolb TM, Lichy J, Newhouse JH: Comparison of the performance of screening mammography, physical examination, and breast US and evaluation of factors that influence them: An analysis of 27,825 patient evaluations. Radiology 225:165-175, 2002. Radiological Society of North America.)

TABLE 4.—Sensitivity of Modalities in Women With Differing Hormonal Status

Modality	Premenopausal	Percentage of Women Postmenopausal not Receiving HRT	Postmenopausal Receiving HRT
Mammography*	66.7 (40/60)	80.4 (119/148)	84.2 (32/38)
PE*	38.3 (23/60)	25.0 (37/148)	21.0 (8/38)
US†	71.4 (35/49)	82.2 (60/73)	62.5 (15/24)

Note: Data in parentheses are numbers used to calculate the percentages.
*Women with both fatty and dense breasts.
†Only women with dense breasts (BI-RADS category 2-4).
Abbreviations: HRT, Hormone replacement therapy; PE, physical examination.
(Courtesy of Kolb TM, Lichy J, Newhouse JH: Comparison of the performance of screening mammography, physical examination, and breast US and evaluation of factors that influence them: An analysis of 27,825 patient evaluations. Radiology 225:165-175, 2002. Radiological Society of North America.)

cantly less sensitive in dense breasts (Table 2) and in women 49 years of age or younger (Table 3); these effects were independent. Hormonal status (independent of breast density) had no effect on the effectiveness of the screening modalities (Table 4). The combination of mammography and US was significantly more sensitive than the combination of mammography and PE (97% vs 74%).

Conclusion.—Mammography is a highly sensitive method for detecting breast cancer in women with fatty breasts but not for detecting tumors in dense breasts. Performing screening US in women with dense breasts improves the detection of breast cancer compared with mammography and PE alone. The sensitivity of mammography is also lower in older women.

Screening US is also significantly more effective than PE in women of all ages with dense breasts, and performing US in conjunction with mammography improves the sensitivity of cancer detection compared with mammography and PE (from 75% to 97%). Screening US can detect cancers similar in size and stage to those detected by mammography and can detect smaller and earlier-stage cancers than PE can detect.

▶ What is the role of US in breast cancer screening? This observational study (n = 11,130 women) from Columbia-Presbyterian Medical Center, New York, presents a careful analysis of the sensitivity, specificity, negative predictive value, positive predictive value, and accuracy of breast cancer screening of asymptomatic women by mammography, US, and PE. Generally, the conclusions are similar to other studies and are becoming accepted in clinical practice. It is clear that US is a useful complement to mammography in women of any age with mammographically dense breast. Not surprisingly, US is more useful in women 49 years of age or younger. In the present study, the sensitivity of US was 78.6% as compared to mammography at 58.0%. Palpation (PE) was the least effective screening method. However, it is well documented elsewhere that some palpable cancers will not be detected by mammography.[1,2] In a clinically reassuring statement, the authors conclude, "Hormonal status has no significant effect on effectiveness of screening independent of breast density."

W. H. Hindle, MD

References

1. Edeiken S: Mammography in the symptomatic woman. *Cancer* 63:1412-1414, 1989.
2. Seidman H, Gelb SK, Silverberg E, et al: Survival experience in the breast cancer detection demonstration project. *CA Cancer J Clin* 37:258-290, 1987.

SUGGESTED READING

Lewin JM, D'Orsi CJ, Hendrick RE, et al: Clinical comparison of full-field digital mammography and screen-film mammography for detection of breast cancer. *AJR* 179:671-677, 2002.

▶ This report from the University of Colorado Health Sciences Center, Denver, covers 6736 imaging examinations of women aged 40 and older. The screening effectiveness of digital mammography was compared with the traditional film mammography. Additional imaging evaluation was recommended in 1467 cases. Cancers were detected in 23% (42/181) of the biopsies performed. Nine cancers were detected only with digital mammography and 15 were detected only with film mammography. Eighteen (43%, 18/42) were detected by both modalities. The authors conclude, "No significant difference in cancer detection was observed between digital mammography and screen-film mammography. Digital mammography resulted in fewer recalls than did screen-film mammography."

Sickles et al[1] at the University of California Medical Center, San Francisco, studied 47,798 screening and 13,286 diagnostic mammographic examinations (1997-2001). The recall rate (4.9% vs 7.1%), the rate of recommended biopsies (9.9% vs 15.8%), the rate of cancers detected (6.0 vs 3.4 per 1000), and the stage of the cancers (stages 0-1, 5.3 vs 3.0 per 1000) for specialist radiologists (mammographers) were compared to the findings of general radiologists. The results are not unexpected but clearly demonstrate the effectiveness of specialized training and experience in mammography interpretation.

Hou et al[2] and Petrick et al[3] reported on the effectiveness and sensitivity of computer-aided mammographic diagnoses. The Hou study (n = 110) documented improved receiver operating characteristics and sensitivity but no difference in specificity with the assistance of the computer diagnosis. The improvement was greater for community radiologists than for mammographers.[2] In the Petrick study (n = 263), increasing computer-aided diagnosis marker rates yielded higher detection of malignant masses, 77% (120/156) at rates of 0.5 marks per mammogram, 83% (130/156) at 1.0 marks, and 87% (135/156) at 1.5 marks.[3] The authors concluded that such mass-detection algorithms of computer-aided diagnosis ". . .may be useful as a second opinion in mammographic interpretation."

William H. Hindle, MD

References

1. Sickles EA, Wolverton DE, Dee KE: Performance parameters for screening and diagnostic mammography: Specialist and general radiologists. *Radiology* 224:861-869, 2002.
2. Huo Z, Giger ML, Vyborny CJ, et al: Breast cancer: Effectiveness of computer-aided diagnosis-observer study with independent database of mammograms. *Radiology* 224:560-568, 2002.
3. Petrick N, Sahiner B, Chan H-P, et al: Breast cancer detection: Evaluation of a mass-detection algorithm for computer-aided diagnosis–experience in 263 patients. *Radiology* 224:217-224, 2002.

Ernster VL, Ballard-Barbash R, Burlow WE, et al: Detection of ductal carcinoma in situ in women undergoing screening mammography. *J Natl Cancer Inst* 94:1546-1554, 2002.

▶ This analysis of 653,833 mammograms on 540,738 women aged 40 to 84 represents the pooled data from 7 regional registries (1996-1997) in the National Cancer Institute's Breast Cancer Surveillance Consortium. Of the 3266 breast cancers, 82% (2675/3266) were invasive and 18% (591/3266) were ductal carcinoma in situ (DCIS). "Overall, approximately 1 in every 1300 screening mammography examinations leads to a diagnosis of DCIS." The percentage of screening-detected DCIS deceased with age. Contrarily, the percentage rate of DCIS per 1000 screening mammograms increased with age. DCIS was detected at a higher sensitivity (86% [95% confidence interval, 83.2-88.8]) than for invasive cancer (75.1% [95% confidence interval, 73.5-76.8]). The prognosis (and natural history) of screening-detected DCIS remains unknown.

William H. Hindle, MD

Long-term Effects of Mammography Screening: Updated Overview of the Swedish Randomised Trials

Nyström L, Andersson I, Bjurstam N, et al (Umeå Univ, Sweden; Malmö Univ, Sweden; Göteborg Univ, Sweden; et al)
Lancet 359:909-919, 2002   31–16

Background.—The debate continues as to whether screening mammography reduces breast cancer mortality. In the late 1980s, the Swedish Cancer Society began an overview of Swedish trials examining this issue and concluded that screening mammography does reduce the number of deaths due to breast cancer. However, other researchers have raised concerns about the validity of their conclusions. Here, the earlier Swedish overview has been updated to include follow-up data through 1996 and to address the concerns of critics.

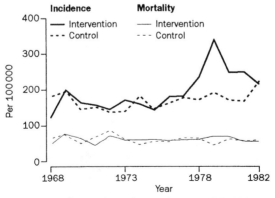

FIGURE 1.—Breast cancer incidence and mortality per 100,000 in 1968-1982 in women randomly assigned to invited group and control group in Östergötland trial. (Courtesy of Nyström L, Andersson I, Bjurstam N, et al: Long-term effects of mammography screening: Updated overview of the Swedish randomised trials. *Lancet* 359:909-919, 2002. Reprinted with permission of Elsevier Science.)

Methods.—Data from 5 Swedish trials have been included: the Malmö Mammographic Screening Trials I and II,[1] the Two-County Trial (only the Östergötland data),[2] the Stockholm Trial,[3] and the Göteborg Trial.[4] These trials have involved 247,010 women 40 to 74 years of age who were randomly assigned to either a control group (117,260 women) or to screening mammography (129,750 women). All women were followed up through December 1996 by record linkage to the Swedish Cancer and Cause of Death Registers. Relative risks for all-cause mortality and breast cancer–specific mortality were calculated for the 2 groups, along with trial-specific and age-specific risks.

Results.—The median follow-up was 15.8 years. In the Two-County Trial, including data only from women in Östergötland did not introduce any significant bias into the analyses (Fig 1), as the incidence of breast cancer and breast cancer mortality before randomization were similar in the screening and control groups. There were 511 deaths due to breast cancer in the screening groups over 1,864,770 person-years of follow-up and 584 deaths

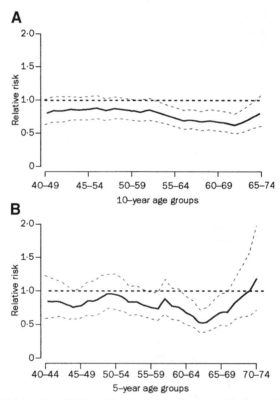

FIGURE 2.—Relative risk and 95% confidence interval, evaluation model, all trials, follow-up until December 1996. A, Consecutive 10-year age groups; B, consecutive 5-year age groups. (Courtesy of Nyström L, Andersson I, Bjurstam N, et al: Long-term effects of mammography screening: Updated overview of the Swedish randomised trials. *Lancet* 359:909-919, 2002. Reprinted with permission of Elsevier Science.)

due to breast cancer in the control groups over 1,688,440 person-years of follow-up.

The risk of breast cancer death was significantly lower in the women undergoing mammography (relative risk, 0.79). This risk was lower regardless of which age groupings were used (5- or 10-year groupings) (Fig 2). For women of all ages combined, the benefit of mammography on cumulative breast cancer mortality began to emerge at about 4 years after randomization (Fig 3), and remained throughout follow-up. The relative reduction in breast cancer mortality was greatest for women who were 60 to 69 years of age at study entry (Fig 4). The age-adjusted relative risk of all-cause mortality associated with screening mammography was 0.98.

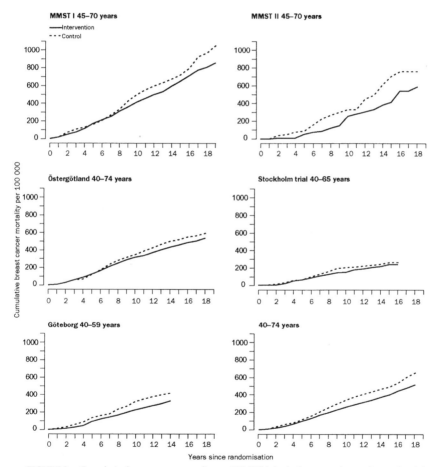

FIGURE 3.—Cumulative breast cancer mortality per 100,000 in invited group and control group by trial and all trials. Evaluation method, follow-up until December 1996. (Courtesy of Nyström L, Andersson I, Bjurstam N, et al: Long-term effects of mammography screening: Updated overview of the Swedish randomised trials. *Lancet* 359:909-919, 2002. Reprinted with permission of Elsevier Science.)

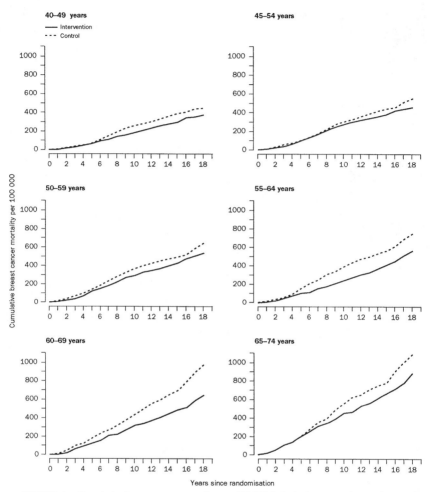

FIGURE 4.—Cumulative breast cancer mortality per 100,000 in invited group and control group in women 40-49, 45-54, 50-59, 55-64, 60-69, and 65-74 years at entry. All trials, evaluation model, follow-up until December 1996. (Courtesy of Nyström L, Andersson I, Bjurstam N, et al: Long-term effects of mammography screening: Updated overview of the Swedish randomised trials. *Lancet* 359:909-919, 2002. Reprinted with permission of Elsevier Science.)

Conclusion.—The benefits of screening mammography on breast cancer death were apparent in each study, and these benefits continue long after randomization. The greatest effect is seen in women 55 to 69 years of age at randomization, and the least effect is seen in women 50 to 54 years of age at randomization.

References

1. Andersson I, Janzon L: Reduced breast cancer mortality in women under age 50: Updated results from the Malmö Mammographic Screening Programs. *J Natl Cancer Ins Mono* 22:63-67, 1997.

2. Tabár L, Fagerberg CJG, Gad A, et al: Reduction in mortality from breast cancer after mass screening with mammography: Randomized trial from the Breast Cancer Screening Working Group of the Swedish National Board of Health and Welfare. *Lancet* 1:829-832, 1985.
3. Frisell J, Glass U, Hellström L, et al: Randomised mammographic screening for breast cancer in Stockholm: First round results and comparison. *Breast Cancer Res Treat* 8:45-54, 1986.
4. Bjurstam N, Björneld L, Duffy SW, et al: The Gothenburg Breast Cancer Screening Trial: Preliminary results on breast cancer mortality for women aged 39-49. *J Natl Cancer Inst Mono* 22:53-55, 1997.

▶ Beginning in 2000, Gotzsche and Olsen began to question the validity of the published randomized clinical trials on the effectiveness of mammography for breast cancer screening and subsequent reduction in breast cancer mortality in the screened group.[1,2] Issues of "inappropriate exclusions, poor randomization, and the excess total mortality in women invited to screening" were raised. Nyström et al reanalyzed the data from 5 Swedish population-based, randomized clinical trials. The reanalysis covers 247,010 women with a median follow-up time of 15.8 years. This study requires careful detailed reading, but the graphs clearly illustrate the effectiveness of screening mammography in all the studies reviewed. Furthermore, the authors conclude, ". . . the recent criticism against the Swedish randomised controlled trials is misleading and scientifically unfounded." Undoubtedly, the debate will continue.

W. H. Hindle, MD

References

1. Gotzsche PC, Olsen O: Is screening for breast cancer with mammography justifiable? *Lancet* 355:129-134, 2000.
2. Olsen O, Gotzsche PC: Cochrane review on screening for breast cancer with mammography. *Lancet* 358:1340-1342, 2001.

The Impact of Organized Mammography Service Screening on Breast Carcinoma Mortality in Seven Swedish Counties: A Collaborative Evaluation
Duffy SW, Tabár L, Chen H-H, et al (Cancer Research UK, London; Falun Central Hosp, Sweden; Natl Taiwan Univ, Taipei; et al)
Cancer 95:458-469, 2002   31–17

Background.—Data from 7 Swedish counties that encompass about 33% of the Swedish female population eligible for screening (ie, 40-69 years of age) were examined to determine the effects of mammography screening on breast cancer mortality.

Methods.—Screening centers in each of the 7 counties (Dalarna, Gävleborg, Södermanland, Uppsala, Värmaland, Västmanland, and Örebro) provided detailed data on the number of women who were invited for screening, the number who underwent screening, and whether each case of breast cancer occurred in an exposed woman (ie, interval cases and those detected by screening combined) or in an unexposed woman (ie, was not in-

TABLE 1.—Nominal Starting Dates, Age Groups Screened, Screening Interval, and Contamination Rates in the Seven Counties

County	Nominal Starting Date	Contamination Before (% Screened)	Contamination After (% Not Screened)	Age Group Screened (yrs)	Screening Interval (yrs)
Dalarna	1978	0.5	25	40-69	1.5-2.75
Gävleborg	1984	0*	16	40-74	2
Södermanland	1990	0.7	23	40-74	2
Uppsala	1989	3	18	40-74	2
Värmland	1994	3	27	50-69	1.5
Västmanland	1989	14	8	40-69	2
Örebro	1989	4	36	40-69†	1.5-2

*Some sporadic screening with very long intervals took place prior to 1984.
†Revised to age 45 to 60 years in 1996.
(Courtesy of Duffy SW, Tabár L, Chen H-H, et al. The impact of organized mammography service screening on breast carcinoma mortality in seven Swedish counties: A collaborative evaluation. *Cancer* 95(3): 458-469. ©2002 American Cancer Society. Reprinted by permission of Wiley-Liss, a subsidiary of John Wiley & Sons, Inc.)

vited or did not attend). Mortality data were obtained from the Regional Oncology Center in Uppsala and the National Cause of Death Register. Statistics Sweden provided annual population data for determining the total number of eligible women living in each county. The numbers of breast cancer deaths and incident tumors were compared between the prescreening epoch (the period before screening became established) and the screening epoch (the period after mammography was widely used).

Because screening mammography was introduced earlier in some counties than in others (Table 1), contamination rates (ie, exposure to screening before the starting date, nonexposure to screening after the starting date) differed among the counties. Total follow-up was 7.5 million person-years. Data were analyzed by Poisson regression analysis and corrected for self-selection bias and lead-time bias as appropriate.

Results.—During the prescreening epoch, there were 5728 incident breast cancers diagnosed and 1169 breast cancer deaths. During the screening epoch, there were 8364 incident breast cancers diagnosed and 875 breast cancer deaths. In all 7 counties combined, compared with the prescreening period, the risk of breast cancer death was 44% lower among women who underwent screening (relative risk, 0.56).

For the 5 counties with 10 years of screening or less, the risk of breast cancer death was 45% lower in the screened women (relative risk, 0.55); for the 2 counties with more than 10 years of screening, the risk of breast cancer death was 43% lower (relative risk, 0.57) (Fig 3). The risk of breast cancer death was also significantly lower when all incident tumors were considered (ie, in both exposed and unexposed women).

For the 5 counties with 10 years of screening or less, the risk of breast cancer death was 18% lower in the screening epoch compared with the prescreening epoch (relative risk, 0.82), and for the 2 counties with 10 years of screening or more, the risk of breast cancer death was 32% lower (relative risk, 0.68) (Table 3). Within the screening epoch, invitation to screening was

FIGURE 3

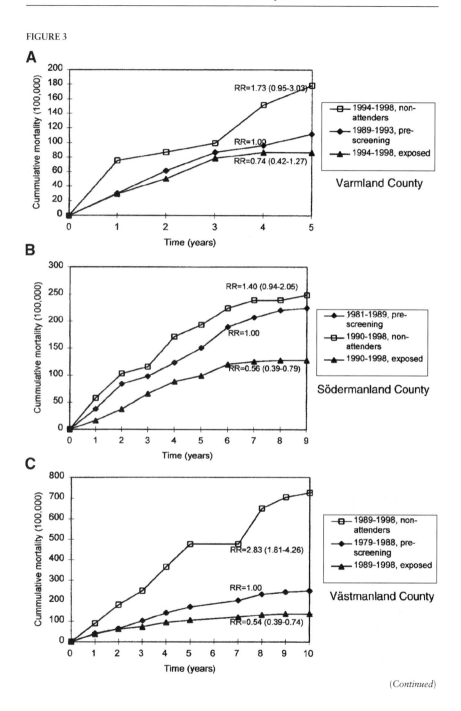

(*Continued*)

FIGURE 3 (cont.)

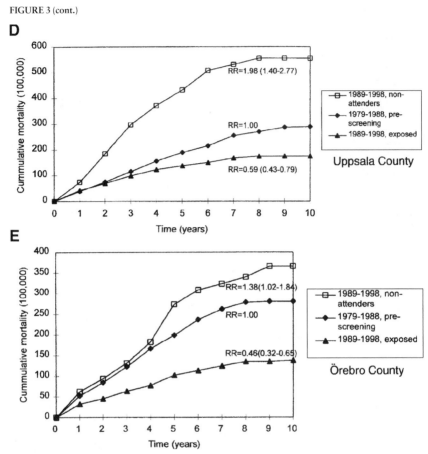

FIGURE 3.—A, Cumulative mortality from breast carcinoma by period for women aged 50 to 69 years in Värmland County. B, Cumulative mortality from breast carcinoma by period for women aged 40 to 60 years in Södermanland County. C, Cumulative mortality from breast carcinoma by period for women aged 40 to 60 years in Västmanland County. D, Cumulative mortality from breast carcinoma by period for women aged 40 to 60 years in Uppsala County. E, Cumulative mortality from breast carcinoma by period for women aged 40 to 60 years in Örebro County. *Abbreviation: RR,* Relative risk. (Courtesy of Duffy SW, Tabár L, Chen H-H, et al. The impact of organized mammography service screening on breast carcinoma mortality in seven Swedish counties: A collaborative evaluation. *Cancer* 95(3): 458-469. ©2002 American Cancer Society. Reprinted by permission of Wiley-Liss, a subsidiary of John Wiley & Sons, Inc.)

associated with a 39% decreased risk of breast cancer death compared with no invitation to screening (relative risk, 0.61) (Table 4).

Conclusion.—Based on data from 7 Swedish counties containing about one third of all Swedish women eligible for mammography screening, organized service screening is associated with a 40% to 45% reduction in the risk of breast cancer death in women who actually undergo screening. Even considering women who are invited for screening but decline, offering screening is associated with a 30% reduction in the risk of breast cancer death. These

TABLE 3.—Comparison of Breast Carcinoma Mortality From Incident Tumors Between the Prescreening and Screening Epochs

County	Epoch	Deaths	Person-years	Rate/100,000	RR (95% CI)
Värmland	Pre	36	159,783	22.5	1.00 (−)
	Screen	37	163,411	22.6	1.00 (0.64-1.59)
Södermanland	Pre	98	396,206	24.7	1.00 (−)
	Screen	79	422,007	18.7	0.76 (0.56-1.02)
Västmanland*	Pre	112	448,442	25.0	1.00 (−)
	Screen	85	470,961	18.0	0.84 (0.64-1.12)
Uppsala	Pre	110	389,156	28.3	1.00 (−)
	Screen	112	471,834	23.7	0.84 (0.65-1.09)
Örebro	Pre	133	476,420	27.9	1.00 (−)
	Screen	108	489,298	22.1	0.79 (0.61-1.02)
All counties with					
≤ 10 years screening†	Pre	489	1,870,007	26.1	1.00 (−)
	Screen	421	2,017,511	20.9	0.82 (0.72-0.94)
Gävleborg	Pre	311	795,110	39.1	1.00
	Screen	219	786,032	27.9	0.71 (0.60-0.85)
Dalarna*	Pre (1)	187	511,629	36.5	1.00 (−)
	Pre (2)	182	516,318	35.2	0.96 (0.78-1.18)
	Screen (1)	138	498,803	27.7	0.76 (0.61-0.95)
	Screen (2)	97	512,984	18.9	0.57 (0.44-0.73)
All counties with					
> 10 years screening†	Pre	680	1,823,057	37.3	1.00 (−)
	Screen	454	1,797,819	25.3	0.68 (0.60-0.77)

Note: Exposed and unexposed women are combined in the screen epoch group.
*Corrected for lead time.
†Adjusted for county.
Abbreviations: RR, Relative risk; *CI,* confidence interval; *Pre,* prescreening epoch; *Screen,* screening epoch.
(Courtesy of Duffy SW, Tabár L, Chen H-H, et al. The impact of organized mammography service screening on breast carcinoma mortality in seven Swedish counties: A collaborative evaluation. *Cancer* 95(3): 458-469. ©2002 American Cancer Society. Reprinted by permission of Wiley-Liss, a subsidiary of John Wiley & Sons, Inc.)

data underscore the efficacy of mammography screening in reducing breast cancer mortality.

▶ This will become a classic landmark collaborative evaluation. Because of the meticulous record keeping of Swedish institutions and the accuracy and completeness of the Swedish mortality data, the mammography studies from Sweden are exemplary and impressive. No other source compares with the quality and quantity of the Swedish screening mammography data. To quote directly from the authors' results, "The mortality reduction for breast cancer in all 7 counties combined for women actually exposed to screening compared with the prescreening period was 44% (relative risk [RR] = 0.56; 95% confidence interval [95% CI], 0.50-0.62)."

This detailed and graphically illustrated (with figures) article presents compelling evidence in support of screening mammography and is a major basis for the American Cancer Society's guideline for annual screening mammography beginning at 40 years of age. To date, adherence to the prompt and systematic application of this guideline is the most potent and effective approach for the reduction in breast cancer mortality. All primary health care providers

TABLE 4.—Comparison of Breast Carcinoma Mortality Between Screened and Unscreened Women Within the Screening Epochs, With Relative Risks and 95% Confidence Intervals

County	Exposure Status	Deaths	Person-years	Rate/100,000	RR (95% CI)*
Värmland	Unscreened	17	43,636	39.0	1.00 (−)
	Screened	20	119,775	16.7	0.72 (0.53-0.98)
Södermanland	Unscreened	34	97,965	34.7	1.00 (−)
	Screened	45	324,042	13.9	0.66 (0.51-0.85)
Västmanland†	Unscreened	26	36,831	70.6	1.00 (−)
	Screened	59	434,130	13.6	0.41 (0.32-0.54)
Uppsala	Unscreened	48	85,598	56.1	1.00 (−)
	Screened	64	386,245	16.6	0.56 (0.44-0.71)
Örebro	Unscreened	68	177,022	38.4	1.00 (−)
	Screened	40	312,276	12.8	0.59 (0.46-0.76)
Gävleborg	Unscreened	49	124,748	39.3	1.00 (−)
	Screened	170	661,284	25.7	0.95 (0.73-1.22)
Dalarna (1988-1997)†	Unscreened	33	62,881	52.5	1.00 (−)
	Screened	64	450,103	14.2	0.54 (0.42-0.69)
All counties	Unscreened	275	628,681	43.7	1.00 (−)
	Screened	462	2,687,855	17.2	0.61 (0.55-0.68)

*The relative risks and 95% confidence intervals were corrected for self-selection bias.
†Also corrected for lead time.
Abbreviations: RR, Relative risk; *CI*, confidence interval.
(Courtesy of Duffy SW, Tabár L, Chen H-H, et al. The impact of organized mammography service screening on breast carcinoma mortality in seven Swedish counties: A collaborative evaluation. *Cancer* 95(3): 458-469. ©2002 American Cancer Society. Reprinted by permission of Wiley-Liss, a subsidiary of John Wiley & Sons, Inc.)

for women should read and understand the impact of the data which are so clearly presented in this article.

W. H. Hindle, MD

SUGGESTED READING

Baseman S, Mouchawar J, Calonge N, et al: Mammography screening matters for young women with breast carcinoma: Evidence of downstaging among 42-49 year old women with a history of previous mammography screening. *Cancer* 97:352-358, 2003.
▶ This study (n = 247) from the University of Colorado Health Sciences Center, Denver, of women aged 42-49 diagnosed with breast cancer compared those who had stages 0 to I cancers to those with stages II to IV. The later stages were 40% in the screened group and 52% in the unscreened group. Thus, the screened group had 30% less later stages. When adjusted for age, year of diagnosis, and family history, the screened group was 0.56 (95% confidence interval, 0.32-0.97) times as likely to have later stage cancers at diagnosis.
Houssami et al[1] at the Sydney-Square Breast Clinic, Sydney, Australia, reported (1994-1996) on 480 consecutive symptomatic women aged 25 to 55 who attended a breast clinic and were evaluated by mammography and US. The sensitivity was 75.8% for mammography and 81.7% for US ($P = .15$, not significant). For women 45 and younger, the sensitivity of sonography was 13.2% (95% confidence interval, 2.1-24.3) more than for mammography. The specificity was 88.0% for both mammography and US. The authors suggest that focused US "may be an appropriate initial imaging examination" for symptomatic women aged 45 and younger.

William H. Hindle, MD

Reference

1. Houssami N, Irwig L, Simpson JM, et al: Sydney breast imaging accuracy study: Comparative sensitivity and specificity of mammography and sonography in young women with symptoms. *AJR* 180:935-940, 2003.

The Pattern of Breast Cancer Screening Utilization and Its Consequences
Michaelson J, Satija S, Moore R, et al (Massachusetts Gen Hosp, Boston; Harvard Med School, Boston)
Cancer 94:37-43, 2002   31–18

Background.—Several randomized, controlled trials have demonstrated that breast cancer screening saves lives. The pattern of screening utilization and its consequences, in terms of the size and time of appearance of invasive breast carcinoma, was examined in a population of women evaluated at a large service screening/diagnostic program over the past decade.

Methods.—A population of 59,899 women who underwent 196,891 mammograms between January 1990 and February 1999 was studied. A total of 604 invasive breast tumors was found. Another 206 invasive breast tumors were found clinically during this period in another 206 women who had no record of a previous mammogram. Additional information was available on screening of women from March 1999 through May 2001.

Findings.—Fifty percent of women who underwent screening did not begin that screening until age 50 years (Fig 1), even though 25% of invasive breast tumors were detected in women who were younger than 50 years. Relatively few women who used screening returned promptly for their annual examinations; by 1.5 years, only 50% of participants had returned. About 25% of invasive breast tumors were identified in women for whom there was no record of a previous screening mammogram. These tumors were larger (median, 15 mm) than the screen-detected tumors (median, 10 mm).

About 30% of the 604 invasive breast tumors in the screening population were identified by means other than mammography; those tumors were also larger (median, 15 mm) than the screen-detected tumors (median, 10 mm). Only 3% of the 604 tumors were identified by nonmammographic criteria within 6 months of the previous negative examination, and only 12% were identified within 1 year. By back-calculating the likely size of each of these tumors at the time of a negative mammogram, it could be determined that most tumors probably emerged as larger, palpable masses not because they were missed at the previous negative mammogram, since most were too small to have been detected, but rather because too much time had been allowed to pass (Figs 4 and 5).

Conclusions.—Many participants did not comply with American Cancer Society recommendations for annual screening beginning at age 40. As a result, nearly 50% of invasive tumors emerged as larger and thus potentially more lethal palpable masses.

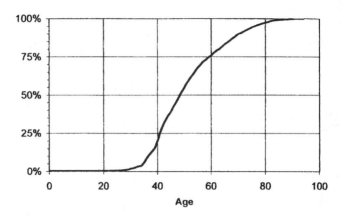

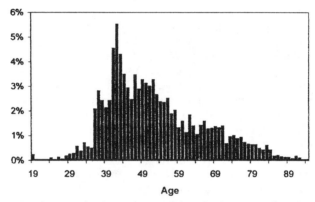

FIGURE 1.—Cumulative age distribution (*bottom*) and age distribution (*top*) for women who underwent their first screening mammograms in 1998. To assess the distribution of women by age when they began screening, 1998 was chosen as a representative year; this made it possible to search the data set for the previous decade to find those women who had no record of a previous mammogram over the past decade. (Courtesy of Michaelson J, Satija S, Moore R, et al: The pattern of breast cancer screening utilization and its consequences. *Cancer* 94(1):37-43. © 2002, American Cancer Society. Reprinted by permission of Wiley-Liss Inc, a subsidiary of John Wiley & Sons, Inc.)

▶ This review of 196,891 mammograms taken on 59,899 women (1990-1999) at the Massachusetts General Hospital Breast Imaging Division, Harvard University Medical School, amply demonstrates that clinicians should improve their efforts and effectiveness for the early detection of breast cancer in their patients. Delay in "annual" mammograms (for example, 50% returned within 18 months and only 60% returned within 24 months) correlated with larger sized cancers at diagnosis. In addition, 50% of the screened women did not begin mammography until after age 50. Furthermore, 25% of the cancers were diagnosed in women who had not previously had a mammogram and the median size was larger (15mm) than the screening-detected cancers (10 mm). There is ample evidence that cancers 10 mm or smaller have approximately 90%, 10-year and longer survival rates when treated.[1-6]

Intervening Cancers

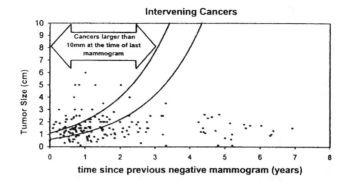

Subsequent Screen Detected Cancers

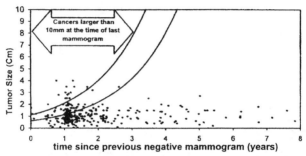

FIGURE 4.—Scatter plots showing the sizes of tumors found after a previous negative mammogram, compared with the time since the previous negative mammogram. Also shown are the theoretical growth curves for tumors measuring 5 mm and 10 mm growing with a doubling time of 130 days. Thus, most of the tumors located below the bottom line were likely to have been 5 mm or smaller at the time of the previous negative mammogram, whereas tumors below the top line were likely to have been 10 mm or smaller at the time of the previous negative mammogram. **Top,** Tumors found by nonmammographic detection in women with a previous negative mammogram (intervening tumors; the results from 2 women who had tumors with time greater than 8 years since the previous negative mammograms were omitted). **Bottom,** Tumors found by mammographic detection in women with a previous negative mammogram (subsequent screen-detected tumors; results from 2 women who had tumors with time greater than 8 years since the previous negative mammograms were omitted). (Courtesy of Michaelson J, Satija S, Moore R, et al: The pattern of breast cancer screening utilization and its consequences. *Cancer* 94(1):37-43. © 2002, American Cancer Society. Reprinted by permission of Wiley-Liss Inc, a subsidiary of John Wiley & Sons, Inc.)

The authors conclude: "Far too many women did not comply with the American Cancer Society recommendations of prompt annual screening from the age of 40 years. Consequently, almost 50% of the invasive tumors emerged as larger and, thus, potentially more lethal, palpable masses." Clinicians and their patients should do better!

W. H. Hindle, MD

References

1. Tabár L, Chen H-H, Duffy SW, et al: A novel method for prediction of long-term outcome of women with T1a, T1b, and 10-14 mm invasive breast cancers: A prospective study. *Lancet* 355:429-433, 2000.
2. Tabár L, Dean PB, Kaufman CS, et al: A new era in the diagnosis of breast cancer. *Surg Oncol Clin N Am* 9:233-277, 2000.

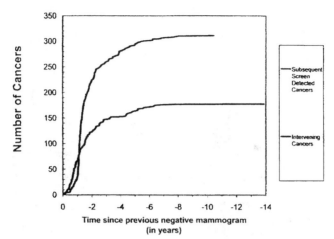

FIGURE 5.—Time since previous negative mammogram, in years, for patients with subsequent screen-detected and intervening tumors. (Courtesy of Michaelson J, Satija S, Moore R, et al: The pattern of breast cancer screening utilization and its consequences. *Cancer* 94(1):37-43. © 2002, American Cancer Society. Reprinted by permission of Wiley-Liss Inc, a subsidiary of John Wiley & Sons, Inc.)

3. Joensuu H, Pylkkanen L, Toikkanan S: Late mortality from pT1N0M0 breast carcinoma. *Cancer* 85:2183-2189, 1999.
4. Lopez MJ, Smart CR: Twenty-year follow-up of minimal breast cancer from the breast cancer detection demonstration project. *Surg Oncol Clin N Am* 6:393-401, 1997.
5. Arnesson LG, Smeds S, Fagerberg G: Recurrence-free survival in patients with small breast cancer. *Eur J Surg* 160:271-276, 1994.
6. Rosen PP, Groshen S, Kinne DW. Survival and prognostic factors in node-negative breast cancer: Results of long-term follow-up studies. *J Natl Cancer Inst Monogr* 11:159-162, 1992.

SUGGESTED READING

Smith RA, Saslow D, Sawyer KA, et al: American Cancer Society Guidelines for Breast Cancer Screening: Update 2003. *CA Cancer J Clin* 53:141-169, 2003.
▶ This definitive statement with 184 references, put together by 6 working groups of recognized experts in their fields, is "must" reading for all providers of women's health care. The recommendation of annual screening mammography and clinical breast examination for women aged 40 years and older is conclusively documented. The controversial considerations and questions that have been raised[1,2] are specifically addressed.[3-6] After 40 years of published research and commentary, it seems unlikely that the basic recommendation will be changed. The American Cancer Society first published this recommendation in 1983.

William H. Hindle, MD

References

1. National Institutes of Health Consensus Development Panel. National Institutes of Health Consensus Development Conference Statement: Breast cancer screening for women ages 40-49, January 21-23, 1997. National Institutes of Health Consensus Development Panel. *J Natl Cancer Inst* 89:1015-1026, 1997.

2. Gotzsche PC, Olsen O: Is screening for breast cancer with mammography justifiable? *Lancet* 355:129-134, 2000.
3. Boyle P: Current situation of screening for cancer. *Ann Oncol* 13:189-198, 2002.
4. Humphrey LL, Helfand M,. Chan BKJ, et al: Breast cancer screening: A summary of the evidence from the U.S. Preventive Services Task Force. *Ann Intern Med* 137:347-360, 2002.
5. Nystrom L, Anderson I, Bjurstam N, et al: Long-term effects of mammography screening: Update overview of the Swedish randomised trials. *Lancet* 359:909-919, 2002.
6. Carney PA, Miglioretti DL, Yankaskas BC, et al: Individual and combined effects of age, breast density, and hormone replacement therapy use on the accuracy of screening mammography. *Ann Intern Med* 138:168-175, 2002.

Moy L, Slanetz PJ, Moore R, et al: Specificity of mammography and US in the evaluation of a palpable abnormality: Retrospective review. *Radiology* 225:176-181, 2002.

▶ This report from the Breast Imaging Center, New York University School of Medicine, New York, and the Department of Breast Imaging, Massachusetts General Hospital, Boston, covers 829 women (1995-1998) who presented with a palpable abnormality and subsequently had negative imaging findings by both mammography and US. Breast cancer was eventually diagnosed in 2.6% of the women. All the cancers were in women with mammographically dense breasts, BI-RADS (Breast Imaging Reporting and Data System) breast composition–density 3 or 4. With 2 years or more of follow-up, no cancers were diagnosed in women with predominately fatty breast tissue. The decreased accuracy of imaging diagnosis of breast cancer in this review appears to be a function of increased mammographic density.

This is important information for clinicians. However, the cardinal rule persists that a dominant palpable breast mass should be definitely diagnosed, either by fine-needle aspiration cytology (with an adequate cellular sample), tissue core-needle histology, or open surgical biopsy histology.

William H. Hindle, MD

Kaiser JS, Helvia MA, Blacklaw RL, et al: Palpable breast thickening: Role of mammography and US in cancer detection. *Radiology* 223:839-844, 2002.

▶ A 1-year experience with 123 consecutive cases of palpable breast thickening is covered in this retrospective review from the Department of Radiology, University of Michigan Health System, Ann Arbor, Mich. Six malignancies (5% or 6/123) were diagnosed, 5 invasive carcinomas, and 1 in situ. The imaging studies of mammography and US resulted in 100% combined negative predictive value. For the invasive cancers, the mammographic sensitivity was 60% (3/5) and the specificity was 94% (102/108). US alone had a sensitivity of 100% (2/2) and a specificity of 96% (65/68). The authors recommend short-term–interval follow-ups, with imaging and clinical examination if a biopsy is not performed. Although the numbers in this review are small, the data are reassuring to clinicians who elect to follow palpable breast thickening that is not a dominant mass. In this editor's opinion, clear explanation to the patient and close follow-up are essential to appropriate management.

William H. Hindle, MD

Randolph WM, Goodwin JS, Mahnken JD, et al: Regular mammography use is associated with elimination of age-related disparities in size and stage of breast cancer at diagnosis. *Ann Intern Med* 137:783-790, 2002.

▶ This retrospective cohort study covers 12,038 women aged 69 years or older who had recently been diagnosed with invasive breast cancer (1995-1996) in the SEER (Surveillance, Epidemiology, and End Results) data bank. When the women aged 69 to 74 were compared to the women older than 74, it was found that the older women had larger tumors and more advanced stages at the time of diagnosis. However, this difference correlated with lack of regular mammography and was not apparent when women in each age group who had annual mammography were compared.

This speaks to the question of when to stop annual screening mammography. For clinicians, the answers seems to be (1) when women in these age groups are unwilling to have mammography or are unwilling to have appropriate treatment if a breast cancer is diagnosed, (2) when there is serious medical co-morbidity, and (3) when the woman's life expectancy is less than 4 years. However, it is imperative that the recommendations for a screening mammogram should be individualized, that the current pertinent information should be given to each woman prior to her decision, and that each woman's life situation and health care wishes be evaluated compassionately.

William H. Hindle, MD

Carney PA, Miglioretti DL, Yankaskas BC, et al: Individual and combined effects of age, breast density, and hormone replacement use on the accuracy of screening mammography. *Ann Intern Med* 138:168-175, 2003.

▶ Data from 7 population-based mammography registries covering 329,495 women aged 40 to 89 formed the basis for this prospective cohort study. During the 1996-1998 study period, 463,372 screening mammograms resulted in 2223 breast cancer diagnoses. The adjusted sensitivity was 62.9% for women with mammographically dense breasts and 87.0% for women with mammographically fatty breasts. The adjusted specificity was 89.1% for the dense breast group and 96.9% for the fatty breast group. The adjusted sensitivity was 68.6% for women aged 40 to 44 and 83.3% for women aged 80 to 89 years.

For women who did not use hormone replacement therapy, the adjusted specificity was 91.4% for the 40 to 44 age group and 94.4% for the 80 to 89 age group. The adjusted specificity for women of all ages who used hormone replacement therapy was 91.7%. These data support the notion that the decreased accuracy of mammography in younger women and in women on hormone replacement therapy is largely a function of increased mammographic density.

William H. Hindle, MD

Postmenopausal Hormone Therapy and Change in Mammographic Density

Greendale GA, Reboussin BA, Slone S, et al (Univ of California, Los Angeles; Wake Forest Univ, Winston-Salem, NC; Univ of Southern California, Los Angeles)

J Natl Cancer Inst 95:30-37, 2003   31–19

Introduction.—The degree of risk associated with mammographic density is greater than the degree of risk associated with nearly all other known breast cancer risk factors. Postmenopausal hormone use is linked with an increase in mammographic density; the magnitude of the increase in density is not known.

Methods.—Between 1989 and 1991, the Postmenopausal Estrogen/ Progestin Intervention Trial enrolled 875 postmenopausal women aged 45 to 64 years from 7 clinical centers. Of these, 571 underwent baseline and 12-month mammograms. Participants were randomly assigned to receive one of the following: daily conjugated equine estrogens (CEE) at 0.625 mg/d, daily CEE and medroxyprogesterone acetate (MPA) at 10 mg/d on days 1 to 12 (CEE+MPA-cyclic), daily CEE and MPA at 2.5 mg/d (CEE+MPA-continuous), daily CEE and micronized progesterone (MP) at 200 mg/d on days 1 to 12 (CEE+MP), or placebo.

Digitized mammograms were analyzed to ascertain the percentage of the left breast composed of dense tissue (ie, mammographic percent density). The effects of treatments on the change in mammographic percent density

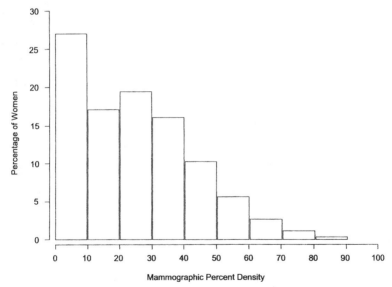

FIGURE 1.—Distribution of the percent density of baseline mammograms (N = 594). (Courtesy of Greendale GA, Reboussin BA, Slone S, et al: Postmenopausal hormone therapy and change in mammographic density. *J Natl Cancer Inst* 95:30-37, 2003. By permission of Oxford University Press.)

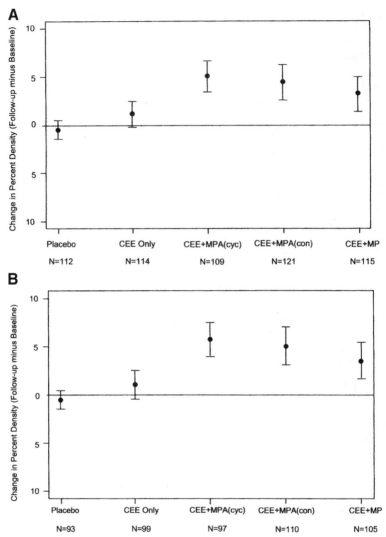

FIGURE 2.—Change in percent density from baseline to 12-month follow-up within individual treatment groups. The mean change in percent density is plotted as a point (**A**) for the entire mammographic density study sample (571 patients) and (**B**) for the participants who adhered to their treatment assignments (504 patients). *Abbreviations: CEE,* Conjugated equine estrogens, 0.625 mg/d; *CEE+MPA(cyc),* CEE, 0.625 mg/d, and medroxyprogesterone acetate, 10 mg/d on days 1-12; *CEE+MPA(con),* CEE, 0.625 mg/d, and MPA, 2.5 mg/d; *CEE+ MP,* CEE, 0.625 mg/day, and micronized progesterone, 200 mg/d on days 1-12. *Error bars* represent 95% confidence intervals. (Courtesy of Greendale GA, Reboussin BA, Slone S, et al: Postmenopausal hormone therapy and change in mammographic density. *J Natl Cancer Inst* 95:30-37, 2003. By permission of Oxford Unniversity Press.)

was evaluated between baseline and 12 months, before and after adjustment for possible confounders.

Results.—The adjusted absolute mean changes in mammographic percent density over 12 months were 4.76% (95% confidence interval [CI],

TABLE 2.—Adjusted Absolute Mean Change and 95% Confidence Intervals in Percent Density From Baseline to Follow-up by Treatment Assignment

Treatment Assignment	N	Adjusted Absolute Mean Change (Follow-up Minus Baseline) in Mammographic Percent Density (95% CI)	P Value*†
Placebo	112	−0.07% (−1.50% to 1.38%)	NA
CEE‡	113	1.17% (−0.28% to 2.62%)	.241
CEE + MPA-cyclic§	109	4.76% (3.29% to 6.23%)	<.001
CEE + MPA-continuous‖	121	4.58% (3.19% to 5.97%)	<.001
CEE + MP¶	114	3.08% (1.65% to 4.51%)	.002

*Model adjusted for baseline percent density, age, body mass index, alcohol use (tertiles), smoking (current versus former/never), level of physical activity (tertiles), 12-month change in body mass index, clinic site, and hysterectomy status (yes/no). Two women with baseline and 12-month mammograms were excluded from the final model after outlier analysis

†P value for *t* test of null hypothesis that mean change in percent density was not different from that of placebo.

‡CEE, conjugated equine estrogens, 0.625 mg/d.

§CEE + MPA-cyclic, CEE, 0.625 mg/d, and medroxyprogesterone acetate, 10 mg/day, on days 1 to12.

‖CEE + MPA-continuous, CEE, 0.625 mg/d, and medroxyprogesterone acetate, 2.5 mg/d.

¶CEE + MP, CEE, 0.625 mg/d, and micronized progesterone, 200 mg;day, on days 1 to 12.

Abbreviations: CEE, Conjugated equine estrogen; MPA, medroxyprogesterone acetate; MP, micronized progesterone; NA, not applicable.

(Courtesy of Greendale GA, Reboussin BA, Slone S, et al: Postmenopausal hormone therapy and change in mammographic density. *J Natl Cancer Inst* 95:30-37, 2003. By permission of Oxford University Press.)

3.29%-6.23%), 4.58% (95% CI, 3.19%-5.97%), and 3.08% (95% CI, 1.65%-4.51%) for women in the CEE+MPA-cyclic, CEE+MPA-continuous, and CEE-MP groups, respectively (Figs 1 and 2 and Table 2). Each of the absolute mean changes was significantly different from the adjusted mean change in mammographic percent density for women in the placebo group, which was −0.07% (95% CI, −1.50%- 1.38%).

Conclusion.—Greater mammographic density was linked with the use of estrogen/progestin combination therapy, regardless of how the progestin was administered, but not with the use of estrogen only.

▶ This study (*n* = 571) of "mammographic percent density" utilized a computer-assisted quantitative method of evaluating digitalized mammographic images of the left breast. The patients were in the Postmenopausal Estrogen/Progestin Intervention trial on randomized treatment with 3 hormone replacement therapy (HRT) regimens, estrogen replacement therapy alone, and placebo. As has been shown in multiple other studies, the mean values of the groups on HRT were elevated compared to the estrogen replacement therapy and placebo groups. However, it is critical to recall that most studies show that only about one fifth of women on HRT manifest increased mammographic density.[1]

Furthermore, the observational correlations of mammographic density with breast cancer risk in most published studies are usually at low epidemiologic levels, that is, "weak association," of relative risk. The biological mechanism of the potential correlation between mammographic density and breast cancer risk is unknown. Fortunately, there is clinical evidence that the increased mammographic density associated with HRT subsides rapidly; for example, within a month of stopping HRT.

In addition, it is well known that increased mammographic density is associated with decreased sensitivity of mammographic breast cancer detection. Clinicians should inform their patients about these potential correlations in their discussions before prescribing HRT.

W. H. Hindle MD

References

1. Greendale GA, Reboussin SA, Sie A, et al: Effects of estrogen and estrogen-progestin on mammographic parenchymal density. *Ann Int Med* 130:262-269, 1999.
2. Boyd NF, Lockwood GA, Byng JW, et al: Mammographic densities and breast cancer risk. *Cancer Epidemiol Biomarkers Prev* 7:1133-1144, 1998.

SUGGESTED READING

Parsons A, Merritt D, Rosen A, et al: Effect of raloxifene on the response to conjugated estrogen vaginal cream or nonhormonal moisturizers in postmenopausal vaginal atrophy. *Obstet Gynecol* 101:346-352, 2003.

▶ This study (n = 187) from the University of South Florida, Tampa, Fla, provides useful information for clinicians. Both the hormonal and nonhormonal vaginal preparations were effective in relieving symptoms, and the therapeutic effects were not interfered with by concurrent raloxifene therapy. In a related raloxifene study (n = 302 for 60 mg per day, 322 for 120 mg per day, and 319 for placebo controls), no differences in sexual desire, frequency of sexual activity, enjoyment, satisfaction, orgasm, or sexual problems were reported between the 2 treatment groups and/or the controls.[1]

William H. Hindle, MD

Reference

1. Modugno F, Ness RB, Ewing S, et al: Effect of raloxifene on sexual function in older postmenopausal women with osteoporosis. *Obstet Gynecol* 101:353-361, 2003.

Physician Specialty Is Significantly Associated With Hormone Replacement Therapy Use
Levy BT, Ritchie JM, Smith E, et al (Univ of Iowa, Iowa City)
Obstet Gynecol 101:114-122, 2003   31–20

Introduction.—Although the use of hormone replacement therapy (HRT) has been encouraged, its current use in the United States is about 38% in postmenopausal women. Many women who begin HRT do not continue treatment. Several reports have indicated that gynecologists feel more strongly than other physicians concerning the preventive role of HRT.

There are no known trials that compare current HRT use in women seen by gynecologists versus family physicians for their annual examination, when controlling for sociodemographics, preventive health behaviors, and co-morbidities. Thus, the characteristics of postmenopausal women seen by gynecologists versus family physicians were examined, along with current HRT use.

Methods.—A cross-sectional survey was performed in 426 postmenopausal women seen for their annual examination at university clinics. Predictors of current HRT use versus never use were examined.

Results.—Overall, 60% of women recruited in family practice clinics and 69% of those in gynecology clinics were current HRT users. Significant positive, multivariable predictors of HRT use were gynecology versus family practice clinic attendance (odds ratio [OR], 2.6; 95% confidence interval [CI], 1.4-4.6), surgical menopause (OR, 2.3; 95% CI, 1.2-4.6), history of depression (OR, 2.3; 95% CI, 1.2-4.7), at least 2 live births (OR, 2.1; 95% CI, 1.1-4.0), and current alcohol use (OR, 1.8; 95% CI, 1.04-3.2) (Table 5).

Significant negative, multivariate predictors included: increasing age (60-70 years vs less than 60 years, OR, 0.4; 95% CI, 0.2-0.8; 70 years or older vs less than 60 years, (OR, 0.4; 95% CI, 0.2-0.9) and history of breast cancer (OR, 0.04; 95% CI, 0.01-0.14). Sociodemographic factors, smoking status, number of self-reported medical disorders, number of prescription medications other than HRT, oral contraceptive use, history of hypertension, and exercise level were examined as covariates and did not enter the model.

The most common reason women reported for currently taking HRT was menopausal symptoms; this was reported more often in women seen by gynecologists than those seen by family practice physicians (Table 2). The most common reasons for ever-users of HRT to discontinue HRT were side effects; there was no significant difference by clinic attended (Table 3).

Conclusion.—Current HRT use rates between clinics were similar and higher than national averages. The adjusted odds of current HRT use among women receiving care from gynecologists was 2.6 times that of women receiving care from family physicians. This difference in practice patterns may reflect physicians' uncertainty concerning the preventive value of HRT.

TABLE 5.—Multivariate Logistic Regression Model of Factors Predicting Current Versus Never Hormone Replacement Therapy Use ($P < .05$)

Variable	OR	95% CI	P
Clinic type			
Gynecology vs family practice	2.6	1.4, 4.6	.002
Menopause type			
Surgical vs natural	2.3	1.2, 4.6	.017
Age group (y)			
60-70 vs <60	0.4	0.2, 0.8	.005
≥70 vs <60	0.4	0.2, 0.9	.024
History of depression	2.3	1.2, 4.7	.018
Alcohol use			
Current vs past/never	1.8	1.04, 3.2	.035
History of breast cancer	0.04	0.01, 0.14	<.001
Live births			
≥2 vs 0-1	2.1	1.1, 4.0	.022

Note: P value is based on 371 current and never users; the 55 past users were excluded from this analysis.
Abbreviation: OR, Odds ratio; *CI*, confidence interval.

(Reprinted with permission from The American College of Obstetricians and Gynecologists courtesy of Levy BT, Ritchie JM, Smith E, et al: Physician specialty is significantly associated with hormone replacement therapy use. *Obstet Gynecol* 101:114-122, 2003.)

TABLE 2.—Reasons for Currently Taking or Not Taking Hormone Replacement Therapy

	Family Practice Clinic ($n = 49$)	Gynecology Clinic ($n = 209$)	$P*$
Reasons for currently taking HRT†			
Menopausal symptoms	50	74	.001
Osteoporosis prevention	57	64	.32
Heart disease prevention	43	53	.26
Beneficial effects on lipids	14	23	.20
Prevention of dry skin	18	19	.81
Bladder infection prevention	9	13	.46
Reasons for not currently taking HRT‡	($n = 29$)	($n = 92$)	
Menopausal symptoms were tolerable	38	26	.23
Worried about the side effects	46	28	.07
Worried about the risk of cancer	38	31	.47
I don't like taking medication	38	24	.15
Physician didn't think I needed them	11	16	.76
Physician never brought this up	14	10	.73

Note: Figures are percentages.
* P values were calculated using Pearson χ^2 on Fisher exact test.
†Only those women who were currently on hormone replacement therapy (*HRT*) answered this question; 8 current HRT users from family practice and 18 from gynecology clinics did not answer this question.
‡Only those women who were either past or never HRT users answered this question; 9 past or never users from family practice and 12 from gynecology clinics did not answer this question.
(Reprinted with permission from The American College of Obstetricians and Gynecologists courtesy of Levy BT, Ritchie JM, Smith E, et al: Physician specialty is significantly associated with hormone replacement therapy use. *Obstet Gynecol* 101:114-122, 2003.)

▶ Recent emphasis on family practice and the gender shift in the obstetrics and gynecology specialty are making meaningful changes in the trends of practice patterns in women's health care, especially for postmenopausal women. This study, from the University of Iowa (1997-1999), documents a greater use of HRT by ob-gyns (69%) compared to family practice physicians (60%). National estimates (1999) of HRT use are at about 38% of postmenopausal women.[1] For both specialties, the negative multivariable predictors were advancing age and history of breast cancer. Fear of breast cancer was given as the reason for stopping HRT by about 5% of patients in both the family practice and ob-gyn setting. It is interesting that the "Hysterectomy rates were not statistically different between the two clinics."

It is imperative that women's health care physicians maintain a current broad perspective on the use, benefits, and risk of HRT. Episodes like the intense media coverage of the curtailment of the HRT arm of the Women's Health Initiative clinical trial unnecessarily alarm patients and distort the balanced discussion of indications and contraindications for HRT and estrogen replacement therapy.

W. H. Hindle, MD

Reference

1. Keating NL, Cleary PD, Rossi AS, et al: Use of hormone replacement therapy by postmenopausal women in the United States. *Ann Intern Med* 130:545-553, 1999.

TABLE 3.—Reported Side Effects and Reasons for Discontinued Use of Hormone Replacement Therapy

	Family Practice Clinic ($n = 65$)	Gynecology Clinic ($n = 271$)	$P*$
Ever experienced the following side effects†			
Weight gain	31	40	.16
Breast tenderness or enlargement	17	36	.004
Water retention/puffiness	14	29	.01
Fear of developing breast cancer	11	16	.30
Decrease in sex drive	15	15	.86
Fear of developing uterine cancer	6	8	.60
Other side effects‡	20	22	.73
Ever discontinued use for the following reasons†	($n = 65$)	($n = 270$)	
Fear of developing breast cancer	6	5	.75
Breast tenderness or enlargement	5	5	>.99
Weight gain	2	4	.48
Fear of developing uterine cancer	6	3	.24
Water retention/puffiness	0	3	.36
Other reasons for discontinued use‡	15	15	.92

Note: Figures are percentages.

*P values were calculated using Pearson χ^2 or Fisher exact test.

†These questions were answered by women who were either current or past users of hormone replacement therapy; 3 women were missing the data for the question pertaining to ever experienced the following side effects, and 4 women were missing the data for the question pertaining to ever discontinued use for the following reasons.

‡Other includes nausea or vomiting, dizziness, increase in migraines, increase in blood pressure, increase in skin irritation/redness, decrease in sex drive, and other.

(Reprinted with permission from The American College of Obstetricians and Gynecologists courtesy of Levy BT, Ritchie JM, Smith E, et al: Physician specialty is significantly associated with hormone replacement therapy use. *Obstet Gynecol* 101:114-122, 2003.)

SUGGESTED READING

Ramakrishnan R, Khan SA, Badve S: Morphological changes in breast tissue with menstrual cycle. *Mod Pathol* 15:1348-1356, 2002.

▶ In this study (n = 73), morphological changes (histologic parameters) of breast tissue surgical specimens from the Northwestern University Medical School, Chicago, were correlated with the stage of the menstrual cycle, based on last menstrual periods and usual cycle length. The results demonstrated a 74% (54/73) correlation of morphological stage with dates (P = .01). Furthermore, of those with simultaneous progesterone levels (31), 80% (25/31) were phase-concordant by progesterone levels and morphology, and 80% (25/31) were concordant by progesterone levels and dates.

The authors summarize, "Women with a high morphologic score were seven times as likely to be in the luteal phase as were women with a low score (odds ratio, 7.1; 95% Confidence Interval)." These data suggest that progesterone may play the dominant role in the multifactorial endocrinologic changes that produce cyclic morphology (and mitotic surges) in the breast ductal epithelium. Hopefully, multiple carefully designed similar studies with much larger numbers will be stimulated by this current "pilot study" to elucidate the endocrinology, physiology, and malignant transformation of the human breast ductal and lobular epithelium.

William H. Hindle, MD

Vassilopoulou-Sellin R, Cohen DS, Hortobagyi GN, et al: Estrogen replacement therapy for menopausal women with a history of breast carcinoma: results of a 5-year prospective study. *Cancer* 95:1817-1826, 2002.

▶ This prospective partially randomized clinical trial (n = 77 and 222 controls) has a mean follow-up of 5 years. The patients had stage I or II breast cancer with at least a 2-year minimum disease-free interval. The treated group received 0.625 mg conjugated equine estrogen for 25 days each month. The disease-free survival was the same for both groups. Thus, with these limited numbers and this limited duration of follow-up, estrogen replacement therapy (ERT) in these selected breast cancer survivors appears to have no adverse effect on disease-free survival. The data are reassuring to clinicians and patients. Furthermore, it is of keen clinical interest that 3.6% (2/56) of the women on ERT developed a contralateral cancer and 13.6% (33/243) of the untreated women developed new or recurrent cancers. If this difference persists with longer follow-up and larger numbers of patients, it merits further investigation.

William H. Hindle, MD

Subject Index

A

Author Index